LEADERSHIP Roles
and MANAGEMENT
Functions in
NURSING
Eleventh Edition
Theory and Application

LEADERSHIP Roles and MANAGEMENT Functions in NURSING

Theory and Application

Eleventh Edition

Carol J. Huston, RN, MSN, DPA, FAAN

Nurse Educator, Consultant, Author, Leader
Interim Executive Director, WellCat Student Health Center
California State University, Chico, California
Past Director/Professor Emerita
School of Nursing, California State University
Chico, California

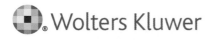 Wolters Kluwer

Philadelphia • Baltimore • New York • London
Buenos Aires • Hong Kong • Sydney • Tokyo

Vice President and Publisher: Julie K. Stegman
Director of Nursing Education and Practice Content: Jamie Blum
Senior Acquisitions Editor: Jonathan Joyce
Associate Development Editor: Phoebe Jordan-Reilly
Editorial Assistant: Devika Kishore
Editorial Coordinator: Erin E. Hernandez
Marketing Manager: Sarah Schuessler
Senior Production Project Manager: Alicia Jackson
Manager, Graphic Arts & Design: Stephen Druding
Art Director, Illustration: Jennifer Clements
Manufacturing Coordinator: Margie Orzech
Prepress Vendor: Aptara, Inc.

11th edition

10 9 8 7 6 5 4 3 2

Printed in Mexico

Library of Congress Cataloging-in-Publication Data available upon request.

ISBN: 978-1-9751-9306-5

shop.lww.com

QUADM0624

A Note About the Language Used in This Book

Wolters Kluwer recognizes that people have a diverse range of identities, and we are committed to using inclusive and nonbiased language in our content. In line with the principles of nursing, we strive not to define people by their diagnoses, but to recognize their personhood first and foremost, using as much as possible the language diverse groups use to define themselves, and including only information that is relevant to nursing care.

We strive to better address the unique perspectives, complex challenges, and lived experiences of diverse populations traditionally underrepresented in health literature. When describing or referencing populations discussed in research studies, we will adhere to the identities presented in those studies to maintain fidelity to the evidence presented by the study investigators. We follow best practices of language set forth by the *Publication Manual of the American Psychological Association, Seventh edition*, but acknowledge that language evolves rapidly, and we will update the language used in future editions of this book as necessary.

I dedicate this book to my newest grandson, Mason.
You are such a wonderful addition to our lives,
and we love you so very much!

Carol J. Huston

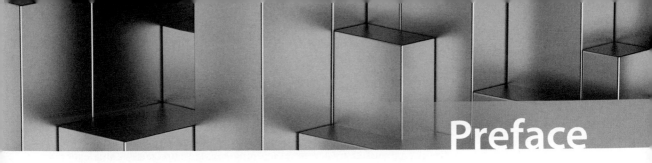

Legacy of *Leadership Roles and Management Functions in Nursing*

This book's philosophy evolved over 40 years of teaching leadership and management. Bessie Marquis (co-author on earlier editions) and I entered academe from the acute care sector of the health care industry, where we held nursing management positions. In our first effort as authors, *Management Decision Making for Nurses: 101 Case Studies*, published in 1987, we used an experiential approach and emphasized management functions appropriate for first- and middle-level managers. The primary audience for this text was undergraduate nursing students.

Our second book, *Retention and Productivity Strategies for Nurse Managers*, focused on leadership skills necessary for managers to decrease attrition and increase productivity. This book was directed at nurse-managers rather than students. The experience of completing research for the second book, coupled with our clinical observations, compelled us to incorporate more leadership content in our teaching and to write this book.

Leadership Roles and Management Functions in Nursing was also influenced by national events in business and finance that led many to believe that a lack of leadership in management was widespread. It became apparent that if managers were to function effectively in the rapidly changing health care industry, enhanced leadership and management skills were needed.

What we attempted to do, then, was to combine these two very necessary elements: leadership and management. We did not see leadership as merely one role of management or management as only one role of leadership. We viewed the two as equally important and necessarily integrated. We attempted to show this interdependence by defining the leadership components and management functions inherent in all phases of the management process. Undoubtedly, a few readers have found fault with our divisions of management functions and leadership roles; however, we felt it necessary to first artificially separate the two components for readers and then to integrate the roles and functions. We do believe strongly that adoption of this integrated role is critical for success in management.

The second concept that shaped this book was our commitment to developing critical thinking skills with the use of experiential learning exercises. We proposed that integrating leadership and management could be accomplished using learning exercises. Far too much academic instruction continues to be conducted in a teacher-lecturer–student-listener format, which is one of the least effective teaching strategies. Few individuals learn best using this style. Instead, most people learn best by methods that utilize concrete, experiential, self-initiated, and real-world learning experiences.

In nursing, theoretical teaching is almost always accompanied by concurrent clinical practice that allows concrete and real-world learning experience. However, the exploration of leadership and management theory may have only limited practicum experience, so learners may have little first-hand opportunity to observe middle- and top-level managers in nursing practice. As a result, novice managers frequently have limited opportunities to practice their skills before assuming their first management position, and their decision making too often reflects trial-and-error methodologies. For us, there was little question that vicarious learning, or learning through mock experience, provided students the opportunity to make significant leadership and management decisions in a safe environment and to learn from the decisions they make.

As a result, we moved away from the lecturer–listener format in our classes, and began using a more Socratic approach, case study debate, and small and large group problem solving instead. Our students, once resistant to the experiential approach, became enthusiastic supporters. We also found this enthusiasm for experiential learning apparent in workshops and seminars for registered nurses. Experiential learning enables management and leadership theory to be fun and exciting, but most importantly, it facilitates retention of didactic material. The research we completed on this teaching approach supports these findings.

Although many leadership and management texts are available, this book meets the need for an emphasis on both leadership and management content and the use of an experiential approach for learning. Included are 279 learning exercises, representing various health care settings and a wide variety of learning modes, to give readers many opportunities to apply theory, resulting in internalized learning. In Chapter 1, guidelines are provided for using the experiential learning exercises and readers are encouraged to use them to supplement the text.

New to This Edition

The first edition of *Leadership Roles and Management Functions in Nursing* presented the symbiotic elements of leadership and management, with an emphasis on problem solving and critical thinking. This 11th edition maintains this precedent with a balanced presentation of a strong theory component along with a variety of real-world scenarios in the experiential learning exercises. This edition also maintains the dual focus of leadership and management.

Content, however, has been added, deleted, and updated in this edition. This edition replaces the American Association of Colleges of Nursing (AACN) *Essentials of Baccalaureate Education and Master's Education* in chapter crosswalks with the AACN *Essentials: Core Competencies for Professional Nursing Education* (2021). In addition, the American Nurses Association (ANA) *Scope and Standards of Practice* have been updated in the crosswalks to reflect the new *Standards of Practice* and *Standards of Professional Performance* released in 2021.

In addition, there is new content on appreciative leadership and appreciative inquiry, supply chain management, academic integrity as an ethical issue, health care reform, ransomware attacks on health care organizations, workplace violence, and drug diversion/reentry to work as part of substance use disorder in nursing. The impact of the COVID-19 pandemic also permeates this new edition including the need for transformative thinking and action, dynamic priority setting, and advocacy for patient and worker safety, as well as the unprecedented fiscal challenges leader-managers faced while determining how to most appropriately (and ethically) allocate physical and human resources in a time of significant human and physical resource shortages.

In addition, new learning exercises have been added that take place in outpatient/community settings and other new learning exercises reinforce the need for a permeation of social justice, diversity, inclusion, and equity in the workplace. Learning exercises have also been added to address some of the new leadership and management challenges experienced as part of the COVID-19 pandemic. Quality and safety, interprofessional collaboration/team building, technology in health care, the promotion of healthy workplaces and civility, and change management continue to be emphasized.

This edition then retains the strengths of earlier editions, reflecting content and application exercises appropriate to the issues faced by nurse leader-managers as they practice in an era increasingly characterized by limited resources and emerging technologies. The 11th edition also includes a continued focus to include current research and theory to ensure accuracy of the didactic material.

Finally, Bessie Marquis is no longer listed as a co-author of this textbook. Bessie retired from book authorship several editions ago; however, her contributions to the content in this book and to me personally, as a mentor and colleague, will forever be appreciated. Thank you, Bessie.

The Text

Unit I provides a foundation for the decision-making, problem-solving, and critical-thinking skills as well as management and leadership skills needed to address the management–leadership problems presented in the text.

Unit II covers ethics, legal concepts, and advocacy, which we see as core components of leadership and management decision making.

Units III to VII are organized using the management processes of planning, organizing, staffing, directing, and controlling.

Features of the Text

The 11th edition contains many pedagogical features designed to benefit both the student and the instructor:

- **Examining the Evidence**, appearing in each chapter, depicts new research findings, evidence-based practice, and best practices in leadership and management.
- **Learning Exercises** interspersed throughout each chapter foster readers' critical-thinking skills and promote interactive discussions. Additional learning exercises are also presented at the end of each chapter for further study and discussion.
- **Breakout Comments** are highlighted throughout each chapter, visually reinforcing key ideas.
- **Tables, Displays, Figures, and Illustrations** are supplied liberally throughout the text to reinforce learning as well as to help clarify complex information.
- **Key Concepts** summarize important information within every chapter.

The Crosswalk

A crosswalk is a table that shows elements from different databases or criteria that interface. New to the eighth edition was a chapter crosswalk of content based on the AACN *Essentials of Baccalaureate Education for Professional Nursing Practice* (2008), the AACN *Essentials of Master's Education in Nursing* (2011), the American Organization for Nursing Leadership (AONL) (formerly American Organization of Nurse Executives [AONE]) *Nurse Executive Competencies* (updated September 2015), and the QSEN Institute *Competencies* (2020). For the ninth edition, the revised Standards for Professional Performance from the ANA *Nursing: Scope and Standards of Practice* (2015) were included. This edition replaces the AACN *Essentials of Baccalaureate Education and Master's Education* with the AACN *Essentials: Core Competencies for Professional Nursing Education* (2021) and updates the ANA Nursing Scope and Standards of Practice to reflect the fourth edition published in 2021.

Each chapter in the book notes how content in that chapter draws from or contributes to content identified as essential for baccalaureate and graduate education, for practice as a nurse administrator, and for safety and quality in clinical practice.

Without doubt, some readers will disagree with the author's determinations of which Essential, Competency, or Standard has been addressed in each chapter, and certainly, an argument could be made that most chapters address many, if not all, of the Essentials, Competencies, or Standards in some way. The crosswalks in this book then are intended to note the primary content focus in each chapter, although additional Essentials, Competencies, or Standards may well be a part of the learning experience.

The American Association of Colleges of Nursing: *The Essentials: Core Competencies for Professional Nursing Education*

The Essentials: Core Competencies for Professional Nursing Education was released in 2021 and identified 10 domains that represent the essence of professional nursing practice and the expected competencies for each domain. Domains are broad distinguishable areas of competence that, when considered in the aggregate, contribute to a descriptive framework for the practice of nursing (AACN, 2021). While the domains and competencies are identical for both entry and advanced levels of nursing education, the sub-competencies build from entry into professional nursing practice to advanced levels of knowledge and practice. The new Essentials also feature eight concepts that are central to professional nursing practice and are integrated within and across the domains and competencies. The 10 domains are noted in Table 1.

TABLE 1   AMERICAN ASSOCIATION OF COLLEGES OF NURSING—THE ESSENTIALS: CORE COMPETENCIES FOR PROFESSIONAL NURSING EDUCATION

Domain 1: Knowledge for Nursing Practice
- Integration, translation, and application of established and evolving disciplinary knowledge and ways of knowing, as well as knowledge from other disciplines, including a foundation in liberal arts and natural and social sciences.

Domain 2: Person-Centered Care
- Focuses on the individual within multiple complicated contexts, including family and/or important others. Directs care to be holistic, individualized, just, respectful, compassionate, coordinated, evidence based, and developmentally appropriate.

Domain 3: Population Health
- Spans the health care delivery continuum from public health prevention to disease management of populations and describes collaborative activities with both traditional and nontraditional partnerships for the improvement of equitable population health outcomes.

Domain 4: Scholarship for Nursing Practice
- The generation, synthesis, translation, application, and dissemination of nursing knowledge to improve health and transform nursing care.

Domain 5: Quality and Safety
- Employment of established and emerging principles of safety and improvement science. As core values of nursing practice, enhance quality and minimize risk of harm to patients and providers through both system effectiveness and individual performance.

Domain 6: Interprofessional Partnerships
- Intentional collaboration across professions and with care team members, patients, families, communities, and other stakeholders to optimize care, enhance the health care experience, and strengthen outcomes.

Domain 7: Systems-Based Practice
- Responding to and leading within complex systems of health care. Coordinating resources to provide safe, quality, and equitable care to diverse populations.

Domain 8: Information and Health Care Technologies
- Information and communication technologies and informatics processes are used to provide care, gather data, form information to drive decision making, and support professionals as they expand knowledge and wisdom for practice. Informatics processes and technologies are used to manage and improve the delivery of safe, high-quality, and efficient health care services in accordance with best practice and professional and regulatory standards.

Domain 9: Professionalism
- Formation and cultivation of a sustainable professional nursing identity, accountability, perspective, collaborative disposition, and comportment that reflects nursing's characteristics and values.

Domain 10: Personal, Professional, and Leadership Development
- Participation in activities and self-reflection that foster personal health, resilience, well-being, lifelong learning, and support the acquisition of nursing expertise and assertion of leadership.

Source: American Association of Colleges of Nursing. (2021). *The essentials: Core competencies for professional nursing education.* https://www.aacnnursing.org/Portals/42/AcademicNursing/pdf/Essentials-2021.pdf

TABLE **AMERICAN ORGANIZATION FOR NURSING LEADERSHIP NURSE EXECUTIVE COMPETENCIES**

1. Communication and relationship building
  - Communication and relationship building includes effective communication, relationship management, influencing behaviors, diversity, community involvement, medical/staff relationships, and academic relationships.

2. Knowledge of the health care environment
  - Knowledge of the health care environment includes clinical practice knowledge, delivery models and work design, health care economics and policy, governance, evidence-based practice/outcome measurement and research, patient safety, performance improvement/metrics, and risk management.

3. Leadership
  - Leadership skills include foundational thinking skills, personal journey disciplines, systems thinking, succession planning, and change management.

4. Professionalism
  - Professionalism includes personal and professional accountability, career planning, ethics, and advocacy.

5. Business skills
  - Business skills include financial management, human resource management, strategic management, and information management and technology.

The American Organization for Nursing Leadership *Nurse Executive Competencies*

In 2004 (updated in 2015), the AONL (formerly AONE) published a paper describing skills common to nurses in executive practice regardless of their educational level or titles in different organizations. Although these *Nurse Executive Competencies* differ depending on the leader's specific position in the organization, the AONL suggested that managers at all levels must be competent in the five areas noted in Table 2 (AONL, AONE, 2015). These competencies suggest that nursing leadership/management is as much a specialty as any other clinical nursing specialty, and as such, it requires proficiency and competent practice specific to the executive role.

The American Nurses Association *Standards of Professional Performance*

In 2021, the fourth edition of *Nursing: Scope and Standards of Practice* was published. This edition included 6 standards of practice and 18 standards of professional performance. Collectively, they represented the *Standards of Professional Nursing Practice* that all registered nurses, regardless of role, population, specialty, and setting, are expected to perform competently. Because the *Standards of Practice* describe a competent level of nursing practice demonstrated by the nursing process and thus cross all aspects of nursing care, only the *Standards of Professional Performance* have been included in the crosswalk of this book (Table 3). The *Standards of Professional Performance* describe a competent level of behavior in the professional role, including activities related to ethics, advocacy, respectful and equitable practice, communication, collaboration, leadership, education, scholarly inquiry, quality of practice, professional practice evaluation, resource stewardship, and environmental health.

The Quality and Safety Education for Nurses Competencies

Using the Institute of Medicine (2003) competencies for nursing, the QSEN Institute (2020) defined six prelicensure and graduate quality and safety competencies for nursing (Table 4) and proposed targets for the knowledge, skills, and attitudes to be developed in nursing programs for each of these competencies. Led by a national advisory board and distinguished faculty, the QSEN Institute pursues strategies to develop effective teaching approaches to assure that future graduates develop competencies in patient-centered care, teamwork and collaboration, evidence-based practice, quality improvement, safety, and informatics.

TABLE **AMERICAN NURSES ASSOCIATION NURSING ADMINISTRATION STANDARDS OF PROFESSIONAL PERFORMANCE**

Standard 7. Ethics
- The registered nurse integrates ethics in all aspects of practice.

Standard 8. Advocacy
- The registered nurse demonstrates advocacy in all roles and settings.

Standard 9. Respectful and Equitable Practice
- The registered nurse practices with cultural humility and inclusiveness.

Standard 10. Communication
- The registered nurse communicates effectively in all areas of professional practice.

Standard 11. Collaboration
- The registered nurse collaborates with the health care consumers and other key stakeholders.

Standard 12. Leadership
- The registered nurse leads within the profession and practice settings.

Standard 13. Education
- The registered nurse seeks knowledge and competence that reflects current nursing practice and promotes futuristic thinking.

Standard 14. Scholarly Inquiry
- The registered nurse integrates scholarship, evidence, and research findings into practice.

Standard 15. Quality of Practice
- The registered nurse contributes to quality nursing practice.

Standard 16. Professional Practice Evaluation
- The registered nurse evaluates one's own and others' nursing practice.

Standard 17. Resource Stewardship
- The registered nurse utilizes appropriate resources to plan, provide, and sustain evidence-based nursing services that are safe, effective, financially responsible, and use judiciously.

Standard 18. Environmental Health
- The registered nurse practices in a manner that advances environmental safety and health.

Source: American Nurses Association (2021). *Nursing: Scope and standards of practice* (4th ed.).

TABLE **QUALITY AND SAFETY EDUCATION FOR NURSES COMPETENCIES**

Patient-centered care
- Definition: Recognize the patient or designee as the source of control and full partner in providing compassionate and coordinated care based on respect for patient's preferences, values, and needs.

Teamwork and collaboration
- Definition: Function effectively within nursing and interprofessional teams, fostering open communication, mutual respect, and shared decision making to achieve quality patient care.

Evidence-based practice
- Definition: Integrate best current evidence with clinical expertise and patient/family preferences and values for delivery of optimal health care.

Quality improvement
- Definition: Use data to monitor the outcomes of care processes and use improvement methods to design and test changes to continuously improve the quality and safety of health care systems.

Safety
- Definition: Minimize the risk of harm to patients and providers through both system effectiveness and individual performance.

Informatics
- Definition: Use information and technology to communicate, manage knowledge, mitigate error, and support decision making.

Source: QSEN Institute. (2020). *Competencies.* http://qsen.org/competencies/

Student and Faculty Resources Available

Leadership Roles and Management Functions in Nursing, 11th edition, has ancillary resources designed with both students and instructors in mind.

Student Resources Available

- **Glossary**—The glossary contains definitions of important terms in the text.
- **Journal Articles**—Twenty-five full articles from Wolters Kluwer journals are provided for additional learning opportunities.
- **Learning Objectives** from the textbook are available in Microsoft Word for your convenience.

Instructor's Resources Available

- **Competency Maps** pull together the mapping provided in the crosswalk feature for each chapter, showing how the book content integrates key competencies for practice.
- An **Image Bank** lets you use the photographs and illustrations from this textbook in your PowerPoint slides or as you see fit in your course.
- An **Instructor's Guide** includes information on experiential learning and guidelines on how to use the text for various types of learners and in different settings as well as information on how to use the various types of Learning Exercises included in the text.
- **PowerPoint Presentations** provide an easy way for you to integrate the textbook with your students' classroom experience, either via slide shows or handouts. Audience response questions are integrated into the presentations to promote class participation and allow you to use iClicker technology.
- **Sample Syllabi** provide guidance for structuring your leadership and management course and are provided for two different course lengths: 8 and 15 weeks.
- **Strategies for Effective Teaching** offer creative approaches for engaging students.
- A **Test Generator** lets you put together exclusive new tests from a bank containing 750 questions to help you in assessing your students' understanding of the material. Test questions link to chapter learning objectives.
- Access to all student resources.

Comprehensive, Integrated Digital Learning Solutions

We are delighted to offer an expanded suite of digital solutions to support instructors and students using *Leadership Roles and Management Functions in Nursing*, 11th edition. This textbook is embedded into Lippincott CoursePoint, an integrated digital learning solution that builds on the features of the text with proven instructional design strategies.

Lippincott
CoursePoint

Our prelicensure solution, **Lippincott CoursePoint**, is a rich learning environment that drives course and curriculum success to prepare students for practice. Lippincott CoursePoint is designed for the way students learn. The solution connects learning to real-life application by integrating content from *Leadership Roles and Management Functions in Nursing* with video cases, interactive modules, and journal articles. Ideal for active, case-based learning, this powerful solution helps students develop higher-level cognitive skills and asks them to make decisions related to simple-to-complex scenarios.

Lippincott CoursePoint for Leadership and Management features the following:

- **Leading content in context:** Digital content from *Leadership Roles and Management Functions in Nursing* is embedded in our Powerful Tools, engaging students and encouraging interaction and learning on a deeper level.
  - The complete eBook provides students with anytime, anywhere access on multiple devices.
  - Full online access to *Stedman's Medical Dictionary for the Health Professions and Nursing* ensures students work with the best medical dictionary available.
- **Powerful tools to maximize class performance:** Additional course-specific tools provide case-based learning for every student.
  - **Video Cases** help students anticipate what to expect as a nurse, with detailed scenarios that capture their attention and integrate clinical knowledge with leadership and management concepts that are critical to real-world nursing practice. By watching the videos and completing related activities, students will flex their problem-solving, prioritizing, analyzing, and application skills to aid both in NCLEX preparation and in preparation for practice.

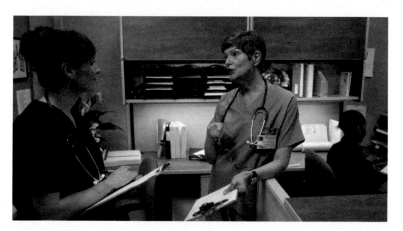

- **Interactive Modules** help students quickly identify what they do and do not understand, so they can study smartly. With exceptional instructional design that prompts students to discover, reflect, synthesize, and apply, students actively learn. Remediation links to the digital textbook are integrated throughout.
  - **Curated Collections of Journal Articles** are provided via *Lippincott NursingCenter*, Wolters Kluwer's premier destination for peer-reviewed nursing journals. Through integration of CoursePoint and NursingCenter, students will engage in how nursing research influences practice.
- **Data to measure students' progress:** Student performance data provided in an intuitive display lets instructors quickly assess whether students have viewed interactive modules and video cases outside of class as well as see students' performance on related NCLEX-style quizzes, ensuring students are coming to the classroom ready and prepared to learn.

To learn more about Lippincott CoursePoint, please visit: http://www.nursingeducation-success.com/coursepoint

Closing Note

It is my hope and expectation that the content, style, and organization of this 11th edition of *Leadership Roles and Management Functions in Nursing* will be helpful to those students who want to become skillful, powerful, visionary leaders and managers.

Carol J. Huston, RN, MSN, DPA, FAAN

REFERENCES

American Association of Colleges of Nursing. (2008). *The essentials of baccalaureate education for professional nursing practice.* http://www.aacnnursing.org/Portals/42/Publications/BaccEssentials08.pdf

American Association of Colleges of Nursing. (2011). *The essentials of master's education in nursing.* http://www.aacnnursing.org/Portals/42/Publications/MastersEssentials11.pdf

American Association of Colleges of Nursing. (2021). *The essentials: Core competencies for professional nursing education.* https://www.aacnnursing.org/Portals/42/AcademicNursing/pdf/Essentials-2021.pdf

American Nurses Association. (2015). *Nursing: Scope and standards of practice* (3rd ed.).

American Nurses Association. (2021). *Nursing: Scope and standards of practice* (4th ed.).

American Organization for Nursing Leadership. (AONL, AONE, 2015). *AONE nurse executive competencies.* https://www.aonl.org/sites/default/files/aone/nec.pdf

Institute of Medicine. (2003). *Health professions education: A bridge to quality.* The National Academies Press.

QSEN Institute. (2020). *Competencies.* http://qsen.org/competencies/

Contents

UNIT VII   Roles and Functions in Controlling   599

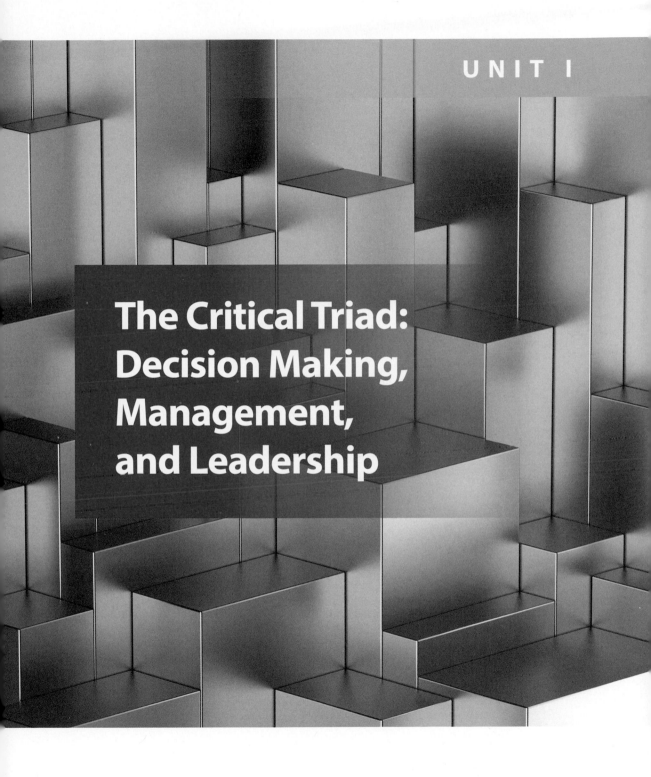

The Critical Triad: Decision Making, Management, and Leadership

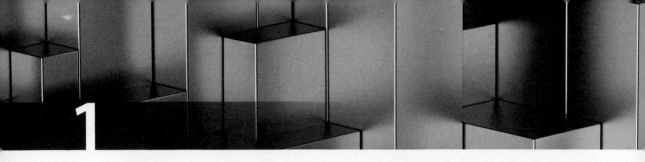

Decision Making, Problem Solving, Critical Thinking, and Clinical Reasoning: Requisites for Successful Leadership and Management

… again and again, the impossible problem is solved when we see that the problem is only a tough decision waiting to be made.—**Robert H. Schuller**

… in any moment of decision, the best thing you can do is the right thing, the next best thing is the wrong thing, and the worst thing you can do is nothing.—**Theodore Roosevelt**

… If we start with the attitude that different viewpoints are additive rather than competitive, we become more effective because our ideas or decisions are honed and tempered by that discourse.—**Edwin Catmull, President of Pixar and Walt Disney Animation Studios**

CROSSWALK

This chapter addresses:

- **AACN Essentials Domain 1:** Knowledge for nursing practice
- **AACN Essentials Domain 4:** Scholarship for nursing practice
- **AACN Essentials Domain 5:** Quality and safety
- **AACN Essentials Domain 7:** Systems-based practice
- **AACN Essentials Domain 8:** Information and health care technologies
- **AACN Essentials Domain 10:** Personal, professional, and leadership development
- **AONL Nurse Executive Competency 1:** Communication and relationship building
- **AONL Nurse Executive Competency 3:** Leadership
- **ANA Standard of Professional Performance 13:** Education
- **ANA Standard of Professional Performance 14:** Scholarly inquiry
- **QSEN Competency:** Informatics
- **QSEN Competency:** Evidence-based practice

LEARNING OBJECTIVES

The learner will:

- differentiate between problem solving, decision making, critical thinking, clinical reasoning, and elastic thinking
- describe how case studies, simulation, and problem-based learning can be used to improve the quality of decision making
- explore strengths and limitations of using intuition and heuristics as adjuncts to problem solving and decision making
- identify characteristics of successful decision makers

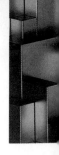

- use a *PICO* (patient or population, intervention, comparison, and outcome) format to search for current best evidence or practices to address a problem
- identify strategies the new nurse might use to promote evidence-based practice
- select appropriate models for decision making in specific situations
- describe the importance of individual variations in the decision-making process
- identify critical elements of decision making
- identify strategies that help decrease individual subjectivity and increase objectivity in decision making
- explore personal propensity for risk taking in decision making
- discuss the effect of organizational power and values on individual decision making
- differentiate between the economic man and the administrative man in decision making
- select appropriate management decision-making tools that would be helpful in making specific decisions

Introduction

Decision making is often thought to be synonymous with management and is one of the criteria on which management expertise is judged. Much of any manager's time is spent critically examining issues, solving problems, and making decisions. The quality of the decisions they make is a factor that often weighs heavily in their success or failure.

Decision making, then, is both an innermost leadership activity and the core of management. This chapter explores the primary requisites for successful management and leadership: decision making, problem solving, and critical thinking. Also, because decision making, problem solving, and critical thinking are learned skills that improve with practice and consistency, an introduction to established tools, techniques, and strategies for effective decision making is included. This chapter also introduces the learning exercise as an approach for vicariously gaining skill in management and leadership decision making. Finally, evidence-based decision making is introduced as an imperative for both personal and professional problem solving.

Decision Making, Problem Solving, Critical Thinking, Clinical Reasoning, and Elastic Thinking

Decision making is a complex, cognitive process often defined as choosing a particular course of action. This implies that doubt exists about several courses of action and that a choice is made to eliminate uncertainty.

Problem solving is part of decision making and is a systematic process that focuses on analyzing difficult situations. Problem solving always includes a decision-making step. Many educators use the terms *problem solving* and *decision making* synonymously, but there is a small, yet important, difference. Although decision making is the last step in the problem-solving process, it is possible for decision making to occur without the full analysis required in problem solving. Problem solving attempts to identify the root problem in situations, so much time and energy are spent on identifying the real problem.

Decision making, on the other hand, is usually triggered by a problem but does not focus on eliminating the underlying problem. For example, if a person decided to handle a conflict when it occurred but did not attempt to identify what caused the conflict, only decision-making skills would be used. The decision maker might later choose to address the actual cause of the conflict or might decide to do nothing at all about the problem. The decision has been made *not* to problem solve.

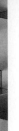

This alternative may be selected because of a lack of energy, time, or resources. In some situations, this is an appropriate decision. For example, assume that a nursing supervisor has a staff nurse who has been frequently absent over the last 3 months. Normally, the supervisor would feel compelled to intervene. However, the supervisor has reliable information that the nurse will be resigning soon. Because the problem will soon no longer exist, the supervisor *decides* the time and energy needed to correct the problem are not warranted.

Critical thinking, sometimes referred to as *reflective thinking*, is related to evaluation and has a broader scope than decision making and problem solving. Dictionary.com (2022) defines critical thinking as "disciplined thinking that is clear, rational, open minded, and informed by evidence" (para. 1). Critical thinking also involves reflecting on the meaning of statements, examining the offered evidence and reasoning, and forming judgments about facts.

> Insight, intuition, empathy, and the willingness to act are components of critical thinking.

Whatever definition of critical thinking is used, most agree that it is more complex than problem solving or decision making, involves higher-order reasoning and evaluation, and has both cognitive and affective components. Insight, intuition, empathy, and the willingness to act are additional components of critical thinking. These same skills are necessary to some degree in decision making and problem solving. See Display 1.1 for additional characteristics of a critical thinker.

Nurses today must have higher-order thinking skills to identify patient problems and to direct clinical judgments and actions that result in positive patient outcomes. When nurses integrate and apply different types of knowledge to weigh evidence, critically think about arguments, and reflect on the process used to arrive at a diagnosis, *clinical reasoning* has occurred. Thus, clinical reasoning uses both knowledge and experience to make decisions at the point of care.

Elastic thinking, a type of creative thinking, differs from step-by-step analytical or linear thinking models in that it arises from what scientists call "bottom-up" processes (Mlodinow, 2018). In this mode, individual neurons fire in complex fashion, with valuable input from the brain's emotional centers rather than the brain's high-level executive structures. Because this kind of processing is nonlinear, it can produce creative ideas that would not have arisen in the step-by-step progression of analytical thinking. This allows decision makers to solve novel problems and overcome the neural and psychological barriers that can impede us from considering new ways of solving problems.

Linear decision-making and problem-solving models as well as elastic thinking are needed by leader-managers, depending on how well defined or structured a problem is. Indeed, Mlodinow notes that the way an issue is framed has a profound influence on the way it is solved (Henni, 2021).

DISPLAY 1.1   CHARACTERISTICS OF A CRITICAL THINKER

Open to new ideas	Flexible	Creative
Intuitive	Empathetic	Insightful
Energetic	Caring	Willing to take action
Analytical	Observant	Outcome directed
Persistent	Risk taker	Willing to change
Assertive	Resourceful	Knowledgeable
Communicative	"Outside-the-box" thinker	Circular thinker

Vicarious Learning to Increase Problem-Solving and Decision-Making Skills

Decision making, one step in the problem-solving process, is an important task that relies heavily on critical thinking and clinical reasoning skills. How do people become successful problem solvers and decision makers? Although successful decision making can be learned through life experience, this trial-and-error method leaves much to chance. Some people are not successful in problem solving and decision making because they have not been taught how to reason insightfully from multiple perspectives.

Moreover, information and new learning may not be presented within the context of real-life situations, although this is changing. For example, nurse educators strive to see that the elements of clinical reasoning are embedded throughout the nursing curricula. In addition, time is included for meaningful reflection on decisions that are made and the outcomes that result. Such learning can occur in both real-world settings and through vicarious learning, where students problem solve and make decisions based on simulated situations that are made real to the learner.

Research by Ahmady and Shahbazi (2020) supports this assertion, noting that structured, social problem-solving training can improve cognitive problem-solving, critical-thinking, and decision-making skills. Nursing education then should consider the addition of new creative teaching strategies in addition to traditional education methods.

Case Studies, Simulation, and Problem-Based Learning

Case studies, simulation, and problem-based learning (PBL) are some of the strategies that have been developed to vicariously improve problem solving and decision making. *Case studies* may be thought of as stories that impart learning. They may be fictional or include real persons and events, be relatively short and self-contained for use in a limited amount of time or be longer with significant detail and complexity for use over extended periods of time.

Case studies, particularly those that unfold or progress over time, are becoming much more common in nursing education because they provide a more interactive learning experience for students than the traditional didactic approach. Indeed, an integrative review by Hammad and Khalaf (2020) suggests the use of case-based learning facilitated the development of clinical decision-making skills in nursing students more than lecture-based learning.

Similarly, *simulation* provides learners opportunities for problem solving that have little or no risk to patients or to organizational performance. For example, some organizations are now using computer simulation (known as *discrete event simulation*) to imitate the operation of a real-life system such as a hospital. The learner's actions in the simulation provide insight to the quality of the learner's decision making based on priority setting, timeliness of action, and patient outcomes.

PBL also provides opportunities for individuals to address and learn from authentic problems vicariously. Typically, in PBL, learners meet in small groups to discuss and analyze real-life problems. Thus, they learn by problem solving. The learning itself is collaborative as the teacher guides the students to be self-directed in their learning, and many experts suggest that this type of active learning helps to develop critical-thinking skills.

The Marquis–Huston Critical-Thinking Teaching Model

The desired outcome for teaching and learning decision making and critical thinking in management is an interaction between learners and others that results in the ability to critically examine management and leadership issues. This is a learning of appropriate social/professional behaviors rather than a mere acquisition of knowledge. This type of learning occurs best in groups, using a PBL approach.

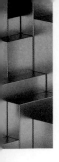

In addition, learners retain didactic material more readily when it is personalized or when they can relate to the material being presented. The use of case studies that learners can identify with assists in retention of didactic materials.

Although formal instruction in critical thinking is important, using a formal decision-making process improves both the quality and consistency of decision making. Many new leaders and managers struggle to make quality decisions because their opportunity to practice making management and leadership decisions is very limited until they are appointed to a management position. These limitations can be overcome by creating opportunities for vicariously experiencing the problems that individuals would encounter in the real world of leadership and management.

The *Marquis–Huston Model for Teaching Critical Thinking* assists in achieving desired learner outcomes (Fig. 1.1). This model comprises four overlapping spheres, each being an essential component for teaching leadership and management. The first is a didactic theory component, such as the material that is presented in each chapter; the second consists of a formalized approach to problem solving and decision making. The third involves some form of a group process, which can be accomplished through large and small groups and classroom discussion. The last sphere entails the material being made real for the learner so that the learning is internalized. This can be accomplished through writing exercises, personal exploration, and values clarification, along with risk taking, as case studies are examined.

This book was developed with the perspective that experiential learning provides valuable mock experiences to apply leadership and management theory. The text includes numerous opportunities for readers to experience the real world of leadership and management through *learning exercises*, including case studies, writing exercises, specific management or leadership problems, staffing and budgeting calculations, group discussion or problem-solving situations, and assessment of personal attitudes and values. Some learning exercises include

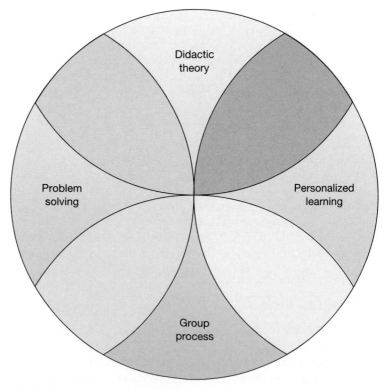

FIGURE 1.1 The Marquis–Huston critical thinking teaching model.

opinions, speculations, and value judgments. All, however, require some degree of critical thinking, problem solving, decision making, or clinical reasoning.

> Experiential learning provides mock experiences that have tremendous value in applying leadership and management theory.

Some of the case studies have been solved (solutions are found at the back of the book) so that readers can observe how a systematic problem-solving or decision-making model can be applied. The author feels strongly, however, that the problem solving suggested in the solved cases should not be considered the only plausible solution or "the right solution" to that learning exercise. Most of the learning exercises in the book have multiple solutions that could be implemented successfully.

Theoretical Approaches to Problem Solving and Decision Making

Farnam Street Media Inc. (2022) suggests that most people don't actually stop to think. They just take their first thought and run with it. That's because many individuals rely on discrete, often unconscious, processes known as *heuristics* to make decisions. Heuristics use trial-and-error methods or a rule-of-thumb approach to problem solving rather than set rules. As such, they are practical mental shortcuts and are not expected to provide perfect or optimal problem solving. They do, however, provide a more immediate solution to the decision at hand. This is particularly true for uncertain or emergent situations where knowledge, time, and resources are limited.

Indeed, clinicians often turn to heuristics to look for general guiding principles to alleviate the ambiguity of clinical diagnostics and decision making related to a lack of high-quality data. For example, Rehana and Huda (2021) suggest that many clinicians use "*anchoring bias*," a type of heuristic that uses an initial source of information as an "anchor" for the basis of decision making. The use of an anchoring bias, however, to reduce ambiguity can lead to medical errors, inappropriate use of resources, and patient harm.

Typically, formal process and structure can benefit the decision-making process, as they force decision makers to be specific about options and to separate probabilities from values. A structured approach to problem solving and decision making increases clinical reasoning and is the best way to learn how to make quality decisions because it eliminates trial and error and focuses the learning on a proven process. A structured or professional approach involves applying a theoretical model in problem solving and decision making. Many acceptable problem-solving models exist, and most include a decision-making step; only four are reviewed here.

> A structured approach to problem solving and decision making increases clinical reasoning.

Traditional Problem-Solving Process

One of the most well-known and widely used problem-solving models is the *traditional problem-solving model*. The seven steps are shown in Display 1.2. (Decision making occurs at step 5.)

Although the traditional problem-solving process is an effective model, its weakness lies in the amount of time needed for proper implementation. This process, therefore, is less effective when time constraints are a consideration. Another weakness is lack of an initial objective-setting step. Setting a decision goal helps to prevent the decision maker from becoming sidetracked.

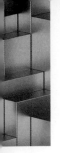

1. Identify the problem.
2. Gather data to analyze the causes and consequences of the problem.
3. Explore alternative solutions.
4. Evaluate the alternatives.
5. Select the appropriate solution.
6. Implement the solution.
7. Evaluate the results.

Managerial Decision-Making Models

To address the weaknesses of the traditional problem-solving process, many contemporary models for management decision making have added an objective-setting step. These models are known as *managerial decision-making models* or *rational decision-making models*. One such model suggested by Decision-making-confidence.com (2006–2022) includes the six steps shown in Display 1.3.

In the first step, problem solvers must identify the decision to be made, who needs to be involved in the decision process, the timeline for the decision, and the goals or outcomes that should be achieved. Identifying objectives to guide the decision making helps the problem solver determine which criteria should be weighted most heavily in making the decision. Most important decisions require this careful consideration of context.

In Step 2, problem solvers must attempt to identify as many alternatives as possible. Alternatives are then analyzed in Step 3, often using some type of *SWOT* (strengths, weaknesses, opportunities, and threats) analysis. Decision makers may choose to apply quantitative decision-making tools, such as decision-making grids and payoff tables (discussed further later in this chapter), to objectively review the desirability of alternatives.

In Step 4, alternatives are rank ordered based on the analysis done in Step 3 so that problem solvers can make a choice. In Step 5, a plan is created to implement desirable alternatives or combinations of alternatives. In the final step, challenges to successful implementation of chosen alternatives are identified and strategies are developed to manage those risks. An evaluation is then conducted of both process and outcome criteria, with outcome criteria typically reflecting the objectives that were set in Step 1.

The Nursing Process

The *nursing process* provides another theoretical system for solving problems and making decisions. Originally a four-step model (assess, plan, implement, and evaluate), diagnosis was delineated as a separate step, and most contemporary depictions of this model now include at least five steps (Display 1.4).

As a decision-making model, the nursing process's greatest strength may be its multiple venues for feedback. The arrows in Figure 1.2 show constant input into the process. When the

1. Determine the decision and the desired outcome (set objectives).
2. Research and identify options.
3. Compare and contrast these options and their consequences.
4. Make a decision.
5. Implement an action plan.
6. Evaluate results.

DISPLAY 1.4 **NURSING PROCESS**

1. Assess
2. Diagnose
3. Plan
4. Implement
5. Evaluate

---

decision point has been identified, initial decision making occurs and continues throughout the process via a feedback mechanism.

Although the process was designed for nursing care and accountability, it can easily be adapted as a theoretical model for solving leadership and management problems. Table 1.1 shows how closely the nursing process parallels the decision-making process.

The weakness of the nursing process, like the traditional problem-solving model, is in not requiring clearly stated objectives. Goals should be clearly stated in the planning phase of the process, but this step is frequently omitted or obscured. However, because nurses are familiar with this process and its proven effectiveness, it continues to be recommended as an adapted theoretical process for leadership and managerial decision making.

Integrated Ethical Problem-Solving Model

Another model for effective thinking and problem solving was developed by the National Association of Social Workers (2020, Display 1.5). Although developed primarily for use in solving ethical problems, the model also works well as a general problem-solving model. Like the three models already discussed, this model provides a structured approach to problem solving that includes an assessment of the problem, problem identification, the analysis and selection of the best alternative, and reflection as a means for evaluation.

Many other excellent problem analysis and decision models exist. The model selected should be one with which the decision maker is familiar and one appropriate for the problem to be solved. Using models or processes consistently will increase the likelihood that

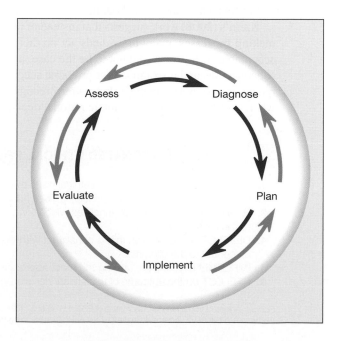

FIGURE 1.2 Feedback mechanism of the nursing process.

TABLE **1.1** COMPARING THE DECISION-MAKING PROCESS WITH THE NURSING PROCESS

Decision-Making Process	Simplified Nursing Process
Identify the decision	Assess
Collect data	
Identify criteria for decision	Plan
Identify alternatives	
Choose alternative	Implement
Implement alternative	
Evaluate steps in decision	Evaluate

critical analysis will occur. Moreover, the quality of problem solving and decision making will improve tremendously via a scientific approach.

Intuitive Decision-Making Models

Some theorists suggest that intuition should always be used as an adjunct to empirical or rational decision-making models. Experienced (expert) nurses often report that gut-level feelings (intuition) encourage them to take appropriate strategic action that impacts patient outcomes, although intuition generally serves as an adjunct to decision making founded on a nurse's scientific knowledge base. Intuition then can and should be used in conjunction with evidence-based practice.

This recognition of familiar problems and the use of intuition to identify solutions is a focus of contemporary research on intuitive decision-making research. Klein (2008) developed the *recognition-primed decision (RPD) model* for intuitive decision making in the mid-1980s to explain how people can make effective decisions under time pressure and uncertainty. Considered a part of *naturalistic decision making*, the RPD model attempts to understand how humans make relatively quick decisions in complex, real-world settings such as firefighting and critical care nursing without having to compare options.

Klein's (2008) work suggests that instead of using classical rational or systematic decision-making processes, many individuals act on their first impulse if the "imagined future" looks acceptable. If this turns out not to be the case, another idea or concept can emerge from their subconscious and is examined for probable successful implementation. Thus, the RPD model blends intuition and analysis, but pattern recognition and experience guide decision makers when time is limited, or systematic rational decision making is not possible.

DISPLAY **1.5** INTEGRATED ETHICAL PROBLEM-SOLVING MODEL

1. DETERMINE whether there is an ethical issue or/and dilemma.
2. IDENTIFY the key values and principles involved.
3. RANK the values or ethical principles which—in your professional judgment—are most relevant to the issue or dilemma.
4. DEVELOP an action plan that is consistent with the ethical priorities that have been determined as central to the dilemma.
5. IMPLEMENT your plan, utilizing the most appropriate practice skills and competencies.
6. REFLECT on the outcome of this ethical decision-making process.

Source: Adapted from National Association of Social Workers. (2020). *Essential steps for ethical problem-solving*. https://www.naswma.org/page/100/Essential-Steps-for-Ethical-Problem-Solving.htm

LEARNING EXERCISE 1.1

Applying Scientific Models to Decision Making

You are a registered nurse. Since your graduation 3 years ago, you have worked as a full-time industrial health nurse for a large manufacturing plant. Although you love your family (spouse and one preschool-aged child), you love your job as well because career is very important to you. Recently, you and your spouse decided to have another baby and jointly decided that if you did so, you would reduce your work time and spend more time at home with the children.

Last week, however, the director of human resources told you that the full-time director of health care services for the plant is leaving and that the organization wants to appoint you to the position. You were initially thrilled and excited; however, you found out several days later that you and your spouse are expecting a baby.

Last night, you spoke with your spouse about your career future. Your spouse is an attorney whose practice has suddenly gained momentum. Although the two of you have shared child rearing equally until this point, your spouse is not sure how much longer this can be done if the law practice continues to expand. If you take the position, which you would like to do, it would mean full-time work and more management responsibilities. You want the decision you and your spouse reach to be well-thought-out, as it has far-reaching consequences and concerns many people.

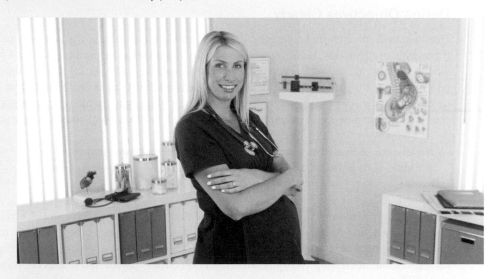

ASSIGNMENT:

Determine what you should do. Examine both the individual aspects of decision making and the critical elements in making decisions. Make a plan including a goal, a list of information, and data that you need to gather and areas where you may be vulnerable to poor decision making. Examine the consequences of each alternative available to you.

After you have made your decision, get together in a group (four to six people) and share your decisions. Were they the same? How did you approach the problem solving differently from others in your group? Was a rational systematic problem-solving process used, or was the chosen solution based more on intuition? How many alternatives were generated? Did some of the group members identify alternatives that you had not considered? Was a goal or objective identified? How did your personal values influence your decision?

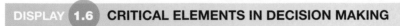

DISPLAY 1.6   CRITICAL ELEMENTS IN DECISION MAKING

1. Define objectives clearly.
2. Gather data carefully.
3. Take the time necessary.
4. Use an evidence-based approach.
5. Generate numerous alternatives.
6. Think logically.
7. Choose and act decisively.

Critical Elements in Problem Solving and Decision Making

Because decisions may have far-reaching consequences, some problem solving and decision making must be of high quality. Using a scientific approach alone for problem solving and decision making does not, however, ensure a quality decision. Special attention must be paid to other critical elements. The elements in Display 1.6, considered crucial in problem solving, must occur if a high-quality decision is to be made.

Define Objectives Clearly

Decision makers often forge ahead in their problem-solving process without first determining their goals or objectives. However, it is especially important to determine goals and objectives when problems are complex. Even when decisions must be made quickly, there is time to pause and reflect on the purpose of the decision. A decision that is made without a clear objective in mind or a decision that is inconsistent with one's philosophy is likely to be a poor-quality decision. Sometimes, the problem has been identified, but the wrong objectives are set.

> If a decision lacks a clear objective or if an objective is not consistent with the individual's or organization's stated philosophy, a poor-quality decision is likely.

For example, it would be important for the decision maker in Learning Exercise 1.1 to determine whether the most important objective is career advancement, having more time with family, or meeting the needs of their spouse. None of these goals is more "right" than the others, but not having clarity about which objective is paramount makes decision making very difficult.

Gather Data Carefully

Because decisions are based on knowledge and information available to the problem solver at the time the decision must be made, one must learn how to process and obtain accurate information. The acquisition of information begins with identifying the problem or the occasion for the decision and continues throughout the problem-solving process. Often, the information is unsolicited, but most information is sought actively.

Clear (n.d.) warns, however, that many people experience confirmation bias in their data gathering. *Confirmation bias* refers to our tendency to search for and favor information that confirms our beliefs while simultaneously ignoring or devaluing information that contradicts our beliefs (Clear, n.d.). The more someone believes they know something, the more they filter and ignore information to the contrary. Thus, people negate new information if it does not validate their perceptions or ideas.

| DISPLAY **1.7** | **QUESTIONS TO EXAMINE IN DATA GATHERING** |

1. What is the setting?
2. What is the problem?
3. Where is it a problem?
4. When is it a problem?
5. Who is affected by the problem?
6. What is happening?
7. Why is it happening? What are the causes of the problem? Can the causes be prioritized?
8. What are the basic underlying issues? What are the areas of conflict?
9. What are the consequences of the problem? Which is the most serious?

In addition, acquiring information always involves people, and no tool or mechanism is infallible to human error. Questions that should be asked in data gathering are shown in Display 1.7.

In addition, human values tremendously influence our perceptions. Therefore, as problem solvers gather information, they must be vigilant that their own preferences and those of others are not mistaken for facts. Managers who become experts at acquiring adequate, appropriate, and accurate information will have a head start in becoming expert decision makers and problem solvers.

Facts can be misleading if they are presented in a seductive manner, if they are taken out of context, or if they are past-oriented.

Take the Time Necessary

Most current problem-solving and decision-making theories argue that human decision making is largely based on quick, automatic, and intuitive processes. Although trivial decisions can be made fairly quickly, slower, more controlled deliberation is needed when outcomes may have significant consequences.

In fact, most people need to actually schedule time to think. Although some people might think more than a few minutes is a waste of time, this viewpoint is shortsighted and flawed. Although it might take 30 minutes to come to the same conclusion that you might come to in 5 minutes, you'll have a better idea of the nuances of the situation, including which variables matter the most, and you'll make fewer mistakes if you take the time to really think about it (Farnam Street Media Inc., 2022).

Use an Evidence-Based Approach

To gain knowledge and insight into managerial and leadership decision making, individuals must reach outside their current knowledge in solving the problems presented in this text. Some data-gathering sources include textbooks, periodicals, experts in the field, colleagues, and current research. Indeed, most experts agree that the best practices in nursing care and decision making are also *evidence-based practices* (Ford & Graves, 2023).

Although there is no one universally accepted definition for an *evidence-based* approach, most definitions suggest the term can be used synonymously with *research based* or *science based*. Others suggest that *evidence based* means that the approach has been reviewed by experts in the field using accepted standards of empirical research and that reliable evidence exists that the approach or practice works to achieve the desired outcomes. Typically, a *PICO* (patient or population, intervention, comparison, and outcome) format is used in evidence-based practice to guide the search for the current best evidence to address a problem.

DISPLAY **1.8**	**STRATEGIES FOR THE NEW NURSE TO PROMOTE EVIDENCE-BASED BEST PRACTICE**

1. Keep abreast of the evidence—subscribe to professional journals and read widely.
2. Use and encourage use of multiple sources of evidence.
3. Use evidence not only to support clinical interventions but also to support teaching strategies.
4. Find established sources of evidence in your specialty—do not reinvent the wheel.
5. Implement and evaluate nationally sanctioned clinical practice guidelines.
6. Question and challenge nursing traditions and promote a spirit of risk taking.
7. Dispel myths and traditions not supported by evidence.
8. Collaborate with other nurses locally and globally.
9. Interact with other disciplines to bring nursing evidence to the table.

Source: Reprinted from Ford, C. D., & Graves, B. A. (2023). Evidence-based practice. In C. J. Huston (Ed.), *Professional issues in nursing: Challenges and opportunities* (6th ed., pp. 67–77). Wolters Kluwer.

Given that human lives are often at risk, nurses, then, should feel compelled to use an evidence-based approach in gathering data to make decisions regarding their nursing practice. Yet, Ford and Graves (2023) suggest that many practicing nurses feel they do not have the time, access, or expertise needed to search and analyze the research literature to answer clinical questions. In addition, many nurses may not have been exposed to formal research courses. Findings from research studies may also be technical, difficult to understand, and even more difficult to translate into practice. Strategies the new nurse might use to promote evidence-based practice are shown in Display 1.8.

> Evidence–based decision making and evidence–based practice should be viewed as imperatives for all nurses today as well as for the profession in general.

It is important to recognize that the implementation of evidence-based best practices is not just an individual, staff nurse–level pursuit (Ford & Graves, 2023). Too few nurses understand what best practices and evidence-based practice are about, and many organizational cultures do not support nurses who seek out and use research to change long-standing practices rooted in tradition rather than in science. Administrative support is needed to access the resources; provide the support personnel; and sanction the necessary changes in policies, procedures, and practices for evidence-based data gathering to be a part of every nurse's practice (Ford & Graves, 2023). This approach to care is even being recognized as a standard expectation of accrediting bodies such as The Joint Commission as well as an expectation for Magnet hospital designation.

Generate Numerous Alternatives

The definition of decision making implies that there are at least two choices in every decision. Unfortunately, many problem solvers limit their choices to two when many more options usually are available. Remember that one alternative in each decision should be the choice to do nothing. When examining decisions to be made by using a formal process, it is often found that the status quo is the right alternative.

> The greater the number of alternatives that can be generated, the greater the chance that the final decision will be sound.

Several techniques can help to generate more alternatives. Because everyone thinks uniquely, increasing the number of people working on a problem increases the number of alternatives that can be generated.

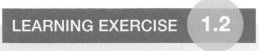

LEARNING EXERCISE 1.2

Possible Alternatives in Problem Solving

In the personal-choice scenario presented in Learning Exercise 1.1, some of the following alternatives could have been generated:

- Do not take the new position.
- Hire a full-time housekeeper and take the position.
- Ask your spouse to quit working.
- Have an abortion.
- Ask one of the parents to help.
- Take the position and do not hire childcare.
- Take the position and hire childcare.
- Have your spouse reduce the law practice and continue helping with childcare.
- Ask the director of human resources if you can work 4 days a week and still have the position.
- Take the position and wait and see what happens after the baby is born.

ASSIGNMENT:

How many of these alternatives did you or your group generate? What alternatives did you identify that are not included in this list?

Brainstorming is another frequently used technique. The goal in brainstorming is to think of all possible alternatives, even those that may seem "off-target." By not limiting the possible alternatives to only apparent ones, people can break through habitual or repressive thinking patterns and allow new ideas to surface. Although most often used by groups, people who make decisions alone also may use brainstorming.

Think Logically

During the problem-solving process, one must draw inferences from information. An *inference* is part of deductive reasoning. People must carefully think through the information and the alternatives. Faulty logic at this point may lead to poor-quality decisions. People think illogically in many ways, but four common ways are:

1. *Overgeneralizing:* This type of "crooked" thinking occurs when one believes that because *A* has a particular characteristic, every other *A* also has the same characteristic. This kind of thinking is exemplified when stereotypical statements are used to justify arguments and decisions.
2. *Affirming the consequences:* In this type of illogical thinking, one decides that if *B* is good and one is currently doing *A*, then *A* must not be good. For example, if a new method is heralded as the best way to perform a nursing procedure and the nurses on your unit are not using that technique, it is illogical to assume that the technique currently used in your unit is wrong or bad.
3. *Arguing from analogy:* This thinking applies a component that is present in two separate concepts and then states that because *A* is present in *B*, then *A* and *B* are alike in all respects. An example of this would be to argue that because intuition plays a part in clinical and managerial nursing, then any characteristic present in a good clinical nurse also should be present in a good nurse-manager. However, this is not necessarily true; a skilled nurse-manager does not necessarily possess all the same skills as a skilled nurse-clinician.

4. *Both-sidesing:* Both-sidesing occurs when someone or something presents two sides as equally valid when one in fact is wrong (Prasad, 2021). Thus, it gives false equivalence to a flawed idea. For instance, a debate on whether the earth is round or flat would be both-sidesing.

Various tools have been designed to assist managers with the important task of analysis. Several of these tools are discussed in this chapter. In analyzing possible solutions, individuals may want to look at the following questions:

1. What factors can you influence? How can you make the positive factors more important and minimize the negative factors?
2. What are the financial implications of each alternative? What are the political implications? Who else will be affected by the decision, and what support is available?
3. What are the weighting factors?
4. What is the best solution?
5. What are the means of evaluation?
6. What are the consequences of each alternative?

Choose and Act Decisively

It is not enough to gather adequate information, think logically, select from among many alternatives, and be aware of the influence of one's values. In the final analysis, one must act. Many individuals delay acting because they do not want to face the consequences of their choices (e.g., if managers granted all employees' requests for days off, they would have to accept the consequences of dealing with short staffing).

> Many individuals choose to delay acting because they lack the courage to face the consequences of their choices.

It may help the reluctant decision maker to remember that even though decisions often have long-term consequences and far-reaching effects, they are not usually cast in stone. Often, judgments found to be ineffective or inappropriate can be changed. By later evaluating decisions, managers can learn more about their abilities and where the problem solving was faulty. However, decisions must continue to be made, although some are of poor quality, because through continued decision making, people develop improved decision-making skills.

Individual Variations in Decision Making

If each person receives the same information and uses the same scientific approach to solve problems, an assumption could be made that identical decisions would result. However, in practice, this is not true. Because decision making involves perceiving and evaluating, and people perceive by sensation and intuition and evaluate their perception by thinking and feeling, individuality inevitably plays a part in decision making. Because everyone has different values and life experiences, and each person perceives and thinks differently, different decisions may be made given the same set of circumstances. No discussion of decision making would, therefore, be complete without a careful examination of the role of the individual in decision making.

Sex

Research suggests that sex may play a role in how individuals make decisions, although some debate continues as to whether these differences are more gender role based than biologic

EXAMINING THE EVIDENCE 1.1

Source: From University of Sydney. (2021, June 2). Revealed: Men and women do think and act differently. Retrieved July 9, 2021, from https://www.sydney.edu.au/news-opinion/news/2021/06/02/revealed-men-and-women-do-think-and-act-differently.html

Gender and Decision Making

This study of more than 50,000 participants in 97 samples, published in the Proceedings of the National Academy of Sciences of the United States of America (PNAS), found that men make more extreme choices and decisions than women, with both positive and negative outcomes. Indeed, men were much more likely than women to "be at the extreme ends of the behavioral spectrum, either acting very selfishly or very altruistically, very trusting or very distrusting, very fair or very unfair, very risky or very risk averse and were either very short-term or very long-term focused" (para 4).

The researchers suggested the differences might have evolutionary roots, but also offered alternative explanations for the existence of what is often referred to as "greater male variability." For example, parental investment theory suggests that men must deviate from the average to stand out and be attractive to women to reproduce, whereas women are able to attract sexual partners without deviating from the average. Another explanation suggests that there are norms and expectations of acceptable gendered behavior and that men's extreme behaviors are socially constructed and reinforced, whereas women may feel socially constrained from displaying the same level of decision-making variability as men.

sex based. Recent research on economic decision making found, however, that men were more likely to make extreme choices and decisions than women (University of Sydney, 2021). Researchers suggested the differences might have evolutionary roots, but also noted alternative explanations for the existence of what is often referred to as greater male variability (see Examining the Evidence 1.1).

Values

Individual decisions are based on each person's value system. No matter how objective the criteria, value judgments will always play a part in a person's decision making, either consciously or subconsciously. The alternatives are generated, and the final choices are limited by each person's value system. For some, certain choices are not possible because of a person's beliefs. Because values also influence perceptions, they invariably influence information gathering, information processing, and outcomes. Values also determine which problems in one's personal or professional life will be addressed or ignored.

> No matter how objective the criteria, value judgments will always play a part in a person's decision making, either consciously or subconsciously.

Life Experience

Each person brings to the decision-making task, past experiences that include education and decision-making experience. The more mature the person and the broader their background, the more alternatives they can identify. Each time a new behavior or decision is observed that possibility is added to the person's repertoire of choices.

In addition, people vary in their desire for autonomy. People seeking autonomy likely have much more experience at making decisions than those who fear autonomy. Likewise, having made good or poor decisions in the past will influence a person's decision making.

Individual Preference

With all the alternatives a person considers in decision making, one alternative may be preferred over another. The decision maker, for example, may see certain choices as involving greater personal risk than others and therefore may choose the safer alternative. Physical, economic, and emotional risks and time and energy expenditures are types of personal risks and costs involved in decision making. For example, people with limited finances or a reduced energy level may decide to select an alternative solution to a problem that would not have been their first choice had they been able to overcome limited resources.

Brain Hemisphere Dominance and Thinking Styles

Our way of evaluating information and alternatives on which we base our final decision constitutes a thinking skill. Individuals think differently. Some think systematically—and are often called analytical thinkers—whereas others think more intuitively. About 40 years ago, researchers first began arguing that most people have either right- or left-brain hemisphere dominance. They suggested that analytical, linear, *left-brain thinkers* process information differently from creative, intuitive, *right-brain thinkers*. Left-brain thinkers were supposed to be better at processing language, logic, and numbers, whereas right-brain thinkers excelled at nonverbal ideation and creativity.

Some researchers, including Nobel Prize winner Roger Sperry, suggested that there were actually four different thinking styles based on brain dominance. Ned Herrmann, a researcher in critical thinking and whole-brain methods, also suggested that there are four brain hemispheres and that decision making varies with brain dominance (12 Manage: The Executive Fast Track, 2022). For example, Herrmann suggested that individuals with upper-left-brain dominance truly are analytical thinkers who like working with factual data and numbers. These individuals deal with problems logically and rationally. Individuals with lower-left-brain dominance are highly organized and detail oriented. They prefer a stable work environment and value safety and security over risk-taking.

In addition, researchers suggested that individuals with upper-right-brain dominance were big picture thinkers who looked for hidden possibilities and were futuristic in their thinking. They were thought to frequently rely on intuition to solve problems and are willing to take risks to seek new solutions to problems. Individuals with lower-right-brain dominance experienced facts and problem solved in a more emotional way than the other three types. They were sympathetic, kinesthetic, and empathetic and focused more on interpersonal aspects of decision making (12 Manage: The Executive Fast Track, 2022).

Newer research suggests, however, that any discussion of the existence of left- or right-brain dominance may be too simplistic, even with the subdivisions proposed by Herrmann or Sperry. Cherry (2020) agrees, suggesting that recent research has shown that the brain is not nearly

LEARNING EXERCISE 1.3

Thinking Styles

In small groups, discuss individual variations in thinking. Did some individuals identify themselves as more intuitive thinkers or more linear thinkers? Did group members self-identify with one or more of the four thinking styles noted by Herrmann (12 Manage: The Executive Fast Track, 2022)? Did gender seem to influence thinking style or brain hemisphere dominance? What types of thinkers were represented in group members' families? Did most group members view variances in a positive way?

as dichotomous as once thought. For example, abilities in subjects such as math are strongest when both halves of the brain work together. Indeed, both sides of the brain collaborate to perform a broad variety of tasks. Cherry (2020) notes that it is true that some brain functions occur in one or the other side of the brain (language tends to be on the left and attention more on the right), but people don't tend to have a stronger left- or right-sided brain network.

> New evidence suggests the existence of left- or right-brain dominance may be an oversimplification.

Overcoming Individual Vulnerability in Decision Making

How do people overcome subjectivity in making decisions? This can never be completely overcome nor should it. After all, life would be boring if everyone thought alike. However, managers and leaders must become aware of their own vulnerabilities and recognize how they influence and limit the quality of their decision making. Using the following suggestions will help decrease individual subjectivity and increase objectivity in decision making.

Values

Being confused and unclear about one's values may affect decision-making ability. Successful problem solvers then must periodically examine their values and have a conscious awareness of the values on which their decisions are based. This awareness is an essential component of decision making and critical thinking. Values clarification exercises are included in Chapter 7.

Life Experience

It is difficult to overcome inexperience when making decisions. However, a person can do some things to decrease this area of vulnerability. First, use available resources, including current research and literature, to gain a fuller understanding of the issues involved. Second, involve other people, such as experienced colleagues, mentors, trusted friends, and experts, to act as sounding boards and advisors. Third, analyze decisions later to assess their success. By evaluating decisions, people learn from mistakes and can overcome inexperience.

Individual Preference

Overcoming this area of vulnerability involves self-awareness, honesty, and risk-taking. The need for self-awareness was discussed previously, but it is not enough to be self-aware; people also must be honest with themselves about their choices and their preferences for those choices. In addition, the successful decision maker must take some risks. Nearly every decision has some element of risk, and most decisions involve consequences and accountability.

> Those who can do the right but unpopular thing and who dare to stand alone will emerge as leaders.

Individual Ways of Thinking

People making decisions alone are frequently handicapped because they are not able to understand problems fully or make decisions from both analytical and intuitive perspectives. However, most organizations include both types of thinkers and proactively seek out a diverse group of thinkers when solving problems and making decisions. Using group process and talking management problems over with others also helps to ensure that both intuitive and analytical approaches are used in solving problems and making decisions.

Decision Making in Organizations

The beginning of this chapter emphasized the need for managers and leaders to make quality decisions. The effect of the individual's values and preferences on decision making was discussed, but it is important for leaders and managers to also understand how the organization influences the decision-making process. Because organizations are made up of people with differing values and preferences, there is often conflict in organizational decision dynamics.

Effect of Organizational Power

Powerful people in organizations are more likely to have decisions made (by themselves or their subordinates) that are congruent with their own preferences and values. On the other hand, people wielding little power in organizations must always consider the preference of the powerful. In organizations, choice is constructed and constrained by many factors, and therefore, choice is not equally available to all people.

In addition, not only do the preferences of the powerful influence decisions of the less powerful but the powerful also can inhibit the preferences of the less powerful. This occurs because individuals who remain and advance in organizations are those who feel and express values and beliefs congruent with the organization. Therefore, a balance must be found between the limitations of choice posed by the power structure within the organization and totally independent decision making that could lead to organizational chaos.

> The ability of the powerful to influence individual decision making in an organization often requires adopting a private personality and an organizational personality.

For example, some might believe they would have made a different decision had they been acting on their own, but they went along with the organizational decision. This "going along" constitutes a decision. People choose to accept an organizational decision that differs from their own preferences and values. The concept of power in organizations is discussed in more detail in Chapter 13.

Rational and Administrative Decision Making

For many years, it was widely believed that most managerial decisions were based on a careful, scientific, and objective thought process and that managers made decisions in a rational manner. In the late 1940s, Herbert A. Simon's work revealed that most managers made many decisions that did not fit the objective rationality theory. Simon (1965) delineated two types of management decision makers: the "*economic man*" and the "*administrative man.*"

Managers who are successful decision makers often attempt to make rational decisions, much like the economic man described in Table 1.2. Because they realize that restricted knowledge and limited alternatives directly affect a decision's quality, these managers gather as much information as possible and generate many alternatives. Simon (1965) believed that the "economic model of man," however, was an unrealistic description of organizational decision making. The complexity of information acquisition makes it impossible for the human brain to store and retain the amount of information that is available for each decision. Because

TABLE **COMPARING THE "ECONOMIC MAN" WITH THE "ADMINISTRATIVE MAN"**

Economic	Administrative
Decisions are made in a rational manner	Decisions made are "good enough"
Decision maker has complete knowledge of the problem or decision situation	Complete knowledge is not possible, so knowledge is always fragmented
All possible alternatives are considered	Because consequences of alternatives occur in the future, they are impossible to predict accurately
A rational system of ordering preference of alternatives is used	Some alternatives are considered, but not all possible ones
Decisions are selected that maximize utility	Final choice is "satisficing" rather than maximizing

Source: Based on Simon, H. A. (1965). *The shape of automation for man and management*. Harper & Row.

of time constraints and the difficulty of assimilating large amounts of information, most management decisions are made using the administrative man model of decision making.

> Most management decisions are made by using the "administrative man" model of decision making.

The administrative man never has complete knowledge and generates fewer alternatives. Simon (1965) argued that the administrative man carries out decisions that are only *satisficing*, a term used to describe decisions that may not be ideal but result in solutions that have adequate outcomes. These managers want decisions to be "good enough" so that they "work," but they are less concerned that the alternative selected is the optimal choice. The "best" choice for many decisions is often found to be too costly in terms of time or resources, so another less costly but workable solution is found.

Clear (n.d.) agrees, suggesting that although researchers and economists believed for some time that humans always made logical, well-considered decisions, more current research suggests that a wide range of mental errors often derail our thinking. Sometimes, we make logical decisions, but there are many times when we make emotional, irrational, and confusing choices.

Annie Duke (2018), a well-known poker player, suggests this occurs because we often must make quick decisions with limited information. This means that mistakes, emotions, and poor choices are common. Judging the quality of our decision making on outcome alone then can be short sighted and counterproductive. Duke notes that sometimes, we make the best choice based on the information available, but other information is hidden. Other times, we choose a path with a high likelihood of success, but it fails. Still, other times, we make a decision that works, but other choices would have been better. So, decision making becomes less about being good or bad and more about "calibrating among all the shades of gray" (Duke, 2018, p. 34).

Decision-Making Tools

There is always some uncertainty in making decisions. However, management analysts have developed tools, which provide some order and direction in obtaining and using information or are helpful in selecting who should be involved in making the decision. Because there are so many decision aids, this chapter presents selected technology that would be most helpful to beginning- or middle-level managers, including decision grids, payoff tables, decision trees, consequence tables, logic models, and program evaluation and review technique (PERT). It is important to remember, though, that any decision-making tool always requires a person to make a final decision and that all such tools are subject to human error.

Alternative	Financial effect	Political effect	Departmental effect	Time	Decision
#1					
#2					
#3					
#4					

FIGURE 1.3 A decision grid.

Decision Grids

A *decision grid* allows one to visually examine the alternatives and compare each against the same criteria. Although any criterion may be selected, the same criteria are used to analyze each alternative. An example of a decision grid is depicted in Figure 1.3. When many alternatives have been generated or a group or committee is collaborating on the decision, these grids are particularly helpful to the process. This tool, for instance, would be useful when changing the method of managing care on a unit or when selecting a candidate to hire from a large interview pool. The unit manager or the committee would evaluate all the alternatives available using a decision grid. In this manner, every alternative is evaluated using the same criteria. It is possible to weigh some of the criteria more heavily than others if some are more important. To do this, it is usually necessary to assign a number value to each criterion. The result would be a numeric value for each alternative considered.

Payoff Tables

The decision aids known as *payoff tables* have a cost–profit–volume relationship and are very helpful when some quantitative information is available, such as an item's cost or predicted use. To use payoff tables, one must determine probabilities and use historical data, such as a hospital census and a report on the number of operating procedures performed. To illustrate, a payoff table might be appropriately used in determining how many participants it would take to make an in-service program break even in terms of costs.

   If the instructor for the class costs $500, the educational department would need to charge each of the 20 participants $25 for the class, but for 40 participants, the class would cost only $12.50 each. Attendance data from past classes and the number of nurses potentially available to attend help to determine probable class size and thus how much to charge for the class. Payoff tables do not guarantee that a correct decision will be made, but they assist in visualizing data.

Decision Trees

Because decisions are often tied to the outcome of other events, management analysts have developed *decision trees*.

   The decision tree in Figure 1.4 compares the cost of hiring regular staff with the cost of hiring temporary employees. Here, the decision is whether to hire extra nurses at regular salary to perform outpatient procedures on an oncology unit or to have nurses available to the unit on an on-call basis and pay them on-call and overtime wages. The possible consequences of a decreased volume of procedures and an increased volume must be considered. Initially, costs

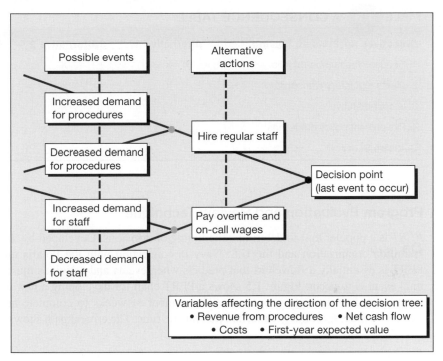

FIGURE 1.4 A decision tree.

would increase in hiring a regular staff, but, over a longer time, this move would mean greater savings if the volume of procedures does not dramatically decrease.

Consequence Tables

Consequence tables demonstrate how various alternatives create different consequences. A consequence table lists the objectives for solving a problem down one side of a table and rates how each alternative would meet the desired objective.

For example, consider this problem: "The number of patient falls has exceeded the benchmark rate for two consecutive quarters." After a period of analysis, the following alternatives were selected as solutions:

1. Provide a new educational program to instruct staff on how to prevent falls.
2. Implement a night check to ensure that patients have side rails up and beds in low position.
3. Implement a policy requiring direct patient observation by sitters on all confused patients.

The decision maker then lists each alternative opposite the objectives for solving the problem, which for this problem might be (a) reduces the number of falls, (b) meets regulatory standards, (c) is cost-effective, and (d) fits present policy guidelines. The decision maker then ranks each desired objective and examines each of the alternatives through a standardized key, which allows a fair comparison between alternatives and assists in eliminating undesirable choices. It is important to examine long-term effects of each alternative as well as how the decision will affect others. See Table 1.3 for an example of a consequence table.

Logic Models

Logic models are schematics or pictures of how programs are intended to operate. The schematic typically includes resources, processes, and desired outcomes and depicts exactly what the relationships are between the three components.

TABLE **1.3** **A CONSEQUENCE TABLE**

Objectives for Problem Solving	Alternative 1	Alternative 2	Alternative 3
1. Reduces the number of falls	X	X	X
2. Meets regulatory standards	X	X	X
3. Is cost-effective		X	X
4. Fits present policy guidelines			X
Decision Score			

Program Evaluation and Review Technique

PERT is a popular tool to determine the timing of decisions. Developed by the Booz–Allen–Hamilton organization and the U.S. Navy in connection with the Polaris missile program, PERT is essentially a flowchart that predicts when events and activities must take place if a final event is to occur. Figure 1.5 shows a PERT chart for developing a new outpatient treatment room for oncology procedures. The number of weeks to complete tasks is listed in optimistic time, most likely time, and pessimistic time. The critical path shows something that

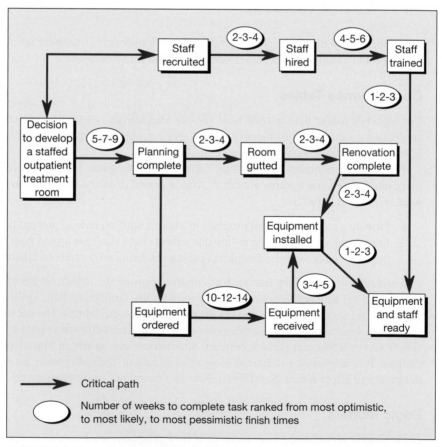

FIGURE 1.5 Example of a program evaluation and review technique flow diagram.

must occur in the sequence before one may proceed. PERT is especially helpful when a group of people is working on a project. The flowchart keeps everyone up-to-date, and problems are easily identified when they first occur. Flowcharts are popular, and many people use them in their personal lives.

Pitfalls in Using Decision-Making Tools

A common flaw in making decisions is to base decisions on first impressions. This then typically leads to confirmation biases. So, even the use of consequence tables, decision trees, and other quantitative decision tools will not guarantee a successful decision. It is also human nature to focus on an event that leaves a strong impression, so individuals may have preconceived notions or biases that influence decisions. Too often, managers allow the past to unduly influence current decisions.

> Many of the pitfalls associated with management decision-making tools can be reduced by choosing the correct decision-making style and involving others when appropriate.

Although there are times when others should be involved, it is not always necessary to involve others in decision making, and frequently, a manager does not have time to involve a large group. However, it is important to separate those decisions that need the input of others from those that a manager can make alone.

Integrating Leadership Roles and Management Functions in Decision Making

This chapter has discussed effective decision making, problem solving, critical thinking, clinical reasoning, and elastic thinking as requisites for being a successful leader and manager. The successful decision maker possesses courage, energy, and creativity and is aware of the need for sensitivity in decision making. Leaders recognize the appropriate people to include in decision making and to use a suitable theoretical model for the decision situation.

Managers who make quality decisions are effective administrators. The manager should develop a systematic, scientific approach to problem solving that begins with a fixed goal and ends with an evaluation step. Decision tools exist to help make more effective decisions; however, leader-managers must remember that such tools are not foolproof and that they often do not adequately allow for the human element in management. In addition, managers should strive to make decisions that reflect research-based best practices and nursing's scientific knowledge base. Yet, the role of intuition as an adjunct to quality decision making should not be overlooked.

The integrated leader-manager understands the significance that sex and gender, personal values, life experience, preferences, willingness to take risks, brain hemisphere dominance, and thinking styles have on selected alternatives in making the decision. The critical thinker pondering a decision is aware of the areas of vulnerability that hinder successful decision making and will expend efforts to avoid the pitfalls of faulty logic and data gathering.

Both managers and leaders understand the impact that the organization has on decision making and that some of the decisions that will be made in the organization will be only "satisficing." However, leaders will strive to problem solve adequately to reach optimal decisions as often as possible.

Key Concepts

- Successful decision makers are self-aware, courageous, sensitive, energetic, and creative.
- The rational approach to problem solving begins with a fixed goal and ends with an evaluation process.
- Naturalistic decision making blends intuition and analysis, but pattern recognition and experience guide decision makers when time is limited or systematic rational decision making is not possible.
- Evidence-based nursing practice integrates the best evidence available to achieve desirable outcomes.
- Typically, a PICO format is used in evidence-based practice to guide the search for the current best evidence to address a problem.
- The successful decision maker understands the significance that sex and gender; personal, individual values; life experience; preferences; willingness to take risks; brain hemisphere dominance; and predominant thinking style have on alternative identification and selection.

- Left- and right-brain dominance may be an oversimplification in terms of how individuals think.
- The critical thinker is aware of areas of vulnerability that hinder successful decision making and makes efforts to avoid the pitfalls of faulty logic when gathering data.
- The act of making and evaluating decisions increases the expertise of the decision maker.
- There are many models for improving decision making. Using a systematic decision-making or problem-solving model reduces heuristic trial-and-error or rule-of-thumb methods and increases the probability that appropriate decisions will be made.
- Two major considerations in organizational decision making are how power affects decision making and whether management decision making needs to be only "satisficing."
- Management science has produced many tools to help decision makers make better and more objective decisions, but all are subject to human error, and many do not adequately consider the human element.

Additional Learning Exercises and Applications

LEARNING EXERCISE 1.4

Assessing Personal Decision Making

ASSIGNMENT:

Write a two- to three-page response to one of the following prompts:

A. Identify a poor decision that you recently made because of faulty data gathering. Have you ever made a poor decision because necessary information was intentionally or unintentionally withheld from you?

B. Describe the two best decisions that you have made in your life and the two worst. What factors assisted you in making the wise decisions? What elements of critical thinking went awry in your poor decision making? How would you evaluate your decision-making ability?

C. Examine the process that you used in your decision to become a nurse. Would you describe it as fitting a profile of the economic man or the administrative man?

D. Do you typically use a problem-solving or decision-making model to solve problems? Have you ever used an intuitive model? Think of a critical decision that you have made in the last year. Describe what theoretical model, if any, you used to assist you in the process. Did you enlist the help of others in solving the problem?

LEARNING EXERCISE 1.5

Sharing Workload

You are a staff nurse on a small telemetry unit. The unit is staffed at a ratio of one nurse for every four patients, and the charge nurse is counted in this staffing. There is also a full-time unit secretary and monitor technician to assist at the desk. The charge nurse is responsible for making the daily staffing assignments.

Although you recognize that the charge nurse needs to reduce her patient care assignment to perform the charge nurse duties, you have grown increasingly frustrated that she normally assigns herself only one patient, if any, and these patients always have the lowest acuity level on the floor. This has placed a disproportionate burden on the other nurses, who often feel the assignment they are being given may be unsafe. The charge nurse is your immediate supervisor. She has not generally been responsive to concerns expressed by the staff to her about this problem.

ASSIGNMENT:

Decide what the problem is in this scenario and who owns it. Identify at least five alternatives for action and select which one you believe will have the greatest likelihood of successful implementation. How did differences in power and status influence the alternatives you identified? What outcomes must be achieved for you to feel that the choice you made was a good one?

LEARNING EXERCISE 1.6

Considering Critical Elements in Decision Making

You are a college senior and president of your student nursing organization. You are on the committee to select a slate of officers for the next academic year. Several of the current officers will be graduating, and you want the new slate of officers to be committed to the organization. Some of the brightest members of the junior class involved in the organization are not well liked by some of your friends in the organization.

ASSIGNMENT:

Looking at the critical elements in decision making, compile a list of the most important points to consider in making the decision for selecting a slate of officers. What must you guard against, and how should you approach the data gathering to solve this problem?

LEARNING EXERCISE 1.7

Decision Making and Risk Taking

You are a new graduate nurse just finishing your 3-month probation period at your first job in acute care nursing. You have been working closely with a preceptor; however, they have been gradually transitioning you to more independent practice. You now have your own patient care assignment and have been giving medications independently for several weeks. Today, your assignment included a confused older adult patient with severe coronary disease. Her medications include antihypertensives, antiarrhythmics, and beta-blockers. It was a very busy morning, and you have barely had a moment to reorganize and collect your thoughts.

It is now 2:30 PM, and you are preparing your handoff report. When you review the patient's 2:00 PM vital signs, you note a significant rise in this patient's blood pressure and heart rate. The patient, however, reports no distress. You remember that when you passed the morning medications, the patient was in the middle of her bath and asked that you just set the medications on the bedside table and that she would take them in a few minutes. You meant to return to see that she did but were sidetracked by a problem with another patient.

You now go to the patient's room to see if she, indeed, did take the pills. The pill cup and pills are not where you left them, and a search of the wastebasket, patient bed, and bedside table yields nothing. The patient is too confused to be an accurate historian regarding whether she took the pills. No one on your patient care team noticed the pills.

At this point, you are not sure what you should do next. You are upset that you did not wait to give the medications in person but cannot change this now. You charted the medications as being given this morning when you left them at the bedside. You are reluctant to report this as a medication error because you are still on probation, and you are not sure that the patient did not take the pills as she said she would. Your probation period has not gone as smoothly as you would have liked anyway, and you are aware that reporting this incident will likely prolong your probation, and that a copy of the error report will be placed in your personnel file. The patient's physician is also frequently short-tempered and will likely be agitated when you report your uncertainty about whether the patient received her prescribed medications. The reality is that if you do nothing, it is likely that no one will ever know about the problem.

You do feel responsible, however, for the patient's welfare. The physician might want to give additional doses of the medication if indeed the patient did not take the pills. In addition, the rise in heart rate and blood pressure has only just become apparent, and you realize that her heart rate and blood pressure could continue to deteriorate over the next shift. The patient is not due to receive the medications again until 9:00 PM tonight (b.i.d. every 12 hours).

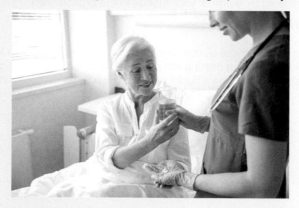

ASSIGNMENT:

Decide how you will proceed. Determine whether you will use a systematic problem-solving model, intuition, or both in making your choices. How did your values, preferences, life experiences, willingness to take risks, and individual ways of thinking influence your decision?

LEARNING EXERCISE   1.8

Determining a Need to Know

You are a nursing student. You were diagnosed as HIV-positive a decade ago. You are now in a committed relationship, and your partner is aware of your HIV status. You have experienced relatively few side effects from the antiretroviral drugs you take, and you appear to be healthy. You have not shared your sexual preferences, past sexual history, or HIV status with any of your classmates, primarily because you do not feel that it is their business and because you fear being ostracized in the local community.

Today, in the clinical setting, one of the students accidentally stuck themselves with a needle right before injecting it into a patient. Laboratory follow-up was ordered to ensure that the patient was not exposed to any blood-borne disease from the student. Tonight, for the first time, you recognize that no matter how careful you are, there is at least a small risk that you could inadvertently expose patients to your bodily fluids and thus to some risk.

ASSIGNMENT:

Decide what you will do. Is it necessary to share your HIV status with the school? With future employers? With patients? What determines whether there is "a need to tell" and a "need to know"? What objective weighted most heavily in your decision?

LEARNING EXERCISE   1.9

Using a Flowchart for Project Management

Think of a project that you are working on; it could be a dance, a picnic, remodeling your bathroom, or a semester schedule of activities in a class.

ASSIGNMENT:

Draw a flowchart, inserting at the bottom the date that activities for the event are to be completed. Working backward, insert critical tasks and their completion dates. Refer to your flowchart throughout the project to see if you are staying on target.

LEARNING EXERCISE   1.10

Addressing a Communication Gap

You are a new graduate nurse just finishing your 3-month probation period at your first job in acute care nursing. Your usual assignment is to be a team leader for eight patients, with one licensed practical nurse/licensed vocational nurse and one nursing assistant on your team. Today, your assignment included a confused older adult patient. You requested, during work assignments with your team, that the nursing assistant pay attention to this patient's intake and output (I & O) as you feel he may need some intravenous fluids if his I & O remain poor. You asked the nursing assistant to notify you if there was a significant change, so you could notify the physician. It was a very busy day, and you have barely had a moment to reorganize and collect your thoughts.

(continues on page 30)

LEARNING EXERCISE 1.10

Addressing a Communication Gap (continued)

It is now 2:30 PM, and you are preparing your end-of-shift report. When you review the patient's 2:00 PM I & O sheet, you note a significant drop in intake, and the total output for the shift is only 90 mL. You meant to check the I & O sheet during the day but kept getting sidetracked by problems with other patients. However, you are also upset that the nursing assistant did not keep you informed of this condition.

You now go to the patient's room and assess the patient and find his vital signs and other findings similar to this morning's assessment. You check with the nursing assistant to make sure the I & O recorded for the day is accurate, and you call the physician to obtain an order to begin intravenous fluids. When you ask the nursing assistant why they did not report the significant drop in output to you, they say, "I forgot."

At this point, you are not sure what you should do next. You feel you should handle this yourself and not go to the charge nurse. You are a new nurse and do want to get started on the wrong foot by speaking too harshly to the nursing assistant, yet you feel this lack of following instructions cannot go unanswered. The reality is that if you do nothing, it is likely that no one else will ever know about the problem.

The doctor did not seem upset when you called about the drop in output, and just ordered the fluids, but the need to start the intravenous line and give report caused you to work overtime. By the time you finished your shift, the nursing assistant had gone home and you are left to spend your evening at home pondering what, if anything, you should do to follow up on this tomorrow.

ASSIGNMENT:

Decide how you will proceed. Determine whether you will use a systematic problem-solving model, intuition, or both in making your choices. How did your values, preferences, life experiences, willingness to take risks, and individual ways of thinking influence your decision?

LEARNING EXERCISE 1.11

Returning to School for a Bachelor of Science in Nursing Degree

You have been a registered nurse (RN) for 5 years. Right after high school, you became a licensed vocational nurse (LVN) and after 6 years decided to attend a local LVN to associate degree in nursing program at a local community college. You have become increasingly interested in attending a university to complete requirements for your Bachelor of Science in Nursing (BSN) degree. You are still undecided; some of your friends are urging you to do this, and others ask why you need the degree.

Not only must you make up your mind about pursuing this option, you must choose from an on-campus or online program. The regional university is 60 miles away and would require significant amounts of driving if you chose the on campus program, but you know you learn best in a traditional classroom environment.

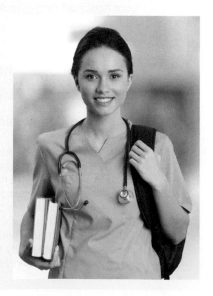

The university also offers an online program that would require only four Saturdays of attendance each semester for the theory courses but you would need to commute for clinical courses anyway. Both options have pros and cons.

Make a payoff table, calculating chances for advancement and salary increase weighed against the cost of your new degree. Decide if it makes economic sense to get a BSN degree.

Then create a pay off table to determine whether to enroll in the on campus or online program.

ASSIGNMENT:

Create a decision grid for the two alternatives, weighting the same criteria for each, using such things as cost, travel, quality of campus life, reputation and quality of the university, and so on. Assign each of your criteria a weighted score for the value that you personally place on it. What did your final grid look like and what was your final decision?

REFERENCES

Ahmady, S., & Shahbazi, S. (2020). Impact of social problem-solving training on critical thinking and decision making of nursing students. *BMC Nursing, 19*(1), 94. https://doi.org.mantis.csuchico.edu/10.1186/s12912-020-00487-x

Cherry, K. (2020, April 10). *Left brain vs. right brain dominance: Is the analytical-creative separation true or false?* Retrieved July 6, 2021, from https://www.verywellmind.com/left-brain-vs-right-brain-2795005

Clear, J. (n.d.). *5 Common mental errors that sway you from making good decisions.* http://jamesclear.com/common-mental-errors?__s=qs5np5qs1thadcasrdsr

Decision-making-confidence.com. (2006–2022). *Six step decision making process.* Retrieved February 7, 2022, from https://www.decision-making-confidence.com/six-step-decision-making-process.html

Dictionary.com. (2022). Critical thinking. In *Dictionary.com Unabridged dictionary.* Retrieved February 7, 2022, from http://www.dictionary.com/browse/critical-thinking?s=t

Duke, A. (2018). *Thinking in bets: Making smarter decisions when you don't have all the facts.* Portfolio/Penguin.

Farnam Street Media Inc. (2022). *Your first thought is rarely your best thought: Lessons on thinking.* Retrieved February 7, 2022, from https://fs.blog/2018/02/first-thought-not-best-thought/

Ford, C. D., & Graves, B. A. (2023). Evidence-based practice. In C. J. Huston (Ed.), *Professional issues in nursing: Challenges and opportunities* (6th ed., pp. 67–77). Wolters Kluwer.

Hammad, B. M., & Khalaf, I. A. (2020). How does case-based learning strategy influence nursing students' clinical decision-making ability in critical care nursing education? An integrative review. *Middle East Journal of Nursing, 14*(2), 3–8.

Henni, Y. (2021, April 4). *Elastic thinking: How it can help you solve your biggest challenges.* Medium. Retrieved February 7, 2022, from https://dr-younes-henni.medium.com/elastic-thinking-is-your-gateway-to-more-innovative-ideas-7cea5bc3a7cd

Klein, G. (2008). Naturalistic decision making. *Human Factors, 50*, 456–460.

Mlodinow, L. (2018). Your elastic mind. *Psychology Today, 51*(2), 92–100.

National Association of Social Workers. (2020). *Essential steps for ethical problem-solving.* https://www.naswma.org/page/100/Essential-Steps-for-Ethical-Problem-Solving.htm

Prasad, V. (2021, August 17). *Seven cognitive distortions poisoning COVID debates.* Medpage Today. Retrieved August 18, 2021, from https://www.medpagetoday.com/opinion/vinay-prasad/94074?xid=nl_mpt_DHE_2021-08-18&eun=g1619680d0r&utm_source=Sailthru&utm_medium=email&utm_campaign=Daily%20Headlines%20Top%20Cat%20HeC%20%202021-08-18&utm_term=NL_Daily_DHE_dual-gmail-definition

Rehana, R. W., & Huda, N. (2021, May). A common heuristic in medicine: Anchoring. *Annals of Medical and Health Sciences Research, 11*(5), 1461–1463. https://www.amhsr.org/articles/a-common-heuristic-in-medicine-anchoring.pdf

Simon, H. A. (1965). *The shape of automation for man and management.* Harper & Row.

12 Manage: The Executive Fast Track. (2022). Whole brain model (Herrmann). Retrieved February 7, 2022, from https://www.12manage.com/methods_herrmann_whole_brain.html

2

Classical Views of Leadership and Management

*…management is efficiency in climbing the ladder of success; leadership determines whether the ladder is leaning against the right wall.—**Stephen R. Covey***

*…no executive has ever suffered because his subordinates were strong and effective.—**Peter Drucker***

*…leadership is a choice, not a position.—**Stephen R. Covey***

CROSSWALK

This chapter addresses:

- **AACN Essentials Domain 1:** Knowledge for nursing practice
- **AACN Essentials Domain 4:** Scholarship for nursing practice
- **AACN Essentials Domain 6:** Interprofessional partnerships
- **AACN Essentials Domain 7:** Systems-based practice
- **AACN Essentials Domain 9:** Professionalism
- **AACN Essentials Domain 10:** Personal, professional, and leadership development
- **AONL Nurse Executive Competency 1:** Communication and relationship building
- **AONL Nurse Executive Competency 2:** A knowledge of the health care environment
- **AONL Nurse Executive Competency 3:** Leadership
- **ANA Standard of Professional Performance 11**: Collaboration
- **ANA Standard of Professional Performance 12:** Leadership
- **ANA Standard of Professional Performance 13:** Education
- **QSEN Competency:** Teamwork and collaboration

LEARNING OBJECTIVES

The learner will:

- identify similarities and differences between leadership and management
- differentiate between leadership roles and management functions
- discuss the historical evolution of management theory
- correlate management theorists with their appropriate theoretical contributions to management science
- define the components of the management process
- discuss the historical evolution of leadership theory
- correlate leadership theorists with their appropriate theoretical contributions to leadership science
- identify common leadership styles and describe situations in which each leadership style could be used appropriately
- differentiate between authoritative, democratic, and laissez-faire leadership styles
- delineate variables suggested in situational and contingency theories

- describe the differences between interactional and transformational leadership theories
- identify contextual factors impacting the relationship between leaders and followers based on full-range leadership theory
- analyze why full-range leadership models suggest leaders must have skills in transformational leadership, transactional leadership, and laissez-faire leadership
- recognize that the integration of both leadership and management skills is critical to the long-term viability of contemporary health care organizations

Introduction

The relationship between leadership and management continues to prompt debate, although there clearly is a need for both. Leadership is viewed by some as one of management's many functions; others maintain that leadership requires more complex skills than management and that management is only one role of leadership. Still, others suggest that management emphasizes *control*—control of hours, costs, salaries, overtime, use of sick leave, inventory, and supplies—whereas leadership increases productivity by building teams, empowering workers, and maximizing *effectiveness*.

If a manager guides and directs workers and a leader empowers them, it could be said that every manager should be a leader. Indeed, Duggal (2021) notes that being a manager and a leader at the same time is a viable concept. But being a phenomenal leader does not guarantee that the person will be an exceptional manager and vice versa. This is because the manager has the responsibility to carry out the four important functions of management in an organization: planning, organizing, leading, and controlling. While most managers tend to be leaders, this is the case only if they also adequately carry out the leadership responsibilities of management, which include communication, motivation, providing inspiration and guidance, and encouraging employees to rise to a higher level of productivity (Duggal, 2021).

In addition, Duggal (2021) notes that while the terms *leadership* and *management* are often used interchangeably, a primary difference between them is that leaders don't necessarily hold or occupy a management position. In other words, leaders don't have to have formal authority to direct others in the organization; they can hold any position in the organization. There are, however, commonly recognized distinctions between leaders and managers and those differences must be understood and recognized so that an organization can leverage each to the fullest (Display 2.1). Display 2.2 contrasts traditional components of leadership and management.

So which is more important—good leadership or good management? The answer varies depending on the situation (situational leadership). We are all aware of individuals in leadership positions who cannot manage and individuals in management roles who cannot lead.

Unfortunately, some managers aren't very good at leading people. This may occur because the processes that determine and shape leaders often produce people who behave differently from what some employees desire. In addition, managers may be promoted into roles based on tenure or previous managerial roles—with little consideration for whether they possess the humanistic skills and qualities of good leadership. Paradoxically, some leaders lack the organization and structured thinking to bring ideas to fruition or to achieve productivity goals. In addition, they may perceive themselves to be more inspiring than they are.

In the end, both leadership and management skills are needed for organizational success. Leadership without management results in chaos and failure for both the organization and the individual. Thus, in the face of significant change, *both* sound management and strong leadership skills are essential to the long-term viability of today's health care

DISPLAY 2.1 DISTINCTIONS BETWEEN LEADERS AND MANAGERS (DUGGAL, 2021)

1. A leader invents or innovates whereas a manager organizes.
2. A manager relies on control whereas a leader inspires trust.
3. A leader asks the questions "what" and "why," whereas a manager leans more toward the questions "how" and "when."
4. Managers have subordinates and leaders gain followers, which implies that managers create a circle of power whereas leaders create a circle of influence.
5. Unlike managers, leaders are followed because of their personality, behavior, and beliefs.
6. Managers control groups to accomplish a specific goal. Leaders motivate, influence, and enable others to contribute to the success of an organization.
7. Inspiration and influence separate leaders from managers—not control and power.
8. Managers count value, and in doing that, sometimes cut down on the value by disabling or otherwise countering ideas and people who add value. Leaders, however, focus on working to generate a certain value that is over and above that which the team creates—and are as much creators of value as their followers.
9. Managers have a greater formal responsibility and accountability for rationality and control than leaders.
10. Leadership inspires change; management manages transformation.

organizations, and most organizations need both kinds of skills and aptitudes to secure enduring success.

This chapter first artificially differentiates between management and leadership, focusing on theory development in each field of study. A chronologic view of the development of management and leadership theory is provided, although the author recognizes that boundaries are blurred between the two since much of the work done by later management theorists and early leadership theorists overlaps. This chapter concludes with a discussion of how closely integrated leadership and management must actually be for individuals in contemporary leadership or management roles.

DISPLAY 2.2 A COMPARISON OF TRADITIONAL MANAGEMENT AND LEADERSHIP COMPONENTS

Managers
- Are assigned a position or title by an organization
- Have a legitimate source of power due to delegated authority that accompanies their position
- Have specific duties and responsibilities they are expected to carry out including establishing work rules, processes, standards, and operating procedures
- Build strategic visions and break them down into plans for workers to follow
- Emphasize control, decision making, decision analysis, and results/productivity
- Manipulate people, the environment, money, time, and other resources to achieve the goals of the organization
- Direct willing and unwilling subordinates

Leaders
- Often do not have delegated, tangible, or formal power over others but obtain power through other means, such as influencing or inspiring others
- Have a wider variety of roles than managers
- Focus on group process, information gathering, feedback, and empowering others
- May or may not be part of the formal hierarchy of the organization
- Emphasize interpersonal relationships
- Take interest in their followers' success, enabling them to reach their goals
- Direct willing followers

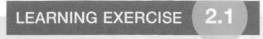

LEARNING EXERCISE   2.1

Leadership Roles and Management Functions

In small or large groups, discuss your views of management and leadership. Do you believe they are the same or different? If you believe that they are different, do you think that they have the same importance for the future of nursing? Do you feel that one is more important than the other? How can novice nurse-managers learn important management functions and develop leadership skills?

Management

Merriam-Webster Dictionary (2022) defines management as "the conducting or supervising of something" or the "judicious use of means to accomplish an end" (para. 1). This definition implies that management is the process of leading and directing all or part of an organization through the deployment and manipulation of resources.

Historical Development of Management Theory

Management science, like nursing, develops a theory base from many disciplines, such as business, psychology, sociology, and anthropology. Because organizations are complex and varied, theorists' views of what successful management is and what it should be have changed repeatedly in the last 100 years.

> Theorists' views of what successful management is and what it should be have changed repeatedly in the last 100 years.

Scientific Management (1900 to 1930)

Frederick W. Taylor, the "father of scientific management," was a mechanical engineer in the Midvale and Bethlehem Steel plants in Pennsylvania in the late 1800s. Frustrated with what he called "systematic soldiering," where workers achieved minimum standards doing the least amount of work possible, Taylor postulated that if workers could be taught the "one best way to accomplish a task," productivity would increase. Borrowing a term coined by Louis Brandeis, a colleague of Taylor's, Taylor called these principles *scientific management*. The four overriding principles of scientific management as identified by Taylor (1911) are:

1. Traditional "rule of thumb" means of organizing work must be replaced with scientific methods. In other words, by using time and motion studies and the expertise of experienced workers, work could be scientifically designed to promote greatest efficiency of time and energy.
2. A scientific personnel system must be established so that workers can be hired, trained, and promoted based on their unique technical competence and abilities.
3. Workers should be able to view how they "fit" into the organization and how they contribute to overall organizational productivity. This provides common goals and a sharing of the organizational mission. Thus, Taylor advocated the use of financial incentives as a reward for work accomplished, and workers were reimbursed according to their level of production rather than by an hourly wage.
4. The relationship between managers and workers should be cooperative and interdependent, and the work should be shared equally. Their roles, however, were not the same.

Human Relations Management (1930 to 1970)

During the 1920s, worker unrest developed. The Industrial Revolution had resulted in great numbers of relatively unskilled laborers working in large factories on specialized tasks. Thus, management scientists and organizational theorists began to look at the role of worker satisfaction in production. This *human relations era* developed the concepts of participatory and humanistic management, emphasizing people rather than machines.

Mary Parker Follett (1926) was one of the first theorists to suggest basic principles of what today would be called *participative decision making* or *participative management*. In her essay "The Giving of Orders," Follett espoused her belief that managers should have authority with, rather than over, employees. Thus, solutions could be found that satisfied both sides without having one side dominate the other.

The human relations era also attempted to correct what was perceived as the major shortcoming of the bureaucratic system—a failure to include the "human element." Studies done at the Hawthorne Works of the Western Electric Company near Chicago between 1927 and 1932 played a major role in this shifting focus. The studies, conducted by Elton Mayo and his Harvard associates, began as an attempt to look at the relationship between light illumination in the factory and productivity.

Mayo and his colleagues discovered that when management paid special attention to workers, productivity was likely to increase, regardless of the environmental working conditions. This *Hawthorne effect* indicated that people respond to the fact that they are being studied, attempting to increase whatever behavior they feel will continue to warrant the attention. Mayo (1953) also found that informal work groups and a socially informal work environment were factors in determining productivity, and Mayo recommended more employee participation in decision making.

Douglas McGregor (1960) reinforced these ideas by theorizing that managerial attitudes about employees (and, hence, how managers treat those employees) can be directly correlated with employee satisfaction. He labeled this *Theory X* and *Theory Y*. Theory X managers believe that their employees are basically lazy, need constant supervision and direction, and are indifferent to organizational needs. Theory Y managers believe that their workers enjoy their work, are self-motivated, and are willing to work hard to meet personal and organizational goals.

Chris Argyris (1964) supported McGregor (1960) and Mayo (1953) by saying that managerial domination causes workers to become discouraged and passive. He believed that if self-esteem and independence needs are not met, employees will become discouraged and troublesome or may leave the organization. Argyris stressed the need for flexibility within the organization and employee participation in decision making.

The human relations era of management science brought about a great interest in the study of workers. Many sociologists and psychologists took up this challenge, and their work in management theory contributed to our understanding of worker motivation, which is discussed in Chapter 18.

Table 2.1 summarizes the development of management theory up to 1970. By the late 1960s, however, there was growing concern that the human relations approach to management

LEARNING EXERCISE   2.3

Management Skills Assessment

Recall times when you have been a manager. This does not only mean a nursing manager. Perhaps you were a head lifeguard or an evening shift manager at a fast-food restaurant. During those times, do you think you were a good manager? Did you involve others in your management decision making appropriately? How would you evaluate your decision-making ability? Make a list of your management strengths and a list of management skills that you felt you were lacking.

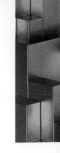

TABLE 2.1	THE DEVELOPMENT OF MANAGEMENT THEORY 1900 TO 1970
Theorist	**Theory**
Taylor	Scientific management
Weber	Bureaucratic organizations
Fayol	Management functions
Gulick	Activities of management
Follett	Participative management
Mayo	Hawthorne effect
McGregor	Theories X and Y
Argyris	Employee participation

was not without its problems. Most people continued to work in a bureaucratic environment, making it difficult to always apply a participatory approach to management. The human relations approach was also time-consuming and sometimes resulted in unmet organizational goals. In addition, not every employee liked working in a less structured environment. This resulted in a greater recognition of the need to intertwine management and leadership than ever before.

Leadership

Despite its relatively new addition to the English language, the word *leadership* has many meanings and there is no single definition broad enough to encompass the total leadership process. To examine the word *leader*, however, is to note that leaders lead. Leaders are those individuals who take risks, attempt to achieve shared goals, and inspire others to action. Those individuals who choose to follow a leader do so by choice, not because they must. Stoner (2022) notes then that leadership impact depends on the ability to influence people, not the ability to command, coerce, or manipulate. Thus, a job title alone does not make a person a leader. Only a person's behavior determines whether they hold a leadership role. The manager is the person who brings things about—the one who accomplishes, has the responsibility, and conducts. A leader is the person who influences and guides direction, opinion, and course of action.

> "How do you recognize a leader? It's not by their location. A leader can be out in front, in the middle, or following behind. You recognize a leader by the response of their followers" (Stoner, 2022).

Other characteristics of leaders include the following:

- Leaders often do not have delegated authority but obtain their power through other means, such as influence.
- Leaders have a wider variety of roles than do managers.
- Leaders may or may not be part of the formal organization.
- Leaders focus on group process, information gathering, feedback, and empowering others.
- Leaders emphasize interpersonal relationships.
- Leaders direct willing followers.
- Leaders have goals that may or may not reflect those of the organization.

Display 2.3 includes a list of common leadership roles.

DISPLAY 2.3	COMMON LEADERSHIP ROLES	
Decision maker	Coach	Forecaster
Communicator	Counselor	Influencer
Evaluator	Teacher	Creative problem solver
Facilitator	Critical thinker	Change agent
Risk taker	Buffer	Diplomat
Mentor	Advocate	Role model
Energizer	Visionary	Innovator
Priority setter	Director	Encourager

It is important also to remember that all it takes to stop being a leader is to have others stop following you. Leadership then is more dynamic than management, and leaders do make mistakes that can result in the loss of their followers. For example, Zenger and Folkman (2021), using 360-degree feedback data from over 87,000 leaders across the globe, identified six fatal flaws that derail leaders (Display 2.4). Although these flaws seem obvious, many ineffective leaders are unaware that they exhibit these behaviors.

Historical Development of Leadership Theory (1900 to Present)

Because strong management skills were historically valued more than strong leadership skills, the scientific study of leadership did not begin until the 20th century. Early works focused on broad conceptualizations of leadership, such as the traits or behaviors of the leader. Contemporary research focuses more on leadership as a process of influencing others within an organizational culture and the interactive relationship of the leader and follower. To better understand newer views about leadership, it is necessary to look at how leadership theory has evolved over the last century.

> Like management theory, leadership theory has been dynamic; that is, what is "known" and believed about leadership continues to change over time.

The Great Man Theory/Trait Theories (1900 to 1940)

The *Great Man theory* and *trait theories* were the basis for most leadership research until the mid-1940s. The Great Man theory asserts that some people are born to lead, whereas others are born to be led. It also suggests that great leaders will arise when the situation demands it. Trait theories assume that some people have certain characteristics or personality traits that make them better leaders than others. To determine the traits that distinguish great leaders, researchers studied the lives of prominent people throughout history. The effect of followers and the impact of the situation were ignored. Although trait theories have obvious

DISPLAY 2.4	SIX FATAL LEADERSHIP FLAWS

1. The inability to inspire and motivate others
2. Not practicing self-development by asking for feedback
3. Poor teamwork and collaboration
4. A failure to develop others
5. The inability to communicate powerfully and prolifically
6. Not building and maintaining positive relationships with others

Source: Adapted from Zenger, J., & Folkman, J. (2021, May 3). *6 Fatal flaws that kill a leader's effectiveness.* Zenger Folkman. https://zengerfolkman.com/articles/6-fatal-flaws-that-kill-a-leaders-effectiveness/

DISPLAY 2.5 CHARACTERISTICS ASSOCIATED WITH LEADERSHIP

Intelligence	Creativity	Interpersonal skills
Knowledge	Cooperativeness	Tact
Judgment	Alertness	Diplomacy
Decisiveness	Self-confidence	Prestige
Oral fluency	Personal integrity	Social participation
Emotional intelligence	Emotional balance and control	Charisma
Independence	Risk taking	Collaborative priority setting
Personable	Critical thinking	Resilience
Skilled communicator	Ability	
Adaptability	Able to enlist cooperation	

shortcomings (e.g., they neglect the impact of others or the situation on the leadership role), they are worth examining. Many of the characteristics identified in trait theories (Display 2.5) are still used to describe successful leaders today.

Contemporary opponents of trait theories argue, however, that leadership skills can be developed, not just inherited. That is not to say that some people don't have certain characteristics or personality traits that may make it easier for them to lead. For example, Huston (2018) notes that some people, even at very young ages, are more fearless. Others are just naturally more outgoing; they're more curious; they take more risks. But not all leaders need to be gregarious by nature. There's room for quiet leadership. In fact, some of the most effective leaders are individuals who didn't seek out that role—they simply grew into it because they stepped forth to do what had to be done when no one else would (Huston, 2018).

> Perhaps leaders are both born and made that way.

Behavioral Theories (1940 to 1980)

During the human relations era, many behavioral and social scientists studying management also studied leadership. For example, McGregor's (1960) theories had as much influence on leadership research as they did on management science. As leadership theory developed, researchers moved away from studying what traits the leader had and examined what they did—the leader's style of leadership.

A breakthrough occurred when Lewin (1951) and White and Lippitt (1960) isolated common *leadership styles*. Later, these styles came to be called authoritarian, democratic, and laissez-faire.

The *authoritarian* leader is characterized by the following behaviors:

- Strong control is maintained over the work group.
- Others are motivated by coercion.
- Others are directed with commands.
- Communication flows downward.
- Decision making does not involve others.
- Emphasis is on difference in status ("I" and "you").
- Criticism is punitive.

Authoritarian leadership results in well-defined group actions that are usually predictable, reducing frustration in the work group and giving members a feeling of security. Productivity is usually high, but creativity, self-motivation, and autonomy are reduced. Authoritarian leadership is frequently found in very large bureaucracies such as the armed forces.

The *democratic* leader exhibits the following behaviors:

- Less control is maintained.
- Economic and ego awards are used to motivate.
- Others are directed through suggestions and guidance.
- Communication flows up and down.
- Decision making involves others.
- Emphasis is on "we" rather than I and you.
- Criticism is constructive.

In other words, democratic leaders seek input from their followers and include them in decision making whenever possible. This makes them feel valued and creates an investment in the outcome of what is being determined.

Democratic leadership, appropriate for groups who work together for extended periods, promotes autonomy and growth in individual workers. Democratic leadership is particularly effective when cooperation and coordination between groups are necessary. Studies have shown, however, that democratic leadership may be less efficient quantitatively than authoritative leadership.

> Because many people must be consulted, democratic leadership takes more time and, therefore, may be frustrating for those who want decisions made rapidly.

The *laissez-faire* leader is characterized by the following behaviors:

- Takes a hands-off approach.
- Is permissive, with little or no control.
- Motivates by support when requested by the group or individuals.
- Provides little or no direction.
- Uses upward and downward communication between members of the group.
- Disperses decision making throughout the group.
- Places emphasis on the group.
- Does not criticize.

Because it is nondirected leadership, the laissez-faire style can be frustrating; group apathy and disinterest can occur. However, when all group members are highly motivated and self-directed, this leadership style can result in much creativity and productivity. Laissez-faire leadership is appropriate when problems are poorly defined, and brainstorming is needed to generate alternative solutions.

LEARNING EXERCISE 2.4

Leadership Skills Assessment

In groups or individually, list additional characteristics that you believe an effective leader possesses. Which leadership characteristics do you have? Do you believe that you were born with leadership skills, or have you consciously developed them during your lifetime? If so, how did you develop them?

Define your predominant leadership style (authoritarian, democratic, or laissez-faire). Ask those who work with you if in their honest opinion this is indeed the leadership style that you use most often. What style of leadership do you work best under? What leadership style best describes your present or former managers?

For some time, theorists believed that leaders had a predominant leadership style and used it consistently. During the late 1940s and early 1950s, however, theorists began to believe that most leaders did not generally fit any one style but rather fell somewhere on a continuum between authoritarian and laissez-faire. They also came to believe that leaders moved dynamically along the continuum in response to each new situation. This recognition was a forerunner to what is known as *situational* or *contingency* leadership theory.

Situational and Contingency Leadership Theories (1950 to 1980)

The idea that leadership style should vary according to the situation or the individuals involved was first suggested almost 100 years ago by Mary Parker Follett (1926), one of the earliest management consultants and among the first to view an organization as a social system of contingencies. Her ideas, published in a series of books between 1896 and 1933, were so far ahead of their time that they did not gain appropriate recognition in the literature until the 1970s. Her *law of the situation*, which said that the situation should determine the directives given after allowing everyone to know the problem, was *contingency leadership* in its humble origins.

Fiedler's (1967) *contingency approach* reinforced these findings, suggesting that no one leadership style is ideal for every situation. Fiedler felt that the interrelationships between the group's leader and its members were most influenced by the manager's ability to be a good leader. The task to be accomplished and the power associated with the leader's position also were cited as key variables.

In contrast to the continuum from autocratic to democratic, Blake and Mouton's (1964) grid showed various combinations of concern or focus managers had for or on productivity, tasks, people, and relationships. In each of these areas, the leader-manager may rank high or low, resulting in numerous combinations of leadership behaviors. Various formations can be effective depending on the situation and the needs of the worker.

Hersey and Blanchard (1977) also developed a situational approach to leadership. Their tridimensional leadership effectiveness model predicts which leadership style is most appropriate in each situation based on the level of the followers' maturity. As people mature, leadership style becomes less task-focused and more relationship-oriented.

Tannenbaum and Schmidt (1958) built on the work of Lewin (1951) as well as White and Lippitt (1960), suggesting that managers need varying mixtures of autocratic and democratic leadership behavior. They believed that the primary determinants of leadership style should include the nature of the situation, the skills of the manager, and the abilities of the group members.

Although situational and contingency theories added necessary complexity to leadership theory and continue to be applied effectively by managers, by the late 1970s, theorists began arguing that effective leadership depended on an even greater number of variables, including organizational culture, the values of the leader and the followers, the work, the environment, the influence of the leader-manager, and the complexities of the situation. Efforts to integrate these variables are apparent in more contemporary interactional and transformational leadership theories.

This complexity of variables suggests there is likely no "one-size-fits-all" answer to the question of what leadership style is most effective. In the face of ambiguity and complexity, it seems that good leadership is nuanced and requires careful consideration. Blanchard (2022) agrees, noting that the best leadership style is the one that matches the developmental needs of the person the leader is working with. Thus, leadership must be tailored to both the individual and the situation.

Interactional Leadership Theories (1970 to Present)

The basic premise of interactional theory is that leadership behavior is generally determined by the relationship between the leader's personality and the specific situation. Schein (1970), an interactional theorist, was the first to propose a model of humans as complex beings whose working environments were open systems to which they responded. A *system* may be defined as a set of objects, with relationships between the objects and between their attributes. A system is considered open if it exchanges matter, energy, or information with its environment. Schein's model, based on systems theory, had the following assumptions:

- People are very complex and highly variable. They have multiple motives for doing things. For example, a pay raise might mean status to one person, security to another, and both to a third.
- People's motives do not stay constant; instead, they change over time.
- Goals can differ in various situations. For example, an informal group's goals may be quite distinct from a formal group's goals.
- A person's performance and productivity are affected by the nature of the task and by their ability, experience, and motivation.
- No single leadership strategy is effective in every situation.

To be successful, the leader must diagnose the situation and select appropriate strategies from a large repertoire of skills. Hollander (1978) was among the first to recognize that both leaders and followers have roles outside of the leadership situation and that both may be influenced by events occurring in their other roles. With leader and follower contributing to the working relationship and both receiving something from it, Hollander (1978) saw leadership as a dynamic two-way process. According to Hollander, a leadership exchange involves three basic elements:

- The leader, including their personality, perceptions, and abilities
- The followers, with their personalities, perceptions, and abilities
- The situation within which the leader and the followers function, including formal and informal group norms, size, and density

Leadership effectiveness, according to Hollander (1978), requires the ability to use the problem-solving process; maintain group effectiveness; communicate well; demonstrate leader fairness, competence, dependability, and creativity; and develop group identification.

Ouchi (1981) was a pioneer in introducing interactional leadership theory in his application of Japanese style management to corporate America. *Theory Z*, the term Ouchi used for this type of management, is an expansion of McGregor's Theory Y and supports democratic leadership. Characteristics of Theory Z include consensus decision making, fitting employees to their jobs, job security, slower promotions, examining the long-term consequences of management decision making, quality circles, guarantee of lifetime employment, establishment of strong bonds of responsibility between superiors and subordinates, and a holistic concern for the workers (Ouchi, 1981). Ouchi was able to find components of Japanese style management in many successful American companies.

In the 1990s, Theory Z lost its favor with many management theorists. American managers seemed unable to put these same ideas into practice in the United States. Instead, many continued to focus on making workers do what they did not want to do. Although Theory Z is more comprehensive than many of the earlier theories, it too neglects some of the variables that influence leadership effectiveness. It has the same shortcomings as situational theories in inadequately recognizing the dynamics of the interaction between the worker and the leader.

One of the pioneering leadership theorists of this time was Kanter (1977), who developed the theory that the structural aspects of the job shape a leader's effectiveness. She postulated that the leader becomes empowered through both formal and informal systems of the organization. A leader must develop relationships with a variety of people and groups within the organization to maximize job empowerment and be successful. The three major work empowerment structures within the organization are opportunity, power, and proportion. Kanter asserted that these work structures have the potential to explain differences in leader responses, behaviors, and attitudes in the work environment. Kanter (1989), however, perhaps

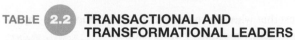

TABLE 2.2	TRANSACTIONAL AND TRANSFORMATIONAL LEADERS	
Transactional Leader	**Transformational Leader**	
Focuses on management tasks	Identifies common values	
Is directive and results oriented	Is a caretaker	
Uses trade-offs to meet goals	Inspires others with vision	
Does not identify shared values	Has long-term vision	
Examines causes	Looks at effects	
Uses contingency reward	Empowers others	

best summarized the work of the interactive theorists by her assertion that title and position authority were no longer sufficient to mold a workforce where subordinates are encouraged to think for themselves, and instead, managers must learn to work synergistically with others.

Transactional and Transformational Leadership

Similarly, Burns (2003), a noted scholar in leader–follower interactions, was among the first to suggest that both leaders and followers have the ability to raise each other to higher levels of motivation and morality. Identifying this concept as *transformational leadership*, Burns maintained that there are two primary types of leaders in management. The traditional manager, concerned with the day-to-day operations, was termed a *transactional leader*. The manager who is committed, has a vision, and can empower others with this vision was termed a *transformational leader*. A composite of the two different types of leaders is shown in Table 2.2.

> Transactional leaders focus on tasks and getting the work done.
> Transformational leaders focus on vision and empowerment.

Similarly, Bass and Avolio (1994) suggested that transformational leadership leads followers to levels of higher morals because such leaders do the right thing for the right reason, treat people with care and compassion, encourage followers to be more creative and innovative, and inspire others with their vision. This new shared vision provides the energy required to move toward the future.

Kouzes and Posner (2017) are perhaps the best-known authors to have furthered the work on transformational leadership in the past decade. Kouzes and Posner suggest that exemplary leaders foster a culture in which relationships between aspiring leaders and willing followers can thrive. This requires the development of the five practices shown in Display 2.6. Kouzes

---

DISPLAY 2.6 KOUZES AND POSNER'S FIVE PRACTICES FOR EXEMPLARY LEADERSHIP

1. Modeling the way: requires value clarification and self-awareness so that behavior is congruent with values
2. Inspiring a shared vision: entails visioning that inspires followers to want to participate in goal attainment
3. Challenging the process: identifies opportunities and taking action
4. Enabling others to act: fosters collaboration, trust, and the sharing of power
5. Encouraging the heart: recognizes, appreciates, and celebrates followers and the achievement of shared goals

Source: From Kouzes, J., & Posner, B. (2017). *The leadership challenge* (6th ed.). Jossey-Bass.

and Posner suggest that when these five practices are employed, anyone can further their ability to lead others to get extraordinary things done.

Although the transformational leader is held as the current ideal, many management theorists sound a warning about transformational leadership. Although transformational qualities are highly desirable, they must be coupled with the more traditional transactional qualities of the day-to-day managerial role. In addition, both sets of characteristics need to be present in the same person in varying degrees. The transformational leader will fail without traditional management skills. Indeed, some leaders are not very visionary or inspiring. While others may be inspiring and passionate, their vision and desired outcomes are flawed.

> Although transformational qualities are highly desirable, they must be coupled with the more traditional transactional qualities of the day–to–day managerial role, or the leader will fail.

Full-Range Leadership Model/Theory

It is this idea that context is an important mediator of transformational leadership that led to the creation of a *full-range leadership model* (FRLM) late in the 20th century. Bass and Avolio (1993) first described a full-range leader as a leader who could apply principles of three specific styles of leadership at any given time: transformational, transactional, and laissez-faire. For example, the full-range leader can empower and inspire others, while enhancing performance to achieve desired outcomes. In addition, the full-range leader appropriately adopts a laissez-faire approach to managing groups when the team is fully capable of doing the work on its own. Thus, full-range leaders evolve and adapt their leadership styles based on which are needed for a given situation.

Leadership Competencies

Just as Fayol (1925) and Gulick (1937) identified management functions, contemporary leadership experts suggest that there are certain competencies (skills, knowledge, and abilities) health care leaders need to be successful. The American College of Healthcare Executives, the American Association for Physician Leadership (formerly the American College of Physician Executives), the American Organization for Nursing Leadership (formerly the American Organization for Nurse Executives), the Healthcare Information and Management Systems Society, the Healthcare Financial Management Association, and the Medical Group Management Association have collaborated to identify leadership competencies, which include leadership skills and behavior, organizational climate and culture, communicating vision, and managing change.

Table 2.3 summarizes the development of leadership theory through the end of the 20th century. Newer (21st century) and emerging leadership theories are discussed in Chapter 3.

Integrating Leadership Roles and Management Functions

Because rapid, dramatic change will continue in nursing and the health care industry, it has grown increasingly important for nurses to develop skills in both leadership roles and management functions. For managers and leaders to function at their greatest potential, the two must be integrated.

Clearly, leadership and management have a symbiotic or synergistic relationship. Every nurse is a leader and manager at some level, and the nursing role requires leadership and management skills. The need for visionary leaders and effective managers in nursing precludes the option of stressing one role over the other. Highly developed management skills are needed to maintain healthy organizations. So too are the visioning and empowerment

TABLE **LEADERSHIP THEORISTS AND THEORIES**

Theorist	Theory
Aristotle	Great Man theory
Lewin and White	Leadership styles
Follett	Law of the situation
Fiedler	Contingency leadership
Blake and Mouton	Task versus relationship in determining leadership style
Hersey and Blanchard	Situational leadership theory
Tannenbaum and Schmidt	Situational leadership theory
Ouchi	Theory Z; a combination of Japanese and American management philosophies and organization values
Kanter	Organizational structure shapes leader effectiveness
Burns	Transactional and transformational leadership
Bass and Avolio	Transformational leadership Full-range leadership theory
Kouzes and Posner	Five practices for exemplary leadership

of subordinates through an organization's leadership team. Because rapid, dramatic change will continue in nursing and the health care industry, it continues to be critically important for nurses to develop skill in both leadership roles and management functions and to strive for the integration of leadership characteristics throughout every phase of the management process.

Key Concepts

- Management functions include planning, organizing, staffing, directing, and controlling. These are incorporated into what is known as the management process.
- Classical or traditional management science focused on production in the workplace and on delineating organizational barriers to productivity. Workers were assumed to be motivated solely by economic rewards, and little attention was given to worker job satisfaction.
- The human relations era of management science emphasized concepts of participatory and humanistic management.
- Three primary leadership styles have been identified: authoritarian, democratic, and laissez-faire.
- Research has shown that the leader-manager must assume a variety of leadership styles, depending on the needs of the worker, the

task to be performed, and the situation or environment. This is known as situational or contingency leadership theory.
- Leadership is a process of persuading and influencing others toward a goal and is composed of a wide variety of roles.
- Early leadership theories focused on the traits and characteristics of leaders.
- Interactional leadership theory focuses more on leadership as a process of influencing others within an organizational culture and the interactive relationship of the leader and follower.
- The manager who is committed, has a vision, and can empower others with this vision is termed a transformational leader, whereas the traditional manager, concerned with the day-to-day operations, is called a transactional leader.

- Full-range leadership theory suggests that context is an important mediator of transformational leadership.
- Full-range leaders evolve and adapt their leadership style based on which leadership styles are needed for a given situation but need transformational, transactional, and laissez-faire leadership skills to be successful.

- Integrating leadership skills with the ability to carry out management functions is necessary if an individual is to become an effective leader-manager.
- The integration of both leadership and management skills is critical to the long-term viability of today's health care organizations.

Additional Learning Exercises and Applications

LEARNING EXERCISE 2.5

When Culture and Policy Clash

You are the nurse-manager of a medical unit. Recently, your unit admitted a 16-year-old East Indian male who has been newly diagnosed with insulin-dependent diabetes. The nursing staff notes the patient is pleasant and cooperative. His large family has been visiting frequently and bringing him food that can compromise his blood glucose levels.

The nursing staff has come to you on two occasions and complained about the family's noncompliance with visiting hours and unauthorized food. Yesterday, two of the family members visited you and complained about hospital visitor policies and what they perceived to be rudeness by two different staff members. You spent time talking to the family, and when they left, they seemed agreeable and understanding. You conclude that the family's social and cultural dietary preferences must be considered while keeping in mind the patient's treatment and the hospital's policies.

Last night, one of the staff nurses told the family that according to hospital policy, only two members could stay (this is true) and if the other family members did not leave, they would call hospital security. This morning, the patient's parents have suggested that they will take him home if this matter is not resolved. The patient's diabetes is still not controlled, and you feel that it would be unwise for this to happen.

ASSIGNMENT:

Leadership is needed to keep this situation from deteriorating further. Divide into groups. Develop a plan of action for solving this problem. First, select three desired objectives for solving the problem and then proceed to determine what you would do that would enable you to meet your objectives. Be sure that you clarify who you consider your followers to be and what you expect from each of them.

Then, list at least five management functions and five leadership roles that you could delineate in this scenario. How would you divide the management functions and leadership roles? For example, you might say that having the nurse-manager adhere to hospital policy was a management function and that counseling staff was a leadership role.

EXAMINING THE EVIDENCE 2.1

Source: From Boyden (2021, July 7). Global research finds lack of alignment in leadership and talent jeopardises post-pandemic growth. https://news.yahoo.com/global-research-finds-lack-alignment-030600388.html

The Need for Leadership Alignment in a Post-Pandemic World

Boyden, a leadership and talent advisory firm with more than 75 offices in over 45 countries, completed a global study in the second quarter of 2021 among senior executives worldwide. The study sought to explore the business outlook among CEOs, boards, and other senior leaders, as well as talent trends, priorities, and investments in the wake of the COVID-19 pandemic through 2022.

Overall, study findings revealed a lack of alignment in talent to strategy, the need for a different skills matrix on the board, and a lack of alignment across leadership teams. While 77% of respondents were extremely confident or confident in their organization's growth potential, just 47% were extremely confident or confident in having the right talent to align to strategy. For industrial and consumer companies, this dropped to 42% and 41%, respectively. Half of all respondents described their business approach in 2022 as one of growth or expansion mode and just over a quarter, 26%, as a learning or transformation opportunity; this bullish approach versus lack of talent alignment was noted to jeopardize postpandemic growth and reinvention.

Respondents were, however, reinventing talent: 74% were extremely likely or likely to invest in leadership development for high potentials; 66% to hire new leadership talent; and 65% to redeploy or retrain existing people. In a pandemic-disrupted work environment, 51% were considering new approaches to measuring performance with the top driver being a desire to tie culture and behaviors to business objectives.

LEARNING EXERCISE 2.6

Leadership Challenges for Health Care Leaders Post-Pandemic

Research by Boyden (2021) revealed a post-pandemic lack of confidence by businesses globally in their organization's ability to align talent with strategy, a need for a different skills matrix on the board, and a lack of alignment across leadership teams (see Examining the Evidence 2.1). Stephens (2021), however, suggests the term "positive but guarded" typifies the current optimistic yet cautious stance that has evolved because of COVID-19 wreaking havoc on American business, with health care not excluded.

Siwicki (2020) concurs, noting the major issues facing health care executives post-pandemic included profitably merging virtual and in-person care, capitalizing on new consumer- and clinician-facing digital health tools, and building a resilient and responsive supply chain for long-term health post–COVID-19 pandemic. Indeed, Siwicki notes that in 2020, many health care organizations saw their financial plans obliterated, patient behaviors radically shift, and virtual care explode.

Carroll (2021) suggests these challenges will persist into the future and adds that rapid increases in lifestyle disease, skills shortages, the acceleration of science and medical device technology, and cutbacks in funding and resources will be additional challenges health care executives will face by 2025. In addition, Carroll notes that health care organizations will witness more change in the scientific and technologic world of health care in the next 10 years than in the last 25.

ASSIGNMENT:

Interview the CEO or top nursing executive at a local health care agency. Ask them what they perceive to be the top five leadership challenges encountered by health care leaders today. Then ask them to identify five management challenges. Did these health care leaders differentiate between leadership and management challenges? Did they feel that the leadership or management challenges were greater? Did they feel that the pandemic impacted or altered the challenges they identified?

LEARNING EXERCISE   2.7

Quiet at Night?

You are the night shift charge nurse on a busy surgical unit in a large, urban teaching hospital. Surgeries occur around the clock, and frequently, noise levels are higher than desired because of the significant number of nurses, physicians, residents, interns, and other health care workers who gather at the nurses' station or in the halls outside of patient rooms. Today, the unit manager has come to you because the hospital's score on the Centers for Medicare and Medicaid Services' *Hospital Consumer Assessment of Healthcare Providers and Systems* (HCAHPS) survey for the category *Always Quiet at Night* falls far below the desired benchmark. She has asked you to devise a plan to address this quality-of-care issue. The management goal in this situation is to achieve an HCAHPS score on *Always Quiet at Night* that meets the accepted best practices benchmark, thus assuring that patients get the rest they need to promote their recovery. The leadership goal is to foster a shared commitment among all health care professionals working on the unit to achieve the *Always Quiet at Night* goal.

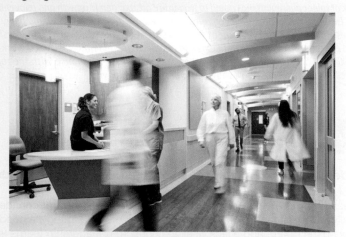

ASSIGNMENT:

1. Identify five management strategies you might use to address the problem of excessive noise on the unit at night. For example, your list might include structural environmental changes or work redesign.
2. Then identify five leadership strategies you might use to promote buy-in of the Quiet at Night initiative by all health care professionals on the unit. How will you inspire these individuals to work with you in achieving this critically important goal? What incentives might you use to reward behavior conducive to meeting this goal?
3. Discuss whether you feel this goal could be achieved by employing only the management strategies you identified. Could it be achieved only with the implementation of leadership strategies for team building?

LEARNING EXERCISE 2.8

Leadership as a New Nurse

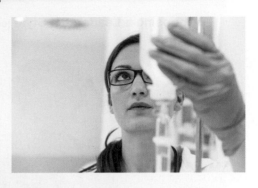

Sally Jones is a 36-year-old new registered nurse (RN) who graduated 6 months ago from a community college with an associate degree in nursing. Sally worked her way through school as a licensed practical nurse in a pediatric unit of a local hospital. After passing her NCLEX-RN examination, she moved to a larger city and was hired to work the evening shift on the pediatric unit as a primary care nurse. Her patient load is usually six pediatric patients, and she has a nursing assistant working under her supervision.

Sally has been bothered recently by discrepancies regarding the credits of intravenous (IV) solutions given in handoff report. For example, she was told at report yesterday that 150 mL remained in one patient's bag of IV solution, but upon making initial patient rounds, she found the IV machine beeping and had to hurriedly replace the bag. At the previous hospital where she had worked, it was a unit policy that all pediatric patients have their IV solutions observed by both oncoming and outgoing primary nurses at shift change so such discrepancies could be discovered and corrected prior to departure of the outgoing shift. She feels this was a good policy and would like to see a similar policy implemented at her new place of employment.

ASSIGNMENT:

If you were Sally, what would you do in this situation? Answer the following questions to help decide what to do.
1. Is it appropriate for a new nurse to take a leadership role in addressing this problem?
2. What are some possible steps you could take in correcting this situation?
3. Would a followership role be better suited to solve this issue?
4. Should you act alone or involve others?

LEARNING EXERCISE 2.9

Choosing a Leadership Style

You are a team leader with one licensed practical nurse/licensed vocational nurse (LPN/LVN) and one nursing assistant on your team. You also share the unit clerical person with two other team leaders and the charge nurse. You have found the LPN/LVN to be a seasoned team member and very reliable. The nursing assistant is young and very new and seems a bit disorganized but is a very willing team member. At various times, you will be directing these three individuals during your workday, that is, asking them to do things, supervising their work, and so on.

(continues on page 52)

LEARNING EXERCISE 2.9

Choosing a Leadership Style (continued)

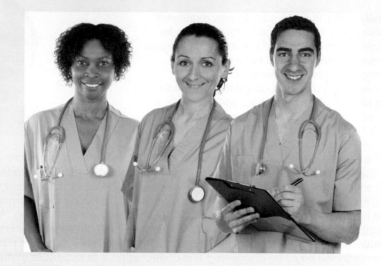

ASSIGNMENT:

What leadership style (authoritative, democratic, or laissez-faire) should you use with each person, or would it be the same with all three? Would you be justified in using only one leadership style? If an emergency occurred, would your leadership style change or remain the same? Discuss solutions to this scenario in class.

LEARNING EXERCISE 2.10

Prescription Misuse and the Opioid Crisis

The National Institute on Drug Abuse (2020) noted that increases in prescription drug misuse over the last 15 years are reflected in increased emergency room visits, overdose deaths associated with prescription drugs, and treatment admissions for prescription drug use disorders, the most severe form of which is an addiction.

ASSIGNMENT:

Assume you are an office nurse in a small family practice. The physicians in the practice have recently attempted to alter their prescribing patterns to address a clearly mounting national problem. Sharp restrictions on opioid prescribing alone, however, will not solve the prescription drug epidemic. Because you have so much direct contact with patients in the practice, you want to be a part of the solution. Identify at least three leadership roles and three management functions that might allow you, as a member of the interprofessional team, to help address the problem. What interprofessional collaboration might be needed to help you implement these leadership roles and management functions?

REFERENCES

Argyris, C. (1964). *Integrating the individual and the organization*. Wiley.

Bass, B. M., & Avolio, B. J. (1993). Transformational leadership: A response to critiques. In M. M. Chemers & R. Ayman (Eds.), *Leadership theory and research: Perspectives and directions* (pp. 49–80). Academic Press.

Bass, B. M., & Avolio, B. J. (Eds.). (1994). *Improving organizational effectiveness through transformational leadership*. Sage.

Blake, R. R., & Mouton, J. S. (1964). *The managerial grid*. Gulf.

Blanchard, K. (2022). *Are you a directive or supportive leader?* Retrieved February 7, 2022, from https://resources.kenblanchard.com/ebooks/are-you-a-directive-or-supportive-leader

Boyden. (2021, July 7). *Global research finds lack of alignment in leadership and talent jeopardises post-pandemic growth*. Retrieved July 10, 2021, from https://news.yahoo.com/global-research-finds-lack-alignment-030600388.html

Burns, J. M. (2003). *Transforming leadership*. Grove/Atlantic.

Carroll, J. (2021). *Keynote: Healthcare 2025—The transformative trends that will really define our future*. Retrieved July 10, 2021, from https://jimcarroll.com/keynote_topics/industry-healthcare/page/2/?_ga=2.6260214.432415825.1625942511-933984731.1625942511

Duggal, N. (2021, December 15). *Leadership vs management: Understanding the key difference*. Simplilearn. https://www.simplilearn.com/leadership-vs-management-difference-article

Fayol, H. (1925). *General and industrial management*. Pittman and Sons.

Fiedler, F. (1967). *A theory of leadership effectiveness*. McGraw-Hill.

Follett, M. P. (1926). The giving of orders. In H. C. Metcalf (Ed.), *Scientific foundations of business administration* (pp. 29–37). Williams & Wilkins.

Gulick, L. (1937). Notes on the theory of the organization. In L. Gulick & L. Urwick (Eds.), *Papers on the science of administration* (pp. 3–13). Institute of Public Administration.

Hersey, P., & Blanchard, K. (1977). *Management of organizational behavior: Utilizing human resources* (3rd ed.). Prentice-Hall.

Hollander, E. P. (1978). *Leadership dynamics: A practical guide to effective relationships*. The Free Press.

Huston, C. (2018). *The road to leadership*. Sigma Theta Tau.

Kanter, R. M. (1977). *Men and women of the corporation*. Basic Books.

Kanter, R. M. (1989). The new managerial work. *Harvard Business Review, 67*(6), 85–92.

Kouzes, J., & Posner, B. (2017). *The leadership challenge* (6th ed.). Jossey-Bass.

Lewin, K. (1951). *Field theory in social sciences*. Harper & Row.

Mayo, E. (1953). *The human problems of an industrialized civilization*. Macmillan.

McGregor, D. (1960). *The human side of enterprise*. McGraw-Hill.

Merriam-Webster. (2022). Management. In *Merriam-Webster.com dictionary*. Retrieved February 7, 2022, from https://www.merriam-webster.com/dictionary/management

National Institute on Drug Abuse. (2020, June). *Misuse of prescription drugs research report overview*. Retrieved July 20, 2021, from https://www.drugabuse.gov/publications/research-reports/misuse-prescription-drugs/overview

Ouchi, W. G. (1981). *Theory Z: How American business can meet the Japanese challenge*. Addison-Wesley.

Schein, E. H. (1970). *Organizational psychology* (2nd ed.). Prentice-Hall.

Siwicki, B. (2020, December 16). *Here are the major issues facing healthcare in 2021, according to PwC*. Healthcare IT News. Retrieved July 11, 2021, from https://www.healthcareitnews.com/news/here-are-major-issues-facing-healthcare-2021-according-pwc

Stephens, S. (2021, May 11). *Here's what's happening in healthcare leadership in 2021*. Health eCareers. https://www.healthecareers.com/article/healthcare-news/heres-whats-happening-in-healthcare-leadership-in-2021

Stoner, J. L. (2022). *How to recognize a leader*. Seapoint Center for Collaborative Leadership. http://seapointcenter.com/how-to-recognize-a-leader/?utm_source=AAL±Clients±and±Alumni&utm_campaign=f9ca67881d-Noteworthy_July_2017_AAL_Subscribers&utm_medium=email&utm_term=0_71cff7fbd0-f9ca67881d-432678093

Tannenbaum, R., & Schmidt, W. (1958). How to choose a leadership pattern. *Harvard Business Review, 36*, 95–102.

Taylor, F. W. (1911). *The principles of scientific management*. Harper & Row.

White, R. K., & Lippitt, R. (1960). *Autocracy and democracy: An experimental inquiry*. Harper & Row.

Zenger, J., & Folkman, J. (2021, May 3). *6 Fatal flaws that kill a leader's effectiveness*. Zenger Folkman. https://zengerfolkman.com/articles/6-fatal-flaws-that-kill-a-leaders-effectiveness/

3

Twenty-First Century Thinking About Leadership and Management

*… No institution can possibly survive if it needs geniuses or supermen to manage it. It must be organized in such a way as to be able to get along under a leadership composed of average human beings.—**Peter Drucker***

*… It is better to lead from behind and to put others in front, especially when you celebrate victory when nice things occur. You take the front line when there is danger. Then people will appreciate your leadership.—**Nelson Mandela***

*… The leaders of tomorrow will face ever-changing team structures, with more remote workers and more diverse skill sets than ever before.—**Catherine Wong***

CROSSWALK

This chapter addresses:

- **AACN Essentials Domain 1:** Knowledge for nursing practice
- **AACN Essentials Domain 4:** Scholarship for nursing practice
- **AACN Essentials Domain 6:** Interprofessional partnerships
- **AACN Essentials Domain 7:** Systems-based practice
- **AACN Essentials Domain 9:** Professionalism
- **AACN Essentials Domain 10:** Personal, professional, and leadership development
- **AONL Nurse Executive Competency 1:** Communication and relationship building
- **AONL Nurse Executive Competency 2:** A knowledge of the health care environment
- **AONL Nurse Executive Competency 3:** Leadership
- **ANA Standard of Professional Performance 10:** Communication
- **ANA Standard of Professional Performance 11:** Collaboration
- **ANA Standard of Professional Performance 12:** Leadership
- **ANA Standard of Professional Performance 13:** Education
- **QSEN Competency:** Teamwork and collaboration

LEARNING OBJECTIVES

The learner will:

- analyze how current and future paradigm shifts in health care affect the leadership skills that are needed by nurses in the coming decade
- compare strengths-based leadership, which focuses on the development or empowerment of workers' strengths, with the traditional management practices of identifying problems, improving underperformance, and addressing weaknesses and obstacles
- identify Level 5 leadership skills (as espoused by Jim Collins), which differentiate great companies from good companies

- identify the characteristics of a servant leader and suggest strategies for encouraging a service inclination in others
- describe situations where followers (agents) might not be inherently motivated to act in the best interest of the principal (leader or employer)
- explore elements of human and social capital, which impact resource allocation in organizations
- describe components of emotional intelligence, which promote the development of productive work teams
- identify characteristics of authentic leadership and discuss the consequences to the leader–follower relationship when leaders are not authentic
- identify contemporary nurse-leaders who exemplify thought leadership and the innovative ideas they have suggested
- describe why quantum leaders need flexibility in responding to the complex relationships that exist between environment and context in work settings
- describe complexities that exist in the relationship between followers and leaders
- provide examples of the 21st-century shift from industrial age leadership to relationship age leadership
- develop insight into personal leadership strengths

Introduction

Throughout history, nursing has been required to respond to changing technologic, environmental, and social forces. In the last decade alone, a growing older-adult population, health care reform, reductions in federal and state government reimbursement as well as commercial insurance, new quality imperatives such as value-based purchasing and pay for performance, and an imperative for sustainability, have resulted in major redesigns of most health care organizations. In addition, the focus of care shifted from acute care hospitals to community and outpatient settings, innovation and technologic advances such as artificial intelligence (AI) transformed the workplace, and organizational cultures increasingly focused on externally regulated, safety-driven, customer-focused care.

These new managerial challenges required nurse administrators who were knowledgeable, skilled, and competent in all aspects of management. In addition, there was a greater emphasis on the business of health care, with nurse managers being involved in the fiscal management of their respective departments. Managers were also expected to be skilled communicators, organizers, and team builders and to be visionary and proactive in preparing for emerging new threats such as ransomware attacks, domestic terrorism, and biologic warfare.

The recent COVID-19 pandemic also significantly impacted health care organizations. Short-term and long-term supply chain shortages of personal protective equipment (PPE), medications, and vaccines were rampant. In addition, health care organizations struggled with how best to both ensure worker safety and maintain an adequate workforce, and telehealth and other virtual care strategies changed the health care landscape by altering not only where care could be provided, but who could provide it.

In addition, Tirakyan (2021) noted that the pandemic and its associated technologic advances brought about innovative changes in the ways organizations communicated and were managed. For example, leaders needed to develop skills in virtual team management. Since this was a relatively new way of working and communicating for many, organizational challenges related to managing a virtual workforce resulted in unpredictability and the need for different communication platforms. Transitions were required in workforce management tools and service strategies. Indeed, some of the transformational changes wrought by digital technology during the pandemic will transform how health care is provided and managed long after the pandemic is contained. Schwantes (2022) goes so far as to suggest that nearly everything will look different in the wake of the COVID-19 pandemic—including the face of leadership. Thus, the pandemic provided innumerable challenges as well as a profound opportunity to reexamine the way we lead and work (Schwantes, 2022).

All this dynamic change in health care has brought about a need for leader-managers to continually learn new roles and develop new skills. As a result, the need for highly developed leadership skills has never been greater. At the national level, nursing leaders and managers are actively involved in determining how best to implement greatly needed health care reform, ensure worker and patient safety, and address health care worker shortages. At the organizational and unit levels, leader-managers are being directed to address health care worker shortages, inadequate numbers of qualified top-level nursing administrators, unionization, intensified efforts to legislate minimum staffing ratios and eliminate mandatory overtime, and the need for civil and productive work environments.

Moreover, ensuring successful recruitment, creating shared governance models, and maintaining high-quality practice depend on successful interprofessional team building, another critical leadership skill in contemporary health care organizations. This challenging and changing health care system requires leader-managers to use their scarce resources appropriately and to be visionary and proactive in planning for challenges yet to come.

In confronting these new and expanding responsibilities and demands, many leader-managers turned to the experts for tools or strategies to meet these expanded role dimensions. What they found was new and innovative thinking about how best to manage organizations and lead people as well as some reengineered interactive leadership theories from the later 20th century. This chapter explores this contemporary thinking about leadership and management, with specific attention given to emergent 21st-century thinking.

New Thinking About Leadership and Management

Given current health care system and organizational complexity, many 21st-century nurses need to improve and add to their leadership/management skill toolbox. In addition, they are required to embrace new roles in new settings. Some leader-managers, however, will undoubtedly try to use a traditional top-down hierarchical approach in leading and managing others but will likely find that it no longer works well, if at all. Instead, they must seek out more participatory, transdisciplinary, and collaborative models that are not easy to develop.

For example, new research on leadership, including *full-range leadership theory* (see Chapter 2), is rediscovering the importance of organizational context, levels of analysis, and potential boundary conditions on transformational leadership. Indeed, much current research focuses on the complexity of the relationship between the leader and the follower, and builds on the interactive leadership theories developed in the latter part of the 20th century. As a result, concepts such as strengths-based leadership, Level 5 Leadership, servant leadership, principal agent theory, human and social capital theory, emotional intelligence (EI), authentic leadership, thought leadership, rebel leadership, agile leadership, reflective thinking and practice, and quantum leadership have emerged as part of the leader-manager's repertoire for the 21st century.

Strengths-Based Leadership and the Positive Psychology Movement

Strengths-based leadership, which grew out of the positive psychology movement (which began in the late 1990s), focuses on the development or empowerment of strengths as opposed to weaknesses or areas of needed growth. Thus, strengths-based leadership is part of the development of *positive organizational scholarship*, which focuses on successful performance that exceeds the norm and embodies an orientation toward strengths and developing collective efficacy.

The importance of strengths-based leadership in organizations was noted in seminal research undertaken by Rath and Conchie (2008) with over 40,000 personal interviews with leaders from around the world and 20,000 interviews with followers to ask *why* they follow a leader. They found that effective leaders invest in their strengths and use them to their advantage. E. Williams (2021) agrees, noting that strengths-based leadership shifts a leader's focus from obstacles to possibilities so that instead of trying to improve deficits, they try to capitalize on available resources, such as people, systems, and tools, to maximize organizational productivity.

In addition, Rath and Conchie (2008) found that the most effective leaders surround themselves with the right people—people who have different strengths than they do. This typically requires leaders to create teams that have a balance of strengths in the following four leadership domains:

1. **Strategic thinking:** Effective leaders keep everyone focused on a long-term future.
2. **Influence:** Effective leaders can sell ideas, develop political support, and get people to rally behind a project or an initiative.
3. **Relationship building:** Effective leaders can unite a group of disparate individuals into a team that works toward a common goal.
4. **Execution:** Effective leaders know how to get things done by translating plans into action.

Finally, Rath and Conchie (2008) found that the most effective leaders understand their followers' needs. The researchers asked followers to choose three words that best describe the contribution that a leader makes to their life. Many of them used the same words to describe what they seek from their leaders. The four most common responses follow:

1. **Trust:** Nothing happens without a sense of trust between leaders and followers.
2. **Compassion:** Followers want to know that their leaders care about them.
3. **Stability:** Followers want leaders they can depend on.
4. **Hope:** Followers want to feel positive about their prospects.

Effective leaders then understand their followers' needs as well as strengths and engage them in activities that allow these strengths to grow and for employees to be empowered and successful. The three basic tenets of strengths-based leadership are shown in Display 3.1.

Appreciative Leadership and Appreciative Inquiry

Like strengths-based leadership, *appreciative leadership* focuses on the recognition of strengths in others and then, using relational processes and methods, builds upon these strengths to collectively make things happen. Thus, it is about recognizing potential in others and supporting them to accomplish more. Similarly, *appreciative inquiry* involves asking followers what they want to accelerate and grow, with the realization that what we appreciate, appreciates (Godwin, 2021). Asking questions that help inspire possibility and inviting new thinking helps people and organizations forward in times of uncertainty.

Malloch and Porter-O'Grady (2022) note that appreciative leadership is a newer model of relationship-based and partnership-driven approaches to leadership and is imperative to meet the demands of today's complex network-structured health systems. Appreciative leaders

---

DISPLAY 3.1   THREE BASIC TENETS OF STRENGTHS-BASED LEADERSHIP SKILLS (E. WILLIAMS, 2021)

1. Successful leaders invest in their employees' strengths.
2. Successful leaders gather the right people to form teams that consist of people who complement each other.
3. Successful leaders work to understand and respond to their employees' needs.

DISPLAY 3.2   JIM COLLINS'S LEVEL 5 LEADERSHIP

Level 1: Highly Capable Individual

Leader makes high-quality contributions to their work, possesses useful levels of knowledge, and has the talent and skills needed to do a good job.

Level 2: Contributing Team Member

Leader uses knowledge and skills to help the team succeed and works effectively, productively, and successfully with other people in the group.

Level 3: Competent Manager

Leader is able to organize a group effectively to achieve specific goals and objectives.

Level 4: Effective Leader

Leader is able to galvanize a department or organization to meet performance objectives and achieve a vision.

Level 5: Great Leader

Leader has all of the abilities needed for the other four levels, plus a unique blend of humility and will that is required for true greatness.

Source: Adapted from Collins, J. (2001). Level 5 leadership: The triumph of humility and fierce resolve. *Harvard Business Review*, 79(1), 66–76.

---

recognize the value and role of every participant upon which the organization depends to grow and thrive (Malloch & Porter-O'Grady, 2022).

Level 5 Leadership

The concept of *Level 5 leadership* was developed by Jim Collins and published in his classic book, *Good to Great: Why Some Companies Make the Leap . . . and Others Don't* (Collins, 2001). Collins (2001) studied 1,435 companies to determine what separates great companies from good companies. What he found was that five levels of leadership skill (Display 3.2) may be present in any organization. Truly great organizations, however, typically have leaders who possess the qualities found in all five levels. Thus, not only do Level 5 leaders have the knowledge to do the job, they also have team-building skills and can help groups achieve shared goals. They also demonstrate humility and seek success for the team, rather than for self-serving purposes, a core component of another 21st-century leadership theory known as *servant leadership*. In addition, Level 5 leaders know when to ask for help, accept responsibility for the errors they or their team make, and are incredibly disciplined in their work.

Level 5 leaders also possess qualities found in the four other levels of leadership that Collins (2001) identified. It is not necessary to pass sequentially through each individual level before becoming a Level 5 leader, but the leader must have the skills and capabilities found in each level of the hierarchy to be a top-performing leader (Mind Tools Content Team, 2022).

Servant Leadership

Although Greenleaf (1977) developed the idea of servant leadership more than 45 years ago, it continues to greatly influence leadership thinking in the 21st century. In more than four decades of working as director of leadership development at AT&T, Greenleaf noticed that most successful managers lead differently from traditional managers. These managers, who he termed *servant leaders*, put serving others, including employees, customers, and the community, as the number one priority.

This choice between personal advantage and organizational advantage speaks to the heart of servant leadership since servant leaders focus on the betterment of their subordinates. For

EXAMINING THE EVIDENCE 3.1

Source: From Lee, A., Lyubovnikova, J., Tian, A. W., & Knight, C. (2020). Servant leadership: A meta-analytic examination of incremental contribution, moderation, and mediation. *Journal of Occupational & Organizational Psychology, 93*(1), 1–44.

Servant Leadership

Servant leadership as an approach to understanding leadership has attracted significant empirical attention. To further understand and develop the servant leadership construct, the researchers completed a quantitative meta-analysis based on 130 independent studies.

- *Study findings included: Servant leadership has predictive validity in terms of individual-level organizational citizen behavior, individual-level creativity, and team-level performance, over other leadership approaches, and therefore, organizations would benefit by developing their current leaders into servant leaders.*
- *Organizations should aim to place servant leaders into influential positions: Training programs and selection profiles and processes need to be aligned and developed to capture the attitudes and behaviors associated with servant leadership inside and outside the organization.*
- *Servant leaders should seek to create a culture that positively promotes the development of trust, fairness, and high-quality leader–follower relationships, as these conditions collectively enable the effects of servant leadership to be transmitted into desirable follower outcomes.*

example, Allen (2021) notes that for employees, having a manager who cares about their motivation helps them think about what makes them want to exchange part of their life to contribute to the organization. They can consider whether they are truly committed to producing the results required and if they can personally define what success looks like in this role.

Another distinguishing feature of servant leadership is the proposition that servant leaders develop followers who also engage in serving behaviors (Wu et al., 2021). This is because servant leaders foster collaboration, teamwork, and collective activism. Servant leaders also seek to elevate those in their charge, supporting the development of the people they lead and nurturing their career growth (M. Williams, 2021).

In addition, recent research suggests that servant leadership has predictive validity in terms of individual-level organizational citizen behavior, individual-level creativity, and team-level performance, over other leadership approaches such as transformational leadership, authentic leadership (AL), and EI (Lee et al., 2020) (see Examining the Evidence 3.1). Organizations benefit then by developing their current leaders into servant leaders. Other defining qualities of servant leadership are shown in Display 3.3.

DISPLAY 3.3   DEFINING QUALITIES OF SERVANT LEADERS

1. The ability to listen on a deep level and to truly understand
2. The ability to keep an open mind and hear without judgment
3. The ability to deal with ambiguity, paradoxes, and complex issues
4. The belief that honestly sharing critical challenges with all parties and asking for their input is more important than personally providing solutions
5. Being clear on goals and good at pointing the direction toward goal achievement without giving orders
6. The ability to be a servant, helper, and teacher first and then a leader
7. Always thinking before reacting
8. Choosing words carefully so as not to damage those being led
9. The ability to use foresight and intuition
10. Seeing the big picture and sensing how people and relationships are connected

LEARNING EXERCISE 3.1

Creating a Service Inclination

An important part of servant leadership is the servant leader's ability to create a service inclination in others. In doing so, more leaders are created for the organization.

ASSIGNMENT:

Identify servant leaders who you have worked with. Did they motivate followers to be service oriented? If so, what strategies did they use? Does servant leadership result in a greater number of leaders within an organization? If so, why do you think that this happens?

Ken Blanchard, author of *Servant Leadership in Action: How You Can Achieve Great Relationships and Results*, notes, however, that although servant leadership is about leading from the ground up, it still requires leadership and that aspect is often forgotten (Kruse, 2018). Servant leaders must still create and communicate their vision, direction, and goals. Followers must be clear about what the leader is trying to accomplish as well as their values and goals. Once that is clear, the pyramid can be turned upside down so that the leader can begin to help followers live according to the vision of values and goals and be successful.

> By positively influencing those they serve and fostering consistent growth and development in their followers, servant leaders multiply leaders. For this reason, it is an infinite process that produces maximum influence and impact (Axe, 2022).

For example, Trojani (2018) shared a story about the first time President John F. Kennedy visited National Aeronautics and Space Administration's headquarters and met a janitor mopping the floor. When President Kennedy asked him what he was doing, he replied, "I'm helping to put a man on the moon." President Kennedy provided the vision, but the janitor felt empowered to do his part to achieve the goal.

LEARNING EXERCISE 3.2

Servant Leadership in Nursing and Medicine

ASSIGNMENT:

Write a one-page essay that addresses the following:
1. Both nursing and medicine are service-oriented professions. Do you believe there are inherent differences in service inclination between individuals who choose nursing for a profession rather than medicine?
2. Do you believe that nursing education fosters a greater service inclination than medical education?
3. Do you believe the fact that the majority of the nursing profession identifies as female influences nursing's propensity to be service-oriented?

LEARNING EXERCISE 3.3

The Agent's Motives

You are a team leader for 10 patients on a busy medical unit. Your team includes Lori, a licensed vocational nurse, passing medications and assisting with patient treatments, and Tom, an experienced certified nursing assistant, who provides basic care such as monitoring vital signs, ambulating patients, and assisting with hygiene. On several occasions in the past, Tom has failed to report significant changes in patients' vital signs to you until considerable time had elapsed or you discovered them yourself. Despite confronting Tom about the need to report these changes and the specific vital sign parameters that need to be reported, this behavior has continued. You have become concerned that patient harm might occur if this pattern of behavior continues.

ASSIGNMENT:

Identify possible motives that Tom (the agent) may have for failing to share this information with you (the principal). What incentives might you employ to modify his behavior?

Principal Agent Theory

Principal agent theory, which first emerged in the 1960s and 1970s, is another interactive leadership theory being actively explored in the 21st century. The *principal agent problem* occurs when one person (the *agent*) can make decisions on behalf of another person (the *principal*). When this happens, there are issues of moral hazard and conflicts of interest.

Such issues arise because not all followers (*agents*) are inherently motivated to act in the best interest of the leader or employer (*principal*). This is because followers may have an informational (expertise or knowledge) advantage over the leader as well as their own preferences, which may deviate from the principal's preferences. The risk then is that agents will pursue their own objectives or interests instead of those of their principal.

Principals then must identify and provide agents with appropriate incentives to act in the organization's best interest. For example, consumers with good health insurance and small out-of-pocket expenses may have little motivation to act prudently in accessing health care resources because payment for services used will come primarily from the insurer. The insurer then must create incentives for agents to access only needed services.

Another example might be end-of-shift overtime. Although most employees do not intentionally seek or want to work overtime after a long and busy shift, the reality is that doing so typically results in financial rewards. Employers then must either create incentives that reward employees who are able to complete their work in the allotted shift time or create disincentives for those who do not.

Human and Social Capital Theory

The traditional view of employees as costs is now obsolete. Instead, employees are now viewed as assets or capital that can be developed and nurtured. *Human capital* refers to the collective skills, knowledge, or other intangible assets of individuals that can be used to create economic value for the employees, their employers, or their community (Dictionary.com, 2022, para. 1). For example, formal educational attainment generally increases human capital because the returns are in the form of wage, salary, or other compensation. Human capital can be viewed, however, from an organizational perspective as well. In this case, human capital would refer to the group's collective knowledge or experience.

> Human capital can refer to a group's collective knowledge, skills, and abilities.

Social capital is defined as social relationships and networks, based on reciprocity and trust, that facilitate mutually beneficial coordination and cooperation (Kida et al., 2021). For example, organizations that encourage employees to view the workplace as a community where people feel accepted and appreciated are building social capital. Workplace social capital then is embedded within the relationships between members and can be a vital management resource (Kida et al., 2021).

Human capital theory suggests that individuals or organizations will invest in education and professional development if they believe that such an investment will have a future payoff. For example, a health care organization that provides tuition reimbursement allowing nurses to return to school to earn higher degrees is likely doing so in anticipation that a more highly educated nursing staff will result in increased quality of care and higher retention rates—both of which should translate into higher productivity and financial return.

Investing in human capital development has been identified as a leadership trend shaping contemporary organizations (Deloitte, 2021). Leaders and companies who recognize the long-term benefit of focusing on human capital development and take a vested interest in helping employees thrive in all areas of their lives (not just work) will create more engagement, productivity, and overall happier employees. Indeed, research done by Deloitte (2021) highlighted well-being as a critical priority for employees, with burnout impacting morale, productivity, and overall retention. Leadership must infuse well-being into the structure of work, allowing employees to weigh in on the flexibility and programming that will empower them and make them successful. Only then can organizations be proactive in creating a desirable employee experience and in accommodating their workforce in a strategic manner instead of remaining reactive.

Emotional Intelligence

Another leadership theory that has gained prominence in the 21st century is that of EI (also known as "emotional quotient" or EQ). Broadly defined, *EI* refers to the ability to perceive, understand, and control one's own emotions as well as those of others. Gabriel (2018) suggests that it's our EI that gives us the ability to read our instinctive feelings and those of others. It also allows us to understand and label emotions as well as express and regulate them.

Gabriel (2018) suggests that many people overestimate their EI because they think it is the ability or tendency to be nice. It's not. Instead, it is about being empathetic, being able to look at situations from alternative points of view, being open minded, bouncing back from challenges, and pursuing goals despite challenges. Some proponents of EI have suggested that having EI may be even more critical to leadership success than intellectual intelligence (IQ).

In their original work on EI in 1990, Mayer and Salovey (1997) suggested that EI consists of three mental processes:

- Appraising and expressing emotions in the self and others
- Regulating emotion in self and others
- Using emotions in adaptive ways

In 1997, they further refined EI into four mental abilities: Perceiving/identifying emotions, integrating emotions into thought processes, understanding emotions, and managing emotions.

Goleman (1998), in his best seller *Working with Emotional Intelligence*, built on this work by identifying five components of EI: self-awareness, self-regulation, motivation, empathy, and social skills.

Goleman (1998) argued that every person has a rational thinking mind and an emotional feeling mind and that both influence action. The goal, then, in EI is *emotional literacy*—being self-aware about one's emotions and recognizing how they influence subsequent action. Unlike Mayer and Salovey (1997), who suggested that EI develops with age, Goleman argued that EI could be learned, although he too felt that it improves with age. This does not mean, however, that we need to grow older to improve this skill set. Practice, reflection, and feedback can improve EI at any age.

Authentic Leadership

Another emerging leadership theory for the contemporary leader-manager's arsenal is *authentic leadership* (also known as *congruent leadership*). Authentic leadership suggests that to lead, leaders must be true to themselves and their values and act accordingly. *Integrity* is conformance between what leaders profess and how they actually act (Kador, 2018).

It is important to remember that authentic or congruent leadership theory differs somewhat from more traditional transformational leadership theories, which suggest that the leader's vision or goals are often influenced by external forces and that there must be at least some "buy-in" of that vision by followers (see Chapter 2).

> In authentic leadership, it is the leaders' principles and their conviction to act accordingly that inspire followers.

Sostrin (2017) suggests that sustaining an enduring alignment between your values and your actions is vital for leadership success.

> *It's what lets you be you and it serves as a bond of integrity that enables your followers to trust you. Increase the alignment between your values and behaviors by understanding what makes you tick—defining the specific values that animate you—then making them apparent to your clients and teams. This integrity will produce a more consistent, authentic expression of who you are in the moments that matter* (para. 7).

Authenticity then breeds trust, which is a crucial element in the workplace as well as between leaders and their followers.

LEARNING EXERCISE 3.4

Emotions and Decision Making

Think back on a recent decision you made that was more emotionally laden than usual. Were you self-aware about what emotions were influencing your thinking and how your emotions might have influenced the course(s) of action you chose? Were you able to objectively identify the emotions that others were experiencing and how these emotions may have influenced their actions?

DISPLAY 3.4 **QUESTIONS TO ASK IN ASSESSING TRUSTWORTHINESS AS AN AUTHENTIC LEADER**

1. Do I act with integrity?
2. Do I welcome ideas and opinions different from my own?
3. Do I appreciate employees who are willing to bring bad news to my attention?
4. Do I admit my own mistakes?
5. Do I always tell the truth, even if it is inconvenient?
6. Do I publicly encourage suggestions from everyone on the team, from the top performers to the most junior employees, and then do I listen to the contributions with equal respect?

Source: From Kador, J. (2018). *Are you a trusted leader?* Retrieved July 11, 2021, from https://chiefexecutive.net/are-you-a-trusted-leader

---

Forbes Coaches Council (2018a) suggests that unfortunately, "leaders have long gotten away with vocally supporting policies and procedures, but their actions say otherwise. That tide will turn. With so much light being shed on unacceptable behavior in all workplaces, leaders must begin to understand they need to not only hold their teams accountable for proper behavior but hold themselves accountable as well" (para. 7).

The reality, though, is that authentic leadership is not easy. It takes great courage to be true to one's convictions when external forces or peer pressure encourage one to do something one feels morally would be inappropriate. For example, there is little doubt that some nurse-leaders experience intrapersonal value conflicts between what they believe to be morally appropriate and a need to deliver results in a health care system increasingly characterized by pay for performance and rewarded by cost containment.

Trust between leaders and followers—essential to authentic leadership—may also take time to develop. Although Kador (2018) notes that trust can occur very quickly under the right circumstances, generally, it takes time as well as a lifelong commitment to self-reflection. Trust is also easier to experience than to precisely measure (Kador, 2018). Five questions one might use to assess one's trustworthiness as an authentic leader are shown in Display 3.4.

Finally, one must not be so idealistic as to assume that all leaders strive to be authentic. Indeed, many are flawed, at least at times. Leaders may be deceitful and trustworthy, greedy

---

LEARNING EXERCISE 3.5

Inconsistency in Word and Action

There are many examples of internationally or nationally recognized leaders who have lost their followers because of their actions being inconsistent with personally stated convictions. An example might be a world-class athlete and advocate for healthy lifestyles who is found to be using steroids to enhance physical performance. Or it might be a political figure who preaches morality and becomes involved in an extramarital affair or a religious leader who promotes celibacy and then becomes involved in a sex scandal.

ASSIGNMENT:

Think of a leader who espoused one message and then acted in a different manner. How did it affect the leader's ability to be an effective leader? How did it change how you personally felt about that leader? Do you feel that leaders who have lost their "authenticity" can ever regain the trust of their followers?

and generous, and cowardly and brave. To assume that all good leaders are good people is foolhardy and makes us blind to the human condition. Future leadership theory may well focus on why leaders behave badly and why followers continue to follow bad leaders.

Thought Leadership and Rebel Leadership

Another relatively new leadership theory to emerge in the 21st century is that of *thought leadership*, which applies to a person who is recognized among their peers for innovative ideas and who demonstrates the confidence to promote those ideas. Thus, thought leadership refers to any situation in which one individual convinces another to consider a new idea, product, or way of looking at things. Ideas put forth by thought leaders typically are future oriented and make a significant impact. In addition, they are generally problem oriented, which increases their value to both individuals and organizations.

Thought leaders then challenge the status quo and attract followers not by any promise of representation or empowerment but by their risk taking, passion, and vision in terms of being innovative. Huston (2020) agrees, noting that vision is one of the hallmarks of leadership since visioning is about movement toward a goal, betterment, growth, or success. Thus, visions communicate possibilities and solutions to both current problems and future challenges, especially when there is an action component.

For example, in her book, *Rebel Talent: Why It Pays to Break the Rules at Work and in Life*, Gino (2018) argues companies should encourage employees to pursue core strengths of novelty, curiosity, perspective, diversity, and authenticity because success is often linked with breaking rules and breaking traditions (Nobel, 2018). Gino suggests that business leaders should strive for and encourage rebellion in their workplaces because when people break rules to explore new ideas and create positive change, everyone benefits (Nobel, 2018). Gino's eight principles of rebel leadership are shown in Display 3.5.

Organizations can also be thought leaders. For example, Blue Cross and Blue Shield were early thought leaders in the development of private health insurance in the late 1920s. Johnson & Johnson launched the *Discover Nursing* campaign earlier this decade to champion the nursing profession and promote the recruitment and retention of nurses. Thought leaders in the coming decade will likely focus on enduring issues that continue to be of critical importance to nursing and health care and address new, emerging problems of significance. For example, thought leadership is still greatly needed in identifying and adopting innovative safety and quality improvement approaches that reduce the risk of harm to patients and health care workers and to address the significant waste and carbon footprint that is a part of many health care systems. In addition, the threat of an international nursing shortage continues to loom, and an inadequate number of innovative solutions have been suggested for addressing an ongoing nursing faculty shortage.

DISPLAY 3.5   **BECOMING A THOUGHT LEADER: FRANCESCA GINO'S EIGHT PRINCIPLES OF REBEL LEADERSHIP**

1. Seek out the new.
2. Encourage constructive dissent.
3. Open conversations—don't close them.
4. Reveal yourself—and reflect.
5. Learn everything—then forget everything.
6. Find freedom in constraints.
7. Lead from the trenches.
8. Foster happy accidents (mistakes may unlock a breakthrough).

Source: From Gino, F. (2018). *Rebel talent: Why it pays to break the rules at work and in life*. HarperCollins.

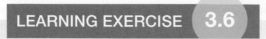

LEARNING EXERCISE 3.6

Technologic Innovation and Thought Leadership

Technologic innovations continue to change the face of health care, and the pace of such innovations continues to increase exponentially. For example, wireless communication, computerized charting, and the barcode scanning of medications have all greatly affected the practice of nursing.

ASSIGNMENT:

Choose at least one of the following technologic innovations and write a one-page report on how this technology is expected to impact nursing and health care in the coming decade. See if you can identify the thought leader(s) credited with developing these technologies and explore the process that they used to both develop and market their innovations.

- Biometrics to ensure patient confidentiality
- Computerized physician order entry
- Point-of-care testing
- Bluetooth technology
- Electronic health records
- Artificial intelligence
- Robotic surgery
- Nursebots (prototype nurse robots)
- Genetic and genomic testing

Agile Leadership

Another newer leadership theory is *agile leadership*, a term borrowed from the software world. Agile leaders have the ability (and agility) to think in many ways so that they can be flexible, adaptable, and fast in their decision making (Forbes Coaches Council, 2018b). The Center for Agile Leadership (2022) concurs, noting that agile leaders are inclusive, democratic leaders who exhibit a greater openness to ideas and innovations. With a passion for learning, a focus on developing people, and a strong ability to define and communicate a desired vision, they possess the tools necessary to inspire others and become an agent for change within any organization.

Agile leaders also listen deeply and ask powerful questions to gain insights and make the right decision to help the organization move forward through problems. They quickly adapt to situations as they come along and are flexible and open to change and growth (Forbes Coaches Council, 2018b).

In addition, agile leaders demonstrate agility with their employees. Indeed, agile leadership was proposed to meet the needs of the millennial workforce, which has different needs, different wants, and different motivators than any generation before it (Center for Agile Leadership, 2022). People like to be communicated with and recognized differently. It is never a one-size-fits-all model. When agile leaders show how much they value their team's contribution by understanding and being what they need, productivity and engagement rise (Forbes Coaches Council, 2018b).

Reflective Thinking and Practice

Other leadership theories that have gained prominence in the past decade are those of *reflective thinking and practice*. Metevier (2021, para 10) defines reflective thinking as "a form

1. How can you bring the power of reflection to bear on your day-to-day work?
2. How could you amplify the effectiveness of your decision making and empower your teams to step up and participate in the decision-making process?

Source: From Sherwood, G. D., & Horton-Deutsch, S. (2015). *Reflective organizations. On the front lines of QSEN & reflective practice implementation*. Nursing Knowledge International.

of self analysis that creates a more valuable experience of consciousness by revealing what is truly important in life." A primary requirement is radical honesty to avoid self-deception. Reflective practice is a learning process that means taking our experiences as an initial point for our learning, learning from those experiences, and taking actions that reflect the new perspectives taken (NursingAnswers.net, 2021).

Sherwood and Horton-Deutsch (2015) emphasize the need for reflective thinking and practice in today's chaotic health care environment since it requires nurse-leaders to be nimble, flexible, and responsive to change. "The need for change arises from the awareness that current practices or processes aren't working—that results are not the desired outcomes" (p. xiii). Thus, the goal for nurse-leaders must be to become so agile that they are able to continually adapt, reflect on progress and setbacks, and adjust their course as needed (Sherwood & Horton-Deutsch, 2015).

Sherwood and Horton-Deutsch (2015) also suggest that reflection provides an opportunity to apply theory from all ways of knowing and learning as an extension of evidence-based practices and research. It also allows individuals to learn from experience by considering what they know, believe, and value within the content of current situations and then to reframe to develop future responses or actions. Sherwood and Horton-Deutsch suggest two questions nurse-leaders can use to increase their reflective practice (Display 3.6).

Quantum Leadership

Quantum leadership is another relatively new leadership theory that is being used by leader-managers to better understand dynamics of environments, such as health care. This theory, which emerged in the 1990s, builds on transformational leadership and suggests that leaders must work together with subordinates to identify common goals, exploit opportunities, and empower staff to make decisions for organizational productivity to occur. This is especially true during periods of rapid change and needed transition.

Building on quantum physics, which suggests that reality is often discontinuous and deeply paradoxical, quantum leadership suggests that the environment and context in which people work is complex and dynamic and that this has a direct impact on organizational productivity. The theory also suggests that change is constant. Today's workplace is a highly fluid, flexible, and mobile environment, and this calls for an entirely innovative set of interactions and relationships as well as the leadership necessary to create them (Albert et al., 2022).

> Quantum leadership suggests that the environment and context in which people work is complex and dynamic and that this has a direct impact on organizational productivity.

Because the health care industry is characterized by rapid change, the potential for intra-organizational conflict is high. Albert et al. (2022) suggest that because the unexpected is becoming the normative, the quantum leader must be able to address the unsettled space between present and future and resolve these conflicts appropriately. In addition, they suggest that the ability to respond to the dynamics of crisis and change is not only an inherent leadership skill but must now also be inculcated within the very fabric of the organization and its operation.

Transition From Industrial Age Leadership to Relationship Age Leadership to Build Employee Engagement

In considering all these emerging leadership theories, it becomes apparent that a paradigm shift has taken place early in the 21st century—a transition from *industrial age leadership* to *relationship age leadership.* Industrial age leadership focused on productivity and traditional top-down hierarchy management structures. Relationship age leadership is grounded upon a leader's genuine investment in the personal and professional development of their followers. Servant leadership, appreciative leadership, AL, reflective thought and practice, human and social capital, and EI are all relationship-centered theories that address the complexity of the leader–follower relationship.

> A paradigm shift has taken place in the 21st century—a transition from industrial age leadership to relationship age leadership.

Relationship age leadership books and articles currently abound in the literature. One of best-selling author Stephen Covey's *10 Key Principles About Life* is that that human growth and prosperity rest on the immutable principles of love, honesty, kindness, hard work, gratitude, patience, perseverance, forgiveness, loyalty, generosity, and faith. These principles are unchanged through the ages and apply to all mankind. Covey notes then that it is essential to strike a balance between production and production capabilities. Production means the ability to work productively and get results, and production capabilities are the ability to maintain efficiency. The balance between production and production capabilities is efficiency. You cannot indefinitely produce (i.e., achieve short-term results) while neglecting your productive capabilities or burnout may occur (Gallery of Thoughts, 2021).

Fred Kofman, a leader development expert from Google, agrees, suggesting that many employers are trying to attract the new generation with the same technologies that attracted the past generation (*Should Leadership Feel*, 2018). The result is abysmal levels of *engagement. Employee engagement* in the United States, which is probably one of the highest in the world, is about 30%. So, 70% of the people either don't care or dislike their jobs and the people they work for, the people they work with, the places where they work, and the customers they are supposed to serve (*Should Leadership Feel*, 2018).

Indeed, Tamara McCleary, speaker, author, and business expert, suggests that employee engagement is the key to relationship building in the 21st century (Edmonds, 2018). To build this engagement, McCleary invests time, energy, and passion into caring about employees. She also constantly checks to see whether her plans, decisions, and actions are building relationships effectively, and she refines those actions if they don't (Edmonds, 2018). McCleary's three-step action plan for engaging employees to build relationships is shown in Display 3.7.

Yet, the leader-manager in contemporary health care organizations cannot and must not focus solely on relationship building. Ensuring productivity and achieving desired outcomes are essential to organizational success. The key, then, likely lies in integrating the two paradigms.

DISPLAY 3.7 TAMARA McCLEARY'S THREE STEPS FOR ENGAGING EMPLOYEES THROUGH RELATIONSHIP BUILDING

1. Invest the time. Pay attention to more than just results. Connect with people at all levels in the organization every day. Learn their names and their passions. Learn what gets in their way of cooperative teamwork and top performance. Act to reduce those frustrations.
2. Get the data. Don't just monitor performance metrics—monitor data that indicates how happy employees are working in your organization. Use reliable data, like turnover, exit interviews, service levels, and more. Also try to measure other satisfaction metrics, like the degree of trust, the frequency of proactive problem solving, etc.
3. Evaluate the progress of employee engagement, service, and results. Embrace proactive relationship management and pay close attention to my "big three"—engagement, service, and results. If the results are not what you want, refine your approaches, then monitor the impact. Keep those practices that help.

Source: From Edmonds, S. C. (2018). *To be the best, invest in relationships AND results*. Retrieved July 25, 2021, from http://www.greatleadershipbydan.com/2018/05/to-be-best-invest-in-relationships-and.html

Technical skills and competence seeking must be balanced with the adaptive skills of influencing followers and encouraging their abilities. Performance and results priorities must be balanced with authentic leadership and character. In other words, leader-managers must seek the same tenuous balance between leadership and management that has existed since time began.

LEARNING EXERCISE 3.7

Balancing the Focus Between Productivity and Relationships

You are a top-level nursing administrator in a large, urban medical center in California. As in many acute care hospitals, your annual nursing turnover rate is more than 15%. At this point, you have many unfilled licensed nursing positions, and local recruitment efforts to fill these positions have been largely unsuccessful.

During a meeting with the chief executive officer (CEO) today, you are informed that the hospital vacancy rate for licensed nurses is expected to rise to 20% with the opening of an additional regional hospital in 3 months. The CEO states that you must reduce turnover or increase recruitment efforts immediately or the hospital will have to consider closing units or reducing available beds when the new ratios take effect.

You consider the following "industrial leadership" paradigm options:

1. You could aggressively recruit international nurses to solve at least the immediate staffing problem.
2. You could increase sign-on bonuses and offer other incentives for recruiting new nurses.
3. You could expand the job description for unlicensed assistive personnel and licensed vocational nurses to relieve the registered nurses of some of their duties.
4. You could make newly recruited nurses sign a minimum 2-year contract upon hire.

You also consider the following "relationship leadership" paradigm options:

1. You could hold informal meetings with current staff to determine major variables affecting their current satisfaction levels and attempt to increase those variables that increase worker satisfaction.
2. You could develop an open-door policy in an effort to be more accessible to workers who wish to discuss concerns or issues about their work environment.
3. You could implement a shared governance model to increase worker participation in decision making on the units in which they work.
4. You could make daily rounds on all the units in an effort to get to know your nursing staff better on a one-to-one basis.

(continues on page 70)

LEARNING EXERCISE 3.7

Balancing the Focus Between Productivity and Relationships (continued)

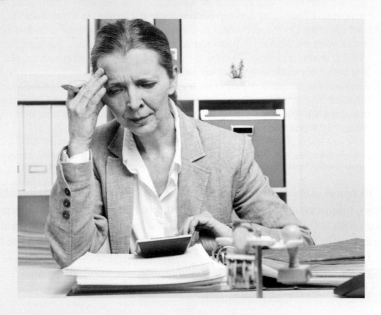

ASSIGNMENT:

● ● ● ● ● ● ● ●

Decide which of the options you would select. Rank order them in terms of what you would do first. Then look at your list. Did it reflect more of the industrial leadership paradigm or a relationship leadership paradigm? What inferences might you draw from your rank ordering in terms of your leadership skills? Do you think that your rank ordering might change with your age? Your experience?

Integrating Leadership Roles and Management Functions in the 21st Century

Seemingly insurmountable problems, a lack of resources to solve these problems, and individual apathy have been and will continue to be issues that contemporary leader-managers face. Effective leadership is critical to organizational success in the 21st century. Becoming a better leader-manager begins with a highly developed understanding of what leadership and management are and how these skills can be developed. The problem is that these skills are dynamic, and what we know and believe to be true about leadership and management changes constantly in response to new research and visionary thinking.

Contemporary leader-managers, then, are challenged not only to know and be able to apply classical leadership and management theory but also to keep abreast of new insights, new management decision-making tools, and new research in the field. It is more important than ever that leader-managers be able to integrate leadership roles and management functions and that some balance be achieved between industrial age leadership and relationship age leadership skills. Leading and managing in the 21st century promises to be more complex than ever before, and leader-managers will be expected to have a greater skill set. The key to organizational success will likely be having enough highly qualified and visionary leader-managers to steer the course.

Key Concepts

- Many new leadership and management theories have emerged in the 21st century to explain the complexity of the leader–follower relationship and the environment in which work is accomplished and goals are achieved.
- *Strengths-based leadership* focuses on the development or empowerment of workers' strengths as opposed to identifying problems, improving underperformance, and addressing weaknesses and obstacles.
- *Appreciative leadership* focuses on recognizing potential in others and supporting them to accomplish more.
- *Level 5 leadership* is characterized by knowledge, team-building skills, the ability to help groups achieve goals, humility, and the empowerment of others through servant leadership.
- *Servant leadership* is a contemporary leadership model that puts serving others as the priority.
- Followers can and do influence leaders in both positive and negative ways.
- *Principal agent theory* suggests that followers may have an informational (expertise or knowledge) advantage over the leader as well as their own preferences, which may deviate from those of the principal. This may lead to a misalignment of goals.
- *Human capital* represents the capability of the individual. Social capital represents what a group can accomplish together.

- *Emotional intelligence* refers to the ability to use emotions effectively and is considered by many to be critical to leadership and management success.
- *Authentic leadership* suggests that to lead, leaders must be true to themselves and their values and act accordingly.
- *Thought leadership* refers to any situation whereby one individual convinces another to consider a new idea, product, or way of looking at things.
- Thought leaders attract followers not by any promise of representation or empowerment but by their risk-taking and vision in terms of being innovative.
- Agile leaders have the ability (and agility) to think in many ways so that they can be flexible, adaptable, and fast in their decision making.
- *Reflective thinking* is a form of honest self-analysis that creates a more valuable experience of consciousness by revealing what is truly important in life.
- *Reflective practice* entails using personal experiences as an initial point for learning, learning from those experiences, and taking actions that reflect new perspectives gained.
- *Quantum leadership* suggests that the environment and context in which people work are complex and dynamic, having a direct impact on organizational productivity.
- A transition has occurred in the 21st century from industrial age leadership to relationship age leadership.

Additional Learning Exercises and Applications

LEARNING EXERCISE 3.8

Reflecting on Emotional Intelligence in Self

Do you feel that you have emotional intelligence? Do you express appropriate emotions such as empathy when taking care of patients? Are you able to identify and control your own emotions when you are in an emotionally charged situation?

ASSIGNMENT:

Describe a recent emotional experience. Write two to four paragraphs reporting how you responded in this experience. Were you able to read the emotions of the other individuals involved? How did you respond, and were you later able to reflect on this incident?

LEARNING EXERCISE 3.9

Self-Regulation and Emotional Intelligence

You have just come from your 6-month performance evaluation as a new charge nurse in a long-term care facility. Although the director of nursing stated that he was very pleased in general with how you are performing in this new role, one area that he suggested you work on was to learn to be calmer in hectic clinical situations. He suggested that your anxiety could be transmitted to patients, coworkers, and subordinates who look to you to be their role model. He feels that you are especially anxious when staffing is short and that at times you vent your frustrations to your staff, which only adds to the general anxiety level on the unit.

ASSIGNMENT:

Create a specific plan of 6 to 10 things you can do to bolster your emotional intelligence in terms of self-regulation during stressful times.

LEARNING EXERCISE 3.10

Human and Social Capital

Examine the institution in which you work or go to school. Assess both the human capital and social capital present. Which is greater? Which do you believe contributes most to this institution's ability to accomplish its stated mission and goals?

LEARNING EXERCISE 3.11

Assessing Emotional Intelligence

You have just completed your first year as a registered nurse and have begun to think about applying for the next charge position that opens on your unit. You really like your unit manager and one of the charge nurses. However, a couple of the charge nurses are rather rude and not very empathetic when they are harried and overworked. At times, the charge nurses are very frustrated, the team members pick up their frustration, and the unit becomes chaotic. You feel that although these nurses are great clinicians, they are not effective charge nurses. You know that you do not want to be like them should you be promoted. You would love to emulate your manager who is calm, supportive, and well grounded emotionally. She is an excellent role model of a person with emotional intelligence, something you are not sure you have.

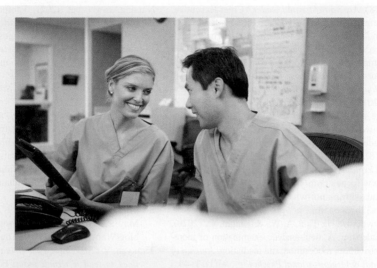

ASSIGNMENT:

Decide what you can do to determine your emotional intelligence and identify at least three strategies you could use to reduce any deficiencies.

REFERENCES

Albert, N. M., Pappas, S., Porter-O'Grady, T., & Malloch, K. (2022). *Quantum leadership: Creating sustainable value in health care* (6th ed.). Jones & Bartlett.

Allen, D. (2021, July 8). *5 Elements of servant leadership.* The Enterprisers Project. https://enterprisersproject.com/article/2021/7/servant-leadership-5-elements

Axe, J. (2022, February 3). *Servant leadership: The ultimate key to a healthy business.* Leaders. https://leaders.com/articles/leadership/servant-leadership/

Center for Agile Leadership. (2022). *Agileadership™.* Retrieved February 7, 2022, from https://centerforagileleadership.com/agileadership/

Collins, J. (2001). *Good to great: Why some companies make the leap … and others don't.* HarperCollins.

Deloitte. (2021). *A public sector perspective: Human capital trends 2021.* Making the shift from "survive to thrive." Retrieved July 12, 2021, from https://www2.deloitte.com/us/en/pages/public-sector/articles/human-capital-trends-government-perspective.html

Dictionary.com. (2022). Human capital. In *Dictionary.com Unabridged dictionary.* Retrieved February 7, 2022, from http://www.dictionary.com/browse/human-capital

Edmonds, S. C. (2018). *To be the best, invest in relationships AND results.* Retrieved July 12, 2021, from http://www.greatleadershipbydan.com/2018/05/to-be-best-invest-in-relationships-and.html

Forbes Coaches Council. (2018a). *14 Leadership trends that will shape organizations in 2018.* Forbes. Retrieved July 12, 2021, from https://www.forbes.com/sites/forbescoachescouncil/2018/01/30/14-leadership-trends-that-will-shape-organizations-in-2018/#4ab51515307e

Forbes Coaches Council. (2018b). *What does it mean to be an agile leader?* Forbes. Retrieved July 11, 2021, from https://www.forbes.com/sites/forbescoachescouncil/2018/06/29/what-does-it-mean-to-be-an-agile-leader/#70a4987e4db4

Gabriel, E. (2018, July 26). *Understanding emotional intelligence and its effects on your life.* CNN. Retrieved February 7, 2022, from https://www.cnn.com/2018/04/11/health/improve-emotional-intelligence/index.html

Gallery of Thoughts. (2021, April 16). *10 Key Stephen Covey's principles about life.* https://www.galleryot.com/2021/04/stephen-covey-principles.html#:~:text=By%20the%20lighthouse%20principle%2C%20Covey%20meant%20the%20eternal,and%20it%20would%20be%20foolish%20to%20fight%20it

Gino, F. (2018). *Rebel talent: Why it pays to break the rules at work and in life.* HarperCollins.

Godwin, L. (2021, March 15). *Leading in a constantly changing world requires a reinvention mindset: Applying appreciative inquiry to modern leadership.* Training Industry. Retrieved September 18, 2021, from https://trainingindustry.com/articles/leadership/leading-in-a-constantly-changing-world-requires-a-reinvention-mindset-applying-appreciative-inquiry-to-modern-leadership/

Goleman, D. (1998). *Working with emotional intelligence.* Bantam Books.

Greenleaf, R. K. (1977). *Servant leadership: A journey into the nature of legitimate power and greatness.* Paulist Press.

Huston, C. J. (2020). The road to positive work cultures. Chapter 10. *Be passionate and purposeful in looking to the future.* Indianapolis, IN: Sigma Theta Tau International.

Kador, J. (2018). *Are you a trusted leader?* Chief Executive. https://chiefexecutive.net/are-you-a-trusted-leader

Kida, R., Togari, T., Yumoto, Y., & Ogata, Y. (2021). The association between workplace social capital and authentic leadership, structural empowerment and forms of communication as antecedent factors in hospital nurses: A cross-sectional multilevel approach. *Journal of Nursing Management, 29*(3), 508–517.

Kofman, F. (2018). *Should leadership feel more like love?* Knowledge at Wharton. Retrieved May 29, 2022 from https://knowledge.wharton.upenn.edu/article/google-adviser-leadership-should-feel-more-like-love/

Kruse, K. (2018). *Servant leadership is not what you think: Ken Blanchard explains.* Forbes. Retrieved July 11, 2021, from https://www.forbes.com/sites/kevinkruse/2018/04/09/servant-leadership-is-not-what-you-think-ken-blanchard-explains/#a32b7366a5fc

Lee, A., Lyubovnikova, J., Tian, A. W., & Knight, C. (2020). Servant leadership: A meta-analytic examination of incremental contribution, moderation, and mediation. *Journal of Occupational & Organizational Psychology, 93*(1), 1–44.

Malloch, K., & Porter-O'Grady, T. (2022). *Appreciative leadership: Building sustainable partnerships for health.* Jones & Bartlett Learning.

Mayer, J. D., & Salovey, P. (1997). What is emotional intelligence? In P. Salovey & D. Sluyter (Eds.), *Emotional development and emotional intelligence: Educational implications* (pp. 3–31). Basic Books.

Metivier, A. (2021, December 23). *Reflective thinking: 5 powerful thought strategies for improving your life.* Magnetic Memory Method. https://www.magneticmemorymethod.com/reflective-thinking/

Mind Tools Content Team. (2022). *Level 5 leadership. Achieving "greatness" as a leader.* Emerald Works Limited. Retrieved February 7, 2022, from http://www.mindtools.com/pages/article/level-5-leadership.htm

Nobel, C. (2018). *How to be a rebel leader.* Harvard Business School. Retrieved July 12, 2021, from https://hbswk.hbs.edu/item/how-to-be-a-rebel-leader

NursingAnswers.net. (2021, February 25). *Defining reflective practice and identifying advantages and implications nursing essay.* Retrieved August 24, 2021 from https://nursinganswers.net/reflections/defining-reflective-practice-and-identifying-advantages-and-implications-nursing-essay.php?vref=1

Rath, T., & Conchie, B. (2008). *Strengths based leadership.* Gallup Press.

Schwantes, M. (2022). *6 Habits of 'rebel leadership' that most of us rarely practice.* Inc. https://www.inc.com/marcel-schwantes/rebel-leadership-habits.html

Sherwood, G. D., & Horton-Deutsch, S. (2015). *Reflective organizations. On the front lines of QSEN & reflective practice implementation.* Indianapolis, IN: Sigma Theta Tau International.

Sostrin, J. (2017). *Who you are is how you lead.* Retrieved May 29, 2022, from https://www.strategy-business.com/blog/Who-You-Are-Is-How-You-Lead

Tirakyan, V. (2021, June 22). *Virtual leadership: 5 best practices to lead a virtual team.* Forbes. Retrieved July 11, 2021 from https://www.forbes.com/sites/forbesbusinesscouncil/2021/06/22/virtual-leadership-5-best-practices-to-lead-a-virtual-team/?sh=3a88a2bd1f06

Trojani, S. (2018). *5 Ways leaders are different to managers.* World Economic Forum. https://www.weforum.org/agenda/2018/02/5-ways-leaders-different-managers-stefano-trojani/

Williams, E. (2021). *The benefits of strengths-based leadership.* Training Industry. Retrieved July 11, 2021 from https://trainingindustry.com/articles/leadership/the-benefits-of-strengths-based-leadership/

Williams, M. (2021). *A business case for servant leadership principles.* https://www.markwwilliams.com/2021/03/08/servant-leadership/

Wu, J., Liden, R. C., Liao, C., & Wayne, S. J. (2021). Does manager servant leadership lead to follower serving behaviors? It depends on follower self-interest. *Journal of Applied Psychology, 106*(1), 152–167.

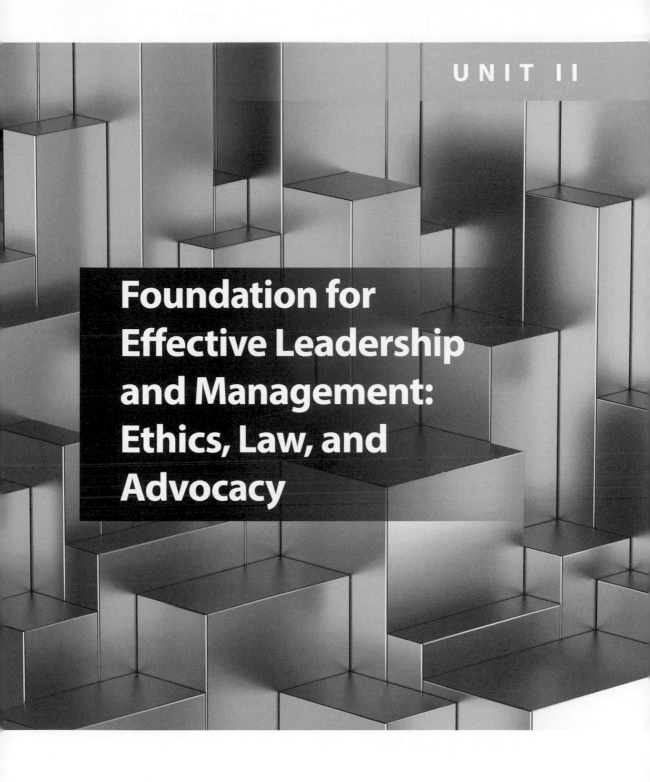

Foundation for Effective Leadership and Management: Ethics, Law, and Advocacy

4

Ethical Issues

*… When organizations go astray ethically, it is usually due to a lack of ethical competence, not bad people.—**John Hooker***

*… All my growth and development led me to believe that if you really do the right thing, and if you play by the rules, and if you've got good enough, solid judgment and common sense, that you're going to be able to do whatever you want to do with your life.—**Barbara Jordan***

*… Ethics is knowing the difference between what you have a right to do and what is right to do.—**Potter Stewart***

CROSSWALK

This chapter addresses:

- **AACN Essentials Domain 1:** Knowledge for nursing practice
- **AACN Essentials Domain 2:** Person-centered care
- **AACN Essentials Domain 4:** Scholarship for nursing practice
- **AACN Essentials Domain 6:** Interprofessional partnerships
- **AACN Essentials Domain 7:** Systems-based practice
- **AACN Essentials Domain 9:** Professionalism
- **AACN Essentials Domain 10:** Personal, professional, and leadership development
- **AONL Nurse Executive Competency 3:** Leadership
- **AONL Nurse Executive Competency 4:** Professionalism
- **ANA Standard of Professional Performance 7:** Ethics
- **ANA Standard of Professional Performance 8:** Advocacy
- **ANA Standard of Professional Performance 9:** Respectful and equitable practice
- **ANA Standard of Professional Performance 11:** Collaboration
- **ANA Standard of Professional Performance 12:** Leadership
- **ANA Standard of Professional Performance 16:** Professional practice evaluation
- **ANA Standard of Professional Performance 17:** Resource stewardship
- **QSEN Competency:** Patient-centered care

LEARNING OBJECTIVES

The learner will:

- define ethics and ethical dilemmas
- differentiate between moral indifference, moral uncertainty, moral conflict, moral distress, and moral outrage
- compare and contrast the utilitarian, duty-based, rights-based, and intuitionist frameworks for ethical decision making
- use a systematic problem-solving or decision-making model to determine appropriate action for select ethical problems
- identify and define nine different principles of ethical reasoning

- demonstrate self-awareness regarding the ethical frameworks and ethical principles that most strongly influence their personal decision making
- role-model ethical decision making congruent with national and international Codes of Ethics and current professional standards
- describe how differences in personal, organizational, subordinate, and patient obligations increase the risk of intrapersonal conflict in ethical decision making
- evaluate the quality of ethical problem solving in terms of both outcome and the process used to make the decision
- describe the limitations of using outcome as the sole criterion for the evaluation of ethical decision making
- identify strategies leader-managers can use to promote ethical behavior as the norm
- distinguish between legal and ethical obligations in decision making

Introduction

Unit II examines ethical, legal, and legislative issues affecting leadership and management as well as professional advocacy. This chapter focuses on applied ethical decision making as a critical leadership role for managers. Chapter 5 examines the impact of legislation and the law on leadership and management, and Chapter 6 focuses on advocacy for patients and subordinates and for the nursing profession in general.

Ethics is the systematic study of what a person's conduct and actions should be regarding self, other human beings, and the environment; it is the justification of what is right or good and the study of what a person's life and relationships should be, not necessarily what they are. Ethics is a system of moral conduct and principles that guide a one's actions regarding right and wrong, oneself, and society at large. Applied ethics requires the application of normative ethical theory to everyday problems.

> Ethics is concerned with doing the right thing, although it is not always clear what that is.

Society helps define the purposes of various institutions, and the purposes, in turn, help ensure that the institution fulfills specific functions. However, the specific values and norms in any institution determine the focus of its resources and shape its organizational life. The values of people within institutions influence actual management practice. Due to this set of complex interactions, arriving at appropriate ethical management decisions can be a difficult task.

In addition, the normative ethical theory for each profession arises from the purpose of the profession. The values and norms of the nursing profession, therefore, provide the foundation and filter from which ethical decisions are made. Nursing management ethics, however, are distinct from clinical nursing ethics. Though significant research exists regarding ethical dilemmas and moral distress experienced by staff nurses in clinical roles, less research exists regarding the ethical distress experienced by nursing managers. The nurse-manager may not have as clearly defined a foundation for ethical reasoning.

Further, because management is a discipline and not a profession, its purpose is not as clearly defined as medicine or law; therefore, the norms that guide ethical decision making are less clear. The manager's ethical obligation is tied to the organization's purpose, and the purpose of the organization is linked to the function that it fills in society and the constraints society places on it. In addition, organizational values influence managerial norms and values. In this way, the responsibilities of the nurse-manager emerge from a complex set of interactions.

Nursing management ethics are also distinct from other areas of management. Although there are many similar areas of responsibility between nurse-managers and non–nurse-managers, many leadership roles and management functions are specific to nursing. These differences require the nurse-manager to deal with obligations and ethical dilemmas that are not encountered in non-nursing management.

Because personal, organizational, subordinate, and consumer responsibilities also differ, there is great potential for nursing managers to experience intrapersonal conflict about the appropriate course of action. Multiple advocacy roles and accountability to the profession further increase the likelihood that all nurse-managers will be faced with ethical dilemmas in their practice.

> Nurses are often placed in situations where they are expected to be agents
> for patients, physicians, and the organization simultaneously, all of which
> may have conflicting needs, wants, and goals.

Therefore, to make appropriate ethical decisions the manager must have knowledge of ethical principles and frameworks, use a professional approach that eliminates trial and error and focuses on proven decision-making models, and use available organizational processes to assist in making such decisions. Such organizational processes include institutional review boards (IRBs), ethics committees, and professional codes of ethics. Using a systematic approach and proven ethical tools and technology allows managers to make better decisions and increases the probability that they will feel confident about the decisions they have made. Leadership roles and management functions associated with ethics are shown in Display 4.1.

Moral Issues Faced by Nurses

Despite 2021 Gallup Poll findings that showed Americans ranked nursing as the most honest ethical profession for the 19th consecutive year (Oakland University News), ethical issues are commonplace in nursing. Peter (2018) agrees, noting that "nurses' moral lives are growing in complexity given rapid changes that are the result of scientific advances, a growing business ethos, and technologic processes aimed at standardizing patient care. At times, nurses believe that they cannot respond adequately to the ethical issues that they encounter because of their enormity and nurses' responsibility to continue to care for patients despite the obstacles" (para. 1).

There are many terms used to describe these moral issues including *moral indifference*, *moral uncertainty*, *moral conflict*, *moral distress*, *moral outrage*, and *ethical dilemmas*. *Moral indifference* occurs when an individual questions why morality in practice is even necessary. *Moral uncertainty* or *moral conflict* occurs when an individual is unsure which moral principles or values apply and perhaps even what the moral problem is.

On the other hand, *moral distress* occurs when the individual knows the right thing to do, but organizational constraints make it difficult to take the right course of action. Examples of these types of values conflicts include continuing what the nurse feels is unnecessary treatment for a patient or witnessing inadequate pain relief because a provider fails to order adequate medication (Saver, 2021). Signs and symptoms of moral distress include feelings of anger, frustration, hopelessness, isolation, and suicidality (Mooney, 2021). Practitioners may also feel belittled, unimportant, or unintelligent and may contemplate leaving their jobs or their profession altogether.

The American Nurses Association (ANA, 2021) agrees, noting that moral distress can make nurses feel powerless, anxious, and even depressed. This occurs because nurses often experience not only the joy of providing care, but also the suffering and stress that sickness can cause patients and families. Thus, the intimate nature of the nurse–patient relationship can contribute to the prevalence of moral distress (ANA, 2021).

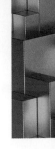

DISPLAY **4.1**	**LEADERSHIP ROLES AND MANAGEMENT FUNCTIONS ASSOCIATED WITH ETHICS**

Leadership Roles

1. Is self-aware regarding own values and basic beliefs about the rights, duties, and goals of human beings
2. Accepts that some ambiguity and uncertainty must be a part of all ethical decision making
3. Accepts that negative outcomes occur in ethical decision making despite high-quality problem solving and decision making
4. Demonstrates risk taking in ethical decision making
5. Role models ethical decision making, which is congruent with current national and international Codes of Ethics and professional standards
6. Clearly communicates expected ethical standards of behavior
7. Role models behavior that eliminates theory–practice–ethics gaps and promotes ethical behavior as the norm
8. Promotes patients' self-determination and informed decision making
9. Collaborates with others to protect human rights and promote social justice
10. Assures that nurses are represented on interprofessional teams addressing ethical risks, benefits, and outcomes

Management Functions

1. Uses a systematic approach to problem solving and decision making when faced with management problems with ethical ramifications
2. Identifies outcomes in ethical decision making that should always be sought or avoided
3. Uses established ethical frameworks to clarify values and beliefs
4. Applies principles of ethical reasoning to define what beliefs or values form the basis for decision making
5. Is aware of legal precedents that may guide ethical decision making and is accountable for possible liabilities should they go against the legal precedent
6. Continually reevaluates the quality of personal ethical decision making based on the process of decision making or problem solving used
7. Constantly assesses levels of moral uncertainty, moral distress, and moral outrage in subordinates and intervenes as necessary to protect quality patient care and workers' well-being
8. Establishes systems whereby ethical issues impacting stakeholders (health care consumers, workers, community, etc.) can be addressed and resolved
9. Recognizes and rewards ethical conduct of subordinates
10. Takes appropriate action when subordinates demonstrate unethical conduct

Moral outrage occurs when a person witnesses the immoral act of another but feels powerless to stop it. The most difficult of all moral issues is termed a *moral* or *ethical dilemma*, which is being forced to choose between two or more undesirable alternatives. For example, a nurse might experience a moral or ethical dilemma if they were required to provide care or treatments that conflicted with their own religious beliefs. In this case, the nurse would likely experience an intrapersonal moral conflict about whether their values, needs, and wants could or should supersede those of the patient. Because ethical dilemmas are so difficult to resolve, many of the learning exercises in this chapter are devoted to addressing this type of moral issue.

> Individual values, beliefs, and personal philosophy play a major role in the moral or ethical decision making that is part of the daily routine of all nurses as well as managers.

How do managers decide what is right and what is wrong? What does the manager do if no right or wrong answer exists? What if all solutions generated seem to be wrong? Remember that the way managers approach and solve ethical issues is influenced by their values and basic beliefs about the rights, duties, and goals of all human beings. Self-awareness, then, is a vital leadership role in ethical decision making, just as it is in so many other aspects of management.

No rules, guidelines, or theories exist that cover all aspects of the ethical problems that managers face. However, it is the manager's responsibility to understand the ethical problem-solving process, to be familiar with ethical frameworks and principles, and to know ethical professional codes and standards. These tools will assist managers in effective problem solving and prevent ethical failure within their organizations. Critical thinking occurs when managers can engage in an orderly process of ethical problem solving to determine the rightness or wrongness of different courses of action.

Ethical Frameworks for Decision Making

Ethical frameworks guide individuals in solving ethical dilemmas. These frameworks do not solve the ethical problem but assist the manager in clarifying personal values and beliefs. Four of the most used ethical frameworks are utilitarianism, duty-based reasoning, rights-based reasoning, and intuitionism (Table 4.1).

> Ethical frameworks do not solve ethical problems, but they do assist decision makers in clarifying personal values and beliefs.

The *teleologic* theory of ethics is also called *utilitarianism* or *consequentialist* theory. Using an ethical framework of utilitarianism encourages decision making based on what provides the greatest good for the greatest number of people. In doing so, the needs and wants of the individual are diminished. Utilitarianism also suggests that the end can justify the means. For example, a manager using a utilitarian approach might decide to use travel budget money to send many staff to regional workshops rather than to fund one or two people to attend a national conference. Another example would be an insurance program that meets the needs of many but refuses coverage for expensive organ transplants. In Learning Exercise 4.6, the organization uses utilitarianism to justify lying to employee applicants because their hiring would result in good for many employees by keeping several units in the hospital open.

Deontologic ethical theory judges whether the action is right or wrong regardless of the consequences and is based on the philosophy of Immanuel Kant in the 18th century. Primarily, this theory uses both duty-based reasoning and rights-based reasoning as the basis for its philosophy. *Duty-based reasoning* is an ethical framework stating that some decisions must be made because one has a duty to do something or to refrain from doing something. In Learning Exercise 4.5, the supervisor feels a duty to hire the most qualified person for the job, even if the personal cost is high.

TABLE 4.1 **ETHICAL FRAMEWORKS**

Framework	Basic Premise
Utilitarian (teleologic)	Decisions are made with the goal of providing the greatest good for the greatest number of people
Rights based (deontologic)	Individuals have basic inherent rights that should not be interfered with during decision making
Duty based (deontologic)	Decisions are made because one has a duty to do something or to refrain from doing something
Intuitionist (deontologic)	Issues are weighed on a case-by-case basis to determine relative goals, duties, and rights

Rights-based reasoning is based on the belief that some things are a person's just due (i.e., everyone has basic claims, or entitlements, with which there should be no interference). Rights are different from needs, wants, or desires. The supervisor in Learning Exercise 4.5 believes that both applicants have the right to fair and impartial consideration of their applications. In Learning Exercise 4.6, Sam believes that all people have the right to truth and, in fact, that he has the duty to be truthful.

The *intuitionist framework* allows the decision maker to review each ethical problem or issue on a case-by-case basis, comparing the relative weights of goals, duties, and rights. This weighting is determined primarily by intuition—what the decision maker believes is right for that specific situation. Recently, some ethical theorists have begun questioning the appropriateness of intuitionism as an ethical decision-making framework because of the potential for subjectivity and bias. Yet, many of the cases solved in this chapter involve some degree of decision making by intuition.

Other more recent theories of ethical philosophy include *ethical relativism* and *ethical universalism*. Ethical relativism suggests that individuals make decisions based only on what seems right or reasonable according to their value systems or cultures. Conversely, ethical universalism holds that ethical principles are universal and constant, and that ethical decision making should not vary because of individual circumstances or cultural differences.

Principles of Ethical Reasoning

Both teleologic and deontologic theorists have developed a group of moral principles that are used for ethical reasoning. These principles of ethical reasoning further explore and define what beliefs or values form the basis for decision making. Respect for people is the most basic and universal ethical principle. The major *ethical principles* stemming from this basic principle are discussed in Display 4.2.

Autonomy (Self-Determination)

A form of personal liberty, *autonomy*, is also called freedom of choice or accepting the responsibility for one's choice. Rosenberg (2021) notes that autonomy means that patients can make independent decisions. This means that nurses should be sure patients have all the information they need to make a decision about their medical care. Examples of nurses fostering patient autonomy include obtaining informed consent from the patient for treatment, accepting the situation when a patient refuses a medication, and maintaining confidentiality.

The legal right of *self-determination* supports autonomy. For example, progressive discipline recognizes the autonomy of the employee. The employee has the choice to meet organizational expectations or to be disciplined further. If the employee's continued behavior

---

DISPLAY 4.2 ETHICAL PRINCIPLES

Autonomy: All people have the right of self-determination and freedom of choice
Beneficence: Actions are taken to promote good
Nonmaleficence: Actions are taken to avoid harm
Paternalism: One individual assumes the right to make decisions for another
Utility: The good of the many outweighs the wants or needs of the individual
Justice: In pursuit of fairness, "equals" should be treated equally, and "unequals" should be treated according to their differences
Veracity: Human beings must always tell the truth
Fidelity: Everyone has a moral obligation to keep promises
Confidentiality: Privileged information must be kept private

warrants termination, the principle of autonomy says that the employee has made the choice to be terminated because of their actions, not by the manager's. Therefore, nurse-managers must be cognizant of the ethical component present whenever an individual's decisional capacity is in question. To take away a person's right to self-determination is a serious but sometimes necessary action.

Beneficence (Doing Good)

This principle states that the actions one takes should be done to promote good. The concept of *nonmaleficence*, which is associated with *beneficence*, says that if one cannot do good, then one should at least do no harm. For example, if a manager uses this ethical principle in planning performance appraisals, they are much more likely to offer feedback during a performance appraisal that can promote employee growth. Another example would be providing a standard of care that minimizes risk or prevents negligent patient care (Rosenberg, 2021).

It is not always clear, however, if a nurse's actions are beneficent or maleficent. For example, Ganz et al. (2018) point out that cardiopulmonary resuscitation is the default procedure during cardiopulmonary arrest. If a patient does not want cardiopulmonary resuscitation, then a "do-not-resuscitate" order must be documented. Sometimes, this order is not given, even if meaningful recovery is not likely. This situation then can lead to a *slow code*, defined as an ineffective resuscitation, where not all resuscitation procedures are performed or are done slowly (Ganz et al., 2018). Some nurses perceive slow codes to be a beneficent ethical alternative, but this contradicts most legal and ethical opinions expressed in the literature.

Paternalism

Paternalism occurs when one person assumes the authority to decide for another. In clinical nursing, care providers may become paternalistic when they believe the patient's judgment is impaired or that they have knowledge the patient does not have. Because *paternalism* limits freedom of choice, however, most ethical theorists believe that paternalism is justified only to prevent a person from coming to harm. In this way, this principle is related to beneficence.

Unfortunately, paternalism is present in nursing management as well as clinical decision making. For example, some managers use the principle of paternalism in subordinates' career planning. In doing so, managers assume that they have greater knowledge of what an employee's short- and long-term goals should be than the employee does.

> The most fundamental universal principle is respect for people.

Utility

This principle reflects a belief in utilitarianism—what is best for the common good outweighs what is best for the individual. Utility justifies paternalism as a means of restricting individual freedom. Managers who use the principle of utility need to be careful not to become so focused on desired group outcomes that they become less humanistic.

Justice (Treating People Fairly)

This principle states that equals should be treated equally and that unequals should be treated according to their differences. For example, Haden (2017) suggests that if two people have the same relative position in an organization and the same level of responsibility, then *justice* is treating them the same in terms of resources, expectations, rewards, and other factors necessary for them to succeed. However, if one person has significantly different responsibilities than another—that is, they are unequal—then the just leader must treat them as unequals.

LEARNING EXERCISE   **4.1**

Are Some People More Equal Than Others?

Research suggests that individuals with health insurance in this country have better access to health care services and enjoy better health care outcomes than those who do not. This does not mean, however, that all individuals with health insurance receive "equal treatment." Medicaid recipients (generally low income) often report that although they have public insurance, many private providers refuse to accept them as patients. Patients enrolled in managed care suggest that their treatment options are more limited than those offered through traditional private insurance because of the use of gatekeepers, required authorizations, and queuing. Some individuals, with lower cost insurance plans under the *Patient Protection and Affordable Care Act*, suggest that high out-of-pocket costs for copayments and deductibles continue to restrict their choice to access needed care.

ASSIGNMENT:

Using the ethical principle of justice, determine whether health care in this country should be a right or a privilege. Are the uninsured and the insured "unequals" that should be treated according to their differences? Does the type of health insurance that one has also create a system of unequals? If so, are the unequals being treated according to their differences?

Haden (2017) also argues that justice is giving each person their due. From this perspective, justice is defined by the leader's responsibility to give each follower what rightfully belongs to them, whether that right is determined by nature or by contract.

The principle of justice is frequently applied when there are scarcities of or competition for resources or benefits. The manager who uses the principle of justice will work to see that pay raises reflect consistent performance and time in service. Nurses demonstrate this when making impartial medical decisions related to limited resources or new treatments regardless of patients' economic status, ethnicity, sexual orientation, or other considerations (Rosenberg, 2021).

Gebreheat and Teame (2021) note that amid the COVID-19 pandemic, health professionals were often challenged to apply autonomy, justice, beneficence, and nonmaleficence in taking care of clients. For example, health workers who were required to work without adequate personal protective equipment placed not only to themselves but their families and other clients at risk of infection. Thus, it violated "no harm to others" or the "nonmaleficence" ethical principle.

Justice was also an ethical challenge during the pandemic in terms of the fair allocation of medical resources. Justice implies fairness in medical decision making. But, during the COVID-19 pandemic, nurses were forced to make difficult decisions about various ethically ambiguous issues, such as which patients should be given scarce intensive care unit beds and receive mechanical ventilation or extracorporeal membrane oxygenation (Gebreheat & Teame, 2021).

In addition, a significant number of nurses faced moral distress during the pandemic because of having to restrict many patients from having end-of-life communication with their families (Gebreheat & Teame, 2021). While patients normally have the autonomy to decide who should be involved in taking care of or visiting them during a stay in the hospital, nurses were not capable of fulfilling many patients' will and wishes.

Other issues that caused nurses moral distress included the obligation to provide care for patients regardless of diagnosis (even when doing so put nurses at risk of contracting COVID-19 themselves), and the tension between the need for self-care and a sense of duty to provide care for others (see Examining the Evidence 4.1).

EXAMINING THE EVIDENCE 4.1

Source: From Alloubani, A., Khater, W., Akhu–Zaheya, L., Almomani, M., & Alashram, S. (2021, May 7). Nurses' ethics in the care of patients during the covid-19 pandemic. *Frontiers in Medicine.* https://www.frontiersin.org/articles/10.3389/fmed.2021.589550/full

Nurses' Ethics During the COVID-19 Pandemic

This study explored ethical issues experienced by nurses in caring for patients during the coronavirus disease 2019 (COVID-19) pandemic. A descriptive qualitative approach was used and a purposive sample of 10 nurses working with patients with COVID-19 was recruited.

Three major themes emerged from the data analysis. The first theme was the obligation of nurses to provide care for patients regardless of their medical diagnosis. This theme included three subthemes: nurses should always be available for patients; patients with COVID-19 have the right to be cared for; and patients should be treated as if they were family members. Participants reported it was their duty to care for patients regardless of medical condition or diagnosis and expressed that this was part of their professional ethics, which are framed by standards of human rights.

The second theme was the ethical dilemma faced by nurses of whether to care for patients or protect themselves from the virus. Although all study participants voluntarily participated in the care of patients with COVID-19, they nonetheless believed that nurses should not be forced to provide care for COVID-19 patients. The researchers noted that nurses themselves should be actively involved in the development and implementation of policies related to the quality of care, especially during exceptional circumstances such as the pandemic. Nurses' capabilities of providing patient care should be acknowledged at all organizational levels, and their concerns should be heard and addressed.

The third theme was the responsibility of nurses to care for themselves. As frontline health care providers, participants believed they needed to protect themselves to avoid contracting the virus. Thus, they believed that they were obligated to have sufficient knowledge and to protect themselves appropriately. They considered this to be part of their accountability as nurses.

Nickitas (2021) notes that the degree of nurses' moral injury and the true impact on the mental and emotional well-being of nurses from the pandemic may not be known for some time. There may be long-lasting emotional, social, and spiritual effects from requiring nurses to act at times in conflict with their moral values and the duty to care during a pandemic crisis. Gebreheat and Teame (2021, p. 1034) agree, noting that "the overall consequences of such gaps have left a scar on the history of the modern nursing profession."

Veracity (Truth Telling)

This principle is used to explain how people feel about the need for truth telling or the acceptability of deception. For example, a manager who believes that deception is morally acceptable if it is done with the objective of beneficence may tell all rejected job applicants that they were highly considered whether they had been or not.

Fidelity (Keeping Promises)

Fidelity refers to the moral obligation individuals have to be faithful to their commitments and promises. Breaking a promise is believed by many ethicists to be wrong regardless of the consequences. In other words, even if there were no far-reaching negative results of someone breaking a promise, it is still wrong because it would render that person's making of any future promise meaningless. However, there are times when keeping a promise (fidelity) may not be in the best interest of the party to whom one has made a promise. Although nurses have multiple fidelity duties (to patient, physician, organization, profession, and self) that at times may be

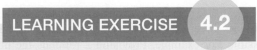

LEARNING EXERCISE 4.2

Weighing Veracity and Nonmaleficence

You are a second-year nursing student. During the first year of the nursing program, you formed a close friendship with Susan, another nursing student, and the two of you spend many of your free evenings and weekends together doing fun things. The only thing that irritates you about your friend is that she is incredibly messy. When you go to her home, you usually see dirty dishes piled in the sink, dog hair over all the furniture, clothing strewn all over the apartment, and uneaten pizza or other half spoiled food sitting on the floor. You attempt to limit your time at her apartment because it bothers you so much, so it has not affected your friendship.

Today, when Susan and you are sitting at the dining table in your apartment, your current roommate tells you that she is unexpectedly vacating her lease at the end of the month. Susan becomes excited and shares that her lease will end at the end of this month as well and suggests how much fun it would be if the two of you could move in together. She immediately begins talking about when she could move in, where she would locate her furniture in the apartment, and where her dog might stay when the two of you are completing clinical practicums. Although you value Susan's friendship and really enjoy the time you spend together, living with someone as untidy as Susan is not something you want to do. Unfortunately, your current lease does not preclude pets or subleases.

ASSIGNMENT:

Decide how you will respond to Susan. Will you tell her the truth? Are your values regarding veracity stronger or weaker than your desire to cause no harm to Susan's feelings (nonmaleficence)?

in conflict, the ANA *Code of Ethics for Nurses With Interpretive Statements* is clear that the nurse's primary commitment is to the patient (ANA, 2015).

Confidentiality (Respecting Privileged Information)

The obligation to observe the privacy of another and to hold certain information in strict confidence is a basic ethical principle and a foundation of both medical and nursing ethics. However, similar to how deception may sometimes be more ethical than truth-telling, there are times when the mandate against disclosing information must be overridden. For example, health care managers are required by law to report certain cases, such as drug use or misuse in employees, elder abuse, and child abuse.

Codes of Ethics and Professional Standards

Professional ethics relate to the values held by a profession. A *professional code of ethics* then is a set of principles, established by a profession, to guide the individual practitioner. The first Code of Ethics for Nurses was adopted by the ANA in 1950 and has been revised six times since then, most recently in 2015. This code outlines the important general values, duties, and responsibilities that flow from the specific role of being a nurse. Although not legally binding, the code functions as a guide to the highest ethical practice standards for nurses and as an aid for moral thinking.

The ANA (2015) *Code of Ethics for Nurses With Interpretive Statements* has nine statements. The professional issues in the first three statements are concerned with protection of clients' rights and safety; those in the next three pertain to promoting healthy work cultures and self-care. The social issues of the last three statements of the code relate to the nurse's obligations to society and the profession. For example, Provision 2 reminds the nurse that their primary commitment is to the patient, whether an individual, family, group, community, or population. Provisions 5 and 6 focus on ethical issues related to the boundaries of duty and loyalty. Provisions 7 to 9 focus on the nurse's ethical duties beyond individual patient encounters and suggest that the nurse has an obligation to address social justice/human rights issues through direct action and involvement in health policy as well as a responsibility to contribute to nursing knowledge through scholarly inquiry and research.

> Professional codes of ethics function as a guide to the highest standards of ethical practice for nurses. They are not legally binding.

LEARNING EXERCISE 4.3

Family Values

You are the evening shift charge nurse of the postanesthesia care unit (PACU). You have just admitted a 32-year-old woman who, 2 hours ago, was thrown from the passenger seat of a car. She was rushed to the emergency department and subsequently to surgery, where she had cranial burr holes placed and an intracranial monitor inserted. No further cranial exploration was attempted because the patient sustained extensive and massive neurologic damage. She will probably not survive your shift. The plan is to hold her in the PACU for 1 hour and, if she is still alive, transfer her to the intensive care unit.

Shortly after receiving the patient, you are approached by the evening house supervisor, who says that the patient's sister is pleading to be allowed into the PACU. Normally, visitors are not allowed into the PACU when patients are being held there only temporarily, but occasionally, exceptions are made. Tonight, the PACU is empty except for this patient. You decide to bend the rules and allow the young woman's sister to come in. The visiting sister is near collapse; you realize she was driving the car when it crashed. As the visitor continues to speak to the comatose patient, her behavior and words make you begin to wonder if she is indeed the patient's sister.

Within 15 minutes, the house supervisor returns and states, "I have made a terrible mistake. The patient's family just arrived, and they say that the visitor we just allowed into the PACU is not a member of the family but is the patient's girlfriend. They are very angry and demand that this woman not be allowed to see the patient."

You approach the visitor and confront her gently about the information that you have just received. She looks at you with tears streaming down her face and says, "Yes, it is true. Mary and I have been together for 6 years. Her family disowned her because of it, but we were everything to each other. She has been my life, and I have been hers. Please, please let me stay. I will never see her again. I know the family will not allow me to attend the funeral. I need to say my goodbyes. Please let me stay. It is not fair that they have the legal right to be family when I have been the one to love and care for Mary."

ASSIGNMENT:

1. Review the ANA (2018). *Position Statement—Nursing Advocacy for LGBTQ+ Populations* available at https://www.nursingworld.org/~49866e/globalassets/practiceandpolicy/ethics/nursing-advocacy-for-lgbtq-populations.pdf
2. Decide what you will do. Recognize that your own value system will play a part in your decision. List several alternatives that are available to you. Identify which ethical frameworks or principles most affected your decision making.

Practitioners may also find ethical guidance in examining the International Council of Nurses (ICN) Code of Ethics for Nurses, which was revised in 2021 (ICN, 2021). This Code provides a guide for action based on social values and needs and has served as the standard for nurses worldwide since it was first adopted in 1953.

Another document that may be helpful specifically to the nurse-manager in creating and maintaining an ethical work environment is *Nursing Administration: Scope and Standards of Practice* (ANA, 2016) published by the ANA. These standards delineate professional standards in management ethics. For example, one standard suggests that managers must advocate for compassionate systems of care delivery that preserve and protect health care consumers', families', and employees' dignity, rights, values, belief, and autonomy. Another standard notes that managers must collaborate with other health professionals and the public to protect human rights, promote health diplomacy, enhance cultural sensitivity and congruence, and reduce health disparities. Yet another suggests that nurse managers must integrate principles of social justice into nursing and policy.

Ethical Problem Solving and Decision Making

Some of the difficulty people have in making ethical decisions can be attributed to a lack of formal education about problem solving. Other individuals lack the thinking skills or risk taking needed to solve complex ethical problems. Some nurses erroneously use decision-making outcomes as the sole basis for determining the quality of the decision making. Although decision makers should be able to identify desirable and undesirable outcomes, outcomes alone cannot be used to assess the quality of the problem solving.

Many variables affect outcome, and some of these are beyond the control or foresight of the problem solver. In fact, even the most ethical courses of action can have undesirable and unavoidable consequences. That is why using outcome alone to determine the quality of problem solving can be so dangerous. Ethical problem solving should be evaluated in terms of both outcome and the process used to make the decision. The best possible decisions stem from structured problem solving, adequate data collection, and examination of multiple alternatives—even if outcomes are less than desired.

> If a structured approach to problem solving is used, data gathering is adequate, and multiple alternatives are analyzed, even with an undesirable outcome, the nurse should accept that the best possible decision was made at that time with the information and resources available.

In addition, Mortell (2012) suggests that some decision making by nurses reflects a *theory–practice–ethics gap*. In other words, nurses often fail to ensure that theory and practice are integrated despite their duty to do so. For example, Mortell notes that noncompliance exists in hand hygiene among practitioners despite ongoing infection prevention education and training; easy access to facilities such as washbasins; antiseptic/alcohol hand gels that are convenient, effective, and skin- and user-friendly; and organizational recognition and support for clinicians in hand washing and hand gel practices. Thus, despite nurses having knowledge of best practices based on current research, they continue to fail to achieve the required and desired compliance in hand hygiene. Mortell concludes that more emphasis should be placed on clinicians' moral and ethical obligations as part of training and orientation, and that organizations must continue to emphasize the duty of care toward patients in nurses' decision making.

Kearney and Penque (2012) provide another example of a theory–practice–ethics gap in their suggestion that although nurses recognize that checklists can reduce episodes of patient harm by ensuring that procedures are being carried out appropriately, some providers will indicate that an intervention has been undertaken when it has not. This occurs because of an increasing emphasis and reliance on documentation that demands that "all boxes must be ticked" to ensure complete care has been provided (as illustrated by the popular nursing mantra "If it wasn't documented, it wasn't done"). Kearney and Penque suggest then that checklists present a context for ethical decision making in that when providers do not take ethics into account, checklists could perpetuate rather than prevent unsafe practices or errors.

The Traditional Problem-Solving Process

Although not recognized specifically as an ethical problem-solving model, one of the oldest and most frequently used tools for problem solving is the traditional problem-solving process. This process, which is discussed in Chapter 1, consists of seven steps, with the actual decision being made at step 5 (review the seven steps under "Traditional Problem-Solving Process" section in Chapter 1). Although many individuals use at least some of these steps in their decision making, they frequently fail to generate an adequate number of alternatives or to evaluate the results—two essential steps in the process.

LEARNING EXERCISE 4.4

A Nagging Uneasiness

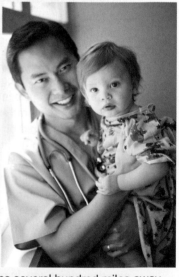

You are a nurse on a pediatric unit. One of your patients is a 15-month-old girl with a diagnosis of failure to thrive. The mother says that the child is emotional, cries a lot, and does not like to be held. You have been taking care of the child for 2 days since her admission, and she has smiled and been receptive to being held by you. She has also eaten well. There is something about the child's reaction to the mother's boyfriend (who is not the child's biologic father) that bothers you. The child appears to draw away from him when he visits. The mother is very young and seems to be rather immature but appears to care about the child.

This is the second hospital admission for this child. Although you were not on duty for the first admission 6 weeks ago, you check the records and see that the child was admitted with the same diagnosis. While you are on duty today, the child's biologic father (the ex-husband of the child's mother) calls and asks about her condition. He lives several hundred miles away and requests that the child be hospitalized until the weekend (it is Wednesday) so that he can "check things out." He tells you that he believes the child is mistreated. He says he is also concerned about his ex-wife's 4-year-old child from another marriage and is attempting to gain custody of that child in addition to his own child. From what little the father said, you are aware that the divorce was bitter and that the mother has full custody. Because of Health Insurance Portability and Accountability Act, you tell the father that you cannot provide any information about the child.

You talk with the physician at length. He says that after the last hospitalization, he requested that the community health agency and Child Protective Services call on the family. Their subsequent report to him was that the 4-year-old child appeared happy and well and that the 15-month-old child appeared clean, although somewhat underweight. There was no evidence to suggest child abuse. However, the community health agency plans to continue following the children. He says that the mother has been good about keeping doctor appointments and has kept the children's immunizations up to date. The pediatrician proceeds to write an order for discharge. He says that although he also feels uneasy, continued hospitalization is not justified, and Medicaid will not pay for additional days. He also says that he will follow up once again with Child Protective Services to make another visit.

When the mother and her boyfriend come to take the baby home, the baby clings to you and refuses to go to the boyfriend. She also seems reluctant to go to the mother. All during the discharge, you are extremely uneasy. When you see the car drive away, you feel very sad.

After returning to the unit, you talk with your supervisor, who listens carefully and questions you at length. Finally, she says, "It seems as if you have nothing concrete on which to act and are only experiencing feelings. I think you would be risking a lot of trouble for yourself and the hospital if you acted rashly at this time. Accusing people with no evidence and making them go through a traumatic experience is something I would hesitate to do."

You leave the supervisor's office still troubled. She did not tell you that you must do nothing, but you believe that she would disapprove of further action on your part. The doctor also felt strongly that there was no reason to do more than was already being done. The child will be followed by community health nurses. Perhaps the ex-husband was just trying to make trouble for his ex-wife and her new boyfriend. You would certainly not want anyone to have reported you or created problems regarding your own children. You remember how often your 5-year-old child bruised himself when he was that age. You go about your duties and try to shake off your feeling. What should you do?

ASSIGNMENT:

1. Solve the case in small groups by using the traditional problem-solving process. Identify the problem and several alternative solutions to solve this ethical dilemma. What should you do and why? What are the risks? How does your value system play a part in your decision? Justify your solution. After completing this assignment, solve the second part of this assignment below.

2. Assume that this was a real case. Twenty-four hours after the child's discharge, she is readmitted with critical head trauma. Police reports indicate that the child suffered multiple skull fractures after being thrown up against the wall by her mother's boyfriend. The child is not expected to live. Does knowing the outcome change how you would have solved the case? Does the outcome influence how you feel about the quality of your group's problem solving?

The Nursing Process

Another problem-solving model not specifically designed for ethical analysis, but appropriate for it, is the nursing process. Most nurses are aware of the nursing process and the cyclic nature of its components of assessment, diagnosis, planning, implementation, and evaluation (see Fig. 1.2). However, most nurses do not recognize its use as a decision-making tool. The cyclic nature of the process allows for feedback to occur at any step and for the process to repeat until adequate information is gathered to make a decision. It does not, however, require clear problem identification. Learning Exercise 4.5 shows how the nursing process might be used as an ethical decision-making tool.

The Moral Decision-Making Model

Crisham (1985) developed a model for ethical decision making incorporating the nursing process and principles of biomedical ethics. This model is especially useful in clarifying ethical problems that result from conflicting obligations. This model is represented by the mnemonic MORAL as shown in Display 4.3. Learning Exercise 4.6 demonstrates the MORAL modeling in solving an ethical issue.

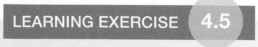

LEARNING EXERCISE   4.5

One Applicant Too Many

The reorganization of the public health agency has resulted in the creation of a new position of community health liaison. A job description has been written, and the job opening has been posted. As the chief nursing executive of this agency, it will be your responsibility to select the best person for the position. Because you are aware that all hiring decisions are made with some subjectivity, you want to eliminate as much personal bias as possible. Two people have applied for the position; one of them is a close friend.

Analysis

Assess: As the chief nursing executive, you have a responsibility to make personnel decisions as objectively as you can. This means that the hiring decision should be based solely on which employee is best qualified for the position. You do recognize, however, that there may be a personal cost in terms of the friendship.

Diagnose: You diagnose this problem as a potential intrapersonal conflict between your obligation to your friend and your obligation to your employer.

Plan: You must plan how you are going to collect your data. The tools you have selected are applications, resumés, references, and personal interviews.

Implement: Both applicants are contacted and asked to submit resumés and three letters of reference from recent employers. In addition, both are scheduled for structured formal interviews with you and two of the board members of the agency. Although the board members will provide feedback, you have been reserved the right to make the final hiring decision.

Evaluate: As a result of your plan, you have discovered that both candidates meet the minimum job requirements. One candidate, however, clearly has higher level communication skills, and the other candidate (your friend) has more experience in public health and is more knowledgeable regarding the resources in your community. Both employees have complied with the request to submit resumés and letters of reference; they are of similar quality.

Assess: Your assessment of the situation is that you need more information to make the best possible decision. You must assess whether strong communication skills or public health experience and familiarity with the community would be more valuable in this position.

Plan: You plan how you can gather more information about what the employee will be doing in this newly created position.

Diagnose: If the job description is inadequate in providing this information, it may be necessary to gather information from other public health agencies with a similar job classification.

Evaluate: You now believe that excellent communication skills are essential for the job. The candidate who had these skills has an acceptable level of public health experience and seems motivated to learn more about the community and its resources. This means that your friend will not receive the job.

Assess: Now, you must assess whether a good decision has been made.

Plan: You plan to evaluate your decision in 6 months, basing your criteria on the established job description.

Implement: You are unable to implement your plan because this employee resigns unexpectedly 4 months after she takes the position. Your friend is now working in a similar capacity in another state. Although you correspond sometimes, the relationship has changed because of your decision.

Evaluate: Did you make a good decision? This decision was based on a carefully thought-out process, which included adequate data gathering and a weighing of alternatives. Variables beyond your control resulted in the employee's resignation, and there was no apparent reason for you to suspect that this would happen. The decision to exclude or minimize personal bias was a conscious one, and you were aware of the possible ramifications of this choice. The decision making appears to have been appropriate.

DISPLAY 4.3 THE MORAL DECISION-MAKING MODEL

*M*assage the dilemma: Collect data about the ethical problem and who should be involved in the decision-making process.

*O*utline options: Identify alternatives and analyze the causes and consequences of each.

*R*eview criteria and resolve: Weigh the options against the values of those involved in the decision. This may be done through a weighting or grid.

*A*ffirm position and act: Develop the implementation strategy.

*L*ook back: Evaluate the decision making.

Source: From Crisham, P. (1985). Moral: How can I do what's right? *Nursing Management, 16*(3), 42A–42N.

LEARNING EXERCISE 4.6

Little White Lies

Sam is the nurse recruiter for a metropolitan hospital that is experiencing an acute nursing shortage. He has been told to do or say whatever is necessary to recruit professional nurses so that the hospital will not have to close several units. He also has been told that his position will be eliminated if he does not produce a substantial number of applicants in the nursing career days to be held the following week. Sam loves his job and is the sole provider for his family. Because many organizations are experiencing severe personnel shortages, the competition for employees is keen. After his third career day without a single prospective applicant, he begins to feel desperate. On the fourth and final day, Sam begins making many promises to potential applicants regarding shift preference, unit preference, salary, and advancement that he is not sure he can keep. At the end of the day, Sam has a lengthy list of interested applicants but also feels a great deal of intrapersonal conflict.

Massage the Dilemma

In a desperate effort to save his job, Sam finds he has taken action that has resulted in high intrapersonal value conflict. Sam must choose between making promises he likely cannot keep and losing his job. This has far-reaching consequences for all involved. Sam has the ultimate responsibility for knowing his values and acting in a manner that is congruent with his value system. The organization is, however, involved in the value conflict in that its values and expectations conflict with those of Sam. Sam and the organization have some type of responsibility to these applicants, although the exact nature of this responsibility is one of the values in conflict. Because this is Sam's problem and an intrapersonal conflict, he must decide the appropriate course of action. His primary role is to examine his values and act in accordance.

Outline Options

Option 1. Quit his job immediately. This would prevent future intrapersonal conflict, provided that Sam becomes aware of his value system and behaves in a manner consistent with that value system in the future. It does not, however, solve the immediate conflict about the action Sam has already taken. This action takes away Sam's livelihood.

Option 2. Do nothing. Sam could choose not to be accountable for his own actions. This will require Sam to rationalize that the philosophy of the organization is in fact acceptable or that he has no choice regarding his actions. Thus, the responsibility for meeting the needs and wants of the new employees is shifted to the organization. Although Sam will have no credibility with the new employees, there will be only a negligible impact on his ability to recruit at least on a short-term basis. Sam will continue to have a job and be able to support his family.

(continues on page 92)

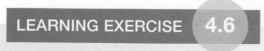

LEARNING EXERCISE 4.6

Little White Lies (continued)

Option 3. If after value clarification, Sam has determined that his values conflict with the organization's directive to do or say whatever is needed to recruit employees, he could approach his superior and share these concerns. Sam should be very clear about what his values are and to what extent he is willing to compromise them. He also should include in this meeting what, if any, action should be taken to meet the needs of the new employees. Sam must be realistic about the time and effort usually required to change the values and beliefs of an organization. He also must be aware of his bottom line if the organization is not willing to compromise.

Option 4. Sam could contact each of the applicants and tell them that certain recruitment promises may not be possible. However, he will do what he can to see that the promises are fulfilled. This alternative is risky. The applicants will probably be justifiably suspicious of both the recruiter and the organization, and Sam has little formal power at this point to fulfill their requests. This alternative also requires a time and energy commitment by Sam and does not prevent the problem from recurring.

Review the Options

In value clarification, Sam discovered that he valued truth telling. Alternative 3 allows Sam to present a recruiting plan to his supervisor that includes a bottom line that this value will not be violated.

Affirm Position and Act

Sam approached his superior and was told that his beliefs were idealistic and inappropriate in an age of severe worker shortages. Sam was terminated. Sam did, however, believe that he made an appropriate decision. He did become self-aware regarding his values and attempted to communicate these values to the organization in an effort to work out a mutually agreeable plan.

Look Back

Although Sam was terminated, he knew that he could find some type of employment to meet his immediate fiscal needs. He did become self-aware regarding his values and used what he had learned in this decision-making process, in that he planned to evaluate more carefully the recruitment philosophy of the organization in relation to his own value system before accepting another job.

Working Toward Ethical Behavior as the Norm

The concerns about ethical conduct in American institutions are documented by many national news articles. Many individuals believe that organizational and institutional ethical failure has become the norm and wonder what has gone wrong.

Unethical organizational behavior, however, cannot simply be excused by nurses because it is normalized. Nor should nurses be silent when they observe unethical behavior simply because they are not sure how to respond. Woods (2021) agrees, noting that nurses are charged with the task of meeting the care-based health needs of humankind in an ethically mindful fashion.

Unfortunately, many nurses report feeling they have gaps in ethical competence and confidence to recognize and skillfully address ethical issues with effective communication and advocacy skills (Rushton et al., 2021). Some fear reprisal, ridicule, or shame, which can lead to patterns of silence and avoidance. As a result, some nurses conform to the decisions of others, creating moral dissonance within themselves by acting contrary to their own ethical standards (Rushton et al., 2021).

This inappropriate ethical conformance has also been observed in educational settings. Indeed, in recent years, cases of cheating, including large-scale cheating at elite colleges, have become front-page headlines (Pittman, 2023). In December 2020, the U.S. Military Academy at West Point was rocked by the news of some 73 cadets cheating on a calculus final exam conducted online in May during the Academy's closure for the pandemic. Despite the Academy's honor code, the cheating occurred and was discovered by professors grading the exams who noted irregularities in the work submitted by students. Some reviewers viewed the incident as an example of the school's honor code working; however, the cheating came to light not because students reported themselves in accordance with the honor code, but due to observant grading by the faculty (Shepherd, 2020).

Cheating is a concern in any academic discipline; however, it is of particular concern to nursing educators because nurses hold the well-being and health of their patients in their hands. Lapses of integrity can have grave consequences for patients. Consequently, nursing educators and leaders must inculcate the highest standards of honesty and integrity in students to create a culture of trustworthiness in the nurses who graduate from their programs. Although there isn't a great deal of data that define the link between academic integrity and professional integrity, there is some evidence, beyond the intuitive, that there is a correlation (Pittman, 2023).

Nursing practice can be challenging, but the privilege of licensure should compel nurses (and nursing students) to behave in an ethical manner and to confront behavior when it is not ethical. Leader-managers, then, have a responsibility to create a climate in their organizations in which ethical behavior is not only the expectation but also the norm. The actions shown in Display 4.4 can help leader-managers in ethical problem solving.

Separate Legal and Ethical Issues

Although they are not the same, separating legal and ethical issues is sometimes difficult. Legal controls are generally clear and philosophically impartial; ethical controls are much less clear and more individualized. In many ethical issues, courts have made a decision that may guide managers in their decision making. Often, however, these guidelines are not comprehensive, or they differ from the manager's own philosophy. Managers must be aware of established legal standards and cognizant of possible liabilities and consequences for actions that go against the legal precedent.

> In general, legal controls are clearer and philosophically impartial; ethical controls are much less clear and individualized.

Legal precedents are frequently overturned later and often do not keep pace with the changing needs of society. In addition, certain circumstances may favor an illegal course of action as the "right" thing to do. If someone were transporting their severely ill spouse to the hospital, it might be morally correct for them to disobey traffic laws. Therefore, the manager should think of the law as a basic standard of conduct, whereas ethical behavior requires a greater examination of the issues involved.

DISPLAY 4.4 STRATEGIES LEADER-MANAGERS CAN USE TO PROMOTE ETHICAL BEHAVIOR AS THE NORM

1. Separate legal and ethical issues.
2. Collaborate through ethics committees.
3. Use institutional review boards appropriately.
4. Role model and encourage ethical behavior.

The manager may confront several particularly sensitive legal–ethical issues, including termination or refusal of treatment, durable power of attorney, abortion, sterilization, child abuse, the use of artificial intelligence (AI), and genetic engineering. Most health care organizations have legal counsel to assist managers in making decisions in such sensitive areas. Because legal aspects of management decision making are so important, Chapter 5 is devoted exclusively to this topic.

Collaborate Through Interprofessional Ethics Committees

The new manager must consult with others when solving sensitive legal–ethical questions because lack of experience may cause a person's own value system to preclude examining all possible alternatives. Many institutions have ethics committees to assist with problem solving in ethical issues. These ethics committees typically are interprofessional and are organized to consciously and reflectively consider significant and often difficult or ambiguous value issues related to patient care or organizational activities. Ethics committees are a core element of collaborative ethical decision making and should include representatives of all stakeholders, including patients when they are involved in the ethical issue.

Use Institutional Review Boards Appropriately

IRBs are primarily formed to protect the rights and welfare of research subjects. They provide oversight to ensure that individuals conducting research adhere to ethical principles. The primary role of the manager regarding IRBs is to make sure that such a board is in place in the organization where the manager works and that any research performed within their sphere of responsibility has been approved by such a board.

Role Model and Encourage Ethical Behavior

Perhaps the most important thing a leader-manager can do to foster an ethical work environment, however, is to role model ethical behavior. Likewise, working as a team with a standard for behavior can promote a positive ethical climate. Other important interventions include encouraging staff to openly discuss ethical issues that they face daily in their practice. This allows subordinates to gain greater perspective on complex issues and provides a mechanism for peer support.

Integrating Leadership Roles and Management Functions in Ethics

Leadership roles in ethics focus on the human element involved in ethical decision making. Leaders are self-aware of their values and basic beliefs about the rights, duties, and goals of human beings. As self-aware and ethical people, they role model confidence in their decision making to subordinates. They also are realists and recognize that some ambiguity and uncertainty must be a part of all ethical decision making. Leaders are willing to take risks in their decision making even though negative outcomes can occur even with quality decision making.

Management roles in ethics often focus on decision making. Because ethical decisions are so complex, and the cost of a poor decision may be high, management functions focus on increasing the chances that the best possible decision will be made at the least possible cost in terms of fiscal and human resources. This usually requires that the manager becomes expert at using systematic approaches to problem solving or decision making, such as theoretical models, ethical frameworks, and ethical principles. By developing expertise, the manager can identify universal outcomes that should be sought or avoided.

The integrated leader-manager recognizes that ethical issues pervade every aspect of leadership and management. Rather than being deterred by the complexity and ambiguity of these issues, the leader-manager seeks counsel as needed, accepts their personal limitations, and makes the best possible decision at that time with the information and resources available.

Health care organizations today need moral leadership as ethics are increasingly involved in health care decision making. For example, Köhler et al. (2021) suggest that emerging technologies such as gene editing and AI now touch upon the fundamental question of what it means to be human; that the innovative use of data and social media to improve public health questions the very notions of privacy and confidentiality; and global events, such as climate change, environmental disasters, and pandemics, have raised concerns about access to resources and their equitable use.

In an era of markedly limited physical, human, and fiscal resources, nearly all decision making by leader-managers involves some ethical component. Indeed, ethics will become an even greater dimension in management decision making in the future due to emerging technologies, regulatory pressures, and competitiveness among health care providers; workforce shortages; an imperative to provide better care at less cost; spiraling costs of supplies and salaries; and the public's increasing distrust of the health care delivery system and its institutions. The complexity of the required ethical decision making for health care leaders and managers cannot be underestimated. Indeed, the American College of Healthcare Executives (2021) notes that it is incumbent upon health care executives to lead in a manner that promotes an ethical culture, affirms the organization's mission and values, sets expectations and accountabilities, and models ethical behavior for their organizations. When organizational resources and guidelines prioritize ethical behavior, the best interests of patients, families, caregivers, the organization, payers, and the community are more likely to be achieved.

Key Concepts

- Ethics is the systematic study of what a person's conduct and actions should be toward self, other human beings, and the environment; it is the justification of what is right or good and the study of what a person's life and relationships should be—not necessarily what they are.
- In an era of markedly limited physical, human, and fiscal resources, nearly all decision making by leader-managers involves some ethical component. Multiple advocacy roles and professional accountability further increase the likelihood that managers will be faced with ethical dilemmas in their practice.
- Many systematic approaches to ethical problem solving are appropriate. These include the use of theoretical problem-solving and decision-making models, ethical frameworks, and ethical principles.
- Outcomes should never be used as the sole criterion for assessing the quality of ethical problem solving because many variables affect outcomes that have no reflection on whether the problem solving was appropriate. Quality, instead, should be evaluated both by the outcome and by the process used to make the decision.

- If a structured approach to problem solving is used, data gathering is adequate, and multiple alternatives are analyzed, regardless of the outcome, the manager should feel comfortable that the best possible decision was made at that time with the information and resources available.
- Four commonly used ethical frameworks for decision making are utilitarianism, duty-based reasoning, rights-based reasoning, and intuitionism. These frameworks do not solve the ethical problem but assist individuals involved in the problem solving to clarify their values and beliefs.
- Principles of ethical reasoning explore and define what beliefs or values form the basis for our decision making. These principles include autonomy, beneficence, nonmaleficence, paternalism, utility, justice, fidelity, veracity, and confidentiality.
- Professional codes of ethics and standards for practice are guides to the highest standards of ethical practice for nurses.
- Sometimes, it is very difficult to separate legal and ethical issues, although they are not the same. Legal controls are generally clear and philosophically impartial. Ethical controls are much more unclear and individualized.

Additional Learning Exercises and Applications

LEARNING EXERCISE 4.7

Everything Is Not What It Seems

You are a perinatal unit coordinator at a large teaching hospital. In addition to your management responsibilities, you have been asked to fill in as a member of the hospital promotion committee, which reviews petitions from clinicians for a step-level promotion on the clinical specialist ladder. You believe that you could learn a great deal on this committee and could be an objective and contributing member.

The committee has been convened to select the annual winner of the Outstanding Clinical Specialist Award. In reviewing the applicant files, you find that one file from a perinatal clinical specialist contains many overstatements and misrepresentations. You know for a fact that this clinician did not accomplish all that she has listed because she is a friend and close colleague. She did not, however, know that you would be a member of this committee and thus would be aware of this deception.

When the entire committee met, several members commented on this clinician's impressive file. Although you were able to dissuade them covertly from further considering her nomination, you are left with many uneasy feelings and some anger and sadness. You recognize that she did not receive the nomination, and thus, there is little real danger regarding the deceptions in the file being used inappropriately at this time. However, you will not be on this committee next year, and if she were to submit an erroneous file again, she could be highly considered for the award. You also recognize that even with the best of intentions and the most therapeutic of communication techniques, confronting your friend with her deception will cause her to lose face and will probably result in an unsalvageable friendship. Even if you do confront her, there is little you can do to stop her from doing the same in future nomination processes other than formally reporting her conduct.

ASSIGNMENT:

Determine what you will do. Do the potential costs outweigh the potential benefits? Be realistic about your actions.

LEARNING EXERCISE 4.8

The Valuable Employee

Gina has been the supervisor of a 16-bed intensive care unit (ICU)/critical care unit (CCU) in a 200-bed urban hospital for 8 years. She is respected and well-liked by her staff. Her unit's staff retention level and productivity are higher than any other unit in the hospital. For the last 6 years, Gina has relied heavily on Mark, her permanent charge nurse on the day shift. He is bright and motivated and has excellent clinical and managerial skills. Mark seems satisfied and challenged in his current position, although Gina has not had any formal career planning meetings with him to discuss his long-term career goals. It would be fair to say that Mark's work has greatly increased Gina's scope of power and has enhanced the reputation of the unit.

Recently, one of the physicians approached Gina about a plan to open an outpatient cardiac rehabilitation program. The program will require a strong leader and manager who is self-motivated. It will not only be a lot of work but will also provide many opportunities for advancement. The physician suggests that Mark would be an excellent choice for the job, although the physician has given Gina full authority to make the final decision.

Gina is aware that Lynn, a bright and dynamic staff nurse from the open-heart surgery floor, also would be very interested in the job. Lynn has been employed at the hospital for only 1 year but has a proven track record and would probably excel in the job. In addition, there is a staffing surplus right now on the open-heart surgery floor because two of the surgeons have recently retired. It would be difficult and time-consuming to replace Mark as charge nurse in the ICU/CCU.

ASSIGNMENT:

What process should this supervisor pursue to determine who should be hired for the position? Should the position be posted? When does the benefit of using transfers/ promotions as a means of reward outweigh the cost of reduced productivity?

LEARNING EXERCISE   4.9

To See or Not to See

For the last few days, you have been taking care of Mr. Cole, a 38-year-old patient with end-stage cystic fibrosis. You have developed a caring relationship with Mr. Cole and his wife. They are both aware of the prognosis of his disease and realize that he has only a short time left to live.

When the doctor made rounds with you this morning, she told the Coles that Mr. Cole could be discharged today if his condition remains stable. They were both excited about the news because they had been urging the doctor to let him go home to enjoy his remaining time surrounded by the people he loves.

When you bring in Mr. Cole's discharge orders to his room to review his medications and other treatments, you find Mrs. Cole assisting Mr. Cole as he coughs up bright red blood. When you confront them, they both beg you not to tell the doctor or chart the incident because they do not want their discharge to be delayed. They believe that it is their right to go home and let Mr. Cole die surrounded by his family. They said that they know that they can leave against their physician's wishes and go home against medical advice, but if they do, their insurance will not pay for home care.

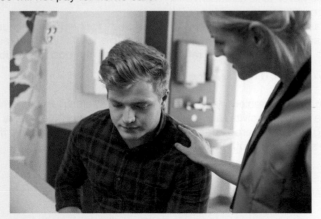

ASSIGNMENT:

What is your duty in this case? What are Mr. Cole's rights? Is it ever justified to withhold information from the physician? Will you chart the incident, and will you report it to anyone? Solve this case, justifying your decision by using ethical principles.

LEARNING EXERCISE 4.10

The Untruthful Employee

You are the registered nurse on duty at a skilled nursing facility. Judy, a 35-year-old, full-time nurse's aide on the day shift, has been with the skilled nursing facility for 10 years. You have worked with Judy on numerous occasions and have found her work to be marginal at best. She tries to be extra friendly with the staff and occasionally brings them small treats that she bakes. She also makes a point of telling everyone how much she needs this job to support her family and how she loves working here. Her daughter has a disability and relies on Judy's hospital-provided health insurance to have her health care needs met.

Most of the other staff seem willing to put up with Judy's poor work habits, but lately, you have felt that her work has shown many serious errors. Things are not reported to you that should have been—intake and output volumes that are in error, strange recordings for vital signs, and so on. She has tried to cover up such errors, with what you suspect are outright lies. She claims to have bathed patients when this does not appear to be the case and has said some patients have refused to eat when you have found that they were willing to eat at your request. Although the chief nursing officer acknowledges that Judy is only a marginally adequate employee, she has been unable to observe directly any of the behaviors that would require disciplinary action and has told you that you must have real evidence of her wrongdoing in order to for her to take action.

During morning report, you made a specific request to Judy that a confused patient assigned to her, Mr. Brown, be assisted to the bathroom, and you told her that someone must remain in the room to assist him when he is up, as he fell last evening. You also told Judy that when in bed, Mr. Brown's side rails were always to be up. Later in the morning, you take Mr. Brown his medication and notice that his side rails are down and after pulling them up and giving him his medicine, you find Judy and talk with her. She denies leaving the side rails down and insisted someone else must have done it. You caution her again about Mr. Brown's needs. Thirty minutes later, you go by Mr. Brown's room and find his bed empty and discover he is in the bathroom unattended. As you are assisting Mr. Brown back to bed, Judy bursts into the room and pales when she sees you with her patient. At first, she denies that she had gotten Mr. Brown up, but when you express your disbelief, she tearfully admits that she left him unattended but states that this was an isolated incident and asks you to forget it. When you reply that her lying about the incident is what most disturbs you, she promises never to lie about anything again. She begs you not to report her to the chief nursing officer, saying she needs her job.

You are torn between wanting to report Judy for her lying because of concerns about patient safety and not wanting to be responsible for getting her fired. You decide to take a break to give yourself time to rationally think over the possible actions you could take.

ASSIGNMENT:

• • • • • • • •

Evaluate this problem. Is this just a simple leadership–management problem that requires some problem solving and a decision or does the problem have ethical dimensions? Using one of the problem-solving models in this chapter, solve this problem. Compare your solution with others in your class.

LEARNING EXERCISE 4.11

Sometimes Things Go Wrong

You have been working as a registered nurse on an orthopedic unit since your graduation from your nursing program 2 years ago. Both the doctors and supervisor respect your work, and you have found it exciting to work with the home health nurses as many of your patients need home health follow-up for physical therapy and other needs following their surgeries.

Mrs. George is an older adult living alone who has recently had bilateral hip replacement. Although she has made good progress, she continues to need quite a bit of assistance with ambulation and uses a walker. Normally, if family members cannot assist them at home, patients with bilateral hip replacements are sent from the hospital to an assisted living facility for several weeks. Mrs. George does not have any immediate family to help her, but she has pleaded with her doctor, you, and the home health nurse to let her go back to her home, which she refers to as a cabin in the "piney woods" to complete her recuperation. The doctor tells you and the home health nurse to work on a plan to see if it is feasible.

The home health nurse reports after her home assessment that with some assistance every day, she could probably manage at home, and although her cabin is not near any neighbor, she does have a telephone. Mrs. George is insistent that she will not go to what she calls "a nursing home" and her insurance will no longer pay for her to stay at the hospital. Eventually, it is decided that *Meals on Wheels* will deliver her daily meals and that a home health nurse will call on her every other day and a physical therapist will visit on the days the home health nurse does not so that she will have at least two people in her home each day.

Although you and the home health nurse and the doctor are a bit uneasy, you feel that you have solved this ethical dilemma (a choice between two negative solutions) and have selected the one that is the least damaging to Mrs. George's quality of life.

Seven days after Mrs. George is discharged, there is a severe storm, which disables most phone lines including Mrs. George's. The storm also causes the flue in her wood stove to overheat in the middle of the night causing a fire. Because she is unable to use her walker fast enough to get outside before the fire consumes the small cabin, Mrs. George dies in the fire.

ASSIGNMENT:

Would you have solved this problem as described? Does knowing the outcome change the way you would solve the problem? Having a negative outcome may or may not mean that the ethical problem solving was faulty. Do you feel the people in this story made a faulty decision? If so, what would you have done differently?

LEARNING EXERCISE 4.12

Shortcuts

Morgan is the charge nurse of the 3:00 PM to 11:00 PM shift on the acute care unit where you have worked for 18 months since your graduation. Your supervisor has asked you if you would like to learn the duties of the relief charge nurse. You were thrilled that she approached you for this position. Because it was a relief position, it was permissible for your supervisor to appoint you and not necessary for you to formally apply for the position.

One day each week, for the last 2 weeks, you have been working with Morgan to learn the responsibilities of the position. There are several things Morgan does that bother you, and you are not sure what you should do. For example, if used supplies were inadvertently not charged to patients at the time of service, Morgan admitted she would just charge them

(continues on page 100)

LEARNING EXERCISE 4.12

Shortcuts (continued)

to whichever patients she thought were likely to have used them. When you questioned Morgan about this, she said, "Well, at the end of the day, the unit needs to make sure that all supplies have been charged for, or the Chief Financial Officer (CFO) will be after all of us. It is one of the charge nurses' responsibilities, and I don't have time to chase everyone down to find the correct patient to charge. Besides, everyone I've charged has insurance so it does not come out of the patient's pocket. Most importantly, we must make sure the hospital gets reimbursed or we won't have our jobs."

In addition, when Morgan does the staffing correlation for the upcoming shift, you notice that she "fudges" a bit and makes sure the night shift is given credit for needing more staff than they need. When questioned, she said, "Oh, we have to take care of each other, better too much staff than not enough."

You think Morgan's actions are unethical, but you do not know what to do about it. It does not directly harm a patient, but you feel uncomfortable about what she is doing.

ASSIGNMENT:

You have many options here including doing nothing. Using the MORAL ethical problem-solving model, solve this case and compare your solution with others in your class.

LEARNING EXERCISE 4.13

Rationing During a Pandemic

During peak waves of the COVID-19 pandemic, some hospitals faced an overwhelming demand for intensive care hospital beds, ventilators, and health care providers. Some states even found themselves having to activate a "crisis standard of care," which led to a sanctioned rationing of these scarce resources.

Some hospitals in the pandemic chose to ration care or equipment based on how likely a patient was to survive, where others chose to treat the sickest patients most aggressively. Others used a first-come, first-served approach, whereas others treated the oldest or most frail patients first.

ASSIGNMENT:

Interview a hospital administrator or a hospital board member who is familiar with the policies put into place during the COVID-19 pandemic that addressed how rationing would occur if it became necessary. Was a rubric developed to determine how care was to be rationed? Were ethics committees a part of that decision making? Was the process transparent to both staff and consumers? Which ethical frameworks or principles appear to have most strongly influenced the decisions made about rationing? Was actual rationing needed? If so, what were the unexpected outcomes of the choices that were made?

REFERENCES

American College of Healthcare Executives. (2021, December 6). *Ethical decision-making for healthcare executives.* https://www.ache.org/about-ache/our-story/our-commitments/ethics/ache-code-of-ethics/ethical-decision-making-for-healthcare-executives

American Nurses Association. (2015). *Code of ethics for nurses with interpretive statements.*

American Nurses Association. (2016). *Nursing administration: Scope and standards of practice* (2nd ed.).

American Nurses Association. (2018). *Position statement—Nursing advocacy for LGBTQ+ populations.* https://www.nursingworld.org/~49866e/globalassets/practiceandpolicy/ethics/nursing-advocacy-for-lgbtq-populations.pdf

American Nurses Association. (2021). Moral distress: What it is and what to do about it. *Healthy Nurse Health Nation.* Retrieved July 20, 2021, from https://engage.healthynursehealthynation.org/blogs/8/531

Crisham, P. (1985). Moral: How can I do what's right? *Nursing Management, 16*(3), 42A–42N.

Ganz, F. D., Sharfi, R., Kaufman, N., & Einav, S. (2019). Perceptions of slow codes by nurses working on internal medicine wards. *Nursing Ethics, 26(6),* 1734–1743. doi:10.1177/0969733018783222

Gebreheat, G., & Teame, H. (2021). Ethical challenges of nurses in COVID-19 pandemic: Integrative review. *Journal of Multidisciplinary Healthcare, 14,* 1029–1035. https://www.ncbi.nlm.nih.gov/pmc/articles/PMC8110276/

Haden, N. K. (2017). *Justice, the outward-looking virtue.* https://9virtues.com/files/Justice-Outward-Looking_Virtue.pdf

International Council of Nurses. (2021, October 20). *Revised ICN Code of Ethics for Nurses reflects lessons learned from the COVID-19 pandemic.* https://www.icn.ch/news/revised-icn-code-ethics-nurses-reflects-lessons-learned-covid-19-pandemic

Kearney, G., & Penque, S. (2012). Ethics of everyday decision making. *Nursing Management, 19*(1), 32–36.

Köhler, J., Alois Reis, A., & Saxena, A. (2021). A survey of national ethics and bioethics committees. *Bulletin of the World Health Organization, 99*(2), 138–147.

Mooney, J. (2021, January). Moral distress: The struggle to uphold ethics in healthcare. *University of Rochester Medical Center.* Retrieved July 20, 2021, from https://www.urmc.rochester.edu/behavioral-health-partners/bhp-blog/january-2021/moral-distress-the-struggle-to-uphold-ethics-in-he.aspx

Mortell, M. (2012). Hand hygiene compliance: Is there a theory-practice-ethics gap? *British Journal of Nursing, 21*(17), 1011–1014.

Nickitas, D. M. (2021, March/April). Confronting the truth and trauma of the COVID-19 pandemic. *Nursing Economics, 39*(2), 57–58.

Oakland University News. (2021, January 22). *Gallup Poll finds nursing is most honest, ethical profession.* Retrieved July 20, 2021, from https://oakland.edu/oumagazine/news/nursing/2021/gallup-poll-finds-nursing-is-most-honest-ethical-profession

Peter, E. (2018). Overview and summary: Ethics in healthcare: Nurses respond. *OJIN: The Online Journal of Issues in Nursing, 23*(1). http://ojin.nursingworld.org/MainMenuCategories/ANAMarketplace/ANAPeriodicals/OJIN/TableofContents/Vol-23-2018/No1-Jan-2018/O-S-Ethics-in-Healthcare.html

Pittman, G. C. (2023). Academic integrity in nursing education, Chapter 19. In C. Huston (Ed.), *Professional issues in nursing: Challenges & opportunities* (6th ed., pp. 274–287). Wolters Kluwer.

Rosenberg, S. (2021). *Why ethics in nursing matters.* Retrieved July 20, 2021, from https://www.snhu.edu/about-us/newsroom/2018/05/ethics-in-nursing

Rushton, C. H., Swoboda, S. M., Reller, N., Skarupski, K. A., Prizzi, M., Young, P. D., & Hanson, G. C. (2021, January). Mindful ethical practice and resilience academy: Equipping nurses to address ethical challenges. *American Journal of Critical Care, 30*(1), e1–e11.

Saver, C. (2021, July/August/September). Managing moral distress. *Georgia Nursing, 81*(3), 14–15.

Shepherd, K. (2020, December 22). More than 70 West Point cadets accused in academy's biggest cheating scandal in decades. *The Washington Post.* Retrieved August 24, 2021, from https://www.msn.com/en-us/news/us/more-than-70-west-point-cadets-accused-in-academy-s-biggest-cheating-scandal-in-decades/ar-BB1c8cPr

Woods, M. (2021). Nursing's essence and the health care needs of humanity. *Nursing Praxis in Aotearoa New Zealand, 37*(1), 12–13.

5

Legal and Legislative Issues

*… It may seem a strange principle to enunciate as the very first requirement in a hospital that it should do the sick no harm.—**Florence Nightingale***

*… Laws or ordinances unobserved, or partially attended to, had better never have been made.—**George Washington, letter to James Madison, March 31, 1787***

*… The best way to get a bad law repealed is to enforce it strictly.—**Abraham Lincoln***

CROSSWALK

This chapter addresses:

- **AACN Essentials Domain 1:** Knowledge for nursing practice
- **AACN Essentials Domain 2:** Person-centered care
- **AACN Essentials Domain 5:** Quality and safety
- **AACN Essentials Domain 7:** Systems-based practice
- **AACN Essentials Domain 8:** Information and health care technologies
- **AACN Essentials Domain 9:** Professionalism
- **AACN Essentials Domain 10:** Personal, professional, and leadership development
- **AONL Nurse Executive Competency 2:** A knowledge of the health care environment
- **AONL Nurse Executive Competency 5:** Business skills
- **ANA Standard of Professional Performance 9:** Respectful and equitable practice
- **ANA Standard of Professional Performance 11:** Collaboration
- **ANA Standard of Professional Performance 12:** Leadership
- **ANA Standard of Professional Performance 13:** Education
- **ANA Standard of Professional Performance 15:** Quality of practice
- **ANA Standard of Professional Performance 16:** Professional practice evaluation
- **ANA Standard of Professional Performance 18:** Environmental health
- **QSEN Competency:** Safety

LEARNING OBJECTIVES

The learner will:

- identify the primary sources of law and how each affects nursing practice
- describe the types (criminal, civil, and administrative) of legal cases nurses may be involved in and differentiate between the burden of proof and the potential consequences for rule breaking in each
- identify specific doctrines used by the courts to define legal boundaries for nursing practice
- correlate the legal authority of nursing practice and the nursing process
- assess their personal need for malpractice insurance as a nurse, weighing the potential risks versus benefits

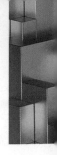

- describe the five elements that must be present for a professional to be held liable for malpractice
- identify strategies nurses can use to reduce their likelihood of being sued for malpractice
- describe the liability nurses, other care providers, and employers share under the concept of joint liability
- identify types of intentional torts as well as strategies nurses can use to reduce their likelihood
- describe appropriate nursing actions to ensure informed consent
- describe the need for patient and family education regarding treatment and end-of-life issues as part of the Patient Self-Determination Act
- describe conditions that must exist to receive liability protection under Good Samaritan laws
- recognize their legal imperative to protect patient confidentiality in accordance with the Health Insurance Portability and Accountability Act of 1996
- identify the role State Boards of Nursing play in professional licensure and discipline
- select appropriate legal nursing actions in sensitive clinical situations
- differentiate between legal and ethical accountability

Introduction

Chapter 4 presented ethics as an internal control of human behavior and nursing practice. Therefore, ethics has to do with actions that people should take, not necessarily actions that they are legally required to take. On the other hand, ethical behavior written into law is no longer just desired; it is mandated. This chapter focuses on the external controls of legislation and law. Since the first mandatory *Nurse Practice Act* was passed in North Carolina in 1903 (Barowski, 2022), nursing has been legislated, directed, and controlled to some extent.

The primary purpose of law and legislation is to protect the patient and the nurse. Laws and legislation define the scope of acceptable practice and protect individual rights. Nurses who are aware of their rights and duties in legal matters are better able to protect themselves against liability or loss of professional licensure.

This chapter presents the primary sources of law and how each affects nursing practice. It emphasizes the nurse's responsibility to proactively establish and revise laws affecting nursing practice. Legal cases involving nurses are presented and the burden of proof and the consequences for criminal, civil, and administrative guilty verdicts are differentiated. The chapter also identifies specific doctrines used by the courts to define legal boundaries for nursing practice and examines the role of state boards in professional licensure and discipline. In addition, the components of malpractice for the individual practitioner and the manager or supervisor are identified. The legal implications of informed consent, medical records, intentional torts, the Patient Self-Determination Act (PSDA), the Good Samaritan Act, and the Health Insurance Portability and Accountability Act (HIPAA) are also examined.

This chapter is not meant to be a complete legal guide to nursing practice. There are many excellent legal textbooks and handbooks that accomplish that function. The primary purpose of this chapter is to emphasize the widely varying and rapidly changing nature of laws and the responsibility that each manager has to keep abreast of legislation and laws affecting both nursing and management practice. Leadership roles and management functions associated with legal and legislative issues are shown in Display 5.1.

| DISPLAY 5.1 | LEADERSHIP ROLES AND MANAGEMENT FUNCTIONS IN LEGAL AND LEGISLATIVE ISSUES |

Leadership Roles

1. Serves as a role model by providing nursing care that meets or exceeds accepted standards of care
2. Practices within the scope of the *Nurse Practice Act*
3. Creates a work environment where each person understands that they have some liability for their own conduct
4. Updates knowledge and skills in the field of practice and seeks professional certification to increase expertise in a specific field
5. Reports substandard nursing care to appropriate authorities following the established chain of command
6. Fosters nurse–patient relationships that are respectful, caring, and honest, thus reducing the possibility of future lawsuits
7. Creates an environment that encourages and supports diversity and sensitivity
8. Prioritizes patient rights and patient welfare in decision making
9. Ensures that patients receive informed consent for treatment
10. Demonstrates vision, risk taking, and energy in applying appropriate legal boundaries for nursing practice

Management Functions

1. Increases knowledge regarding sources of law and legal doctrines that affect nursing practice
2. Ensures that organizational guidelines regarding scope of practice are consistent with the state *Nurse Practice Act*
3. Delegates to subordinates wisely, looking at the manager's scope of practice and that of the individuals they supervise
4. Understands and adheres to institutional policies and procedures
5. Minimizes the risk of product liability by assuring that all staff are appropriately oriented to the appropriate use of equipment and products
6. Monitors subordinates to ensure that they have a valid, current, and appropriate license to practice nursing
7. Uses foreseeability of harm in delegation and staffing decisions
8. Increases staff awareness of intentional torts and assists them in developing strategies to reduce their liability in these areas
9. Provides education for staff and patients on issues concerning treatment and end-of-life issues under the *Patient Self-Determination Act*
10. Protects all patients' rights to confidentiality under the *Health Insurance Portability and Accountability Act*
11. Ensures that patients have reasonable access to information in the medical record, following established organizational processes
12. Secures appropriate background checks for new employees to reduce managerial liability
13. Provides educational and training opportunities for staff on legal issues affecting nursing practice

Sources of Law

The US legal system can be somewhat confusing because there are not only four sources of the law (constitutions, statues, administrative agencies, and court decisions) but also parallel systems at the state and federal levels. A comparison is shown in Table 5.1.

A *constitution* is a system of fundamental laws or principles that govern a nation, society, corporation, or other aggregates of individuals. The purpose of a constitution is to establish the basis of a governing system for the future and the present. The U.S. Constitution establishes the general organization of the federal government and grants and limits its specific powers. Each state also has a constitution that establishes the general organization of the state government and grants and limits its powers.

TABLE 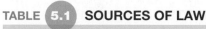 **SOURCES OF LAW**

Origin of Law	Use	Impact on Nursing Practice
The Constitution	The highest law in the United States; interpreted by the U.S. Supreme Court; gives authority to other three sources of the law	Constitutional law has little direct involvement in the area of malpractice.
Statutes	Also called *statutory law* or *legislative law*; laws that are passed by the state or federal legislators and that must be signed by the president or governor	Before 1970s, very few state or federal laws dealt with malpractice. Since the malpractice crisis, many statutes affect malpractice.
Administrative agencies	The rules and regulations established by appointed agencies of the executive branch of the government (governor or president)	State Boards of Nursing and agencies, such as the National Labor Relations Board and health and safety boards significantly impact nursing practice.
Court decisions	Also called *tort law*; this is court mode law, and the courts interpret the statutes and set precedents; in the United States, there are two levels of court: trial court and appellate court	Most malpractice laws are addressed by the courts.

The second source of law is *statutes*—laws that govern. Legislative bodies, such as the U.S. Congress, state legislatures, and city councils, make these laws. Statutes are officially enacted (voted on and passed) by the legislative body and are compiled into codes, collections of statutes, and ordinances. The 51 *Nurse Practice Acts* representing the 50 states and the District of Columbia are examples of statutes. Although Nurse Practice Acts may vary among states, all must be consistent with provisions or statutes established at the federal level.

> The 51 Nurse Practice Acts (one for each state and the District of Columbia) define and limit the practice of nursing, thereby stating what constitutes authorized practice as well as what exceeds the scope of authority.

Boundaries for practice are defined in the Nurse Practice Act of each state. These acts are general in most states to allow for some flexibility in the broad roles and varied situations in which nurses practice. Because this allows for some interpretation, many employers have established guidelines for nursing practice in their own organizations. These guidelines regarding scope of practice cannot, however, exceed the requirements of the state Nursing Practice Acts.

Administrative agencies, the third source of law, are given authority to act by the legislative bodies and create rules and regulations that enforce statutory laws. For example, State Boards of Nursing are administrative agencies set up to implement and enforce the state Nurse Practice Act by writing rules and regulations and by conducting investigations and hearings to ensure the law's enforcement. Administrative laws are valid only to the extent that they are within the scope of the authority granted to them by the legislative body.

The fourth source of law is *court decisions*. Judicial or decisional laws are made by the courts to interpret legal issues that are in dispute. Depending on the type of court involved, judicial or decisional law may be made by a single justice, with or without a jury, or by a panel of justices. In general, initial trial courts have a single judge or magistrate, intermediary appeal courts have three justices, and the highest appeal courts have nine justices.

Types of Laws and Courts

Although many nurses worry primarily about being sued for malpractice, in reality, they may be involved in three different types of court cases: criminal, civil, and administrative

TABLE **5.2** **TYPES OF LAWS AND COURTS**

Type	Burden of Proof Required for Guilty Verdict	Likely Consequences of a Guilty Verdict
Criminal	Beyond a reasonable doubt	Incarceration, probation, and fines
Civil	Based on a preponderance of the evidence	Monetary damages
Administrative	Clear and convincing standard	Suspension or loss of licensure

(Table 5.2). The court in which each is tried, the burden of proof required for conviction, and the resulting punishment associated with each are different.

In *criminal* cases, the individual faces charges generally filed by the state or federal attorney general for crimes committed against an individual or society. In criminal cases, the individual is always presumed to be innocent unless the state can prove guilt beyond a reasonable doubt. Incarceration and even death are possible consequences for being found guilty in criminal matters. Nurses found guilty of intentionally administering fatal doses of drugs to patients would be charged in a criminal court.

In *civil* cases, one individual sues another for money to compensate for a perceived loss. The burden of proof required to be found guilty in a civil case is described as a *preponderance of the evidence*. In other words, the judge or jury must believe that it was more likely than not that the accused individual was responsible for the injuries of the complainant. Consequences of being found guilty in a civil suit are monetary. Most malpractice cases are tried in civil court.

In *administrative* cases, an individual is sued by a state or federal governmental agency assigned the responsibility of implementing governmental programs. State Boards of Nursing are one such type of governmental agency. When an individual violates the state Nurse Practice Act, the Boards of Nursing may seek to revoke licensure or institute some form of discipline. The burden of proof in these cases varies from state to state. When the *clear and convincing standard* is not used, the preponderance of the evidence standard may be used. "Clear and convincing" involves higher burdens of proof than preponderance of evidence but a significantly lower burden of proof than "beyond a reasonable doubt."

> The burden of proof required for conviction as well as the type of punishment given differs in criminal, civil, and administrative cases.

LEARNING EXERCISE **5.1**

Both Guilty and Not Guilty

Think of celebrated cases where defendants have been tried in both civil and criminal courts. What were the verdicts of both trials? If the verdicts were not the same, analyze why this happened. Do you agree that taking away an individual's personal liberty by incarceration should require a higher burden of proof than assessing for monetary damages?

ASSIGNMENT:

Complete a literature search to see if you can find cases where a nurse faced both civil and administrative charges. Were you able to find cases where the nurse was found guilty in a civil court but did not lose their license? Did you find the opposite?

Legal Doctrines and the Practice of Nursing

Two important legal doctrines frequently guide all three courts in their decision making. The first of these, *stare decisis*, means to let the decision stand. *Stare decisis* uses precedents as a guide for decision making. This doctrine gives nurses insight into ways that the court has previously fixed liability in given situations. However, two considerations must exist for *stare decisis* to apply.

> Precedent is often used as a guide for legal decision making.

The first is that the previous case must be within the jurisdiction of the court hearing the current case. For example, a previous Florida case decided by a state court does not set precedent for a Texas appellate court (courts that hear and review appeals from legal cases that have already been heard in lower courts). Although the Texas court may model its decision after the Florida case, it is not compelled to do so. The lower courts in Texas, however, would rely on Texas appellate decisions.

The other consideration is that the court hearing the current case can depart from the precedent and set a landmark decision. Landmark decisions generally occur because societal needs have changed, technology has become more advanced, or following the precedent would further harm an already injured person. *Roe v. Wade*, the 1973 landmark decision to allow a woman to seek and receive a legal abortion during the first two trimesters of pregnancy, is an example. Given the influence of politics, new Texas legislation enacted in 2021, and varying societal views about abortion, this precedent could change again in the future.

The second doctrine that guides courts in their decision making is *res judicata*, which means a "thing or matter settled by judgment." It applies only when a competent court has decided a legal dispute and when no further appeals are possible. This doctrine keeps the same parties in the original lawsuit from retrying the same issues that were involved in the first lawsuit.

When using doctrines as a guide for nursing practice, the nurse must remember that all laws are fluid and subject to change. An example of changing law regarding professional nursing occurred in an Illinois Supreme Court more than a decade ago when the law finally recognized nursing as an independent profession with its own unique body of knowledge. In this case (*Sullivan v. Edward Hospital*, 2004), the Illinois Supreme Court decided that physicians could not serve as expert witnesses regarding nursing standards (FindLaw for Legal Professionals, 2022). This demonstrates how the law is ever-evolving. Laws cannot be static; they must change to reflect the growing autonomy and responsibility desired by nurses.

It is critical that all nurses be aware of and sensitive to rapidly changing laws and legislation that affect their practice. Nurses must also recognize that state laws may differ from federal laws and that legal guidelines for nursing practice in the organization may differ from state or federal guidelines. All nurses must understand the legal controls for nursing practice in their own states. Managers need to be aware of their organizations' specific practice interpretations and ensure that subordinates are aware of the same and follow established practices.

Professional Negligence (Malpractice)

All liability suits involve a plaintiff and a defendant. In malpractice cases, the *plaintiff* is the injured party, and the *defendant* is the professional who is alleged to have caused the injury. *Negligence* is the omission to do something that a reasonable person, guided by the considerations that ordinarily regulate human affairs, would do—or as doing something that a reasonable and prudent person would not do. *Reasonable and prudent* generally means the average judgment, foresight, intelligence, and skill that would be expected of a person with similar training and experience. *Malpractice*—the failure of a person with professional training to act in a reasonable and prudent manner—also is called *professional negligence*.

> Medical Malpractice is a type of lawsuit where a person seeks justice for injury or death caused by a negligent medical provider. A medical provider can be a doctor, surgeon, nurse, or other professionals who cares for patients (Cirrinicione, 2021).

Elements of Malpractice

Five elements must be present for a professional to be held liable for malpractice (Table 5.3).

First, a *standard of care* must have been established that outlines the level or degree of quality considered adequate by a given profession. Standards of care outline the duties a defendant has to a plaintiff or a nurse to a client. These standards represent the skills and learning commonly possessed by members of the profession and generally are the minimal requirements that define an acceptable level of care. Standards of care, which guarantee clients safe nursing care, include organizational policy and procedure statements, job descriptions, and student guidelines.

Second, after the standard of care has been established, it must be shown that the standard was violated—there must have been a *breach of duty*. This breach is shown by calling other nurses who practice in the same specialty area as the defendant to testify as expert witnesses.

Third, the nurse must have had the knowledge or availability of information that not meeting the standard of care could result in harm. This is called *foreseeability of harm*. If the average, reasonable person in the defendant's position could have anticipated the plaintiff's injury as a result of their actions, then the plaintiff's injury was foreseeable.

> Being ignorant is not a justifiable excuse for malpractice, but not having all the information in a situation may impede one's ability to foresee harm.

TABLE 5.3 COMPONENTS OF PROFESSIONAL NEGLIGENCE

Elements of Liability	Explanation	Example: Giving Medications
1. Duty to use due care (defined by the standard of care)	The care that should be given under the circumstances reflects what a reasonably prudent nurse would have done.	A nurse should give medications accurately, completely, and on time.
2. Failure to meet standard of care (breach of duty)	The care that should have been given was not.	A nurse fails to give medications accurately, completely, or on time.
3. Foreseeability of harm	The nurse must have reasonable access to information about whether the possibility of harm exists.	The drug handbook specifies that the wrong dosage or route may cause injury.
4. A direct relationship between failure to meet the standard of care (breach) and injury can be proved.	Patient is harmed because proper care is not given.	Wrong dosage causes the patient to have a convulsion.
5. Injury	Actual harm results to the patient.	Brain injury or other serious complication occurs.

For example, a charge nurse assigns another registered nurse (RN) to care for a critically ill patient. The assigned RN makes a medication error that injures the patient in some way. If the charge nurse had reason to believe that the RN was incapable of adequately caring for the patient or failed to provide adequate supervision, foreseeability of harm is apparent, and the charge nurse also could be held liable. If the charge nurse was available as needed and had good reason to believe that the RN was fully capable, they would be less likely to be held liable.

Many malpractice cases have hinged on whether the nurse was persistent enough in attempting to notify health care providers of changes in a patient's condition or to convince the providers of the seriousness of a patient's condition. Because the nurse has foreseeability of harm in these situations, the nurse who is not persistent can be held liable for failure to intervene because the intervention was below what was expected of them as a patient advocate.

The fourth element is that *failure to meet the standard of care must have the potential to injure the patient*. There must be a provable correlation between improper care and injury to the patient.

The final element is that *actual patient injury* must occur. This injury must be more than transitory. The plaintiff must show that the action of the defendant directly caused the injury, and that the injury would not have occurred without the defendant's actions. It is important to remember here, however, that not taking action is considered an action in such cases.

Being Sued for Malpractice

Historically, physicians were the health care providers most likely to be held liable for patient harm. As nurses have gained authority and autonomy, they have assumed increased responsibility, accountability, and liability for patient outcomes. In addition, as roles have expanded, nurses have begun performing duties traditionally reserved for medical practice. Unfortunately, both the enhanced role of nurses and the increase in the number of insured nurses have led to an increase in the number of liability suits seeking damages from nurses as individuals.

LEARNING EXERCISE 5.2

Who Is Responsible for Harm to This Patient? You Decide

You are a surgical nurse at Memorial Hospital. At 4:00 PM, you receive a patient from the recovery room who has had a total hip replacement. You note that the hip dressings are saturated with blood but are aware that total hip replacements frequently have some postoperative oozing from the wound. There is an order on the chart to reinforce the dressing as needed, and you do so. When you next check the dressing at 6:00 PM, you find the reinforcements saturated and drainage on the bed linen. You call the physician and tell her that you believe the patient is bleeding too heavily. The physician reassures you that the amount of bleeding you have described is not excessive but encourages you to continue to monitor the patient closely. You recheck the patient's dressings at 7:00 and 8:00 PM. You again call the physician and tell her that the bleeding still looks too heavy. She again reassures you and tells you to continue to watch the patient closely. At 10:00 PM, the patient's blood pressure drops precipitously, and the patient goes into shock. You summon the doctor, and she comes immediately.

ASSIGNMENT:

What are the legal ramifications of this case? Using the components of professional negligence outlined in Table 5.3, determine who in this case is guilty of malpractice. Justify your answer. At what point in the scenario should each character have altered their actions to reduce the probability of a negative outcome?

Many nurses now carry individual malpractice insurance. This is a double-edged sword. Nurses need malpractice insurance in basic practice as well as in expanded practice roles. They do incur a greater likelihood of being sued, however, if they have malpractice insurance because injured parties will usually seek damages from as many individuals with financial resources as possible.

In addition, some nurses count on their employer-provided professional liability policies to protect them from malpractice claims and indeed, most employers will answer to allegations against their employees (O'Neill, 2021). Such policies, however, may have limitations. For example, employers may not provide coverage once an employee has terminated employment, even if the situation that led to the complaint occurred while the nurse was employed there, and some employer-provided policies have inadequate limits of liability for the individual employee. In addition, an employer's liability coverage will not cover the nurse for actions related to a state Board of Nursing proceeding (O'Neill, 2021). Nurses then are advised to obtain their own personal liability policy.

Furthermore, nurses who do not have personal liability insurance are typically dependent on the attorney representing their employer and the attorney's priority is to defend the employer. The nurse needs an attorney dedicated solely to their own interests.

How many nurses are being sued and how big are the claims payouts? A study by the Nurses Service Organization (NSO) reported that $90 million was paid out in nursing malpractice claims over a recent 5-year period (Bajaj, 2018). Another recent report noted that the average total ($210,513) incurred from professional liability claims in 2020 was 4% greater than the report issued in 2015 ($201,670) (CNA/NSO, 2020) (see Examining the Evidence 5.1).

EXAMINING THE EVIDENCE 5.1

Source: From CNA/NSO. *Nurse professional liability exposure claim report*, 4th ed. (2020, June). Retrieved February 8, 2022, from https://www.cna.com/web/wcm/connect/f8b73780–0c25–453e–b4cf–b5343da8e374/Nurse-Exposure-Claim-Report-4th-Edition.pdf?MOD=AJPERES

Nurse Professional Liability Claims 2015–2020

This collaborative report published by CNA Financial Corporation, the leading professional liability insurer of nurses and business partners at Nurses Service Organization (NSO), reviewed the professional liability closed claims encountered by CNA/NSO on behalf of insured members from 2015–2020. The 2020 dataset included 455 professional liability closed claims involving registered nurses (RNs), licensed practical nurses (LPNs)/licensed vocational nurses (LVNs), or nursing students that resulted in an indemnity payment of $10,000 or greater.

Of the 455 claims, 86.8% involved RNs, 12.8% involved LPNs/LVNs, and less than 1% involved student nurses. The majority of professional liability closed claims involved nurses who provided direct patient care. Death and pressure injury were the two most common patient injuries, representing half of the closed claims. Claims brought against nurses in leadership roles were due to management or administrative responsibilities, such as hiring or educating staff, as well as making patient care assignments.

Claims asserted against LPNs/LVNs resulted in a higher average total incurred when compared to claims against RNs ($219,871 vs. $208,636). This occurred because of a higher frequency of LPN/LVN claims that settled for more than $250,000. Most of the claims involving LPNs/LVNs occurred in patient homes.

The average incurred claim was $210,513 as compared to $201,670 in 2015. More than half of all claims resulted in an indemnity payment of less than $100,000. The average expenses associated with defending these claims represented more than $20,000 per claim.

Obstetrical nurses experienced the highest average claim cost. Other specialty practice areas that experienced high claim awards were ambulatory surgery, correctional health, and postanesthesia care units.

Over 75% of all nursing malpractice occurs in the hospital setting (Miller & Zois, 2022). Labor and delivery nurses face the most malpractice claims in part because of well-established causal links between certain birth injuries and medical errors, making it the most litigated field of medicine in general (Miller & Zois, 2022). Nurses working in surgery settings have the second-highest incidence of malpractice, followed closely by nurses working in medical units.

It is not just nurses working in acute care settings, however, who experience malpractice claims. Famakinwa (2020) notes that home-based care nurses—including home health, hospice, and palliative care professionals—have seen a steady rise in professional liability claims since 2011. Overall, home-based care accounted for more than 20% of total closed claims against nurses in 2020. This is a sharp increase from 12.4% in 2015 and from 8.9% 9 years ago. In comparison, professional liability for nurses in other areas of aging services—independent living, assisted living, memory care, and skilled nursing—only accounted for 11.2% of claims in 2020 (Famakinwa, 2020).

In particular, malpractice has become a greater concern to advanced practice nurses such as nurse practitioners (NPs) and nurse midwives. Failure to diagnose is the most frequent malpractice allegation asserted against NPs. It accounts for 32.8% of all malpractice claims against NPs (NSO, 2021). Failure to diagnose cancer and failure to diagnose infections account for 50% of failure to diagnose allegations (NSO, 2021). As a result of their increased risk for litigation, NPs pay high costs for their insurance premiums and are subject to strict professional liability (malpractice) insurance requirements.

Avoiding Malpractice Claims

Interactions between nurses and clients that are less businesslike and more personal are more satisfying to both. It has been shown that despite technical competence, nurses who have difficulty establishing positive interpersonal relationships with patients and their families are at greater risk for being sued. Communication that proceeds in a caring and professional manner has been shown repeatedly to be a major reason that people do not sue despite adequate grounds for a successful lawsuit.

In addition, many experts have suggested a need to create safer environments for care so that fewer patients are injured during their care. For example, even though there are unit-dose systems in play, nurse-leaders often look the other way when staff pour all the medications into a soufflé cup and hand them to patients, thus increasing the possibility of medication errors.

Strategies recommended by The Joint Commission, in its 2005 seminal report, *Health Care at the Crossroads* (Joint Commission on Accreditation of Healthcare Organizations, 2005), can be viewed in Display 5.2. The three major areas of focus in the call to action are to prevent injuries, improve communication, and examine mechanisms for injury compensation.

Nurses can reduce the risk of malpractice claims by taking the following actions:

- Practice within the scope of the Nurse Practice Act.
- Observe agency policies and procedures.
- Model practice after established standards by using evidence-based practice.
- Always put patient rights and welfare first.
- Be aware of relevant laws and legal doctrines and combine such with the biologic, psychological, and social sciences that form the basis of all rational nursing decisions.
- Practice within the area of individual competence.
- Upgrade technical skills consistently by attending continuing education programs and seeking specialty certification.

Nurses should also purchase their own liability insurance and understand the limits of their policies. Although this will not prevent a malpractice suit, it should help protect a nurse from financial ruin should there be a malpractice claim.

DISPLAY 5.2 **SUMMARY OF RECOMMENDATIONS FROM THE EXECUTIVE SUMMARY OF *HEALTH CARE AT THE CROSSROADS: STRATEGIES FOR IMPROVING THE MEDICAL LIABILITY SYSTEM AND PREVENTING PATIENT INJURY***

1. Pursue patient safety initiatives that prevent medical injury by
   - Strengthening oversight and accountability mechanisms to better ensure the competencies of physicians and nurses
   - Encouraging appropriate adherence to clinical guidelines to improve quality and reduce liability risk
   - Supporting team development through team training
   - Continuing to leverage patient safety initiatives through regulatory and oversight bodies
   - Building an evidence-based information and technology system that impacts patient safety and pursuing proposals to offset implementation costs
   - Promoting the creation of cultures of patient safety in health care organizations
   - Establishing a federal leadership locus for advocacy of patient safety and health care quality
   - Pursuing "pay-for-performance" strategies that provide incentives to improve patient safety and health care quality
2. Promote open communication between patients and practitioners by
   - Involving health care consumers as active members of the health care team
   - Encouraging open communication between practitioners and patients when adverse events occur
   - Pursuing legislation that protects disclosure and apology from being used as evidence against practitioners in litigation
   - Encouraging nonpunitive reporting of errors to third parties that promote information and data analysis as a basis for developing safety improvement
   - Enacting federal safety legislation that provides legal protection for information reported to patient safety organizations
3. Create an injury compensation system that is patient centered and serves the common good by
   - Conducting demonstration projects of alternatives to medical liability that promote patient safety and transparency and provide swift compensation for injured patients
   - Encouraging continued development of mediation and early-offer initiatives
   - Prohibiting confidential settlements that prevent learning from events
   - Redesigning the National Practitioner Data Bank
   - Advocating for court-appointed, independent expert witnesses to mitigate bias in expert witness testimony

Source: From Joint Commission on Accreditation of Healthcare Organizations. (2005). *Health care at the crossroads: Strategies for improving the medical liability system and preventing patient injury*.

Extending the Liability

In recent years, the concept of *joint liability*, in which the nurse, physician, and employing organization are all held liable, has become the current position of the legal system. This likely reflects the higher level of accountability now present in the nursing profession compared with previous years. Before 1965, nurses were rarely held accountable for their own acts, and hospitals were usually exempt due to *charitable immunity*. However, following precedent-setting cases in the 1960s, employers are now held liable for the nurse's acts under a concept known as *vicarious liability*.

One form of vicarious liability is called *respondeat superior*, which means "the master is responsible for the acts of his servants." *Respondeat superior* applies when an employee causes damages or injuries while working on behalf of their employer (Hale Law Firm, 2022). In such a scenario, the employer would also be liable for the injuries. The theory behind the doctrine is that an employer should be held legally liable for the conduct of employees whose actions they have a right to direct or control.

LEARNING EXERCISE   5.3

Understanding Limitations and Rules

Have you ever been directed in your nursing practice to do something that you believed might be unsafe or that you felt inadequately trained or prepared to do? What did you do? Would you act differently if the situation occurred now? What risks are inherent in refusing to follow the direct orders of a physician or superior? What are the risks of performing a task that you believe may be unsafe?

The difficulty in interpreting *respondeat superior* is that many exceptions exist. The first and most important exception is related to the state in which the nurse practices. In some states, the *doctrine of charitable immunity* applies, which holds that a charitable (nonprofit) hospital cannot be sued by a person who has been injured because of a hospital employee's negligence. Thus, liability is limited to the employee.

Another exception to *respondeat superior* occurs when the state or federal government employs the nurse. The common law rule of *governmental immunity* provides that governments cannot be held liable for the negligent acts of their employees while carrying out government activities. Some states have changed this rule by statute, however, and in these jurisdictions, *respondeat superior* continues to apply to the acts of nurses employed by the state government.

> The purpose of *respondeat superior* is not to shift the burden of blame from the employee to the organization but rather to share the blame, increasing the possibility of larger financial compensation to the injured party.

Some nurses erroneously assume that they do not need to carry malpractice insurance because their employer will probably be sued as well and thus will be responsible for financial damages. Under the doctrine of *respondeat superior*, any employer required to pay damages to an injured person because of an employee's negligence may have the legal right to recover or be reimbursed that amount from the negligent employee.

One rule that all nurses must know and understand is that of *personal liability*, which says that every person is liable for their own conduct. The law does not permit a wrongdoer to avoid legal liability for their own wrongdoing, even though someone else also may be sued and held legally liable. For example, if a manager directs a subordinate to do something that both know to be improper, the injured party can recover damages against the subordinate even if the supervisor agreed to accept full responsibility for the delegation at the time. In the end, each nurse is always held liable for their own negligent practice.

Managers are not automatically held liable for all acts of negligence on the part of those they supervise, but they may be held liable if they were negligent in the supervision of those employees at the time that they committed the negligent acts. Liability for negligence is generally based on the manager's failure to determine which of the patient needs can be assigned safely to a subordinate or the failure to supervise a subordinate adequately for the assigned task (Huston, 2023c). Both the abilities of the staff member and the complexity of the task assigned must be considered when determining the type and amount of direction and supervision warranted.

Hospitals have also been found liable for assigning personnel who were unqualified to perform duties as shown by their evaluation reports. Managers, therefore, need to be cognizant of their responsibilities in assigning and appointing personnel because they could be found liable for ignoring organizational policies or for assigning employees duties that they are not capable of performing. In such cases, though, the employee must provide the supervisor with the information that they are not qualified for the assignment. The manager does have the right to reassign employees as long as they are capable of discharging the anticipated duties of the assignment.

In addition, there has been a push to have more in-depth background checks when health care employees are hired. Indeed, most states now mandate such checks for nursing licensure. At present, except in a few states, personnel directors in hospitals (those making hiring decisions) are required to request information from the National Practitioner Data Bank for those individuals who seek clinical privileges, and many states now require nursing students to be fingerprinted before they can work with vulnerable populations. In the future, hiring someone without an adequate background check, who later commits a crime involving a patient, could be another area of liability for the manager. This is an example of the type of pending legislation with which a manager must keep abreast so that if it becomes law, its impact on future management practices will be minimized.

Incident Reports and Adverse Event Forms

Incident reports or *adverse event forms* are records of unusual or unexpected incidents that occur during a client's treatment. Because attorneys use incident reports to defend the health agency against lawsuits brought by clients, the reports are generally considered confidential communications and cannot be subpoenaed by clients or used as evidence in their lawsuits in most states. (Be sure, however, that you know the law for the state in which you live, as this does vary.) However, incident reports that are inadvertently disclosed to the plaintiff are no longer considered confidential and can be subpoenaed in court. Thus, a copy of an incident report should not be left in the chart. In addition, no entry should be made in the patient's record about the existence of an incident report. The chart should, however, provide enough information about the incident or occurrence so that appropriate treatment can be given.

Intentional Torts

Torts are legal wrongs committed against a person or property, independent of a contract, that render the person who commits them liable for damages in a civil action. Whereas, professional negligence is considered an *unintentional tort*, assault, battery, false imprisonment, invasion of privacy, defamation, and slander are intentional torts. *Intentional torts* are a direct invasion of someone's legal rights. Managers are responsible for seeing that staff members are

---

LEARNING EXERCISE 5.4

Discussing Lawsuits and Liability

In small groups, discuss the following questions:

1. Do you believe that there are unnecessary lawsuits in the health care industry? What criteria can be used to distinguish between appropriate and unnecessary lawsuits?
2. Have you ever advised a friend or family member to sue to recover damages that you believed they suffered because of poor-quality health care? What motivated you to encourage them to do so?
3. Do you think that you will make clinical errors in judgment as a nurse? If so, what types of errors should be considered acceptable (if any) and what types are not acceptable?
4. Do you believe that the recent national spotlight on medical error identification and prevention will encourage the reporting of medical errors when they do occur?

aware of and adhere to laws governing intentional torts. In addition, the manager must clearly delineate policies and procedures about these issues in the work environment.

Nurses can be sued for assault and battery. *Assault* is conduct that makes a person fearful and produces a reasonable apprehension of harm, and *battery* is an intentional and wrongful physical contact with a person that entails an injury or offensive touching. The Thompson & Hiller Defense Firm (2021) notes that actual battery is not necessary to be charged with either first- or second-degree assault and battery. It is only necessary that bodily injury could have resulted.

Unit managers must be alert to patient reports of being handled in a rough manner or reports of excessive force in restraining patients. In fact, performing any treatment without patient's permission or without receiving an informed consent might constitute both assault and battery. In addition, many battery suits have been won based on the use of restraints when dealing with confused patients.

The use of physical restraints also has led to claims of *false imprisonment*. False imprisonment occurs when a person (who doesn't have legal authority or justification) intentionally restrains another person's ability to move freely (FindLaw, 2022). Practitioners are liable for false imprisonment when they unlawfully restrain the movement of their patients.

Unfortunately, the use of restraints continues to be common practice in many health care institutions (especially skilled nursing facilities) despite a growing body of evidence that supports the implementation of alternative strategies to promote resident safety. Physical restraints should be applied only with a physician's direct order. Likewise, the patient who wishes to sign out against medical advice should not be held against their will. This tort also is frequently applicable to involuntary commitments to mental health facilities. Managers in mental health settings must be careful to institutionalize patients in accordance with all laws governing commitment.

Another intentional tort is defamation. *Defamation* is communicating to a third-party false information that injures a person's reputation. When defamation is written, printed, or broadcasted, it is called *libel*. When it is spoken, it is called *slander*. The damages for defamation can be enhanced by how widespread the publication of the defamatory information was.

Other Legal Responsibilities of the Manager

Managers also have some legal responsibility for the quality control of nursing practice at the unit level, including such duties as reporting dangerous understaffing, checking staff credentials and qualifications, and carrying out appropriate discipline. Health care facilities may also be held responsible for seeing that staff know how to operate equipment safely. Sources of liability for managers vary from facility to facility and from position to position.

For example, standards of care as depicted in policies and procedures may pose a liability for the nurse if such policies and procedures are not followed. The chain of command in reporting inadequate care by a physician is another area in which management liability may occur if employees are not taught proper protocols. Managers have a responsibility to see that written protocols, policies, and procedures are followed to reduce liability. In addition, the manager, like all professional nurses, is responsible for reporting improper or substandard medical care, child and elder abuse, and communicable diseases, as specified by the Centers for Disease Control and Prevention.

Individual nurses also may be held liable for *product liability*. Historically, a contractual relationship known as *privity of contract* had to exist for a product liability claim to be filed. This meant that the injured party had to have purchased a product directly from the manufacturer to sue the manufacturer for injury caused by the product (Mascaranhas, 2018). By the 1950s and 1960s, the courts moved away from privity of contract because more wholesalers and retailers were selling products directly to the consumer. In 1963, California became the first state to adopt *strict product liability*, and in 1986, many other states followed (Mascaranhas, 2018).

Essentially, strict liability holds that a product may be held to a higher level of liability than a person. In other words, if it can be proved that the equipment or product had a defect that caused an injury, then it would be debated in court by using all the elements essential for negligence, such as duty and breach. Therefore, equipment and other products fall within the scope of nursing responsibility. Nurses should not use equipment they are unfamiliar with. In addition, if they are aware that equipment is faulty, nurses should refuse to use the equipment. If the fault in the equipment is not readily apparent, risks are low that the nurse will be found liable for the results of its use.

Informed Consent

Many nurses erroneously believe that they have obtained informed consent when they witness a patient's signature on a consent form for surgery or procedure. Strictly speaking, *informed consent* (Display 5.3) can be given only after the patient has received a complete explanation of the surgery, procedure, or treatment and indicates that they understand the risks and benefits related to it.

The information must be in a language that the patient can understand and should be conveyed by the individual who will be performing the procedure. Patients must be invited to ask questions and have a clear understanding of the options as well.

> Informed consent is obtained only after the patient receives full disclosure of all pertinent information regarding the surgery or procedure and only if the patient understands the potential benefits and risks associated with doing so.

Only a competent adult can legally sign the form that shows informed consent. To be considered competent, patients must be capable of understanding the nature and consequences of the decision and of communicating their decision. Spouses or other family members cannot legally sign unless there is an approved guardianship or conservatorship or unless they hold a durable power of attorney for health care. If the patient is younger than 16 years (18 years in some states), a parent or guardian must generally give consent.

In an emergency, the physician can invoke *implied consent*, in which the physician states in the progress notes of the medical record that the patient is unable to sign but that treatment is immediately needed and is in the patient's best interest. Usually, this type of implied consent must be validated by another physician.

DISPLAY 5.3 **GUIDELINES FOR INFORMED CONSENT**

The person(s) giving consent must fully comprehend

1. The procedure to be performed
2. The risks involved
3. Expected or desired outcomes
4. Expected complications or side effects that may occur as a result of treatment
5. Alternative treatments that are available

Consent may be given by

1. A competent adult
2. A legal guardian or an individual holding durable power of attorney
3. An emancipated or married minor
4. A mature minor (varies by state)
5. A parent of a minor child
6. A court order

LEARNING EXERCISE 5.5

Is It Really Informed Consent?

Cory Baxter is a staff nurse in a surgical unit. Shortly after receiving hand-off report, he completes rounds on all his patients. Mrs. Jones is a 36-year-old woman scheduled for a bilateral salpingo-oophorectomy and hysterectomy. Mrs. Jones comments that she is glad she will not be undergoing menopause as a result of this surgery. She elaborates by stating that one of her friends had surgery that resulted in "surgical menopause" and that it was devastating to her. Cory returns to the chart and checks the surgical permit and doctor's progress notes. The operating room permit reads "bilateral salpingo-oophorectomy and hysterectomy," and it is signed by Mrs. Jones. The physician has noted "discussed surgery with patient" in the progress notes.

Cory returns to Mrs. Jones's room and asks her what type of surgery she is having. She states, "I'm having my uterus removed." He phones the physician and relates his information to the surgeon who says, "Mrs. Jones knows that I will take out her ovaries if necessary; I've discussed it with her. She signed the permit. Now, please get her ready for surgery—she is the next case."

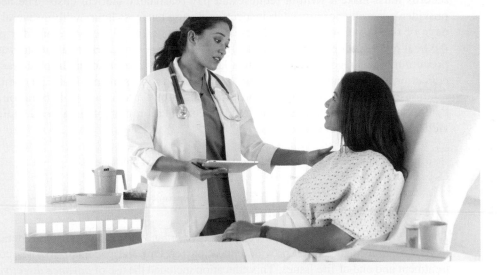

ASSIGNMENT:

Discuss what Cory should do at this point. Why did you select this course of action? What issues are involved here? Be able to discuss legal ramifications of this case.

Nurses frequently seek *express consent* from patients by witnessing patients sign a standard consent form. In express consent, the role of the nurse is to be sure that the patient has received informed consent and to seek remedy if they have not.

Informed consent does pose ethical issues for nurses. Although nurses are obligated to provide teaching and to clarify information given to patients by their physicians, nurses must be careful not to give new information that contradicts information given by the physician, thus interfering in the physician–patient relationship. The nurse is not responsible for explaining the procedure to be performed. The role, rather, is to be a patient advocate by determining their level of understanding and seeing that the appropriate person answers their questions. At times, this can be a cloudy issue both legally and ethically.

Informed Consent for Clinical Research

The intent of informed consent in clinical research is to give patients adequate information, through a full explanation of a proposed treatment, including any possible harms, so that they can make an informed decision. Studies, however, repeatedly suggest that participants often have incomplete understanding of various features of clinical trials and issues associated with written informed consent are common.

Medical Records

One source of information that people seek to help them make decisions about their health care is their medical record. Nurses have a legal responsibility for accurately recording appropriate information in the client's medical record. The alteration of medical records can result in license suspension or revocation.

Although the patient owns the information in that medical record, the actual record belongs to the facility that originally made the record and is storing it. Although patients must have "reasonable access" to their records, the method for retrieving the record varies greatly from one institution to another. In general, a patient who wishes to inspect their records must make a written request and pay reasonable clerical costs. The health care provider generally permits such inspection during business hours within several working days of the inspection request. Nurses should be aware of the procedure for procuring medical records for patients at the facilities where they work. Often, a patient's attempt to procure medical records results from a lack of trust or a need for additional teaching and education. Nurses can do a great deal to reduce this confusion and foster an open, trusting relationship between the patient and their health care providers. Collaboration between health care providers and patients, and documentation thereof, is a good indication of well-provided clinical care.

> If it is not documented in the health care record . . . it did not happen.

The Patient Self-Determination Act

The *PSDA*, enacted in 1991, required health care organizations that received federal funding (Medicare and Medicaid) to provide education for staff and patients on issues concerning treatment and end-of-life issues. This education included the use of *advance directives* (ADs), written instructions regarding desired end-of-life care. Most ADs address the use of dialysis and respirators, if one wants to be resuscitated if breathing or heartbeat stops, tube feeding, and organ or tissue donation (MedlinePlus, 2021). They also likely include a *durable power of attorney* for health care, which names one's *health care proxy*, someone one trusts to make health decisions if one is unable to do so (MedlinePlus, 2021).

The PSDA requires acute care facilities to document on the medical record whether a patient has an AD and to provide written information to patients who do not. However, despite mechanisms within most health care institutions to provide this information, the AD completion rate remains low and many patients do not understand what is included in the AD or whether this is something important they should have. The reality is that many people do not express their wishes about end-of-life treatment before a crisis occurs, at which point they may be unable to do so.

Good Samaritan Laws

Nurses are not required to stop and provide emergency services as a matter of law, although most health care workers feel ethically compelled to stop if they believe they

LEARNING EXERCISE 5.6

Mrs. Brown's Chart

You are a nurse in a multiphysician office that treats oncology patients. Mrs. Brown, a patient seen by Dr. Watson in your office, was recently diagnosed with invasive cancer. She started radiation treatments last week. Her husband attends her radiation treatments and office visits with her and seems to be devoted to her. They both are very interested in her progress.

Although they have asked many questions during the last two office visits and you have given truthful answers, Dr. Watson's interactions have sometimes been a bit short, and you felt that Mr. and Mrs. Brown may have left with unanswered questions. In addition, Dr. Watson has not shared much with them yet about Mrs. Brown's prognosis as he continues to refine his differential diagnosis.

Today, when you walk into Mrs. Brown's examination room, you find Mr. Brown reading her electronic record on the computer tablet that was inadvertently left on the counter in her room. He has a confused and overwhelmed look on his face.

ASSIGNMENT:

Identify several alternatives for action that you have. Discuss what you would do and why. Is there a problem here? What follow-up is indicated? Attempt to solve this learning exercise on your own before reading the sample analysis that follows.

Analysis

The nurse needs to determine the most important goal in this situation. Possible goals include (a) eliminating Mr. Brown's access to the medical record as soon as possible, (b) protecting the privacy of Mrs. Brown, (c) gathering more information, or (d) becoming an advocate for the Browns.

In solving the case, it is apparent that not enough information has been gathered. Mr. Brown has already viewed at least a portion of his wife's electronic medical record. Usually, the danger in patients' families reading a patient's record lies in the direction of their not understanding the information contained within or the patient's privacy being invaded because the patient has not consented to family members' access to their records.

Using this as the basis for rationale, the nurse could use the following approach:

1. Clarify that Mr. Brown has Mrs. Brown's permission to read her records by asking her directly.
2. Ask Mr. Brown if there is anything in the electronic health record that he did not understand or anything that he questions. You may even ask him to summarize what he has read. Clarify the things that are appropriate for the nurse to address, such as terminology, procedures, and nursing care.
3. Refer questions that are inappropriate for the nurse to answer to the physician and let Mr. Brown know that you will help him in talking with the physician regarding the medical plan and prognosis.
4. When finished talking with Mr. Brown, the nurse should secure the electronic health record.
5. The nurse should notify Dr. Watson about the incident and Mr. Brown's concerns and assist the Browns in obtaining the information they have requested.

Conclusion

The nurse first gathered more information before becoming the adversary or advocate. It is possible that the Browns had only simple questions to ask, and that the problem was a lack of communication between staff and their patients rather than a physician–patient communication deficit. Legally, patients have a right to understand what is happening to them, and that should be the basis for the decisions in this case.

can help. *Good Samaritan laws* suggest that health care providers are typically protected from potential liability if they volunteer their nursing skills away from the workplace (generally limited to emergencies), if actions taken are not grossly negligent, and if the health care worker does not exceed their training or scope of practice in performing the emergency services.

Gross negligence would negate Good Samaritan protection since these laws give liability protection only against *ordinary negligence*. Ordinary negligence is the failure to act as a reasonably prudent person or to exercise such care as most people would under the same or similar circumstances (West & Varacallo, 2021).

> Good Samaritan laws apply only if the health care worker does not exceed their training or scope of practice in performing the emergency services.

In addition, protections under Good Samaritan laws vary from state to state. Some states' protections only apply to those with some medical training or background although most extend those protections to all volunteers who provide care without expectation of payment (West & Varacallo, 2021). In some states, the law grants immunity to RNs but does not protect licensed vocational nurses (LVNs) or licensed practical nurses (LPNs). Other states offer protection to anyone who offers assistance, even if they do not have a health care background. Nurses should be familiar with the Good Samaritan laws in their state.

Health Insurance Portability and Accountability Act of 1996

Another area of the law that nurses must understand is the right to confidentiality. Efforts to preserve patient confidentiality increased tremendously with the passage of the HIPAA of 1996 (also known as the Kassebaum–Kennedy Act). Unauthorized release of information or photographs in medical records may make the person who discloses the information civilly liable for invasion of privacy, defamation, or slander. Written authorization by the patient to release information is needed to allow such disclosure.

Many nurses have been caught unaware by telephone calls requesting information about a patient's condition. It is extremely important that the nurse does not give out unauthorized information, regardless of the urgency of the person making the request. In addition, nurses must be careful not to discuss patient information in venues where it can be inadvertently overheard, read, transmitted, or otherwise unintentionally disclosed.

HIPAA essentially represents two areas for implementation. The first is the *Administrative Simplification plan*, and the second area includes the *Privacy Rule*. The Administrative Simplification plan is directed at restructuring the coding of health information to simplify the digital exchange of information among health care providers and to improve the efficiency of health care delivery. The privacy rules are directed at ensuring strong privacy protections for patients without threatening access to care.

The Privacy Rule applies to health plans, health care clearinghouses, and health care providers. It also covers all patient records and other individually identifiable health information. Although there are many components to HIPAA, key components of the Privacy Rule are that direct treatment providers must make a good faith effort to obtain written acknowledgment of the notice of privacy rights and practices from patients. Health care providers also must disclose protected health information to patients requesting their own information or when oversight agencies request the data. Reasonable efforts must be taken, however, to limit the disclosure of personal health information to the minimum information necessary to complete the transaction. There are situations, however, when limiting the information is not required. For example, a minimum of information is not required for treatment purposes because it is clearly better to have too much information than too little. The HIPAA Privacy Rule and Common Rule also require that individuals participating in research studies should be assured privacy, particularly regarding personal health information.

> The Privacy Rule attempts to balance the need for the protection of personal health information with the need to disclose that information for patient care.

Because of the complexity of the HIPAA regulations, it is not expected that only a nurse manager would be responsible for compliance. Instead, it is most important that the manager works with the administrative team to develop compliance procedures. For example, managers must ensure that unauthorized people do not have access to patient charts or medical records and that unauthorized people are not allowed to observe procedures.

It is equally important that managers remain cognizant of ongoing changes to the guidelines and are aware of how rules governing these issues may differ in the state in which they are employed. Some provisions of the Privacy Rules mention "reasonable efforts" toward achieving compliance but being reasonable is provision specific. The American Recovery and Reinvestment Act applies several of HIPAA's security and privacy requirements to business associates and changes data restrictions, disclosure, and reporting requirements.

Legal Considerations of Managing a Diverse Workforce

Diversity has been defined as the differences among groups or between individuals and comes in many forms, including age, gender, religion, customs, sexual orientation, physical size, physical and mental capabilities, beliefs, culture, ethnicity, and skin color. Demographic data from the United States Census Bureau continue to show increased diversification of the US population, a trend that began almost 50 years ago (Huston, 2023b).

As discussed in later chapters, a primary area of diversity is language, including word meanings, accents, and dialects. This language diversity can lead to misunderstandings or a reluctance to ask questions in a diverse workforce. Staff from cultures in which assertiveness is not promoted may find it difficult to disagree with or question others. How the manager handles these manifestations of cultural diversity is of major importance. If the manager's response is seen as discriminatory, the employee may file a complaint with one of the state or federal agencies that oversee civil rights or equal opportunity enforcement. Such things as overt or subtle discrimination are prohibited by Title VII (Civil Rights Act of 1964). Managers have a responsibility to be fair and just. Minority employees may be denied promotions or given unfair assignments due to their differences, which is illegal.

In addition, English-only rules in the workplace may be viewed as discriminatory under Title VII. Such rules may not violate Title VII if employers require English only during certain periods of time. Even in these circumstances, the employees must be notified of the rules and how they are to be enforced.

Managers should be taught how to deal sensitively and appropriately with an increasingly diverse workforce. Enhancing self-awareness and staff awareness of personal cultural biases, developing a comprehensive cultural diversity program, and role modeling cultural sensitivity are some of the ways that managers can effectively avoid many legal problems associated with discriminatory issues. However, it is hoped that future goals for the manager would go beyond compliance with Title VII and move toward understanding of and respect for other cultures.

Professional Versus Institutional Licensure

In general, a *license* is a legal document that permits a person to offer special skills and knowledge to the public in a particular jurisdiction when such practice would otherwise be unlawful. Licensure establishes standards for entry into practice, defines a scope of practice, and allows for disciplinary action. Currently, licensing for nurses is a responsibility of State Boards of Nursing or State Boards of Nurse Examiners, which also provide discipline as necessary. The manager, however, is responsible for monitoring that all subordinates requiring licensure have a valid, appropriate, and current license to practice.

> Professional licensure is a privilege and not a right.

All nurses must safeguard the privilege of licensure by knowing the standards of care applicable to their work setting. Deviation from that standard should be undertaken only when nurses are prepared to accept liability and loss of licensure as the consequences of their actions. Nurses who violate specific norms of conduct, such as securing a license by fraud, performing specific actions prohibited by the Nurse Practice Act, exhibiting unprofessional or illegal conduct, performing malpractice, and abusing alcohol or drugs, may have their licenses suspended or revoked by the licensing boards in all states.

While most nurses fear civil allegations of malpractice, the National Practitioner Data Bank notes that nursing professionals were on average more than 62 times more likely to be involved in an adverse licensing action than a medical malpractice payment in 2019 (Nurse Spotlight, 2021). Professional conduct allegations were the most frequent allegations asserted against nurses, comprising 32.5% of license protection matters (CNA/NSO, 2020; Nurse Spotlight, 2021). Collectively, professional conduct, scope of practice, and documentation error or omission accounted for 67% of all license protection closed matters (CNA/NSO, 2020) (see Examining the Evidence 5.2). Other frequent causes of license revocation are shown in Display 5.4.

EXAMINING THE EVIDENCE 5.2

Sources:

- From Nurse spotlight: Defending your license. (2021, May). *Colorado Nurse, 121*(2), 17–19.
- From CNA/NSO. *Nurse professional liability exposure claim report*, 4th ed. (2020, June). Retrieved February 8, 2022, from https://www.cna.com/web/wcm/connect/f8b73780-0c25-453e-b4cf-b5343da8e374/Nurse-Exposure-Claim-Report-4th-Edition.pdf?MOD=AJPERES

Nurses Facing State Board of Nursing Licensure Review and Discipline 2015–2020

- *The 4th edition of the Nurse Liability Claim Report, published by NSO, in collaboration with CNA Financial Corporation, revealed a total of 1,377 closed license protection matters with payment in the 5-year analysis, with an average defense expense of $5,330.*
- *Professional conduct allegations comprised 32.5% of license protection matters, and were the most frequent allegations asserted against nurses in license protection matters.*
- *Allegations related to failure to maintain minimum standard of nursing practice comprised 58.9% of scope of practice license protection matters.*
- *46.9% of the documentation matters involved an allegation related to fraudulent or falsified patient care or billing records.*
- *Collectively, professional conduct, scope of practice, and documentation error or omission accounted for 67% of all license protection closed matters.*
- *In 45.6% of licensure cases in 2020, the State Board of Nursing decided not to take action. In 15.5% of matters, the nurse received a letter of concern which was considered a "warning" or reprimand. The more serious outcomes included: Probation 12.0%, Surrender 4.8%, Suspension 3.2%, and Revocation 1.5%.*

DISPLAY 5.4 COMMON CAUSES OF PROFESSIONAL NURSING LICENSE SUSPENSION OR REVOCATION

- Professional negligence
- Practicing medicine or nursing without a license
- Obtaining a nursing license by fraud or allowing others to use your license
- Felony conviction for any offense substantially related to the function or duties of a registered nurse
- Participating professionally in criminal abortions
- Failing to follow accepted standards of care
- Not reporting substandard medical or nursing care
- Providing patient care while under the influence of drugs or alcohol
- Giving narcotic drugs without an order
- Falsely holding oneself out to the public or to any health care practitioner as a "nurse practitioner"
- Failing to use equipment safely and responsibly

Typically, suspension and revocation proceedings are administrative. Following a complaint, the Board of Nursing completes an investigation. Most of these investigations reveal no grounds for discipline; however, there are things a nurse should do if they become aware they are being investigated by the board. These are shown in Display 5.5.

If the investigation supports the need for discipline, nurses are notified of the charges and can prepare a defense. At the hearing, which is very similar to a trial, the nurse can present evidence. Based on the evidence, an administrative law judge makes a recommendation to the State Board of Nursing, which makes the final decision. The entire process, from complaint to final decision, may take 2 years or longer. State Board of Nursing disciplinary actions can range from no action against the nurse, up to and including revocation of the nurse's license to practice (Nurse Spotlight, 2021).

Some professionals have advocated shifting the burden of licensure, and thus accountability, from individual practitioners to an institution or agency. Proponents of this move believe that *institutional licensure* would provide more effective use of personnel and greater flexibility. Most professional nursing organizations oppose this move strongly because they believe that it has the potential for diluting the quality of nursing care.

An alternative to institutional licensure has been the development of *certification programs* by the American Nurses Association (ANA). By passing specifically prepared written examinations, nurses can qualify for certification in most nurse practice areas. This voluntary testing

DISPLAY 5.5 ACTIONS A NURSE SHOULD TAKE WHEN BEING INVESTIGATED BY THE BOARD OF NURSING

1. Do not ignore the Board's notification. It won't go away.
2. Do not unnecessarily share news of the complaint with friends and colleagues as it may undermine your credibility.
3. Read employee handbooks/contracts/policy and procedures to determine if you must report the investigation to your employer.
4. Consider contacting an attorney.
5. If a lawyer is needed, hire an experienced one.
6. Carefully consider anything you put in writing.
7. Contact your malpractice insurance provider.
8. If the investigation involves a patient, do not violate HIPAA by copying the patient's medical record.
9. Do not alter the patient's medical record.
10. Be prepared for a lengthy process of investigation.

Source: Extracted from Mackay, T. R. (2018). *What do you mean there's a complaint?! Texas Nursing, 92*(1), 20–22.

program represents professional organizational certification. In addition to ANA certification, other specialties, such as cardiac care, offer their own certification examinations. Many nursing leaders today strongly advocate professional certification as a means of enhancing the profession. However, certification is really only helpful in determining a nurse's continued competence if that nurse is functioning in the areas of their certified competence (Huston, 2023a).

Integrating Leadership Roles and Management Functions in Legal and Legislative Issues

Legislative and legal controls for nursing practice have been established to clarify the boundaries of nursing practice and to protect clients. The leader uses established legal guidelines to role model nursing practice that meets or exceeds accepted standards of care. Leaders also are role models in their efforts to expand expertise in their field and to achieve specialty certification. Perhaps the most important leadership roles in law and legislation are those involving vision, risk taking, and energy. The leader is active in professional organizations and groups that define what nursing is and what it should be in the future. This is an internalized responsibility that must be adopted by many more nurses if the profession is to be a recognized and vital force in the political arena.

Management functions in legal and legislative issues are more directive. Managers are responsible for seeing that their practice and the practice of their subordinates are in accord with current legal guidelines. This requires that managers have a working knowledge of current laws and legal doctrines that affect nursing practice. Because laws are not static, this is an active and ongoing function. The manager has a legal obligation to uphold the laws, rules, and regulations affecting the organization, the patient, and nursing practice.

Managers have a responsibility to be fair and nondiscriminatory in dealing with all members of the workforce, including those whose culture differs from their own. The effective leader goes beyond merely preventing discriminatory charges and instead strives to develop sensitivity to the needs of a culturally diverse staff.

The integrated leader-manager reduces the personal risk of legal liability by creating an environment that prioritizes patient needs and welfare. In addition, caring, respect, and honesty as part of nurse–patient relationships are emphasized. If these functions and roles are truly integrated, the risks of patient harm and nursing liability are greatly reduced.

 Key Concepts

- Sources of law include constitutions, statutes, administrative agencies, and court decisions.
- The burden of proof required to be found guilty and the punishment for the crime varies significantly between criminal, civil, and administrative courts.
- Nurse Practice Acts define and limit the practice of nursing in each state.
- Professional organizations generally espouse standards of care that are higher than those required by law. These voluntary controls often are forerunners of legal controls.

- Legal doctrines such as *stare decisis* and *res judicata* frequently guide courts in their decision making.
- Currently, licensing for nurses is a responsibility of State Boards of Nursing or State Boards of Nurse Examiners. These state boards also provide discipline as necessary.
- Some professionals have advocated shifting the burden of licensure, and thus accountability, from individual practitioners to an institution or agency. Many professional nursing organizations oppose this move.

- Malpractice or professional negligence is the failure of a person with professional training to act in a reasonable and prudent manner. Five components must be present for an individual to be found guilty of malpractice.
- Employers of nurses can now be held liable for an employee's acts under the concept of vicarious liability.
- Each person, however, is liable for their own tortious conduct.
- Managers are not automatically held liable for all acts of negligence on the part of those they supervise, but they may be held liable if they were negligent in supervising those employees at the time that they committed the negligent acts.
- Although professional negligence is considered an unintentional tort, assault, battery, false imprisonment, invasion of privacy, defamation, and slander are intentional torts.

- Consent can be informed, implied, or expressed. Nurses need to understand the differences between these types of consents and use the appropriate one.
- Although the patient owns the information in a medical record, the actual record belongs to the facility that originally made it and is storing it.
- It has been shown that despite good technical competence, nurses who have difficulty establishing positive interpersonal relationships with clients and their families are at greater risk for being sued for malpractice.
- Each nurse should be aware of how laws such as Good Samaritan immunity or legal access to incident reports are implemented in the state in which they live.
- New legislation pertaining to confidentiality (HIPAA) and patient rights (e.g., PSDA) continues to shape nurse–client interactions in the health care system.

Additional Learning Exercises and Applications

LEARNING EXERCISE   5.7

Where Does Your Responsibility Lie?

Mrs. Shin is a 68-year-old patient with liver cancer. She has been admitted to the oncology unit at Memorial Hospital. Her admitting physician has advised chemotherapy, even though her medical opinion is that it will be palliative, not curative. The patient asks her doctor, if there is an alternative treatment to chemotherapy. She replies, "Nothing else has proved to be effective. Everything else is quackery, and you would be wasting your money." After the doctor leaves, the patient and her family ask the nurse providing care if they know anything about alternative treatments. When the nurse indicates some current literature is available, they beg to have that information shared with them.

> *ASSIGNMENT:*
>
> What should the nurse do? What is the nurse's legal responsibility to the patient, the doctor, and the hospital? Using your knowledge of the legal process, the Nurse Practice Act, patients' rights, and legal precedents (look for the case *Tuma v. Board of Nursing*, 1979; The Climate Change and Public Health Law Site, n.d.), explain what you would do if you were the nurse and defend your decision.

LEARNING EXERCISE   5.8

Legal Ramifications for Exceeding One's Duties

You have been the evening charge nurse in the emergency department at Memorial Hospital for the last 2 years. You have two licensed vocational nurses (LVNs) and four registered nurses (RNs) working in your department with you. Your normal staffing is to have two RNs and one LVN on duty Monday to Thursday and one LVN and three RNs on duty during the weekend.

It has become apparent that one of the LVNs, Maggie, resents the recently imposed limitations of LVN duties because she has had 10 years of experience in nursing, including a tour of duty as a medic in the first Gulf War. The emergency department physicians admire her and are always asking her to assist them with any minor wound repair. Occasionally, she has exceeded her job description as an LVN in the hospital, although she has done nothing illegal of which you are aware. You have given her satisfactory performance evaluations in the past, even though everyone is aware that she sometimes pretends to be a "junior physician." You also suspect that the physicians sometimes allow her to perform duties outside her licensure, but you have not investigated this or seen it yourself.

Tonight, you come back from supper and find Maggie suturing a deep laceration while the physician looks on. They both realize that you are upset, and the physician takes over the suturing. Later, the doctor comes to you and says, "Don't worry! She does a great job, and I'll take the responsibility for her actions." You are not sure what you should do. Maggie is a good employee and taking any action will result in unit conflict.

ASSIGNMENT:

What are the legal ramifications of this case? Discuss what you should do, if anything. What responsibility and liability exist for the physician, Maggie, and you? Use appropriate rationale to support your decision.

LEARNING EXERCISE   5.9

To Float or Not to Float

You have been an obstetrical staff nurse at Memorial Hospital for 25 years. The obstetrical unit census has been abnormally low lately, although the patient census in other areas of the hospital has been extremely high. When you arrive at work today, you are told to float to the thoracic surgery unit. This is a specialized unit, and you feel ill prepared to work with the equipment on the unit and the type of patients who are there. You call the staffing office and ask to be reassigned to a different area. You are told that the entire hospital is critically short staffed, that the thoracic surgery unit is four nurses short, and that you are at least as well equipped to handle that unit as the other three staffs who also are being floated. Now, your anxiety level is even higher. You will be expected to handle a normal registered nurse–patient assignment. You also are aware that more than half of the staff on the unit today will have no experience in thoracic surgery. You consider whether to refuse to float. You do not want to place your nursing license in jeopardy, yet you feel conflicting obligations.

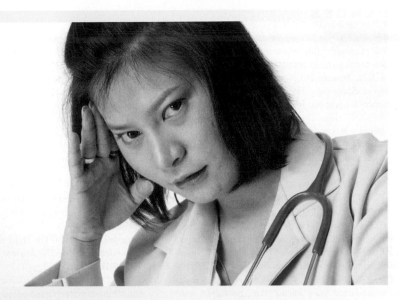

ASSIGNMENT:

To whom do you have conflicting obligations? You have little time to make this decision. Outline the steps that you use to reach your final decision. Identify the legal and ethical ramifications that may result from your decision. Are they in conflict?

LEARNING EXERCISE 5.10

Is It the Nurse's Responsibility to Force the Surgeon to See the Patient?

Jimmy Smith is a 19-year-old male who suffered a severe compound fracture of his tibia today in football practice. He returned from the surgery to set and cast the leg at 4:00 PM today. The 3–11 PM shift reported he was having quite a bit of swelling from the severe trauma that accompanied the fracture, but that the toes on the affected leg were warm and his pedal pulses were good.

By the time Jason Creed, the oncoming registered nurse (RN), received hand-off report at 11:00 PM and went to check on Jimmy, his pedal pulses were slightly diminished and his foot was slightly cool to touch. By 2:00 AM, Jason felt the swelling had increased slightly and he noted that Jimmy's toes were quite cool, although they were not blue.

Jason phones Jimmy's physician, and she was quite upset to be awakened in the middle of the night. She instructed Jason to put ice on the cast and to elevate Jimmy's leg higher to reduce the swelling. She promised she would see Jimmy first thing in the morning. As the night wears on, Jason becomes increasingly alarmed. By the time the night supervisor arrives at 4:00 AM, Jason is so concerned that he asks the night supervisor to check the casted leg. The supervisor does so and rushes out of the room and says, "The circulation in this boy's leg is severely compromised, why haven't you gotten the doctor here to cut the cast?"

ASSIGNMENT:

Has Jason committed malpractice? Has the doctor? What is Jason's responsibility in reporting a patient's condition to the physician? Examine the elements of malpractice. If there is permanent damage to Jimmy's leg, who will be liable for the failure to act soon enough to prevent injury?

REFERENCES

Bajaj, V. (2018). *Can nurses be sued for medical malpractice?* Injury Trial Lawyers. https://getinjuryanswers.com/can-nurses-sued-medical-malpractice/

Barowski, J. (2022, January 26). *Nurse Practice Act: History and overview.* Study.com. https://study.com/learn/lesson/nurse-practice-act-purpose-impact.html

Cirrinicione, L. (2021, July 23). *Understanding medical malpractice.* Murphy & Landon Injury Attorneys. https://www.msllaw.com/2021/07/23/understanding-medical-malpractice/

The Climate Change and Public Health Law Site. (n.d.). *Nurse disciplined for telling patient about alternative treatments (court reverses)—Tuma v. Board of Nursing,* 100 Idaho 74, 593 P.2d 711 (Idaho Apr 17, 1979). http://biotech.law.lsu.edu/cases/pro_lic/Tuma_v_Board_of_Nursing.htm

CNA/NSO. (2020, June). *Nurse professional liability exposure claim report,* 4th ed. https://www.cna.com/web/wcm/connect/f8b73780-0c25-453e-b4cf-b5343da8e374/Nurse-Exposure-Claim-Report-4th-Edition.pdf?MOD=AJPERES

Famakinwa, J. (2020, October 18). *As malpractice claims against home-based care nurses rise, providers must focus on risk management.* Home Health Care News. https://homehealthcarenews.com/2020/10/as-malpractice-claims-against-home-based-care-nurses-rise-providers-must-focus-on-risk-management/

FindLaw. (2022). *What is false imprisonment.* https://injury.findlaw.com/torts-and-personal-injuries/false-imprisonment.html

FindLaw for Legal Professionals. (2022). *Supreme Court of Illinois.* JUANITA SULLIVAN, indiv. and as special adm'r of the estate of Burns Sullivan, deceased, appellant, v. EDWARDHOSPITAL et al., appellees. No. 95409. http://caselaw.findlaw.com/il-supreme-court/1367447.html

Hale Law Firm. (2022). *What is respondeat superior?* https://www.halelawfirm.com/blog/2018/02/what-is-respondeat-superior.shtml

Huston, C. J. (2023a). Assuring provider competence through licensure, continuing education, and certification. In C. J. Huston (Ed.), *Professional issues in nursing: Challenges and opportunities* (6th ed., pp. 288–301). Wolters Kluwer.

Huston, C. J. (2023b). Diversity in the nursing workforce. In C. J. Huston (Ed.), *Professional issues in nursing: Challenges and opportunities* (6th ed., pp. 121–135). Wolters Kluwer.

Huston, C. J. (2023c). Unlicensed assistive personnel and the registered nurse. In C. J. Huston (Ed.), *Professional issues in nursing: Challenges and opportunities* (6th ed., pp. 109–120). Wolters Kluwer.

Joint Commission on Accreditation of Healthcare Organizations. (2005). *Health care at the crossroads: Strategies for improving the medical liability system and preventing patient injury.*

Mascaranhas, C. (2018). The legal nurse consultant's primer on product liability. *The Journal of Legal Nurse Consulting, 29*(1), 18–21.

MedlinePlus. (2021, October 12). *Advance directives.* http://www.nlm.nih.gov/medlineplus/advancedirectives.html

Miller & Zois, Attorneys at Law. (2022). *Nursing malpractice statistics.* https://www.millerandzois.com/nurse-malpractice-statistics.html

Nurse spotlight: Defending your license. (2021, May). Colorado Nurse, *121*(2), 17–19.

Nurses Service Organization. (2021). *Nurse practitioner case study: Failure to diagnose.* Affinity Insurance Services. https://www.nso.com/Learning/Videos/Failure-to-Diagnose-Case-Study

O'Neill, S. P. (2021). Individual nurse liability insurance. *American Nurse Journal, 16*(5), 54–58.

Thompson & Hiller Defense Firm. (2021). *Assault and battery.* https://www.grandstrandlaw.com/assault-and-battery.html

West, B., & Varacallo, M. (2021, September 20). *Good Samaritan laws.* https://www.ncbi.nlm.nih.gov/books/NBK542176/

6

Patient, Subordinate, Workplace, and Professional Advocacy

*… to see what is right, and not do it, is want of courage, or of principles.—**Confucius***

*… in our imperfect state of conscience and enlightenment, publicity and the collision resulting from publicity are the best guardians of the interest in the sick.—**Florence Nightingale***

*… No voice is too soft when that voice speaks for others.—**Janna Cachola***

CROSSWALK

This chapter addresses:

- **AACN Essentials Domain 1:** Knowledge for nursing practice
- **AACN Essentials Domain 2:** Person-centered care
- **AACN Essentials Domain 3:** Population health
- **AACN Essentials Domain 4:** Scholarship for nursing practice
- **AACN Essentials Domain 5:** Quality and safety
- **AACN Essentials Domain 6:** Interprofessional partnerships
- **AACN Essentials Domain 7:** Systems-based practice
- **AACN Essentials Domain 8:** Information and health care technologies
- **AACN Essentials Domain 9:** Professionalism
- **AACN Essentials Domain 10:** Personal, professional, and leadership development
- **AONL Nurse Executive Competency 2:** A knowledge of the health care environment
- **AONL Nurse Executive Competency 3:** Leadership
- **AONL Nurse Executive Competency 4:** Professionalism
- **ANA Standard of Professional Performance 7:** Ethics
- **ANA Standard of Professional Performance 8:** Advocacy
- **ANA Standard of Professional Performance 9:** Respectful and equitable practice
- **ANA Standard of Professional Performance 10:** Communication
- **ANA Standard of Professional Performance 11:** Collaboration
- **ANA Standard of Professional Performance 12:** Leadership
- **ANA Standard of Professional Performance 15:** Quality of practice
- **ANA Standard of Professional Performance 17:** Resource stewardship
- **ANA Standard of Professional Performance 18:** Environmental health
- **QSEN Competency:** Patient-centered care
- **QSEN Competency:** Teamwork and collaboration

LEARNING OBJECTIVES

The learner will:

- identify values central to advocacy
- differentiate between the nurse's responsibility to advocate for patients, for subordinates, for the organization, for the profession, and for self

- identify how a Patient's Bill of Rights protects patients
- differentiate between controlling patient choices and assisting patients to choose
- select an appropriate response that exemplifies advocacy in given situations
- identify entry points for user engagement in the health care system as well as strategies for patient and family engagement in health care
- describe the core concepts of person- and family-centered care
- describe how a manager can advocate for subordinates
- identify ways individual nurses can become advocates for the profession
- identify both the risks and potential benefits of becoming a whistleblower
- specify both direct and indirect strategies to influence legislation that promotes advocacy
- describe strategies nurses can use to successfully interact with the media

Introduction

Advocacy—helping others to grow and self-actualize—is a critically important leadership role. Many of the leadership skills described in the following chapters, such as risk taking, vision, self-confidence, the ability to articulate needs, and assertiveness, are used in the advocacy role. In addition, managers, by their many roles, must be advocates for the profession, subordinates, workplace, and patients. The actions of an *advocate* are to inform others of their rights and to be sure they have adequate information on which to base their decisions. Indeed, the term *advocacy* can be stated in its simplest form as "the act of pleading or arguing in favor of something, such as a cause, idea, or policy; active support" (The Free Dictionary by Farlex, 2003–2021, para. 1).

The American Nurses Association (ANA) believes that advocacy is a pillar of nursing (Ferguson, 2021). Indeed, advocacy has been recognized as one of the most vital and basic roles of the nursing profession since the time of Florence Nightingale. Nurses, as the frontline care providers, often have comprehensive knowledge and a well-rounded perspective about patient care issues, both those of direct care and system issues. When patients in the system are without insurance, are denied care, or do not know how to access appropriate care, nurses should have the knowledge competencies to provide informational guidance regarding these or similar issues.

For example, those who are incarcerated constitute one such vulnerable population, particularly those with opioid addictions. Advocacy groups note that many incarcerated people with opioid addictions in the United States do not have access to what leading medical organizations consider to be the standard of care: medication-assisted treatment (MAT) with methadone, buprenorphine, or naltrexone (Kaleka & Perzhinsky, 2020). Indeed, according to the Substance Abuse and Mental Health Services Administration (SAMHSA), there were 2,700 operational drug courts in the United States as of 2020; however, only 56% offered MAT to participants. In addition, most individuals with substance use disorder (SUD) do not receive treatment while they are incarcerated, or they are forced to withdraw from treatment they were receiving before incarceration. Nurses may be in the best position to advocate for care that represents best practices for this vulnerable population.

Older adults make up another vulnerable population. For example, investigative reporting in 2021 revealed that some understaffed nursing homes are using antipsychotic drugs to reduce staffing needs, even though these drugs can be dangerous for older people with dementia, nearly doubling their chance of death from heart problems, infections, falls, and other ailments (Thomas et al., 2021) (see Examining the Evidence 6.1). In addition, these nursing homes have given residents false diagnoses of schizophrenia to eliminate their need to report the drug use to government oversight agencies.

EXAMINING THE EVIDENCE 6.1

Source: From Thomas, K., Gebeloff, R., & Silver-Greenberg, J. (2021, August 11). Phony diagnoses hide high rates of drugging at nursing homes. *New York Times*. https://www.nytimes.com/ 2021/09/11/health/nursing-homes-schizophrenia-antipsychotics.html?campaign_id=9&emc= edit_nn_20210912&instance_id=40234&tnl=the-morning&regi_id=128435702&segment_ id=68744&te=1&user_id=5959ad8f4f1b62be2691e7495867c967

Advocating for Nursing Home Residents: A Vulnerable Population

Antipsychotic drugs—which for decades have faced criticism as "chemical straitjackets"—can be dangerous for older people with dementia, nearly doubling their chance of death from heart problems, infections, falls, and other ailments. But some understaffed nursing homes use the drugs so that they don't have to hire more staff to care for residents. As a result, the government, concerned with the overuse of these drugs, began publicly disclosing such prescriptions by individual nursing homes in 2012; however, patients with documented schizophrenia and two other mental health conditions were to be excluded from the data. Medicare data revealed that nursing home residents with a schizophrenia diagnosis soared 70 percent after 2012.

As of 2021, one in nine nursing home residents has a schizophrenia diagnosis. In the general population, the disorder afflicts roughly one in 150 people. In May 2021, a report by a federal oversight agency said that nearly one third of long-term nursing home residents with schizophrenia diagnoses in 2018 had no Medicare record of being treated for the condition. In addition, a 2021 New York Times investigation showed that at least 21 percent of nursing home residents—about 225,000 people—are on antipsychotics. The New York Times investigative report concluded that both the government and industry practices are obscuring the true rate of antipsychotic drug use with vulnerable residents.

Other vulnerable groups in health care include under-represented minority populations and the lesbian, gay, bisexual, transgender, and queer (LGBTQ) community. Nurses must increasingly be aware of and advocate for the elimination of racism, discrimination, and implicit bias experienced by these groups in society as well as within the nursing profession. Burke & Nickitas (2023) note that nurses are acknowledging and addressing the problem. For example, in 2021, the ANA launched the *National Commission to Address Racism in Nursing*. The Commission's mission is to set as a scope and standard of practice that nurses confront and mitigate systemic racism within the nursing profession and address the impact racism has on nurses and nursing.

The ANA suggests using the *Nursing: Scope and Standards of Practice Fourth Edition* (2021) as a framework to create a roadmap for action, including the goals to:

- Engage in national discussions within the nursing profession to own, amplify, understand, and change how racism negatively impacts colleagues, families, and communities and the health care system.
- Develop strategies to actively address racism within nursing education, practice, policy, and research, including issues of leadership and the use of power.

"Nurses have a moral and ethical obligation to address all forms of racism and to advocate for policies and laws that promote equity and the delivery of high-quality care to all individuals. This responsibility entails addressing all types of discrimination across such sectors as housing, education, criminal justice, employment, and health care impacting individuals and communities of color (Burke & Nickitas, 2023, p. 371)."

> **Nurses may act as advocates by helping others make informed decisions, by acting as intermediaries in the environment, or by directly intervening on behalf of others.**

DISPLAY 6.1   LEADERSHIP ROLES AND MANAGEMENT FUNCTIONS ASSOCIATED WITH ADVOCACY

Leadership Roles

1. Creates a climate where advocacy and its associated risk taking are valued
2. Seeks fairness and justice for individuals who are unable to advocate for themselves
3. Seeks to strengthen patient and subordinate support systems to encourage autonomous, well-informed decision making
4. Role models the use of patient and family engagement strategies
5. Influences others by providing information necessary to empower them to act autonomously
6. Assertively advocates on behalf of patients and subordinates when an intermediary is necessary
7. Participates in professional nursing organizations and other groups that seek to advance the profession of nursing
8. Role models proactive involvement in health care policy through both formal and informal interactions with the media and legislative representatives
9. Works to establish the creation of a national, legally binding Patient's Bill of Rights
10. Speaks up when appropriate to advocate for health care practices necessary for safety and quality improvement
11. Supports workers who report perceived wrongdoings through whistleblowing
12. Advocates for social justice in addition to individual patient advocacy
13. Appropriately differentiates between controlling patient choices (domination and dependence) and assisting patient choices (allowing freedom)

Management Functions

1. Assures that subordinates and patients have adequate information to make informed decisions
2. Establishes a work climate that prioritizes the rights and values of patients in health care decision making
3. Seeks appropriate consultation when advocacy results in intrapersonal or interpersonal conflict
4. Promotes and protects the workplace safety and health of subordinates and patients
5. Encourages subordinates to bring forth concerns about the employment setting and seeks impunity for whistleblowers
6. Demonstrates the skills needed to interact appropriately with the media and legislators regarding nursing and health care issues
7. Is aware of current legislative efforts affecting nursing practice and organizational and unit management
8. Assures that the work environment is both safe and conducive to professional and personal growth for subordinates
9. Creates work environments that promote subordinate empowerment so that workers have the courage to speak up for patients, themselves, and their profession
10. Takes immediate action when illegal, unethical, or inappropriate behavior occurs that can endanger or jeopardize the best interests of the patient, the employee, or the organization

This chapter examines the processes through which advocacy is learned as well as the ways in which leader-managers can advocate for their patients, subordinates, and the profession. The role of "whistleblower" as an advocacy role is discussed. Specific suggestions for interacting with legislators and the media to influence health policy are also included. Leadership roles and management functions essential for advocacy are shown in Display 6.1. Common areas in which nurses must advocate for patients are shown in Display 6.2.

Becoming an Advocate

Although advocacy is present in all clinical practice settings, the nursing literature contains only limited descriptions of how nurses learn the advocacy role, and some experts have even questioned whether advocacy can be taught at all. Some students learn about the advocacy role as part of ethics or policy content in their nursing education, and although most undergraduate

DISPLAY 6.2	COMMON AREAS REQUIRING NURSE–PATIENT ADVOCACY

1. End-of-life decisions
2. Technologic advances
3. Health care reimbursement
4. Access to health care
5. Transitions in health care
6. Provider–patient conflicts regarding expectations and desired outcomes
7. Withholding of information or blatant lying to patients
8. Insurance authorizations, denials, and delays in coverage
9. Medical errors
10. Patient information disclosure (privacy and confidentiality)
11. Patient grievance and appeals processes
12. Cultural and ethnic diversity and sensitivity
13. Respect for patient dignity
14. Inadequate consents
15. Incompetent health care providers
16. Complex social problems including AIDS, teenage pregnancy, violence, and poverty
17. Aging population

and graduate programs likely include some type of advocacy instruction, the extent or impact of this education is largely unknown. Regardless of how or when advocacy is learned, or the extent to which it is used, there are nursing values central to advocacy (Display 6.3).

> The nursing values central to advocacy emphasize caring, autonomy, respect, and empowerment.

Patient Advocacy

Standard 7 of the ANA (2021) *Nursing: Scope and Standards of Practice* calls for registered nurses to practice ethically. As such, the registered nurse is expected to take appropriate action regarding instances of illegal, unethical, and inappropriate behaviors that can endanger or jeopardize the best interests of the health care consumer or situation; speak up when appropriate to question health care practice when necessary for safety and quality improvement; and advocate for equitable health care consumer care.

This patient advocacy is necessary because disease almost always results in decreased independence, loss of freedom, and interference with the ability to make choices autonomously. In addition, aging, as well as physical, mental, or social disability, may make individuals more vulnerable and in need of advocacy. Thus, advocacy is the foundation and essence of nursing, and nurses have a responsibility to promote human advocacy.

DISPLAY 6.3	NURSING VALUES CENTRAL TO ADVOCACY

1. Every individual has a right to autonomy in deciding what course of action is most appropriate to meet their health care goals.
2. Every individual has a right to hold personal values and to use those values in making health care decisions.
3. All individuals should have access to the information they need to make informed decisions and choices.
4. The nurse must act on behalf of patients who are unable to advocate for themselves.
5. Empowerment of patients and subordinates to make decisions and act on their own is the essence of advocacy.

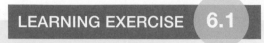

Values and Advocacy

How important a role do you believe advocacy to be in nursing? Do you believe that your willingness to assume this role is a learned value? Were the values of caring and service emphasized in your family or community when you were growing up? Have you identified any role models in nursing who actively advocate for patients, subordinates, or the profession? What strategies might you use as a new nurse to impart the need for advocacy to your peers and to the student nurses who work with you?

These ideas are also reinforced in the ANA (2015) *Code of Ethics for Nurses With Interpretive Statements*. Provision 2 of the *Code* suggests that the nurse's primary commitment is to the patient, whether an individual, family, group, community, or population. Provision 3 suggests that the nurse promotes, advocates for, and protects the rights, health, and safety of the patient.

Patient and Family Engagement

In addition, in 2013, the American Hospital Association (AHA) Committee on Research released a report entitled *Engaging Health Care Users: A Framework for Healthy Individuals and Communities*, suggesting that health care user engagement is a key ingredient in reaching the triple aim of better population health, enhanced patient experience, and lower costs (AHA, 2021). The report argued that hospitals must become more active in their efforts to engage patients and that a continuum for engagement from information sharing to partnerships must exist. The report went on to recommend entry points for user engagement at four different levels of the health care system as shown in Display 6.4.

In addition, the Agency for Healthcare Research and Quality (AHRQ, 2017) developed the *Guide to Patient and Family Engagement in Hospital Quality and Safety* to help patients, families, and health professionals work together as partners to promote improvements in care. The *Guide* (AHRQ, 2017) outlines four strategies hospitals can use to connect with patients and families:

- Encourage patients and family members to participate as advisors.
- Promote better communication among patients, family members, and health care professionals from the point of admission.
- Implement safe continuity of care by keeping the patient and family informed through nurse bedside change-of-shift reports.
- Engage patients and families in discharge planning throughout the hospital stay.

DISPLAY 6.4   ENTRY POINTS FOR USER ENGAGEMENT IN THE HEALTH CARE SYSTEM

- **Individual:** The aim is to increase the skills, knowledge, and understanding of patients and families about what to expect when receiving care.
- **Health care team:** The focus is to promote shared understanding of expectations among patients and providers when seeking care.
- **Organization:** The objective is to encourage partnerships and integrate the patient and family perspective into all aspects of hospital operations.
- **Community:** The emphasis is to expand the focus beyond the hospital setting and find opportunities to improve overall community health.

Source: From American Hospital Association. (2021). *Engaging health care users: A framework for healthy individuals and communities*. http://www.aha.org/research/cor/engaging/index.shtml

LEARNING EXERCISE 6.2

Culture and Decisions

You are a staff nurse on a medical unit. One of your patients, Mr. Dau, is a 56-year-old Hmong immigrant to the United States. He has lived in the United States for 4 years and became a citizen 2 years ago. His English is marginal, although he understands more than he can verbalize. He was admitted to the hospital with sepsis resulting from urinary tract infection. His condition is now stable.

Today, Mr. Dau's physician informed him that his computed tomography scan shows a large tumor in his prostate. The physician wants to do immediate follow-up testing and surgical resection of the tumor to relieve his symptoms of hesitancy and urinary retention. Although the tumor is probably cancerous, the physician believes that it will respond well to traditional oncology treatments. The expectation is that Mr. Dau should recover fully.

One hour later, when you go in to check on Mr. Dau, you find him sitting on his bed with his suitcase packed, waiting for a ride home. He informs you that he is checking out of the hospital. He states that he believes he can make himself better at home with herbs and through prayers by the Hmong shaman. He concludes by telling you, "If I am meant to die, there is little anyone can do." When you reaffirm the hopeful prognosis reported by his physician that morning, Mr. Dau says, "The doctor is just trying to give me false hope. I will either make myself better or prepare to die."

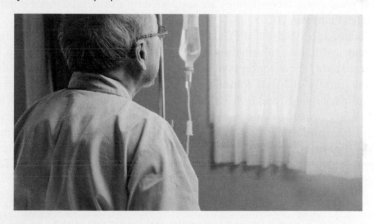

ASSIGNMENT:

What should you do? How can you best advocate for this patient? Is the problem a lack of information? How does culture play a role in the patient's decision? Does a lack of understanding on this patient's part justify paternalism?

Managers also must advocate for patients regarding distribution of resources and the use of technology. The advances in science and limits of financial resources have created new problems and ethical dilemmas. For example, although diagnosis-related groupings may have eased the strain on government fiscal resources, they have also created ethical problems, such as patient dumping, premature patient discharge, and inequality of care.

In addition, Huston (2023b) notes that debates about how best to merge the human element of care (caring) and emerging technology will undoubtedly continue. Health care organizations must consider what technology can best be used in each setting and how it can be used ethically. Nurses must therefore prioritize the improvement of patient care in their technology development agenda while embracing the use of technology as one of the skill sets that will be expected of them in the 21st century (Huston, 2023b).

Person- and Family-Centered Care

The Institute for Healthcare Improvement (2021) defines *patient- and family-centered care* (also known as *patient-centered care*) as putting the patient and the family at the heart of every decision and empowering them to be genuine partners in their care. Planetree agrees, noting that patient-centered care is a "moral imperative" as well as a blueprint for success. Thus, this approach to care humanizes, personalizes, and demystifies the patient experience (Planetree, 2021).

The Institute for Patient- and Family-Centered Care (IPFCC, n.d.) supports the value of patient- and family-centered care, asserting that it is an approach to the planning, delivery, and evaluation of health care that is grounded in mutually beneficial partnerships among health care providers, patients, and families, thus redefining the relationships in health care. Core concepts of patient- and family-centered care are shown in Display 6.5.

Planetree and the IPFCC have been two of the most prominent pioneers in developing and promoting patient- and family-centered care. Planetree is a mission-based, not-for-profit organization that partners with health care organizations around the world and across the care continuum to transform how care is delivered (Planetree, 2021). Guided by foundational principles regarding patient-centered care, Planetree informs policy at a national level, aligns strategies at a system level, guides implementation of care delivery practices at an organizational level, and facilitates compassionate human interactions at a deeply personal level. Their philosophical convictions are supported by a structured process that enables sustainable change (Planetree, 2021).

Founded in 1992, the IPFCC is a not-for-profit organization offering health care providers and institutions information and core guiding concepts related to patient- and family-centered care. These concepts include open visitation; family presence during all procedures; patient, family, and staff communication and collaboration in care plan development, multidisciplinary rounds, and bedside handoffs between nurses; information availability in patient and family resource centers; and the use of patient and family advisors in performance and safety improvement efforts (IPFCC, n.d.). In addition, the model encourages the use of soft colors, lighting, homelike fabrics, and music for patient rooms and common areas as well as opportunities for patients and families to learn about their illness to foster participation in their care.

DISPLAY 6.5 **CORE CONCEPTS OF PATIENT- AND FAMILY-CENTERED CARE**

- Patient care is organized first and foremost around the needs of patients.
- Patient and family perspectives are sought out, and their choices are honored.
- Patient and family knowledge, values, beliefs, and cultural backgrounds are incorporated into the planning and delivery of care.
- Health care providers communicate and share complete, accurate, and unbiased information openly and honestly with patients and families to empower them to be effective partners in their health care decision making.
- Patients and families are encouraged and supported in participating in care and decision making at the level they choose.
- Patients, families, and health care providers collaborate in policy and program development, implementation, and evaluation; in research; in facility design; and in professional education as well as in the delivery of care.
- The voice of the patient and family is represented at both the organizational and policy levels as well as at the health system's strategic planning.
- Health care practitioners listen to and honor patient and family perspectives and choices.

Source: From Planetree. (2021). *History of Planetree*. https://www.planetree.org/certification/about-planetree; Institute for Patient- and Family-Centered Care. (n.d.). *Patient- and family-centered care*. http://www.ipfcc.org/about/pfcc.html

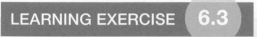

LEARNING EXERCISE 6.3

Changing Organization Cultures to Be Patient and Family Centered

Adoption of patient- and family-centered care often requires changing an organization culture so that patients and families are truly recognized as partners in care, whether at the bedside or at the institutional level in strategic planning. It also requires a reconsideration of many of the rules and barriers often in place that pose obstacles for patients and families to be active participants in care decisions.

ASSIGNMENT:

Select any one of the following rules/procedures/situations common to many hospitals and write a one-page essay outlining why it would not be consistent with a patient- and family-centered care approach. Include in the discussion how the rule/procedure/situation could be changed to better reflect the core concepts shown in Display 6.5.
1. Visiting hours end at 9:00 PM unless someone is willing to "bend the rules."
2. Only one visitor is allowed at a time in the critical care units and then for only 20 minutes every hour.
3. Flat, comfortable sleeping surfaces are not readily available for family members who wish to spend the night in patient rooms.
4. Physicians typically make patient care rounds between 7:00 AM and 8:00 AM before family members have arrived.
5. Handoff report occurs behind closed doors, and family members do not participate.
6. Family lounges are too small to accommodate all visitors during peak visiting hours.
7. Staff complain in handoff report that patients are unwilling to follow the plan of care rather than asking if the patients themselves were involved in determining the plan of care.
8. Dining halls are open only to staff in the middle of the night.

Patient Rights

Until the 1960s, patients had few rights in health care settings. This changed with the adoption of the *Consumer Bill of Rights and Responsibilities*, also known as the *Patient's Bill of Rights* in 1998. This document and subsequent revisions had three key goals: to help patients feel more confident in the US health care system, to stress the importance of a strong relationship between patients and their health care providers, and to emphasize the key role patients play in staying healthy by laying out rights and responsibilities for all patients and health care providers (American Cancer Society, 2022).

Since that time, the National League for Nursing, the AHA, and many other organizations have created documents outlining the rights of patients. Although not legally binding, these documents do guide health care organizations and practitioners in terms of professional expectations for patient advocacy. Some federal laws do exist, though, in terms of patient rights such as the right to get a copy of one's medical records and the right to keep them private (MedlinePlus, 2020).

In addition, with the passage of the *Patient Protection and Affordable Care Act* in 2010, a new Patient's Bill of Rights was established to give greater patient protections in dealing with insurance companies (American Cancer Society, 2022). These protections included the elimination of annual and lifetime coverage limits, provided for choice of physician from a plan's network, allowed individuals to get health insurance in spite of existing medical conditions, allowed children to stay on a parent's policy until age 26 years if they met other requirements, and restricted health insurance companies from being able to rescind (take back) health coverage because of honest mistakes on insurance applications.

LEARNING EXERCISE 6.4

Advocating for a Transgender Patient

You are the charge nurse on a medical unit. Today, during walking rounds, a patient who is a transgender woman tells you that she hears the staff whispering and making fun of her in the hallway outside her room. She says this is hurtful and that although the staff may lack clarity about her gender identity, she does not, and has always known she is a woman. She reports that friends who have come to visit her have also been made to feel uncomfortable.

ASSIGNMENT:

1. How best can you advocate for this patient?
2. What leadership roles could you employ to address the lack of compassion and advocacy for this patient with the staff?
3. What policies should be created to assure compliance with the U.S. Department of Health and Human Services mandate to protect the visitation rights of this patient's friends and significant others?

The government, in its role as the single largest insurer of health care, has also influenced the protection of patient rights by linking reimbursement with patient right provisions. For example, in 2011, the U.S. Department of Health and Human Services mandated that all hospitals that receive Medicare and Medicaid funding must protect the visitation rights of LGBTQ patients. As a result, hospitals must:

(1) inform each patient of their right to receive visitors whom they designate, including a domestic partner, (2) [not] restrict or limit visitation rights based on sexual orientation and gender identity, among other factors, and (3) ensure that all visitors have full and equal visitation rights, consistent with a patient's wishes. A hospital that fails to comply with these new requirements could be terminated from the Medicare program (The Human Rights Campaign, n.d.).

Learning Exercise 6.4 addresses the rights of LGBTQ patients.

There has also been significant progress in patient rights related to the privacy of health care information, including the *Health Insurance Portability and Accountability Act of 1996* (HIPAA). In addition, legislation—the American Recovery and Reinvestment Act of 2009—maintains and expands HIPAA guidelines as they are related to patient health information privacy and security protections.

States have also created bills of rights. In 1994, the Illinois General Assembly (n.d.) established a Medical Patient Rights Act that established certain rights for medical patients and provided a penalty for violations of these rights. California has adopted a similar patient guide pertaining to health care rights and remedies (Display 6.6). These guidelines, however, are not legally binding, although they may influence federal or state funding and certainly should be considered professionally binding.

Some legally binding legislation has been passed, however, to safeguard vulnerable populations. One such legislation, the *Genetic Information Nondiscrimination Act*, is a federal law passed in 2008, making it illegal for health insurers or employers to discriminate against individuals based on their genetic information (Genetics Home Reference, 2021).

Genetics Home Reference (2021) notes that the law has two parts: Title I, which prohibits genetic discrimination in health insurance, and Title II, which prohibits genetic discrimination in employment. Title I makes it illegal for health insurance providers to use or require genetic information to make decisions about a person's insurance eligibility or coverage. This part of the law went into effect on May 21, 2009. Title II makes it illegal for employers to

---

DISPLAY 6.6   LIST OF PATIENT RIGHTS IN CALIFORNIA

In accordance with Section 70707 of the California Administrative Code, patients have a right to:

1. Continuous care, second opinions, referrals, and information
2. Informed consent
3. Medical records and confidentiality
4. Emergency medical care
5. Coverage of preexisting conditions
6. File grievances with your health plan and the Department of Managed Health Care
7. Have your health maintenance organization's (HMO's) decisions independently reviewed and to sue your HMO
8. Appeal and litigate benefit denials under the Employee Retirement Income Security Act (ERISA)

Source: From Consumer Watchdog. (n.d.). *The California patient's guide. Your health care rights and remedies*. http://www.calpatientguide.org/index.html

---

use a person's genetic information when making decisions about hiring, promotion, and several other terms of employment. This part of the law went into effect on November 21, 2009 (para. 2–3).

The Right to Die Movement and Physician-Assisted Suicide

At times, individual rights must be superseded to ensure the safety of all parties involved. It is important, however, for the patient advocate to know the difference between controlling patient choices and assisting patients to choose. Health care professionals often have knowledge that patients do not have but must be careful not to use paternalism at the cost of patient autonomy.

> It is important for the patient advocate to be able to differentiate between controlling patient choices (domination and dependence) and assisting patient choices (allowing freedom).

For example, the right to die movement has gained momentum in the past decade. In 1997, Oregon became the first state to allow terminally ill people to receive lethal doses of medication from their doctors. By mid-2022, six other states (Colorado, Hawaii, Maine, New Jersey, New Mexico, and Washington), as well as the District of Columbia, had adopted a Death with Dignity Statute. California and Vermont passed amendments and enacted legislation instead (Death with Dignity, 2022). Multiple other states are considering legislation for *physician-assisted suicide* (PAS) as well.

Typically, right to die laws apply only to patients who are at least 18 years old, with the capacity to make medical decisions, with a terminal disease expected to result in death within 6 months. The California *End of Life Option Act*, which passed in 2016, requires the patient to make two verbal requests at least 15 days apart and one written request that is signed, dated, and witnessed by two adults (UCSF/UC Hastings Consortium, n.d.). The patient may rescind the request for an aid-in-dying drug at any time and in any manner, and a request for a prescription cannot be made on behalf of a patient through an agent under a power of attorney, an advance health care directive, a conservator, or any other person. Once the prescription is filled, the patient must complete a "Final Attestation for an Aid-in-Dying Drug to End My Life in a Humane and Dignified Manner" form (UCSF/UC Hastings Consortium, n.d.).

In addition, the patient must be the one to physically take the drug, though others can help prepare the drug and sit with the patient. Although the law is silent as to what cause of death should be identified on the death certificate, it does say taking an aid-in-dying drug shall not constitute suicide (UCSF/UC Hastings Consortium, n.d.).

Debates, however, around the impetus for and ethics of PAS continue to rage. Although many proponents characterize the action as a humane end to suffering, others note that advances in pain control and hospice care could alleviate some of the issues that lead terminally ill patients to seek PAS. It is not easy then to help patients and family members make decisions about PAS given the tension that often exists between promoting patient autonomy and the profound sense of loss that occurs when a loved one dies.

Physicians do have the legal right to choose whether they will participate in PAS. Physicians or facilities who do not participate in aid-in-dying must have a written policy that is given to patients, and can't prevent someone from referring patients to a physician who does participate (UCSF/UC Hastings Consortium, n.d.). Physicians who do participate are protected from criminal, civil, and administrative liability if they follow the requirements.

The bottom line is that patients are increasingly aware that they have rights, and as a result, they are more assertive and involved in their health care. They want to know and understand their treatment options and to be participants in decisions about their health care. Leader-managers have a responsibility to see that all patient rights are met, including the right to privacy and personal liberty, which are guaranteed by the Constitution.

Subordinate and Workplace Advocacy

Subordinate advocacy is a neglected concept in management theory but is an essential part of the leadership role. Standard 7 of the ANA (2016) *Nursing Administration: Scope and Standards of Practice* asserts that nurse administrators should advocate for other health care providers (including subordinates) as well as patients, especially concerning issues of health and safety.

For example, *workplace advocacy* is a critical role that managers assume to promote subordinate advocacy. In this type of advocacy, the manager assures that the work environment is both safe and conducive to professional and personal growth for subordinates. For example, managers should assure that Occupational Safety and Health Administration (OSHA) guidelines for worker safety are followed. Educating staff about proper body mechanics and assuring that staffing is adequate for safely ambulating and turning patients can reduce the incidence of back injuries in health care workers. In addition, occupational health and safety must be assured by interventions such as reducing worker exposure to workplace violence, needle sticks, or blood and body fluids. When these working conditions do not exist, managers must advocate to higher levels of the administrative hierarchy to correct the problems.

Workplace advocacy is also needed to address workplace violence, an ever-increasing problem in contemporary society but particularly in the health care system. The National Institute for Occupational Safety and Health (NIOSH, 2021) notes that workplace violence can occur anywhere and at any time, but certain groups of workers are at increased risk, including nurses. Indeed, Kokalias (2021) reported that 73% of nonfatal workplace injuries and illnesses causing days of missed work in health care are connected to workplace violence. In addition, the risk of workplace violence increased during the COVID-19 pandemic—because of stress and uncertainty about the future, resistance to vaccine and masking requirements, and frustration about strict hospital visitation requirements, both on the part of patients and staff.

As a result of this growing problem in health care, The Joint Commission introduced new workplace violence requirements, effective January 1, 2022. These requirements address how to better manage safety and security risks; the need to continually monitor, internally report and investigate incidents related to workplace violence; and how to create a safety culture (The Joint Commission, 2022).

Another area managers must advocate for subordinates is in the establishment of working conditions. Subordinates should be able to expect that their work hours and schedules will be reasonable, that staffing ratios will be adequate to support safe patient care, that wages will be fair and equitable, and that nurses will be allowed participation in organizational decision making.

When the health care industry has faced the crisis of inadequate human resources and nursing shortages, many organizations have made quick, poorly thought-out decisions to find short-term solutions to a long-term and severe problem. New workers have been recruited at a phenomenally high cost; yet the problems that caused high worker attrition were not solved. These decisions must be made carefully, following a thorough examination of the political, social, economic, and ethical costs.

Another way leaders advocate for subordinates is in creating a work environment that promotes risk taking and leadership. For example, administrators should foster work environments that promote subordinate empowerment so that workers have the courage to speak up for patients, themselves, and their profession. In addition, managers must help members of their health care team resolve ethical problems and work effectively with solutions at the unit level.

An organization's commitment to promoting nurse–patient advocacy is critically important. For example, nurses have a unique vantage point in witnessing the human consequences of organizational policies that either impede or promote optimal patient outcomes. Nurses can mediate between providers and patients when treatment recommendations are at odds with patient concerns and beliefs since regular, direct contact with patients and families helps nurses better understand cultural beliefs and potential barriers to successful treatment (The Importance of Nursing Advocacy, 2021).

For example, Shoemark and Foran (2021) note that perioperative patients are made vulnerable by anesthesia when they are temporarily unable to act on their own behalf. Perioperative nurses must be protectors from harm and human rights activists. There are, however, barriers to perioperative nurse advocacy and the creation of a safety culture including hierarchy and communication constraints (see Examining the Evidence 6.2).

Health care administrators then must maintain an effective and efficient chain of command so that nurses know where to report concerns and how to access the chain of command. The following are suggestions for creating an environment that promotes subordinate advocacy:

- Invite collaborative decision making.
- Listen to staff needs.
- Get to know staff personally.

EXAMINING THE EVIDENCE 6.2

Source: From Shoemark, T., & Foran, P. (2021). Identifying barriers to patient advocacy in the promotion of a safety culture: An integrative review. *Journal of Perioperative Nursing, 34*(2), e-36–e-42.

Barriers to Advocacy in Perioperative Nursing

An electronic database search of the literature was conducted to identify barriers to effective patient advocacy in perioperative settings. The study found that preoperative patients expected all the information pertaining to their care would be made available when they arrived. When gaps in information occurred, distrust and fear built, and patient outcomes were negatively impacted.

Nurses perceived themselves as important in filling these gaps to build trust, and by gathering all the necessary information, they put themselves in a position to protect their patients from harm. Through acts of advocacy, nurses execute their responsibility and moral obligation to promote the rights of their patients and to provide the highest standard of safe patient care.

Hierarchy in the perioperative environment, often between nurses and physicians, and a fear of blame, however, impeded nurses from acting in the advocacy role. The researchers noted that the ability of perioperative nurses to speak up on behalf of their patients was paramount in the operating suite where patients are vulnerable and often unable to speak for themselves.

This research highlighted the complexities of the perioperative team environment. Open communication and nonpunitive approaches to risk reporting were recognized as key characteristics influencing the perioperative climate and the establishment of a safety culture.

- Take time to understand the challenges faced by the staff in delivering care.
- Face challenges and solve problems together.
- Support staff as needed.
- Promote shared governance.
- Empower staff.
- Promote nurse autonomy.
- Provide staff with workable systems.

Managers must recognize what subordinates are striving for and the goals and values that subordinates consider appropriate. The leader-manager should be able to guide subordinates toward actualization while defending their right to autonomy. To help nurses deal with ethical dilemmas in their practice, nurse-managers should establish and utilize appropriate support groups, ethics committees, and channels for dealing with ethical problems.

LEARNING EXERCISE 6.5

How Can You Best Advocate?

You are a unit supervisor in a skilled nursing facility. One of your aides, Martha Greenwald, recently reported that she suffered a "back strain" several weeks ago when she was lifting an older adult patient. She did not report the injury at the time because she did not think it was serious. Indeed, she finished the remainder of her shift and has performed all her normal work duties since that time.

Today, Martha reports that she has just left her physician's office and that he has advised her to take 4 to 6 weeks off from work to fully recover from her injury. He has also prescribed physical therapy and electrical nerve stimulation for the chronic pain. Martha is a relatively new employee, so she has not yet accrued enough sick leave to cover her absence. She asks you to complete the paperwork for her absence and that the cost of her treatments be covered as a work-related injury.

When you contact the workers' compensation case manager for your facility, she states that the claim will be investigated; however, with no written or verbal report of the injury at the time it occurred, there is great likelihood that the claim will be rejected.

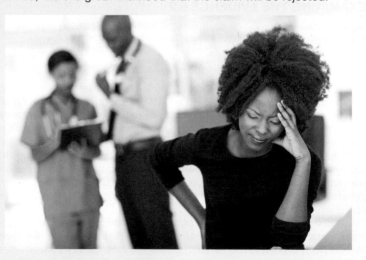

ASSIGNMENT:

How best can you advocate for this subordinate?

Whistleblowing as Advocacy

The public has become much more aware of ethical malfeasance within its institutions and corporate organizations because of various scandals that have occurred in the last 50 years. Wrongdoing does not stop at large corporations or political activity, however; it also occurs within health care organizations. Huston argues that in an era of managed care, declining reimbursements, and the ongoing pressure to remain fiscally solvent, the risk of fraud, misrepresentation, and ethical malfeasance in health care organizations have never been higher. As a result, the need for *whistleblowing* has also likely never been greater.

Huston (2023d) explains that there are two basic types of whistleblowing. *Internal whistleblowing* occurs within an organization, reporting up the chain of command. *External whistleblowing* involves reporting outside the organization such as to the media or elected officials. An example of whistleblowing by a health care provider might be to report inflated practices of documentation and coding that result in elevated cost reimbursement.

Nurses as health care professionals have a responsibility to uncover, openly discuss, and condemn shortcuts, which threaten the clients they serve (Huston, 2023d). It is important, however, to remember that whistleblowing should rarely be considered the first solution to ethically troubling behavior. Indeed, it should be considered only after other prescribed avenues of solving problems have been attempted. The exception is when patients' lives are at stake. In those cases, immediate action must be taken.

In addition, the employee should typically go up the chain of command in reporting concerns, unless the immediate supervisor is the source of the problem. In such a case, the employee might need to skip that level to see that the problem is addressed. Indeed, most whistleblowers would rather raise the issue internally to their manager than take it outside. Thus, companies generally get the opportunity to resolve issues internally—the question is whether they will take this opportunity or miss it.

There are other general guidelines for blowing the whistle that should be followed, including carefully documenting all attempts to address the problem and being sure to report facts and not personal interpretations. These guidelines, as well as others, are presented in Display 6.7.

Unfortunately, although much of the public wants wrongdoing or corruption to be reported, some look on this behavior with distrust, and whistleblowers may be considered disloyal or experience repercussions for their actions, even if the whistleblowing was done with the best of intentions. Indeed, most whistleblowers set out believing that their actions will be welcomed, only to discover that the problems raised go much deeper than they imagined, and the personal consequences can be overwhelming. The whistleblower cannot even trust that other health care professionals, with similar belief systems about advocacy, will value their efforts because the public's feelings about whistleblowers are so mixed (Huston, 2023d).

> Speaking out as a whistleblower is often honored more in theory than in fact.

Leader-managers must be willing to advocate for whistleblowers so that they feel assured that if they are acting within the scope of their expertise, they can seek remedy through appropriate channels without fear of retaliation. Unfortunately, there has been a collective silence in many cases of ethical malfeasance. The reality is that whistleblowing offers no guarantee that the situation will change, or the problem will improve, and the literature is replete with horror stories of negative consequences endured by whistleblowers. For all these reasons, it takes tremendous courage to come forward as a whistleblower. It also takes an exceptional sense of what is right and what is wrong as well as a commitment to follow a problem through until an acceptable level of resolution is reached (Huston, 2023d).

DISPLAY 6.7 **GUIDELINES FOR BLOWING THE WHISTLE**

- Stay calm and think about the risks and outcomes before you act.
- Know your legal rights because laws protecting whistleblowers vary by state.
- First, make sure that there really is a problem. Check resources such as the medical library, the Internet, and institutional policy manuals to be sure.
- Seek validation from colleagues that there is a problem, but do not get swayed by groupthink into not doing anything if you should.
- Follow the chain of command in reporting your concerns whenever possible.
- Confront those accused of the wrongdoing as a group whenever possible.
- Present just the evidence; leave the interpretation of facts to others. Remember that there may be an innocent or good explanation for what is occurring.
- Use internal mechanisms within your organization.
- If internal mechanisms do not work, use external mechanisms.
- Private groups, such as The Joint Commission or the National Committee for Quality Assurance, do not confer protection. You must report to a state or national regulator.
- Although it is not required by every regulatory agency, it is a good rule of thumb to put your complaint in writing.
- Document carefully the problem that you have seen and the steps that you have taken to see that it is addressed.
- Do not lose your temper, even if those who learn of your actions attempt to provoke you.
- Do not expect thanks for your efforts.

Source: From Huston (2023d); American Nurses Association (ANA). (n.d.). *Things to know about whistle blowing.*
https://www.nursingworld.org/practice-policy/workforce/things-to-know-about-whistle-blowing/

Although whistleblower protection has been advocated at the federal level and has passed in some states, many employees are reluctant to report unsafe conditions for fear of retaliation. Nurses should check with their state association to assess the status of whistleblower protection in their state. At present, there is no federal legal protection for whistleblowers in the United States.

Professional Advocacy

Leader-managers also must be advocates for the nursing profession. This type of advocacy has a long history in nursing. It was nurses who pushed for accountability through state Nurse Practice Acts and state licensing, although this was not accomplished until 1903. Advocating for professional nursing is a leadership role.

Joining a profession requires making a personal decision to involve oneself in a system of socially defined roles. Thus, entry into a profession involves a personal and public promise to serve others with the special expertise that a profession can provide, and that society legitimately expects it to provide.

Professional issues are always ethical issues. When nurses find a discrepancy between their perceived role and society's expectations, they have a responsibility to advocate for the profession. At times, individual nurses believe that the problems of the profession are too big for them to make a difference; however, their commitment to their profession obligates them to ask questions and think about problems that affect the profession. They cannot afford to become powerless or helpless or claim that one person cannot make a difference. Often, one voice is all it takes to raise the consciousness of colleagues within a profession. Accepting the challenge to be an advocate for the profession is a choice.

For example, the COVID-19 pandemic brought forth significant and frightening threats to patient and nurse safety. Morin and Baptiste (2020) report that nurses took to the streets (including in front of the White House) to protest the lack of needed personal protective equipment

LEARNING EXERCISE   6.6

Write It Down. How Can You Advocate?

ASSIGNMENT:

Write a two-page essay about one of the following topics:
1. List five things that you would like to change about nursing or the health care system. Prioritize the changes that you have identified. Identify the strategies that you could use individually and collectively as a profession to make the change happen. Be sure that you are realistic about the time, energy, and fiscal resources you have to implement your plan.
2. Do you belong to your state nursing organization or student nursing organization? Why or why not? Make a list of six other things that you could do to advocate for the profession. Be specific and realistic in terms of your energy and commitment to nursing as a profession.

and unsafe working conditions (high patient to nurse staffing ratios). Nurses also engaged in counter-protests, reading the names of nurses who had been infected with or died because of COVID-19, while facing protesters who were rallying for lifting lockdown and stay-at-home orders. Morin and Baptiste (2020) maintain that these nurses should be applauded for taking a stand and for being activists at a time when support from leaders and colleagues may have been limited, or even absent.

> A professional commitment means that people cannot shrink from their duty to question and contemplate problems that face the profession.

Nursing's Advocacy Role in Legislation and Public Policy

A distinctive feature of American society is how citizens can participate in the political process. People have the right to express their opinions about issues and candidates by voting. People also have relatively easy access to lawmakers and policy makers and can make their individual needs and wants known. Theoretically, then, any one person can influence those in policy-making positions. This rarely happens, however; policy decisions are generally focused on group needs or wants.

In addition to active participation in national nursing organizations, nurses can influence legislation and health policy in other ways. Ferguson (2021) labels changing practice barriers with legislation or practice rules as "upstream advocacy." With upstream advocacy, nurses can correct problems before they reach the client, including changes that make things better for the nurse as well. Nurses who want to be directly involved can lobby legislators either in person or by letter. This process may seem intimidating to the new nurse; however, there are many books and workshops available that deal with the subject, and a common format is used.

Personal letters are more influential than form letters, and the tone should be formal but polite. The letter should also be concise (not more than one page). Be sure to address the legislator properly by title. Establish your credibility early in the letter as both a constituent and a health care expert. State your reason for writing the letter in the first paragraph and refer to the specific bill that you are writing about. Then, state your position on the issue and give personal examples as necessary to support your position. Offer your assistance as a resource person for additional information. Sign the letter, including your name and contact information.

DISPLAY 6.8   SAMPLE: A LETTER TO A LEGISLATOR

March 15, 2024
The Honorable John Doe
Member of the Senate
State Capitol, Room _____
City, State, Zip Code

Dear Senator Doe,

I am a registered nurse and member of the American Nurses Association (ANA). I am also a constituent in your district. I am writing in support of SB XXX, which requires the establishment of minimum registered nurse (RN) staffing ratios in acute care facilities. As a staff nurse on an oncology unit in our local hospital, I see firsthand the problems that occur when staffing is inadequate to meet the complex needs of acutely ill patients: medical errors, patient and nurse dissatisfaction, workplace injuries, and perhaps most important, the inability to spend adequate time with and comfort patients who are dying.

I have enclosed a copy of a recent study conducted by John Smith that was published in the January 2023 edition of *Nurses Today*. This article details the positive impact of legislative staffing ratio implementation on patient outcomes as measured by medication errors, patient falls, and nosocomial infection rates.

I strongly encourage you to vote for SB XXX when it is heard by the Senate Business and Professions Committee next week. Thank you for your ongoing concern with nursing and health care issues and for your past support of legislation to improve health care staffing. Please feel free to contact me if you have any questions or would like additional information.

Respectfully,
Nancy Thompson, RN, BSN
Street
City, State, Zip Code
Phone number including area code
E-mail address

Remember to be persistent and write to legislators repeatedly who are undecided on an issue. Display 6.8 presents a format common to letters written to legislators.

Other nurses may choose to monitor the progress of legislation, count congressional votes, and track a specific legislator's voting intents as well as past voting records. Some nurses may choose to join network groups, where colleagues meet to discuss professional issues and pending legislation. Nurses can also influence legislators through social media.

For nurses interested in a more indirect approach to professional advocacy, their role may be to influence and educate the public about nursing and the nursing agenda to reform health care. This may be done by speaking with professional and community groups about health care and nursing issues and by interacting directly with the media. Never underestimate the influence that a single nurse may have even in writing letters to the editor of local newspapers or by talking about nursing and health care issues with friends, family, neighbors, teachers, clergy, and civic leaders.

In addition, there is a need for collective influence to impact health care policy. The need for organized group efforts by nurses to influence legislative policy has long been recognized in this country. In fact, the first state associations were organized expressly for unifying nurses to influence the passage of state licensure laws.

The nursing profession, however, has not yet recognized the full potential of collective political activity. Nurses must exert their collective influence and make their concerns known to policy makers before they can have a major impact on political and legislative outcomes. Because they have been reluctant to become politically involved, nurses have failed to have a strong legislative voice in the past. Legislators and policy makers are more willing to deal with nurses as a group rather than as individuals; thus, joining and supporting professional organizations allow nurses to become active in lobbying for a stronger nurse practice act or for the creation or expansion of advanced nursing roles.

> Nurses must exert their collective influence and make their concerns known to policy makers before they can have a major impact on political and legislative outcomes.

Political action committees (PACs) attempt to persuade legislators to vote in a particular way. Lobbyists of the PAC may be members of a group interested in a specific law or paid agents of the group that wants a specific bill passed or defeated. Nursing must become more actively involved with PACs to influence health care legislation, and PACs provide one opportunity for small donors to feel like they are making a difference.

In addition, professional organizations generally espouse standards of care that are higher than those required by law. Voluntary controls often are forerunners of legal controls. What nursing is and should be depends on nurses taking an active part in their professional organizations. Currently, nursing lobbyists in our nation's capital are influencing legislation on quality of care, access to care issues, patient and health worker safety, health care restructuring, direct reimbursement for advanced practice nurses, and funding for nursing education to be sure that the nursing perspective is heard in health policy issues.

Nursing and the Media

Although registered nurses are among the most knowledgeable, frontline health care providers, their interactions with mainstream media are often limited. This is because too few nurses are willing to interact with the media about vital nursing and health care issues. Often, this is because they believe that they lack the expertise to do so or because they lack self-confidence. This is especially unfortunate because both the media and the public place a high trust in nurses and want to hear about health care issues from a nursing perspective.

The reality is that the responsibility for nursing's image as perceived by the public lies solely on the shoulders of those who claim nursing as their profession. Until nurses can agree on the desired collective image and are willing to do what is necessary to both tell and show the public what that image is, little will change (Huston, 2023a). Nurses should take every opportunity to appear in the media—in newspapers, radio, and television. Nurses should also complete special training programs to increase their self-confidence in working with journalists and other media representatives.

Regardless, the first few media interactions will likely be stressful, just like any new task or learning. The following tips may be helpful to nurses learning to navigate media waters:

- Dress professionally for the interview.
- Remember that reporters often have short deadlines. A delay in responding to a reporter's request for an interview usually results in the reporter looking elsewhere for a source.
- Do not be unduly paranoid that the reporter "is out to get you" by inaccurately representing what you have to say. The reporter has a job to do, and most reporters do their best to be fair and accurate in their reporting.
- Come to the interview prepared with any statistics, important dates and times, anecdotes, or other information you want to share.
- Limit your key points to two or three and frame them as bullet points to reduce the likelihood that you will be misheard or misinterpreted. Brief but concise sound bites are much more quotable than rambling arguments.
- Avoid technical or academic jargon.
- Speak with credibility and confidence but do not be afraid to say that you do not know if asked a question beyond your expertise or which would be better answered by someone else. If you choose not to answer a question, give a brief reason for not wanting to do so rather than simply saying "no comment."

DISPLAY **6.9** **TIPS FOR INTERACTING WITH THE MEDIA**

1. Establish proactive, routine communication with local, regional, and national media to promote cooperation and transparency.
2. Attend media training and/or practice speaking in front of a camera with a microphone.
3. Dress professionally for interviews.
4. Respect and meet the reporter's deadlines.
5. Assume, until proven otherwise, that the reporter will be fair and accurate in their reporting.
6. Have key facts and figures ready for the interview.
7. Limit your key points to two or three and frame them as bullet points.
8. Avoid technical or academic jargon.
9. Speak confidently but do not be afraid to say when you do not have the expertise to answer a question or when a question is better directed to someone else.
10. Avoid being pulled into inflammatory arguments or blame setting and repeat key points if you are pulled off into tangents.
11. Provide the reporter with contact information for follow-up and needed clarifications.

- Avoid being pulled into inflammatory arguments or blame setting. If you feel that you have been baited or that you are being pulled off on tangents, simply repeat the key points you intended to make and refocus the conversation if possible. Remember that you cannot control the questions you are asked, but you can control your responses.
- Be prepared to respond to follow-up media inquiries via e-mail. Provide contact information so that the reporter can reach you if additional information or clarifications are needed. Be aware, however, that most reporters will not allow you to preview their story prior to publication.

These strategies are summarized in Display 6.9.

LEARNING EXERCISE **6.7**

Preparing for a Media Interview

You are the staffing coordinator for a medium-sized community hospital in California. Minimum staffing ratios were implemented in January 2004. Although this has represented an even greater challenge in terms of meeting your organization's daily staffing needs, you believe that the impetus behind the legislative mandate was sound. You also are a member of the state nursing association that sponsored this legislation and wrote letters of support for its passage. The hospital that employs you and the state hospital association fought unsuccessfully against the passage of minimum staffing ratios.

The local newspaper contacted you this morning and wants to interview you about staffing ratios in general as well as how these ratios are impacting the local hospital. You approach your chief nursing officer, and she tells you to go ahead and do the interview if you want but to remember that you are a representative of the hospital.

ASSIGNMENT:

Assume that you have agreed to participate in the interview.
1. How might you go about preparing for the interview?
2. Identify three factual points that you can state during the interview as your sound bites. What would be your primary points of emphasis?
3. Is there a way to reconcile the conflict between your personal feelings about staffing ratios and those of your employer? How would you respond if asked directly by the reporter to comment about whether staffing ratios are a good idea?

Integrating Leadership Roles and Management Functions in Advocacy

Nursing leader-managers recognize that they have an obligation not only to advocate for the needs of their patients, subordinates, and themselves but also to be active in furthering the goals of the profession. To accomplish these types of advocacies, nurses must value autonomy and empowerment.

However, the leadership roles and management functions to achieve advocacy with patients and subordinates and for the profession differ greatly. Advocating for patients requires that the manager create a work environment that recognizes patients' needs and goals as paramount. This means creating a work culture where patients are respected, well informed, and empowered. The leadership role required to advocate for patients is often one of risk taking, particularly when advocating for a client who may be in direct conflict with a provider or institutional goal. Leaders must also be willing to accept and support patient choices that may be different from their own.

Advocating for subordinates requires that the manager create a safe and equitable work environment where employees feel valued and appreciated. When working conditions are less than favorable, the manager is responsible for relaying these concerns to higher levels of management and advocating for needed changes.

The same risk taking that is required in patient advocacy is a leadership role in subordinate advocacy because subordinate needs and wants may conflict with the organization. There is always a risk that the organization will view the advocate as a troublemaker, but this is not an excuse for managers to be complacent in this role. Managers also must advocate for subordinates in creating an environment where ethical concerns, needs, and dilemmas can be openly discussed and resolved.

Advocating for the profession requires that the nurse-manager be informed and involved in all legislation affecting the unit, organization, and the profession. The manager must also be an astute handler of public relations and demonstrate skill in working with the media. It is the leader, however, who proactively steps forth to be a role model and an active participant in educating the public and improving health care through the political process.

 ## Key Concepts

- Advocacy is helping others to grow and self-actualize and is a leadership role.
- Managers, by virtue of their many roles, must be advocates for patients, subordinates, and the profession.
- It is important for the patient advocate to be able to differentiate between controlling patient choices (domination and dependence) and assisting patient choices (allowing freedom).
- Since the 1960s, advocacy groups, professional associations, and states have passed bills of rights for patients. Although these are not legally binding, they can be used to guide professional practice.

- The philosophy of person- and family-centered care suggests that care should be organized primarily around the needs of patients and family members.
- In workplace advocacy, the manager works to see that the work environment is both safe and conducive to professional and personal growth for subordinates.
- Although much of the public wants wrong-doing or corruption to be reported, such behavior is often looked on with distrust, and whistleblowers are often considered disloyal and experience negative repercussions for their actions.

- Leader-managers must be willing to advocate for whistleblowers who speak out about organizational practices that they believe may be harmful or inappropriate.
- Professional issues are ethical issues. When nurses find a discrepancy between their perceived role and society's expectations, they have a responsibility to advocate for the profession.
- If nursing is to advance as a profession, practitioners and managers must broaden their sociopolitical knowledge base to better understand the bureaucracies in which they live.
- Because legislators and policy makers are more willing to deal with nurses as a group rather than as individuals, joining and actively supporting professional organizations allow nurses to have a greater voice in health care and professional issues.
- Nurses need to exert their collective influence and make their concerns known to policy makers before they can have a major impact on political and legislative outcomes.
- Nurses have great potential to educate the public and influence policy through the media because of the public's high trust in nurses and because the public wants to hear about health care issues from a nursing perspective.

Additional Learning Exercises and Applications

LEARNING EXERCISE 6.8

Ethics and Advocacy

You are a new graduate staff nurse in a home health agency. One of your clients is a 23-year-old man with acute schizophrenia who was just released from the local county, acute care, behavioral health care facility, following a 72-hour hold. He has no insurance. His family no longer has contact with him, and he is unable to hold a permanent job. He is nonadherent in taking his prescription drugs for schizophrenia. He is homeless and has been sleeping and eating intermittently at the local homeless shelter; however, he was recently asked not to return because he is increasingly agitated and, at times, violent. He calls you today and asks you "to help him with the voices in his head."

You approach the senior registered nurse (RN) case manager in the facility for help in identifying options for this individual to get the behavioral health care services that he needs. She suggests that you tell the patient to go to Maxwell's Mini Mart, a local convenience store, at 3:00 PM today and wait by the counter. Then she tells you that you should contact the police at 2:55 PM and tell them that Maxwell's Mini Mart is being robbed by your patient so that he will be arrested. She states, "I do this with all of my uninsured mental health patients, since the state Medicaid program offers only limited mental health services and the state penal system provides full mental health services for the incarcerated." She goes on to say that the store owner and the police are aware of what she is doing and support the idea because it is the only way "patients really have a chance of getting better." She ends the conversation by saying, "I know you are a new nurse and don't understand how the 'real world' works, but the reality is that this is the only way I can advocate for patients like this, and you need to do the same for your patients."

ASSIGNMENT:

1. Will you follow the advice of the senior RN case manager?
2. If not, how else can you advocate for this patient?

LEARNING EXERCISE 6.9

Determining Nursing's Entry Level

Grandfathering is the term used to grant certain people working within the profession for a given time or prior to a deadline date the privilege of applying for a license without having to take the licensing examination. Grandfathering clauses have been used to allow licensure for wartime nurses—those with on-the-job training and expertise—even though they did not graduate from an approved school of nursing.

Some professional nursing organizations are once again proposing that the Bachelor of Science in Nursing (BSN) become the entry-level requirement for professional nursing. Some have suggested that as a concession to current associate degree in nursing and diploma-prepared nurses, all nurses who have passed the registered nursing licensure examination before the new legislation, regardless of educational preparation or experience, would retain the title of professional nurse. Nonbaccalaureate-educated nurses after that time would be unable to use the title of professional nurse.

ASSIGNMENT:

Do you believe that the "BSN as entry level" proposal advocates the advancement of the nursing profession? Is grandfathering conducive to meeting this goal? Would you personally support both proposals? Does the long-standing internal dissension about making the BSN the entry level into professional nursing reduce nursing's status as a profession? Do lawmakers or the public understand this dilemma or care about it? How might you personally become more involved in speaking out about or advocating your position?

LEARNING EXERCISE 6.10

How Would You Proceed?

You are a registered nurse case manager for a large insurance company. Sheila Johannsen is a 34-year-old mother of two small children. She was diagnosed with advanced metastatic breast cancer 6 months ago. Traditional chemotherapy and radiation seem to have slowed the spread of the cancer, but the prognosis is not good.

Sheila contacted you this morning to report that she has been in contact with a physician at one of the most innovative medical centers in the country. He told her that she might benefit from an experimental gene therapy treatment; however, she is ineligible for participation in the free clinical trials because her cancer is so advanced. The cost for the treatment is approximately $350,000. Sheila states that she does not have the financial resources to pay for the treatment and begs you "to do whatever you can to get the insurance company to pay; otherwise, I'll die."

You know that the cost of experimental treatments is almost always disallowed by Sheila's insurance company. You also know that even with the experimental treatment, Sheila's probability of a cure is very small.

ASSIGNMENT:

Decide how you will proceed. How can you best advocate for this patient?

LEARNING EXERCISE 6.11

Conflict of Values

You are a case manager in an outpatient disease management program assigned to coordinate the care needs of Sam, a 72-year-old man with multiple chronic health problems. His medical history includes myocardial infarctions, implantation of a pacemaker, open-heart surgery, an inoperable abdominal aneurysm, and repeated episodes of congestive heart failure. Because of his poor health, he cannot operate the small business he owns or work for any length of time at his gardening or other hobbies.

Although Sam has told you that death would be a relief to his nearly constant discomfort and depression, his wife dismisses such talk as "nonsense" and tells Sam that she still needs him and will always do everything in her power to keep him here with her. In deference to his wife's wishes, Sam has not completed any of the legal paperwork necessary to create a durable power of attorney or a living will should he become unable to make his own health care decisions. Today, Sam takes you aside and tells you that he "wants to fill out this paperwork so that no extraordinary means of life support are used," and he "wants you to witness it so that his wife will not know."

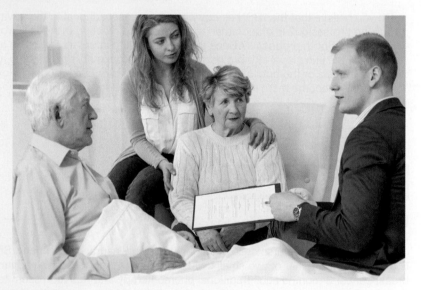

ASSIGNMENT:

Decide what you will do. What is your obligation to Sam? To his wife? To yourself? Whose needs are paramount? How do the ethical principles of autonomy, duty, and veracity intersect or compete in this case?

LEARNING EXERCISE 6.12

Peer Advocacy

You are a nursing student. Like many of the students in your nursing program, sometimes you feel that you study too much and therefore miss out on partying with friends, something many of your college friends do on a regular basis. Today, after a particularly grueling examination, three of your nursing school peers approach you and ask you to go out with them to a party tonight, off campus, which is being cohosted by Matt, another nursing student. Alcohol will be readily available, although not everyone at the party is of legal drinking age, including you and one of your nursing peers (Jenny). Because you really do not want to drink anyway, you agree to be the designated driver.

Almost immediately after you arrive at the party, all three of your nursing peers begin drinking. At first, it seems pretty harmless, but after several hours, you decide the tenor of the party is changing and becoming less controlled and that it is time to take your friends home. Two of your peers agree, but you cannot find Jenny. As you begin searching for her, several partygoers tell you that she has been drinking all night and that she "looked pretty wasted" the last time they saw her. They suggest that you check the bathroom because Jenny said she was not feeling very well.

When you enter the bathroom, you see Jenny slumped in the corner by the toilet. She has vomited all over the floor as well as her clothing and she reeks of alcohol. When you attempt to rouse her, her eyelids flutter but she is unable to wake up or answer any questions. Her breathing seems regular and unlabored, but she is continuing to vomit in her "blacked-out" state. Her skin feels somewhat clammy, and she cannot stand or walk on her own. You are not sure how much Jenny actually had to drink or how long it has been since she "passed out."

You are worried that Jenny is experiencing acute alcohol poisoning but are not very experienced with this sort of thing. The other two nursing students you brought to the party feel that you are overreacting, although they agree that Jenny has had too much to drink and needs to be watched. One of your peers suggests calling an older classmate in the nursing program, who offered just the other day to provide rides to students who have been drinking. You think she might be able to provide some guidance. Another one tells you that she feels Jenny just needs to "sleep it off" and that she will stay with Jenny tonight to make sure she is OK, although she has had a fair amount to drink herself.

You think Jenny should be seen in the local emergency department (ED) for treatment and are contemplating calling for an ambulance. One partygoer agrees with you that Jenny should be seen at the hospital but suggests that you drop Jenny off anonymously at the front door of the ED so "you won't get in any trouble." Matt encourages you not to take her to the ED at all because he is afraid the incident will be reported to the local police because Jenny is a minor and that he could be in "real trouble" for furnishing alcohol to a minor. He argues that this could threaten both his progression and Jenny's in the nursing program. He says that she can just stay at the house tonight and that he will check on her on a regular basis.

To complicate things, you, Jenny, and the other two students you brought to the party live in the college dormitories and they lockdown for the evening in another 30 minutes. It will take you at least 20 minutes to gather the manpower you need to get Jenny down to your car and up to her dormitory room by lockdown, if that is what you decide to do. If you are not inside the dormitories by lockdown, you will need to find another place to spend the evening. In addition, there will likely be someone at the door to the dormitory assigned to turn away students who are clearly intoxicated.

ASSIGNMENT:

Decide what you will do. How do you best advocate for a peer when they are unable to advocate for themselves? Does it matter if the risk is self-induced? How do you weigh the benefits of advocating for one person when it can result in potential harm or risk to another person?

REFERENCES

Agency for Healthcare Research and Quality. (2017). *Guide to patient and family engagement in hospital quality and safety.* Retrieved August 17, 2021, from http://www.ahrq.gov/professionals/systems/hospital/engagingfamilies/index.html

American Cancer Society. (2022). *Patient's Bill of Rights.* Retrieved June 18, 2022 from https://www.cancer.org/treatment/finding-and-paying-for-treatment/managing-health-insurance/patients-bill-of-rights.html

American Hospital Association. (2021). *Engaging health care users: A framework for healthy individuals and communities.* http://www.aha.org/research/cor/engaging/index.shtml

American Nurses Association. (2015). *Code of ethics for nurses with interpretive statements.*

American Nurses Association. (2016). *Nursing administration: Scope and standards of practice* (2nd ed.).

American Nurses Association. (2021). *Nursing: Scope and standards of practice* (4th ed.).

Burke, S. A., & Nickitas, D. M. (2023). Health and public policy: The influence and power of nursing (chapter 25). In C. Huston (Ed.), *Professional issues in nursing: Challenges and opportunities* (6th ed., pp. 370–391). Philadelphia: Wolters Kluwer.

Death with Dignity. (2022). *Resources.* https://deathwithdignity.org/learn/

Eastern Illinois University. (2021, January 27). *The importance of nursing advocacy.* https://learnonline.eiu.edu/articles/rnbsn/importance-of-nursing-advocacy.aspx

Ferguson, S. (2021, April). The building blocks of advocacy: Beyond exceptional advocacy for patients, how do nurses advocate for the profession and better health care? *New Mexico Nurse, 66*(2), 1–5.

The Free Dictionary by Farlex. (2003–2021). Advocacy. Retrieved August 13, 2021, from http://www.thefreedictionary.com/advocacy

Genetics Home Reference. (2021). *What is genetic discrimination?* https://ghr.nlm.nih.gov/primer/testing/discrimination

The Human Rights Campaign. (n.d.). *Hospital visitation guide for LGBTQ families.* https://www.hrc.org/resources/hospital-visitation-guide-for-lgbt-families

Huston, C. J. (2023a). Professional identity and image (chapter 24). In C. J. Huston (Ed.), *Professional issues in nursing: Challenges and opportunities* (6th ed., pp. 353–369). Wolters Kluwer.

Huston, C. J. (2023b). Technology in healthcare (chapter 21). In C. J. Huston (Ed.), *Professional issues in nursing: Challenges and opportunities* (6th ed., pp. 302–318). Wolters Kluwer.

Huston, C. J. (2023c). The nursing profession's historic struggle to increase its power base (chapter 23). In C. J. Huston (Ed.), *Professional issues in nursing: Challenges and opportunities* (6th ed., pp. 338–352). Wolters Kluwer.

Huston, C. J. (2023d). Whistle-blowing in nursing (chapter 17). In C. J. Huston (Ed.), *Professional issues in nursing: Challenges and opportunities* (6th ed., pp. 248–261). Wolters Kluwer.

Illinois General Assembly. (n.d.). *Medical Patient Rights Act.* http://www.ilga.gov/legislation/ilcs/ilcs3.asp?ActID=1525&ChapterID=35

Institute for Healthcare Improvement. (2021). *Person- and family-centered care.* http://www.ihi.org/Topics/PFCC/Pages/Overview.aspx

Institute for Patient- and Family-Centered Care. (n.d.). *Patient- and family-centered care.* http://www.ipfcc.org/about/pfcc.html

The Joint Commission. (2022). *Workplace violence prevention resources.* https://www.jointcommission.org/resources/patient-safety-topics/workplace-violence-prevention/

Kaleka, K., & Perzhinsky, J. M. (2020). The case for medication-assisted treatment: An ethical priority. *Psychiatric Times, 37*(10). Retrieved August 13, 2022 from https://www.psychiatrictimes.com/view/case-medication-assisted-treatment-ethical-priority

Kokalias, A. E. (2021, August 9). *New workplace violence prevention requirements coming in 2022.* https://www.jointcommission.org/resources/news-and-multimedia/blogs/dateline-tjc/2021/08/new-workplace-violence-prevention-requirements-coming-in-2022/

MedlinePlus. (2020, December 2). *Patient rights.* http://www.nlm.nih.gov/medlineplus/patientrights.html

Morin, K. H., & Baptiste, D. (2020). Nurses as heroes, warriors and political activists. *Journal of Clinical Nursing, 29*(15/16), 2733.

National Institute for Occupational Safety and Health. (2021, August). *eNews: Volume 18, Number 12.* Centers for Disease Control and Prevention. https://www.cdc.gov/niosh/enews/enewsv18n12.html

Planetree. (2021). *History of Planetree.* https://www.planetree.org/certification/about-planetree

Shoemark, T., & Foran, P. (2021). Identifying barriers to patient advocacy in the promotion of a safety culture: An integrative review. *Journal of Perioperative Nursing, 34*(2), e-36–e-42.

Thomas, K., Gebeloff, R., & Silver-Greenberg, J. (2021, August 11). Phony diagnoses hide high rates of drugging at nursing homes. *New York Times.* https://www.nytimes.com/2021/09/11/health/nursing-homes-schizophrenia-antipsychotics.html?campaign_id=9&emc=edit_nn_20210912&instance_id=40234&nl=the-morning&regi_id=128435702&segment_id=68744&te=1&user_id=5959ad8f4f1b62be2691e7495867c967

UCSF/UC Hastings Consortium. (n.d.). *Understanding California's end of life option act.* https://health.ucdavis.edu/huntingtons/files/CA-End-of-Life-Options-Act-UCHastings-summary.pdf

Roles and Functions in Planning

7

Organizational Planning

… in the absence of clearly defined goals, we are forced to concentrate on activity and ultimately become enslaved by it.—**Chuck Conradt**

… people buy into the leader long before they buy into the vision.—**Neslyn Watson Druee**

… a goal without a plan is just a wish.—**Antoine de Saint-Exupéry**

CROSSWALK

This chapter addresses:

- **AACN Essentials Domain 1:** Knowledge for nursing practice
- **AACN Essentials Domain 2:** Person-centered care
- **AACN Essentials Domain 4:** Scholarship for nursing practice
- **AACN Essentials Domain 5:** Quality and safety
- **AACN Essentials Domain 6:** Interprofessional partnerships
- **AACN Essentials Domain 7:** Systems-based practice
- **AACN Essentials Domain 8:** Information and health care technologies
- **AACN Essentials Domain 10:** Personal, professional, and leadership development
- **AONL Nurse Executive Competency 2:** A knowledge of the health care environment
- **AONL Nurse Executive Competency 3:** Leadership
- **AONL Nurse Executive Competency 5:** Business skills
- **ANA Standard of Professional Performance 11:** Collaboration
- **ANA Standard of Professional Performance 12:** Leadership
- **ANA Standard of Professional Performance 13**: Education
- **ANA Standard of Professional Performance 14:** Scholarly inquiry
- **ANA Standard of Professional Performance 15:** Quality of practice
- **ANA Standard of Professional Performance 17:** Resource stewardship
- **ANA Standard of Professional Performance 18:** Environmental health
- **QSEN Competency:** Teamwork and collaboration
- **QSEN Competency:** Evidence-based practice

LEARNING OBJECTIVES

The learner will:

- identify contemporary paradigm shifts and trends impacting health care organizations
- analyze social, political, and cultural forces that may affect the ability of 21st-century health care organizations to forecast accurately in strategic planning
- describe how tools such as SWOT analysis and balanced scorecards can facilitate the strategic planning process
- describe the steps necessary for successful strategic planning
- identify barriers to planning as well as actions the leader-manager can take to reduce or eliminate these barriers

- include evaluation checkpoints in organizational planning to allow for midcourse corrections as needed
- discuss the relationship between an organizational mission statement, philosophy, goals, objectives, policies, procedures, and rules
- write an appropriate mission statement, organization philosophy, nursing service philosophy, goals, and objectives for a known or fictitious organization
- discuss appropriate actions that may be taken when personal values conflict with those of an employing organization
- recognize the need for periodic value clarification to promote self-awareness
- reflect on which personal planning style (reactive, inactive, preactive, or proactive) is used most often

Introduction

Planning is critically important to and precedes all other management functions. Without adequate planning, the management process fails, and organizational needs and objectives cannot be met. *Planning* may be defined as deciding in advance what to do; who is to do it; and how, when, and where it is to be done. Therefore, all planning involves choosing among alternatives.

> All planning involves choice: a necessity to choose from among alternatives.

This implies that planning is a proactive and deliberate process that reduces risk and uncertainty. It also encourages unity of goals and continuity of energy expenditure (human and fiscal resources) and directs attention to the objectives of the organization. Adequate planning also provides the manager with some means of control and encourages the most appropriate use of resources.

In effective planning, the manager must identify short- and long-term goals and changes needed to ensure that the unit will continue to meet its goals. Identifying such short- and long-term goals requires leadership skills such as vision and creativity because it is impossible to plan what cannot be dreamed or envisioned.

Likewise, planning requires flexibility and energy—two other leadership characteristics. Yet, planning also requires management skills such as data gathering, forecasting, and transforming ideas into action.

Unit III focuses on several aspects of planning, including organizational planning, planned change, time management, fiscal planning, and career planning. This chapter deals with skills needed by the leader-manager to implement both day-to-day and future organizational planning. In addition, the leadership roles and management functions involved in developing, implementing, and evaluating the planning hierarchy are discussed (Display 7.1).

Visioning: Looking to the Future

Because of health care reform, rapidly changing technology, increasing government involvement in regulating health care, and scientific advances, health care organizations are finding it increasingly difficult to identify long-term needs appropriately and plan accordingly. In fact, most long-term planners find it difficult to plan more than a few years ahead.

> Unlike the 20-year strategic plans of the 1960s and 1970s, most long-term planners today find it difficult to look even 5 years in the future.

DISPLAY 7.1   LEADERSHIP ROLES AND MANAGEMENT FUNCTIONS ASSOCIATED WITH ORGANIZATIONAL PLANNING

Leadership Roles

1. Translates knowledge regarding contemporary paradigm shifts and trends impacting health care into vision and insights, which foster goal attainment
2. Assesses the organization's internal and external environment in forecasting and identifying driving forces and barriers to strategic planning
3. Demonstrates visionary, innovative, and creative thinking in organizational and unit planning, thus inspiring proactive rather than reactive planning
4. Influences and inspires group members to be actively involved in both short- and long-term planning
5. Periodically completes value clarification to increase self-awareness
6. Encourages subordinates toward value clarification by actively listening and providing feedback
7. Communicates and clarifies organizational goals and values to subordinates
8. Encourages subordinates to be involved in policy formation, including developing, implementing, and reviewing unit philosophy, goals, objectives, policies, procedures, and rules
9. Is receptive to new and varied ideas
10. Role models proactive planning methods to followers

Management Functions

1. Is knowledgeable regarding legal, political, economic, and social factors affecting health care planning
2. Demonstrates knowledge of and uses appropriate techniques in both personal and organizational planning
3. Provides opportunities for subordinates, peers, competitors, regulatory agencies, and the general public to participate in organizational planning
4. Coordinates unit-level planning to be congruent with organizational goals
5. Periodically assesses unit constraints and assets to determine available resources for planning
6. Develops and articulates a unit philosophy that is congruent with the organization's philosophy
7. Develops and articulates unit goals and objectives that reflect unit philosophy
8. Develops and articulates unit policies, procedures, and rules that put unit objectives into operation
9. Periodically reviews unit philosophy, goals, policies, procedures, and rules and revises them to meet the unit's changing needs
10. Actively participates in organizational planning, defining, and operationalizing plans at the unit level

The problem is that the health care system is in chaos, as is much of the business world. Traditional management solutions no longer apply, and a lack of strong leadership in the health care system has at times, limited the innovation needed to create solutions to the new and complex problems the future will bring. For example, Herzlinger and Richman (2021) note that the COVID-19 pandemic exposed severe shortcomings in hospital financing. Many hospitals in hotspot areas could not provide an adequate supply of hospital beds; yet, even when filled to capacity, many hospitals suffered severe revenue losses. This should never occur in a well-working market when demand exceeds supply (Herzlinger & Richman, 2021).

Brown (2021, para. 1) agrees, noting that the year 2020 was full of unbelievable statistics and powerful events. "No one predicted the year we experienced—one that jolted the entire world and will impact health care institutions for years to come. We need to thank the workers in our industry and acknowledge the burnout many have felt. At the same time, we need to emerge from crisis mode and plan for uncertainty."

> Health care leaders must remain farsighted to create a transition to the better system of tomorrow, even as they navigate current crises (Herzlinger & Richman, 2021).

Because change can occur so rapidly, managers can easily become focused on short-range plans and miss changes that can drastically alter specific long-term plans. Health care facilities are particularly vulnerable to external social, economic, and political forces; long-range planning, then, must address these changing dynamics. It is imperative, therefore, that long-range plans be flexible, permitting change as external forces assert their impact on health care facilities. Whenever possible, a picture of the future should be used to formulate long-range planning. This process of learning about the future allows us to determine what we want to happen. Identifying what may or could happen allows us to avert, encourage, or direct the course of events.

There are many factors emerging in the rapidly changing health care system that must be incorporated in planning for a health care organization's future. Some emerging paradigms are outlined below:

- Further consolidation of hospitals/systems, medical groups, ancillary services, health plans, and postacute providers is expected.
- The tension between "value" and "volume" has driven growing linkages between expected quality outcomes and reimbursement. Health care organizations must increasingly determine whether value drives volume or whether volume is necessary to achieve value.
- The transformation from *revenue management* to *cost management* will continue as declining reimbursement forces providers to focus on how to maximize limited resources and provide care at less cost.
- *Physician integration*, an interdependence between physicians and health care organizations (typically hospitals) that may involve employment, as well as shared decision making and mutual goal setting, is changing practice patterns and reimbursement patterns as hospitals increasingly assume more of the financial and liability risks for what was historically private physician practice.
- Scientific breakthroughs and technologic advancements in precision diagnostics, precision medicine, patient monitoring, and drug discovery and delivery for targeted therapies will pave the way for patient-centric care and a shift from the field's focus on illness to sustaining health and well-being (American Hospital Association [AHA], 2022a).
- Technology, which facilitates mobility and portability of relationships, interactions, and operational processes, will increasingly be a part of high-functioning organizations. Electronic health records (EHRs) and clinical decision support are examples of such technology because both impact not only what health care data is collected but also how it is used, communicated, and stored.
- The introduction and use of robotic pharmacists will have both positive and negative effects on the entire pharmacy industry (RPH On the Go, 2020).
- The International Classification of Diseases, 10th revision (ICD-10), pricing, information technology (IT), in-patient volumes, physician relationships, and physician recruitment will increasingly become intertwined.
- The rising cost of pharmaceuticals and ongoing drug shortages will continue to be a problem for US hospitals.
- Health care systems will continue to move toward managing populations rather than individuals and will need to integrate long-term care and extended care into their continuum of care.
- The ongoing movement away from illness care to wellness care and the use of disease management programs will continue to reduce the demand for expensive acute care services.
- The use of *complementary and alternative medicine* will increase as public acceptance and demand for these services increase.

- The interdependence of professionals and the need for *interprofessional collaboration* rather than professional autonomy will continue. Thus, the autonomy for all health care professionals will decrease, including managers.
- The shift in framework to the patient as a consumer of cost and quality information will continue. Quality data will be increasingly public, and transparency regarding organizational effectiveness (quality and costs) will be a public expectation. Indeed, new hospital price transparency rules went into effect on January 2021. The Centers for Medicare & Medicaid Services (CMS) believes price disclosure will help the public make more informed decisions about their care, increase market competition, and drive down costs of care (Brown, 2021).
- A transition from continuity of provider to continuity of information will continue.
- The health care team will be characterized by highly educated, multidisciplinary experts. Although this would appear to ease the leadership challenges of managing such a team, it is far easier to build teams of experts than to build expert teams.

In addition, Huston (2023) suggests the following factors will further influence the future of health care:

- Robotic technology and the use of prototype nurse robots called *nursebots* will serve as an adjunct to scarce human resources in the provision of health care.
- *Biomechatronics*, which creates machines that replicate or mimic how the body works, will increase in prominence in the future.
- *Biometrics*, the science of identifying people through physical characteristics such as fingerprints, handprints, retinal scans, voice recognition, and facial structure, will be used to assure targeted and appropriate access to client records.
- Health care organizations will integrate biometrics with "smart cards" (credit card–sized devices with a chip, stored memory, and an operating system) to ensure that an individual presenting a secure ID credential really has the right to use that credential.
- *Point-of-care testing* will improve bedside care and promote more positive outcomes because of more timely decision making and treatment.
- Technology-aided options, such as telehealth, will continue to grow exponentially, resulting in a huge influx of data coming into the health care system. Traditional working hours will be offset by this virtual technology, increasing patient access but making it increasingly difficult for providers to disconnect from all the digital domains (Frieden, 2021).
- The internet will continue to improve Americans' health by enhancing communications and improving access to information for care providers, patients, health plan administrators, public health officials, biomedical researchers, and other health professionals. It will also change how providers interact with patients with consumers increasingly adopting the role of *expert patient*.
- An aging workforce, improving economy, inadequate enrollment in nursing schools to meet projected demand, increased employment of nurses in outpatient or ambulatory care settings, and inadequate long-term pay incentives will lead to new nursing shortages.

Such paradigm shifts and changing trends occur almost constantly. Successful leader-managers stay abreast of the dynamic environments in which health care is provided so that this can be reflected in their planning. The result is proactive or visionary planning that allows health care agencies to function successfully in the 21st century.

For example, the National Institutes of Health (NIH, 2021) released their strategic plan for fiscal years 2021–2025, expanding the definition of integrative health to include whole person health, that is, empowering individuals, families, communities, and populations to improve their health in multiple interconnected domains: biologic, behavioral, social, and environmental. The plan was informed and shaped by an effort to better define and map a path to whole person health by expanding and building on current activities while advancing new research strategies and ideas.

Forces Affecting Health Care

In small groups, identify six additional forces, beyond those identified in this chapter, affecting today's health care system. You may include legal, political, economic, social, or ethical forces. Try to prioritize these forces in terms of how they will affect you as a manager or registered nurse. For at least one of the six forces you have identified, brainstorm how that force would affect your strategic planning as a unit manager or director of a health care agency.

Proactive Planning

Planning has a specific purpose and is one approach to developing strategy. In addition, planning represents specific activities that help achieve objectives; therefore, planning should be purposeful and proactive. Although there is always some crossover between types of planning within organizations, there is generally an orientation toward one of four planning modes: reactive planning, inactivism, preactivism, or proactive planning.

Reactive planning occurs *after* a problem arises. Because there is dissatisfaction with the current situation, planning efforts are directed at returning the organization to a previous, more comfortable state. Frequently, in reactive planning, problems are dealt with separately without integration with the whole organization. In addition, because it is done in response to a crisis, this type of planning can lead to hasty decisions and mistakes.

Inactivism is another type of conventional planning. Inactivists seek the status quo, and they spend their energy preventing change and maintaining conformity. When changes do occur, they occur slowly and incrementally.

A third planning mode is *preactivism*. Preactive planners utilize technology to accelerate change and are future-oriented. Unsatisfied with the past or present, preactivists do not value experience and believe that the future is always preferable to the present.

> Proactive planning is dynamic, and adaptation is considered a key requirement because the environment changes so frequently.

The last planning mode is *interactive* or *proactive planning*. Planners who fall into this category consider the past, present, and future and attempt to plan the future of their organization rather than react to it. Because the organizational setting changes often, adaptability is a key requirement for proactive planning.

One example of recent, successful organizational proactive planning was the hiring and staffing of physician hospitalists by the Texas Health Physicians Group (THPG) in Fort Worth early in the COVID-19 pandemic (Rausch, 2021). Although low patient volumes led some hospitalist

What Is Your Planning Style?

How would you describe your planning? Is your planning more likely to be reactive, inactive, preactive, or proactive? Write a brief essay that describes your most-used planning style. Use specific examples and then share your insights in a group.

groups to cut back on staffing in early 2020, THPG made the decision not to cancel any shifts or cut back on staffing because they did not want their hospitalists to be impacted negatively by things that were out of their control and because future projections suggested patient volumes could increase dramatically and quickly. As hospitals began creating new COVID units and COVID patient volumes increased during the last quarter of 2020, THPG was able to ensure there were adequate physicians available to take care of hospitalized patients.

Another example of proactive planning critical to organizational success is *supply chain management*. Supply chain management refers to managing the flow of products and services to maximize quality, delivery, customer experience, and profitability (IBM, n.d.). In the first step, proactive planners determine the resources required to meet customer demand for an organization's products or services. Then they choose suppliers to provide the goods and services. The next step is organizing the activities required to accept the products or services in terms of delivery logistics and assuring they meet quality standards. Finally, the supply chain manager must receive the products, pay for them, and charge system users to cover their costs (IBM, n.d.).

It was clear when the COVID pandemic began growing in early 2020 that proactive supply chain management had not occurred. While governments and private sector organizations did have disaster plans and stockpiles in place, the pandemic exposed several major supply chain vulnerabilities, including shortages of personal protective equipment (PPE) and testing kits (Mahmoodi et al., 2021). Other shortages included N95 masks, isolation gowns, nitrile gloves, syringes, sharps containers, and some drugs. In some cases, this occurred because of shortages of raw materials or delivery logistics, but often, demand simply exceeded supply. The shortages brought abrupt price increases, an increase in counterfeit products with unacceptable quality levels, and long delays in receiving goods and services. Even the World Health Organization released a statement on March 5, 2020, warning that global supply chain disruptions for PPE left health workers dangerously ill-equipped for handling the pandemic (Mahmoodi et al., 2021).

Mahmoodi et al. (2021) note that proactive planning will be needed to strengthen and stabilize the health care supply chain for the future. Health care organizations and pharmaceutical companies will need to assess which strategies can help them mitigate supply chain disruptions during major emergencies without incurring exorbitant costs. They will need to build redundancy in the supply chain, increase surge capacity, and diversify the supply base. While some organizations will emerge from the pandemic as more agile and innovative, others will "just assume that COVID-19 was a 'one-off' public health crisis and choose to not adjust their proactive supply chain planning—an approach that increases risk and squanders an important learning opportunity" (Mahmoodi et al., 2021, para. 35).

Forecasting

A mistake common to novice managers is a failure to complete adequate proactive planning. Instead, many managers operate in a crisis mode and fail to use available historical patterns to assist them in planning or they fail to examine present clues and projected statistics to determine future needs. In other words, they fail to forecast. *Forecasting* involves trying to estimate how a condition will be in the future. Forecasting takes advantage of input from others, gives sequence in activity, and protects an organization against undesirable changes.

For example, Brown (2021) argues that health care leaders must consider the economic recovery, corporate taxes, and mergers and acquisitions as they develop health care financial forecasts. They must also rethink old processes, timeframes, and assumptions. As a result, many health care organizations are now using shorter timeframes and reforecasting quarterly (Brown, 2021).

The manager who is unwilling or unable to forecast accurately impedes the organization's efficiency and the unit's effectiveness. Increased competition, changes in government reimbursement, and decreased hospital revenues have reduced intuitive managerial decision making. To avoid disastrous outcomes when making future professional and financial plans, managers need to stay well informed about the legal, political, and socioeconomic factors affecting health care.

> Managers who are uninformed about the legal, political, economic, and social factors affecting health care make planning errors that may have disastrous implications for their professional development and the financial viability of the organization.

Strategic Planning at the Organizational Level

Planning has many dimensions. Two of these dimensions are time span and complexity or comprehensiveness. In general, complex organizational plans that involve a long period (usually 3 to 7 years) are referred to as *long-range* or *strategic* plans. However, strategic planning may be done once or twice a year in an organization that changes rapidly. At the unit level, any planning that is at least 6 months in the future may be considered long-range planning.

Unfortunately, many organization leaders focus heavily on short-term goals and expectations. Although this is important, it is equally—if not more—important to emphasize longer-term objectives. Leader-managers who adopt long-term strategies eventually help their organizations become more profitable and have happier employees and shareholders.

Strategic planning at the organizational level then must consider both the short- and long-term goals and needs of the organization. In doing this, strategic planning can forecast the future success of an organization by matching and aligning an organization's capabilities with its external opportunities. For instance, an organization could develop a strategic plan for dealing with a nursing shortage, preparing succession managers in the organization, developing a marketing plan, redesigning workload, developing partnerships, or simply planning for organizational success.

> Strategic planning typically examines an organization's purpose, mission, philosophy, and goals in the context of its external environment.

Some experts suggest, however, that the need for increased operational efficiencies has required a reconfiguration of how strategic planning is done in most health care organizations. Instead of focusing on the external environment and the marketplace, health care organizations need to look closely at their competencies and weaknesses, examine their readiness for change, and identify those factors critical to achieving future goals and objectives.

This assessment should begin with gathering data related to financial performance, human resources, strategy, and service offerings as well as outcomes and results. Feedback from senior leadership, the medical staff, and the board is then needed so that consensus can be obtained from stakeholders regarding the organization's strengths and weaknesses. Then, an action plan can be created that strengthens the organization's infrastructure. The assessment concludes with an evaluation of how well the organization is achieving its goals and objectives and the process begins once again.

SWOT Analysis

There are many effective tools that assist health care organizations in strategic planning. One of the most used is *SWOT analysis*, also known as *TOWs analysis*. SWOT is an acronym for the identification of strengths, weaknesses, opportunities, and threats (Display 7.2). Internal factors, aspects over which an organization has control, generally govern strengths and weaknesses. External factors, influences over which organizations have little to no control, govern opportunities and threats (Sudhakaran, 2020).

DISPLAY 7.2 SWOT DEFINITIONS

Strengths are those *internal* attributes that help an organization to achieve its objectives.
Weaknesses are those *internal* attributes that pose barriers to an organization achieving its objectives.
Opportunities are *external* conditions that promote achievement of organizational objectives.
Threats are *external* conditions that challenge or threaten the achievement of organizational objectives.

The first step in SWOT analysis is to define the desired end state or objective. After the desired objective is defined, the SWOTs are discovered and listed. Decision makers must then decide if the objective can be achieved in view of the SWOTs. If the decision is no, a different objective is selected and the process repeats. An example of an abbreviated SWOT process is shown in Display 7.3, and a brief SWOT analysis is summarized in Examining the Evidence 7.1.

Performed correctly, SWOT analysis allows strategic planners to identify those issues most likely to impact a particular organization or situation in the future and then to develop an appropriate plan for action. Several simple rules, however, should be followed for SWOT analysis to be successful, and these are shown in Display 7.4.

DISPLAY 7.3 EXAMPLE OF ABBREVIATED SWOT PROCESS

Desired End State or Objective: Hospital Z wishes to increase the number of nurses with baccalaureate and graduate degrees in the staffing mix.

Strengths

1. Local schools of nursing offer online baccalaureate and master's degrees at affordable costs for working nurses.
2. Hospital Z offers generous professional development funding opportunities for staff.
3. This objective is in alignment with recommendations cited in the Institute of Medicine's report, *The Future of Nursing: Leading Change, Advancing Health*, that 80% of registered nurses should have baccalaureate or higher degrees by 2020.

Weaknesses

1. Recent high turnover rates have resulted in tight staffing, and requests by nurses for reduced workloads to return to school would be difficult to honor.
2. At present, there is no role differentiation for nurses at Hospital Z based on a nurse's educational level.
3. At present, Hospital Z does not offer a salary differential to nurses with baccalaureate or higher degrees, but another hospital in the immediate area does.

Opportunities

1. Current research evidence suggests that increasing the number of nurses with baccalaureate or higher degrees in the staffing mix would positively impact quality of care.
2. Hospital Z could consider application for Magnet status if more nurses held higher degrees.
3. Increasing the number of nurses with baccalaureate and graduate degrees better prepares them to assume new and emerging professional roles in an increasingly complex health care environment.
4. A review of the literature suggests that nurses with graduate degrees are more likely to report being extremely satisfied with their jobs compared with nurses who hold associate degrees.

Threats

1. Local schools of nursing have impacted enrollments, so not all nurses who want to return to school can be accepted.
2. An impending national nursing shortage could further exacerbate current staffing shortages.
3. Not all nurses are inherently motivated to return to school.

EXAMINING THE EVIDENCE 7.1

Source: From Stoller, J. K. (2021). A perspective on the educational "SWOT" of the Coronavirus pandemic. *Chest, 159*(2), 743–748.

Educational Implications of the COVID-19 Pandemic: A SWOT Analysis

The coronavirus pandemic disrupted clinical practice, health care organizations, and life (weaknesses and threats). As disruptive as the pandemic was to traditional practices—both clinically and educationally—strengths and opportunities were also presented. This paper completed a SWOT analysis (strengths, weaknesses, opportunities, and threats) on the implications for higher education, specifically graduate medical education (GME), related to the coronavirus pandemic.

Clinical benefits (strengths) of the COVID-19 pandemic included the propulsion of clinical innovation, including items such as the development of novel vaccines and accelerated understanding of multiplex ventilation. There were educational strengths as well. These included growing experience with virtual teaching and virtual learning strategies, the invitation to codify best virtual teaching practices, a tightening of alignment between undergraduate and GME (e.g., around virtual interview strategies), and opportunities for both self-reflection and a commitment to act virtuously. In addition, the pandemic accelerated hybrid models for student and trainee onboarding.

Approaches to educating students and other learners, however, changed radically, with the suspension of live teaching in most instances, and a precipitous transition to virtual instruction occurred. There were obvious disadvantages (weaknesses) with the loss of face-to-face interaction (e.g., isolation, risks to camaraderie, loss of hands-on training opportunities, and loss of in-person celebratory events like graduations and end-of-training celebrations). In addition, for some students the home learning environment was distracting (e.g., noise, kids' needs, many competing demands) and not conducive to high-quality learning.

Opportunities included the push to develop novel virtual teaching methods, to develop online methods to showcase medical schools and graduate medical education (GME) programs and to interview when travel was no longer possible, to develop novel vaccines with unprecedented speed, to invent new basic ventilators, and to develop multiplex ventilation strategies.

Threats and challenges were embedded in the weaknesses. Did the pandemic and the precipitous transition to virtual work do irreparable damage to the camaraderie of the learning environment? For those averse to virtual work, either because of technical challenges or the deep need for live interaction with colleagues, result in a loss of program interest or withdrawal?

The researchers concluded that on balance, the pandemic created the opportunity, indeed the necessity, to innovate in practice and in education, making the landscape ripe for creative practice, new mastery, and the concomitant benefits to learners and to educators.

DISPLAY 7.4 SIMPLE RULES FOR SWOT ANALYSIS

- Be objective and reflective about the strengths and weaknesses of your organization. These should reflect consumer perceptions.
- Be inclusive regarding external stakeholders and the broader environment when considering threats and opportunities.
- Organizations and environments continually change; a reassessment of SWOT is needed when major change occurs.
- Be specific about what you want to learn in the SWOT analysis and what motives are driving you to carry out the process.
- Keep SWOT analysis short and simple. Statements should be precise and unambiguous.

Balanced Scorecard

Balanced scorecard, developed by Robert Kaplan and David Norton in the early 1990s, is another tool that is highly assistive in strategic planning. Strategic planners using a balanced scorecard develop *metrics* (performance measurement indicators), collect data, and analyze that data from four organizational perspectives: financial, customers, internal business processes (or simply processes), and learning and growth. Because all the measures are related and are assumed to eventually lead to outcomes, an overemphasis on financial measures is avoided. The scorecard then is "balanced" in its outcomes.

Balanced scorecards also allow organizations to align their strategic activities with the strategic plan. The best balanced scorecards are not a static set of measurements but instead reflect the dynamic nature of the organizational environment. Because the balanced scorecard can translate strategy into action, it is an effective tool for translating an organization's strategic vision into clear and realistic objectives.

Strategic Planning as a Management Process

Although SWOT analysis and balanced scorecard are different, they both can help organizations assess what they do well and what they need to do to continue to be effective and financially sound. Many other strategic planning tools exist as well, although they are not discussed in this text. Regardless of the tool(s) used, strategic planning as a management process generally includes the following steps:

1. Clearly define the purpose of the organization.
2. Establish realistic goals and objectives consistent with the mission of the organization.
3. Identify the organization's external constituencies or stakeholders and then determine their assessment of the organization's purposes and operations.
4. Clearly communicate the goals and objectives to the organization's constituents.
5. Develop a sense of ownership of the plan.
6. Develop strategies to achieve the goals.
7. Ensure that the most effective use is made of the organization's resources.
8. Provide a base from which progress can be measured.
9. Provide a mechanism for informed change as needed.
10. Build a consensus about where the organization is going.

It should be noted, though, that some critics argue that strategic planning is rarely linear nor is it static. Strategic planning instead involves various actions and reactions that are partially planned and partially unplanned. As such, strategic plans must be adaptable and flexible, so they can respond to changes in both internal and external environments.

Who Should Be Involved in Strategic Planning?

Long-range planning for health care organizations historically was accomplished by top-level managers and the board of directors, with limited input from middle-level managers. More contemporary strategies, however, suggest the need to seek input from subordinates from all organizational levels to give the strategic plan meaning and to increase the likelihood of its successful implementation.

All organizations should establish annual strategic planning conferences, involving all departments and levels of the hierarchy; this action should promote increased effectiveness of nursing staff; better communication between all levels of personnel; a cooperative spirit relative to solving problems; and a pervasive feeling that the departments are unified, goal-directed, and doing their part to help the organization accomplish its mission.

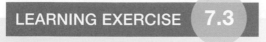

LEARNING EXERCISE 7.3

Making a Long-Term Plan

The human resource manager in the facility where you are a supervisor has just completed a survey of the potential retirement plans of the nursing staff and found that within 5 years, 45% of the staff will probably be retiring. You know that past and present available statistics show that you normally replace 10% to 15% of your staff each year with new hires. You are concerned as you do not know how you will be able to handle this new increase in your need for staff.

ASSIGNMENT:

Make a 5-year, long-term plan that will increase the likelihood of you being able to meet this new demand. Remember that other units within your facility and other health care organizations in your region may also be facing the same problem.

Organizational Planning: The Planning Hierarchy

There are many types of planning; in most organizations, these plans form a hierarchy, with the plans at the top influencing all the plans that follow. As depicted in the pyramid in Figure 7.1, the hierarchy broadens at lower levels, representing an increase in the number of planning components. Planning components at the top of the hierarchy are more general, and lower components are more specific.

Vision and Mission Statements

Vision statements are used to describe future goals or aims of an organization. They are written descriptions that conjure up a picture for all group members of what they want to accomplish together. According to Prichard (2018), the most consequential leaders throughout history were able to both communicate their vision skillfully and personify it: "At the summit of

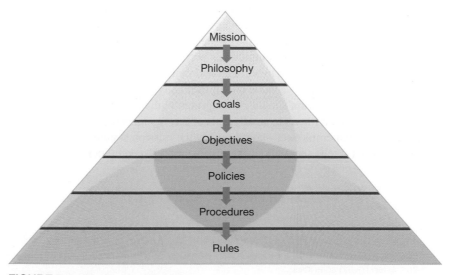

FIGURE 7.1 The planning hierarchy.

DISPLAY 7.5 **SAMPLE VISION STATEMENT**

DISPLAY 7.5 **SAMPLE VISION STATEMENT**

County Hospital will be the leading center for trauma care in the region.

influence, their every action, gesture or word moves into service of their greater cause. This is at once an extraordinary accomplishment, opportunity, and burden. It requires a unity of life and work, of thought and action, an overarching integrity" (para. 17). It is critical, then, that organization leaders recognize that the organization will never be greater than the vision that guides it.

When leaders share strong visions, employees flock to them. These visions permeate the workplace and are manifested in the actions, beliefs, values, and goals of everyone in the organization. In addition, leaders must demonstrate passion when sharing vision, because a person must have both passion and purpose to have influence (Huston, 2020).

A fictional vision statement for a hospital is shown in Display 7.5.

> An organization will never be greater than the vision that guides it.

The *purpose* or *mission statement* is a brief statement (typically no more than three or four sentences) identifying the reason that an organization exists. The mission statement identifies the organization's constituency and addresses its position regarding ethics, principles, and standards of practice.

A well-written mission statement will identify what is unique about the organization. For example, all hospitals want to have high-quality, patient-centered, cost-effective care, but mission statements that include only this verbiage do not differentiate between organizations. The mission statement should clearly drive action if it is to be a template of purpose for the organization. In addition, it can be challenging to meet an ambitious mission in an era of cost-cutting and limited resources; hence, the often-stated adage, "No margin, no mission."

An example of a mission statement for County Hospital, a fictional teaching hospital, is shown in Display 7.6.

The mission statement is of highest priority in the planning hierarchy because it influences the development of an organization's philosophy, goals, objectives, policies, procedures, and rules. Managers employed by County Hospital would have two primary goals to guide their planning: (a) to provide high-quality, evidence-based care and (b) to provide learning opportunities for students in medicine, nursing, and other allied health sciences. To meet these goals, adequate fiscal and human resources would have to be allocated for preceptorships and clinical research. In addition, an employee's performance appraisal would examine the worker's performance in terms of organizational and unit goals.

Mission statements have value only if they truly guide the organization. Actions taken at all levels of the organization should be congruent with the organization's stated mission. Therefore, involving individuals from all levels of the organization in crafting mission statements is crucial. Potential employees should review the mission statement of potential employers and consider what it tells them about the organization's stakeholders and what beliefs and values

DISPLAY 7.6 **SAMPLE MISSION STATEMENT**

County Hospital is a tertiary care facility that provides comprehensive, holistic care to all state residents who seek treatment. The purpose of County Hospital is to combine high-quality, evidence-based care with the provision of learning opportunities for students in medicine, nursing, and allied health sciences.

LEARNING EXERCISE 7.4

No Margin, No Mission?

You are a nurse team leader in Jamestown Hospital, an acute care, for-profit hospital. The mission statement for Jamestown Hospital states that the hospital has two primary purposes: (a) to provide the highest possible quality of care for its clients and (b) to maximize the efficiency and cost-effectiveness of resource utilization in recognition of its obligation to internal and external stakeholders.

Recently, you have become increasingly concerned regarding what you perceive to be the economically motivated, premature discharge of patients with chronic diseases. You know that some patients with diabetes or heart failure yield little, if any, profit for the organization. You are well acquainted with the discharge planner on the unit, and both of you have discussed your concerns with each other, but neither of you have taken any action.

ASSIGNMENT:

Do you feel the dual goal mission statement is in conflict? As a registered nurse, do you feel you can influence the discharge process? How do you plan on handling the conflict you are beginning to feel regarding these early discharges? What alternatives are available to you in deciding what, if anything, to do?

are espoused. Only then can the potential employee determine whether this is an organization they want to work for.

> An organization must truly believe and act on its mission statement; otherwise, the statement has no value.

Organizational Philosophy

The *philosophy* flows from the purpose or mission statement and delineates the set of values and beliefs that guide all actions of the organization. The foundation directs all further planning toward that mission. A statement of philosophy can usually be found in policy manuals at the institution or is available upon request. A philosophy that might be generated from County Hospital's mission statement is shown in Display 7.7.

DISPLAY 7.7 SAMPLE PHILOSOPHY STATEMENT

The board of directors, medical and nursing staff, and administrators of County Hospital believe that human beings are unique due to different genetic endowments; personal experiences in social and physical environments; and the ability to adapt to biophysical, psychosocial, and spiritual stressors. Thus, each patient is considered a unique individual with unique needs. Identifying outcomes and goals, setting priorities, prescribing strategy options, and selecting an optimal evidence-based strategy for care will be negotiated by the patient, physician, and health care team.

As unique individuals, patients provide medical, nursing, and allied health students invaluable diverse learning opportunities. Because the board of directors, medical and nursing staff, and administrators believe that the quality of health care provided directly reflects the quality of the education of its future health care providers, students are welcomed and encouraged to seek out as many learning opportunities as possible. Because high-quality health care is defined by and depends on technologic advances and scientific discovery, County Hospital encourages research as a means of scientific inquiry.

DISPLAY 7.8   SAMPLE NURSING SERVICE PHILOSOPHY

The philosophy of nursing at County Hospital is based on respect for the individual's dignity and worth. We believe that all patients have the right to receive effective, evidence-based nursing care. This care is a personal service that is based on patients' needs and their clinical diseases or conditions.

Recognizing the obligation of nursing to help restore patients to the best possible state of physical, mental, and emotional health and to maintain patients' sense of spiritual and social well-being, we pledge multidisciplinary collaboration in coordinating nursing service with the medical and allied professional practitioners. Understanding the importance of research and teaching for improving patient care, the nursing department will support, promote, and participate in these activities. Using knowledge of human behavior, we shall strive for mutual trust and understanding between nursing service and nursing employees to provide an atmosphere for developing the fullest possible potential of each member of the nursing team. We believe that nursing personnel are individually accountable to patients and their families for the quality and compassion of the patient care rendered and for upholding the standards of care as delineated by the nursing staff.

The *organizational philosophy* provides the basis for developing nursing philosophies at the unit level and for nursing service collectively. Written in conjunction with the organizational philosophy, the *nursing service philosophy* should address fundamental beliefs about nursing and nursing care; the quality, quantity, and scope of nursing services; and how nursing specifically will meet organizational goals. Frequently, the nursing service philosophy draws on the concepts of holistic care, education, and research. The nursing service philosophy in Display 7.8 builds on County Hospital's mission statement and organizational philosophy.

The *unit philosophy*, adapted from the nursing service philosophy, specifies how nursing care provided on the unit will correspond with nursing service and organizational goals. This congruence in philosophy, goals, and objectives among the organization, nursing service, and unit is shown in Figure 7.2.

Although unit-level managers have limited opportunity to help develop the organizational philosophy, they are active in determining, implementing, and evaluating the unit philosophy. In formulating this philosophy, the unit manager incorporates knowledge of the unit's internal and external environments and an understanding of the unit's role in meeting organizational goals. The manager must understand the planning hierarchy and be able to articulate ideas both verbally and in writing. Leader-managers also must be visionary, innovative, and creative in identifying unit purposes or goals so that the philosophy not only reflects current practice but also incorporates a view of the future.

LEARNING EXERCISE   7.5

Developing a Philosophy Statement

Recover Inc., a fictitious for-profit home health agency, provides complete nursing and supportive services for in-home care. Services include skilled nursing, bathing, shopping, physical therapy, occupational therapy, meal preparation, housekeeping, speech therapy, and social work. The agency provides around-the-clock care, 7 days a week, to a primarily underserved rural area in Northern California. The brochure the company publishes says that it is committed to satisfying the needs of the rural community and that it is dedicated to excellence.

ASSIGNMENT:

Based on this limited information, develop a brief philosophy statement that might be appropriate for Recover Inc. Be creative and embellish information if appropriate.

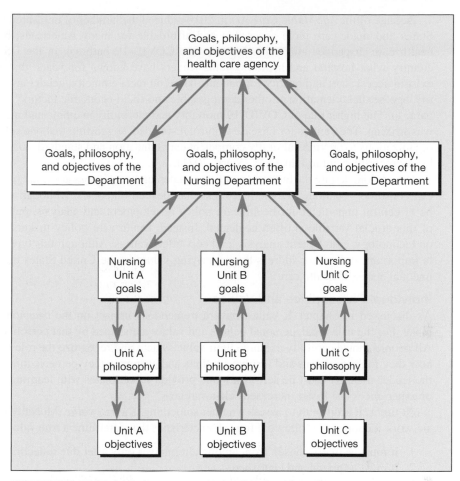

FIGURE 7.2 Philosophical congruence in the planning hierarchy.

Like the mission statement, statements of philosophy in general can be helpful only if they truly direct the work of the organization toward a specific purpose. A department's decisions, priorities, and accomplishments reflect its working philosophy.

> A working philosophy is evident in a department's decisions, in its priorities, and in its accomplishments.

A person should be able to identify exactly how the organization is implementing its stated philosophy by observing members of the staff, reviewing the budgetary priorities, and talking to consumers of health care. The decisions made in an organization make the philosophy visible to all—no matter what is espoused on paper. A philosophy that is not or cannot be implemented is useless.

Societal Philosophies and Values Related to Health Care

Societies and organizations have philosophies or sets of beliefs that guide their behavior. These beliefs that guide behavior are called *values*. Values have an intrinsic worth for a society or an individual. Some strongly held American values are individualism, capitalism, and competition. These values profoundly affected health care policy formation and implementation with the result being a US health care system that historically promoted structured inequalities.

Passage of the *Affordable Care Act* in 2010 reduced the number of uninsured in the United States and made care more accessible and affordable for many Americans, but numerous health care disparities still exist. Indeed, "the COVID-19 outbreak in the US showed the country what hospital and health systems leaders have known for years: that serious gaps exist in access, cost and quality for patients based on race, ethnicity, gender and gender identity, age, sexual orientation or other demographic and socio-economic factors" (AHA, 2022b, para. 1). The higher rate of COVID-19 mortality and morbidity in ethnic and minority groups was striking. The Centers for Disease Control responded, suggesting that one solution was for organizations to provide culturally competent care education and standards to address hidden biases regarding cultural diversity (Stark, 2021).

In addition, despite the highest spending as a percentage of gross domestic product, American consumers continue to experience less than desired outcomes. Although values seem to be of central importance for health care policy development and analysis, public discussion of this crucial variable is often neglected. Instead, health care policy makers tend to focus on technology, cost–benefit analysis, and cost-effectiveness. Although this type of evaluation is important, it does not address the underlying values in the United States that have led to unequal access to health care.

Individual Philosophies and Values

As discussed in Chapter 1, values have a tremendous impact on the decisions that people make. For the individual, personal beliefs and values are shaped by that person's experiences. All people should carefully examine their value system and recognize the role that it plays in how they make decisions and resolve conflicts and even how they perceive things. Therefore, the leader-manager must be self-aware and provide subordinates with learning opportunities or experiences that foster increased self-awareness.

At times, it is difficult to assess whether something is a *true value*. McNally's (1980) classic work identified the following four characteristics that determine a true value:

1. It must be freely chosen from among alternatives only after due reflection.
2. It must be prized and cherished.
3. It is consciously and consistently repeated (part of a pattern).
4. It is positively affirmed and enacted.

If a value does not meet all four criteria, it is a *value indicator*. Most people have many value indicators but few true values. For example, many nurses assert that they value their national nursing organization; yet, they do not pay dues or participate in the organization. True values require that the person take action, whereas value indicators do not. Thus, the value ascribed to the national nursing organization is a value indicator for these nurses and not a true value.

In addition, because our values change with time, periodic clarification is necessary to determine how our values may have changed. Sometimes, values change because of life experiences or newly acquired knowledge. Most of the values we have as children reflect the values of those who raise us. Later, our values are modified by peers and role models. Although they are learned, values cannot be forced on a person because they must be internalized. However, restricted exposure to other viewpoints also limits the number of value choices a person can generate. Therefore, becoming more worldly increases our awareness of alternatives from which we select our values.

Occasionally, however, individual values conflict with those of the organization. Because the philosophy of an organization determines its priorities in goal selection and distribution of resources, nurses need to understand the organization's philosophy. For example, assume that a nurse is employed by County Hospital, which clearly states in its philosophy that teaching is a primary purpose for the hospital's existence. Consequently, medical students are allowed to practice endotracheal intubation on all people who die in

LEARNING EXERCISE 7.6

Reflecting on Your Values

Using what you have learned about values, value indicators, and value clarifications, answer the following questions. Take time to reflect on your values before answering. This may be used as a writing exercise.

1. List three or four of your basic beliefs about nursing.
2. Knowing what you know now, ask yourself, "Do I value nursing? Was it freely chosen from among alternatives after appropriate reflection? Do I prize and cherish nursing? If I had a choice to do it over, would I still choose nursing as a career?"
3. Are your personal and professional values congruent? Are there any values espoused by the nursing profession that are inconsistent with your personal values? How will you resolve resultant conflicts?

the hospital, allowing the students to gain needed experience in emergency medicine. This practice disturbs the nurse a great deal; it is not consistent with their own set of values and thus creates great personal conflict.

Nurses who frequently make decisions that conflict with their personal values may experience confusion and anxiety. This intrapersonal struggle ultimately will lead to job stress and dissatisfaction, especially for the novice nurse who comes to the organization with inadequate values clarification. The choices that nurses make about client care are not merely strategic options; they are moral choices. Internal conflict and burnout may result when personal and organizational values do not mesh.

> When a nurse experiences cognitive dissonance between personal and organizational values, the result may be intrapersonal conflict and burnout.

As part of the leadership role, the manager should encourage all potential employees to read and think about the organization's mission statement or philosophy before accepting the job. The manager should give a copy of the philosophy to the prospective applicant before the hiring interview. The applicant also should be encouraged to speak to employees in various positions within the organization regarding how the philosophy is implemented at their job level. For example, a potential employee may want to determine how the organization feels about cultural diversity and what policies they have in place to ensure that patients who speak different languages have a mechanism for translation as needed.

Finally, new employees should be encouraged to speak to community members about the institution's reputation for care. New employees who understand the organizational philosophy will not only have clearer expectations about the institution's purposes and goals but also have a better understanding of how they fit into the organization.

Although all nurses should have a philosophy comparable with that of their employer, it is especially important for the new manager to have a value system consistent with that of the organization. Institutional changes that closely align with the value system of the nurse-manager will receive more effort and higher priority than those that are not true values or that conflict with the nurse-manager's value system.

> It is unrealistic for managers to accept a position under the assumption that they can change the organization's philosophy to more closely match their personal philosophy.

Managers who take a position with the idea that they can change the organization's philosophy to more closely agree with their own philosophy are likely to be disappointed. Such a change will require extraordinary energy and precipitate inevitable conflict because the organization's philosophy reflects the institution's historical development and the beliefs of those people who were vital in the institution's development.

Goals and Objectives

Goals and objectives are the ends toward which the organization is working. All philosophies must be translated into specific goals and objectives if they are to result in action. Thus, goals and objectives "operationalize" the philosophy.

A *goal* may be defined as the desired result toward which effort is directed; it is the aim of the philosophy. Although institutional goals are usually determined by the organization's highest administrative levels, there is increasing emphasis on including workers in setting organizational goals. Goals, much like philosophies and values, change with time and require periodic reevaluation and prioritization.

Goals, although somewhat broad in nature, should be measurable and ambitious but realistic. Goals also should delineate the desired end product. When goals are not clear, simple misunderstandings may compound, and communication may break down. Organizations usually set long- and short-term goals for services rendered; economics; use of resources, including people, funds, and facilities; innovations; and social responsibilities. Display 7.9 lists sample goal statements.

Although goals may direct and maintain the behavior of an organization, there are several dangers in using goal evaluation as the primary means of assessing organizational effectiveness. The first danger is that goals may conflict with each other, creating confusion for employees and consumers. For example, the need for-profit maximization in health care facilities today may conflict with some stated patient goals or quality goals. The second danger is that publicly stated goals may not truly reflect organizational goals. In addition, some organizational goals may be developed simply as a conduit for individual or personal goals. The final danger is that because goals are inclusive of an entire organization, it is often difficult to determine whether they have been obtained.

Objectives are like goals in that they motivate people to a specific end and are explicit, measurable, observable or retrievable, and obtainable. Objectives, however, are more specific and measurable than goals because they identify how and when the goal is to be accomplished.

Goals usually have multiple objectives that are each accompanied by a targeted completion date. The more specific the objectives for a goal can be, the easier for all involved in goal

---

DISPLAY 7.9 SAMPLE GOAL STATEMENTS

- All nursing staff will recognize the patient's need for independence and right to privacy and will assess the patient's level of readiness to learn in relation to their illness.
- The nursing staff will provide effective patient care relative to patient needs insofar as the hospital and community facilities permit through the use of care plans, individual patient care, and discharge planning, including follow-up contact.
- An ongoing effort will be made to create an atmosphere that is conducive to favorable patient and employee morale and that fosters personal growth.
- The performance of all employees in the nursing department will be evaluated in a manner that produces growth in the employee and upgrades nursing standards.
- All nursing units within County Hospital will work cooperatively with other departments within the hospital to further the mission, philosophy, and goals of the institution.

attainment to understand and carry out specific role behaviors. This is especially important for the nurse-manager to remember when writing job descriptions; if there is little ambiguity in the job description, there will be little role confusion or distortion. Clearly written goals and objectives must be communicated to all those in the organization responsible for their attainment. This is a critical leadership role for the nurse-manager.

Objectives can focus on either the desired process or the desired result. *Process objectives* are written in terms of the method to be used, whereas *result-focused objectives* specify the desired outcome. An example of a process objective might be "100% of staff nurses will orient new patients to the call-light system, within 30 minutes of their admission, by first demonstrating its appropriate use and then asking the patient to repeat said demonstration." An example of a result-focused objective might be "95% postoperative patients will perceive a decrease in their pain levels 10 minutes following the administration of intravenous pain medication." Writing good objectives requires time and practice.

For the objectives to be measurable, they should have certain criteria. There should be a specific time frame in which the objectives are to be completed, and the objectives should be stated in behavioral terms, be objectively evaluated, and identify positive outcomes rather than negative outcomes.

As a sample objective, one of the goals at Mercy Hospital is that "all RNs will be proficient in the administration of intravenous fluids." Objectives for Mercy Hospital might include the following:

- All RNs will complete Mercy Hospital's course "IV Therapy Certification" within 2 weeks of beginning employment. The hospital will bear the cost of this program.
- RNs who score less than 90% on a comprehensive examination in "IV Therapy Certification" must attend the remedial 4-hour course "Review of Basic IV Principles" not more than 1 week after the completion of "IV Therapy Certification."
- RNs who achieve a score of 90% or better on the comprehensive examination for "IV Therapy Certification" after completing "Review of Basic IV Principles" will be allowed to perform IV therapy on patients. The unit manager will establish individualized plans of remediation for employees who fail to achieve this score on the examination.

The leader-manager clearly must be skilled in determining and documenting goals and objectives. Prudent managers assess the unit's constraints and assets and determine available resources before developing goals and objectives. The leader must then be creative and futuristic in identifying how goals might best be translated into objectives and thus implemented. The willingness to be receptive to new and varied ideas is a critical leadership skill. In addition, well-developed interpersonal skills allow the leader to involve and inspire subordinates in goal setting. The final step in the process involves clearly writing the identified goals and objectives, communicating changes to subordinates, and periodically evaluating and revising goals and objectives as needed.

LEARNING EXERCISE 7.7

Writing Goals and Objectives

ASSIGNMENT:

Practice writing goals and objectives for County Hospital based on the mission and philosophy statements in this chapter. Identify three goals and three objectives to operationalize each of these goals.

Policies and Procedures

Policies are plans reduced to statements or instructions that direct organizations in their decision making. These comprehensive statements, derived from the organization's philosophy, goals, and objectives, explain how goals will be met and guide the general course and scope of organizational activities. Thus, policies direct individual behavior toward the organization's mission and define broad limits and desired outcomes of commonly recurring situations while leaving some discretion and initiative to those who must carry out that policy. Although some policies are required by accrediting agencies, many policies are specific to the individual institution, thus providing management with a means of internal control.

Policies also can be implied or expressed. *Implied policies*, neither written nor expressed verbally, have usually developed over time, and follow a precedent. For example, a hospital may have an implied policy that employees should be encouraged and supported in their activity in community, regional, and national health care organizations. Another example might be that nurses who limit their personal leave request to 3 months can return to their former jobs and shifts with no status change.

Expressed policies are delineated verbally or in writing. Most organizations have many written policies that are readily available to all people and promote consistency of action. Expressed policies may include a formal dress code, policy for sick leave or vacation time, and disciplinary procedures.

All organizations need to develop facility-wide policies and procedures to guide workers in their actions. These policies and procedures are ideally developed with input from all levels of the organization. Unfortunately, in many health care organizations, this function falls to isolated *policy and procedure committees*. Involving more individuals in the process, as in a shared governance approach, should increase the quality of the end product and the likelihood that procedures will be implemented as desired.

Although top-level management is more involved in setting organizational policies (usually by policy committees), unit managers must determine how those policies will be implemented on their units. Input from subordinates in forming, implementing, and reviewing policy allows the leader-manager to develop guidelines that all employees will support and follow. Even if unit-level employees are not directly involved in policy setting, their feedback is crucial to its successful implementation. Having uniform policies and procedures developed through collaboration is critical.

In addition, policies and procedures should be evidence-based. The addition of evidence to policies and procedures, however, requires the development of a process that ensures consistency, rigor, and safe nursing practice. Unfortunately, many policies continue to be driven by tradition or regulatory requirements and inadequate evidence exists to guide best practices in policy development.

After policy has been formulated, the leadership role of managers includes the responsibility for communicating that policy to all who may be affected by it. This information should be transmitted in writing and verbally. A policy's perceived value often depends on how it is communicated.

Procedures are plans that establish customary or acceptable ways of accomplishing a specific task and delineate a sequence of steps of required action. Established procedures save staff time, facilitate delegation, reduce cost, increase productivity, and provide a means of control. Procedures identify the process or steps needed to implement a policy and are generally found in manuals at the unit level of the organization.

The manager also has a responsibility to review and revise policies and procedure statements to ensure currency and applicability. Given the current explosion of evidence-based research as well as new regulations, technology, and drugs, keeping policies and procedures current and relevant is a tremendous management challenge.

Because procedural instructions involve elements of organizing, some textbooks place the development of procedures in the organizing phase of the management process. Regardless of where procedural development is formulated, there must be a close relationship with planning—the foundation for all procedures.

Rules

Rules and regulations are plans that define specific action or nonaction. Generally included as part of policy and procedure statements, *rules* describe situations that allow only one choice of action. Rules are fairly inflexible, so the fewer rules, the better. Existing rules, however, should be enforced to keep morale from breaking down and to allow organizational structure. Chapter 25, on discipline, includes a more detailed discussion of rules and regulations.

Overcoming Barriers to Planning

Benefits of effective planning include timely accomplishment of higher-quality work and the best possible use of capital and human resources. Because planning is essential, managers must be able to overcome barriers that impede planning. For successful organizational planning, the manager must remember several points:

- The organization can be more effective if movement within it is directed at specified goals and objectives. Unfortunately, the novice manager frequently forgoes establishing a goal or objective. Setting a goal for a plan keeps managers focused on the bigger picture and saves them from getting lost in the minute details of planning. Just as the nursing care plan establishes patient care goals before delineating problems and interventions, managers must establish goals for their planning strategies that are congruent with goals established at higher levels.
- Because a plan is a guide to reach a goal, it must be flexible and allow for readjustment as unexpected events occur. This flexibility is a necessary attribute for the manager in all planning phases and the management process.
- The manager should include all people and units that could be affected by a plan in the planning process. Although time-consuming, employee involvement in how things are done and by whom increases commitment to goal achievement. Although not everyone will want to contribute to unit or organizational planning, all should be invited. The manager also needs to clearly communicate the goals and specific individual responsibilities to all those responsible for carrying out the plans so that work is coordinated.
- Plans should be specific, simple, and realistic. A vague plan is impossible to implement. A plan that is too global or unrealistic discourages rather than motivates employees. If a plan is unclear, the nurse-leader must restate the plan in another manner or use group process to clarify common goals.
- Know when to plan and when not to plan. Some people devote excessive time to arranging details that might be better left to those who will carry out the plan. Other times, managers erroneously assume that people and events will naturally fall into some desired and efficient method of production.
- Good plans have built-in evaluation checkpoints so that there can be a midcourse correction if unexpected events occur. A final evaluation should always occur at the end of the plan. If goals were not met, the plan should be examined to determine why it failed. This evaluation process assists the manager in future planning.

Integrating Leadership Roles and Management Functions in Planning

Planning requires managerial expertise in health care economics, human resource management, political and legislative issues affecting health care, and planning theory. Planning also requires the leadership skills of being sensitive to the environment, being able to appraise accurately the social and political climate, and being willing to take risks.

The leader-manager must be skilled in determining, implementing, documenting, and evaluating all types of planning in the hierarchy because an organization's leaders are integral to realizing the mission of the organization. Managers then must draw on the philosophy and goals established at the organizational and nursing service levels in implementing planning at the unit level. Initially, managers must assess the unit's constraints and assets and determine the resources available for planning. The manager then draws on their leadership skills in creativity, innovation, and futuristic thinking to problem solve how philosophies can be translated into goals, goals into objectives, and so on down the planning hierarchy. The wise manager will develop the interpersonal leadership skills needed to inspire and involve subordinates in this planning hierarchy. The manager also must demonstrate the leadership skill of being receptive to new and varied ideas.

The final step in the process involves articulating identified goals and objectives clearly; this learned management skill is critical to the success of the planning. If the unit manager lacks management or leadership skills, the planning hierarchy fails.

Key Concepts

- The planning phase of the management process is critical and precedes all other functions.
- Planning is a proactive function required of all nurses.
- A plan is a guide for action in reaching a goal and must be flexible.
- Plans should be specific, simple, and realistic.
- All planning must include an evaluation step and requires periodic reevaluation and prioritization.
- All people and organizational units affected by a plan should be included in the planning.
- Plans must have a time for evaluation built into them so that there can be a midcourse correction if necessary.
- New paradigms and trends emerge continuously, requiring leader-managers to be observant and proactive in organizational strategic planning.
- Because of rapidly changing technology, increasing government regulatory involvement in health care, changing population demographics, and decreasing provider autonomy, health care organizations are finding it increasingly difficult to appropriately identify long-term needs and plan accordingly.
- Organizations and planners tend to use one of the four planning modes: reactive, inactive,

preactive, or proactive. A proactive planning style is always the goal.
- Strategic planning tools such as SWOT analysis and balanced scorecard help planners to identify those issues most likely to impact a particular organization or situation in the future and then to develop an appropriate plan for action.
- All planning in the organizational hierarchy must flow from and be congruent with planning done at higher levels in the hierarchy.
- Planning in the organizational hierarchy typically includes the development of organizational vision and mission statements, philosophies, goals, objectives, policies, procedures, and rules.
- An organizational philosophy that is not or cannot be implemented is useless.
- To avoid ongoing intrapersonal values conflicts, employees should have a philosophy compatible with that of their employer.
- Policies and procedures should be evidence-based.
- Rules are fairly inflexible, so the fewer rules, the better. Existing rules, however, should be enforced to keep morale from breaking down and to provide organizational structure.

Additional Learning Exercises and Applications

Exploring the Impact of Philosophy on Management Action

Susan is the supervisor of the 22-bed oncology unit at Memorial Hospital, a 150-bed hospital. Unit morale and job satisfaction are high, despite a unit occupancy rate of less than 50% in the last 6 months. Patient satisfaction on this unit is as high as or higher than that of any other unit in the hospital.

Susan's personal philosophy is that oncology patients have physical, social, and spiritual needs that are different from other patients. Both the unit and nursing service philosophy reflect this belief. Thus, nurses working in the oncology unit receive additional education, orientation, and socialization regarding their unique roles and responsibilities in working with oncology patients.

At this morning's regularly scheduled department head meeting, the chief nursing officer suggests that because of extreme budget shortfalls and continuing low census, the oncology unit should be closed, and its patients merged with the general medical-surgical patient population. The oncology nursing staff would be reassigned to the medical-surgical unit, with Susan as the unit's co-supervisor.

The idea receives immediate support from the medical-surgical supervisor because of the current staffing shortage on her unit. Susan, startled by the proposal, immediately voices her disapproval and asks for 2 weeks to prepare her argument. Her request is granted.

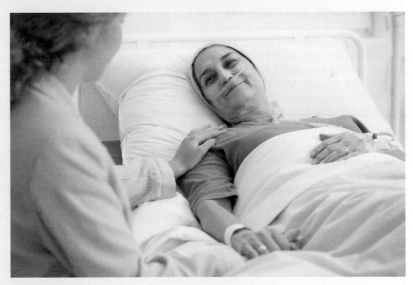

ASSIGNMENT:

What values or beliefs are guiding Susan, the chief nursing officer, and the medical-surgical unit supervisor? Determine an appropriate plan of action for Susan. What impact does a unit or nursing service philosophy have on the actions of management and employees?

LEARNING EXERCISE 7.9

Incremental Goal Setting

Assume that your career goal is to become a nurse-lawyer. You are currently a registered nurse in an acute care facility in a large, metropolitan city. You have your Bachelor of Science in Nursing degree but will need to take at least 12 units of prerequisite classes for acceptance into law school. A law school within commuting distance of your home offers evening classes that would allow you to continue your current day job at least part-time. Quitting your job entirely would be financially unfeasible.

ASSIGNMENT:

Identify at least four objectives that you need to set to achieve your career goal. Be sure that these objectives are explicit, measurable, observable or retrievable, and obtainable. Then identify at least three actions for each objective that delineate how you will achieve them.

LEARNING EXERCISE 7.10

Current Events and Planning

You are a manager in a public health agency. In reading the morning paper before going to work today, you peruse an article about the influx of Hispanic families in your county. This population has increased 10% in the last year alone and is expected to continue to rise. You ponder how this will affect your client population and your agency.

You decide to gather your staff together and develop a strategic plan for dealing with the challenges and opportunities that this change in client demographics may present.

ASSIGNMENT:

In examining the 10 steps listed in development of strategic plans, what are the things that you can personally influence, and what other individuals in the organization should be involved with the strategic plan? Make a list of 10 to 12 strategies that will assist you in planning for this new client population. What other information or data will you need to help you plan? What are some other future developments in your county that could have a positive or negative influence on your plan?

REFERENCES

American Hospital Association. (2022a). *Market insights: Disruptive innovation.* Center for Health Innovation. https://www.aha.org/center/emerging-issues/market-insights/disruptive-innovation

American Hospital Association. (2022b). *Using data to reduce health disparities and improve health equity.* Center for Health Innovation. https://www.aha.org/center/market-insights/leveraging-data/using-data-reduce-health-disparities-and-improve-health-equity

Brown, B. (2021, May 28). *The 2021 healthcare financial forecast: What to expect, how to prepare.* Health Catalyst. https://www.healthcatalyst.com/insights/healthcare-financial-forecast-what-expect-2021/

Frieden, J. (2021, August 12). *Health IT a mixed blessing during the pandemic—Has helped with patient care, but pay attention to the burnout it can cause, experts urge.* MEDPAGE Today. https://www.medpagetoday.com/meetingcoverage/himss/94015?xid=nl_mpt_confroundup_2021-08-18&eun=g8855534d41r

Herzlinger, R., & Richman, B. (2021, June 10). Preparing hospitals for the next pandemic. *Harvard Business Review.* Retrieved March 20, 2022, from https://hbr.org/2021/06/preparing-hospitals-for-the-next-pandemic

Huston, C. J. (2020). *The road to positive work cultures.* Sigma Theta Tau International.

Huston, C. J. (2023). Technology in health care: Opportunities, limitations, and challenges (chapter 21). In C. J. Huston (Ed.), *Professional issues in nursing: Challenges and opportunities* (6th ed., pp. 302–318). Wolters Kluwer.

IBM. (n.d.). *What is supply chain management?* https://www.ibm.com/topics/supply-chain-management

Mahmoodi, F., Blutinger, E., Echazú, L., & Nocetti, D. (2021, February 17). COVID-19 and the health care supply chain: Impacts and lessons learned. *Supply Chain Quarterly.* https://www.supplychainquarterly.com/articles/4417-covid-19-and-the-health-care-supply-chain-impacts-and-lessons-learned

McNally, M. (1980). As individual experience broadens, realistic value systems must be flexible enough to grow: Part 1. *Supervisor Nurse, 11,* 27–30.

National Institutes of Health, U.S. Department of Health and Human Services. (2021, May). *Strategic plan FY 2021–2025.* National Center for Complementary and Integrative Health. https://files.nccih.nih.gov/nccih-strategic-plan-2021-2025.pdf#:~:text=NCCIH%E2%80%99s%20new%20strategic%20plan%20for%20Fiscal%20Years%20%28FY%29,multiple%20interconnected%20domains%3A%20biological%2C%20behavioral%2C%20social%2C%20and%20environmental

Prichard, S. (2018, July 18). *Who are you serving?* https://www.skipprichard.com/who-are-you-serving/

Rausch, S. L. (2021, August 13). HM administrators plan for 2021 and beyond. *The Hospitalist.* https://www.the-hospitalist.org/hospitalist/article/244283/leadership-training/hm-administrators-plan-2021-and-beyond?channel=36604

RPH On the Go. (2020, February 26). Are robotic "pharmacists" a help or a hindrance? https://www.rphonthego.com/blog/are-robotic-pharmacists-a-help-or-a-hindrance/

Stark, J. (2021, May). A vision of culturally competent care. *Case Management Monthly, 18*(5), 5–6.

Sudhakaran, A. (2020, December 24). *Johnson and Johnson SWOT analysis 2021—Comprehensive report.* Pestle Analysis. https://pestleanalysis.com/johnson-and-johnson-swot-analysis/

8

Planned Change

*... The nature of leadership is resistance and change.—**Scott Mabry***

*... I can't understand why people are frightened of new ideas. I'm frightened of old ones.—**John Cage***

*... If you want to make enemies, try to change something.—**Woodrow Wilson***

CROSSWALK

This chapter addresses:

- **AACN Essentials Domain 1:** Knowledge for nursing practice
- **AACN Essentials Domain 2:** Person-centered care
- **AACN Essentials Domain 4:** Scholarship for nursing practice
- **AACN Essentials Domain 6:** Interprofessional partnerships
- **AACN Essentials Domain 7:** Systems-based practice
- **AACN Essentials Domain 10:** Personal, professional, and leadership development
- **AONL Nurse Executive Competency 1:** Communication and relationship building
- **AONL Nurse Executive Competency 2:** A knowledge of the health care environment
- **AONL Nurse Executive Competency 3:** Leadership
- **AONL Nurse Executive Competency 5:** Business skills
- **ANA Standard of Professional Performance 8:** Advocacy
- **ANA Standard of Professional Performance 10:** Communication
- **ANA Standard of Professional Performance 11:** Collaboration
- **ANA Standard of Professional Performance 12:** Leadership
- **ANA Standard of Professional Performance 14:** Scholarly inquiry
- **ANA Standard of Professional Performance 15:** Quality of practice
- **ANA Standard of Professional Performance 17:** Resource stewardship
- **ANA Standard of Professional Performance 18:** Environmental health
- **QSEN Competency:** Teamwork and collaboration

LEARNING OBJECTIVES

The learner will:

- differentiate between planned change and change by drift
- identify the responsibilities of a change agent
- develop strategies for unfreezing, movement, and refreezing
- assess driving and restraining forces for change in given situations
- apply rational–empirical, normative–reeducative, and power–coercive strategies for effecting change
- describe resistance as a natural and expected response to change
- identify and implement strategies to manage resistance to change
- involve all those who may be affected by a change in planning for that change whenever possible

- identify characteristics of aged organizations as well as strategies to keep them ever-renewing
- identify critical features of complex adaptive systems change theory
- describe the impact of chaos and the butterfly effect on both short- and long-term planning
- plan at least one desired personal change

Introduction

Effectively dealing with rapid change while leading increasingly complex organizations toward a preferred future is a critical 21st leadership competency. Bhasin (2020) explains, though, that planning for change and planning for innovation are not the same things. Innovation is a transformative process that requires a significant change.

Some of the forces driving change in contemporary health care include rising health care costs, declining reimbursement, new quality imperatives, workforce shortages, emerging technologies, the dynamic nature of knowledge, the growing older adult population, and pandemic-induced supply chain shortages of both personnel and physical resources. Contemporary health care agencies then must continually institute change to upgrade their structure, promote greater quality, and keep their workers. In fact, most health care organizations find themselves undergoing continual change directed at organizational restructuring, quality improvement, and employee retention.

In most cases, these changes are planned. *Planned change*, in contrast to accidental change or *change by drift*, results from a well-thought-out and deliberate effort to make something happen. Planned change is the deliberate application of knowledge and skills to bring about a change. Successful leader-managers must be well grounded in change theories and be able to apply such theories appropriately.

> Organizational change is constant, and leader-managers must have highly developed skills in change management for 21st-century organizations to grow and thrive.

Many change attempts fail because the approach used to implement the change lacks structure or planning. Indeed, what often differentiates a successful change effort from an unsuccessful one is the ability of the *change agent*—a person skilled in the theory and implementation of planned change—to deal appropriately with conflicted human emotions and to connect and balance all aspects of the organization that will be affected by that change. In organizational planned change, the manager is often the change agent.

In some large organizations today, however, multidisciplinary teams of individuals, representing all key stakeholders in the organization, are assigned the responsibility for managing the change process. In such organizations, this team manages the communication between the people leading the change effort and those who are expected to implement the new strategies. In addition, this team manages the organizational context in which change occurs and the emotional connections essential for any transformation.

But having a skilled change agent alone is not enough. Change is never easy, and regardless of the type of change, all major change brings feelings of achievement and pride as well as loss and stress. Leader-managers must remember that transformational change must become personal for every employee if it is to happen and be maintained (Carucci, 2021). Leader-managers then must use developmental, political, and relational expertise to ensure that needed change is not sabotaged. Strategies for inspiring others to change are shown in Display 8.1.

INSPIRING OTHERS TO CHANGE

1. Mastering how to inspire others hinges on honing leadership skills which evoke feelings of awe and wonder in others.
2. Leaders exercise soft skills (like empathy) to enhance engagement, since empathy facilitates the trust necessary to inspire others. Conversely, hard skills (like hunger and drive) are useful for inspiring by way of example.
3. Employees are likely to be most inspired by leaders who are simultaneously empathetic and driven toward success.
4. In order to master how to inspire people, you must first understand what already inspires them.
5. Lead by example.
6. Set goals and expectations that inspire employees. Rather than set a standard of "good enough," set a standard of "exceptional."
7. Master empathy and focus on relationships.
8. Embrace the process.

Source: Adapted from Robbins, T. (2022). *When you know how to inspire others, you create impactful relationships.* Robbins Research International, Inc. https://www.tonyrobbins.com/business/how-to-inspire-others/

In addition, many good ideas are never realized because of poor timing or a lack of power on the part of the change agent. For example, both organizations and individuals tend to reject outsiders as change agents because they are perceived as having inadequate knowledge or expertise about the status quo and their motives often are not trusted. Therefore, there is more widespread resistance if the change agent is an outsider. The outside change agent, however, tends to be more objective in their assessment, whereas the inside change agent is often influenced by a personal bias regarding how the organization functions.

Likewise, some greatly needed changes are never implemented because the change agent lacks sensitivity to timing. If the organization or the people within that organization have recently undergone a great deal of change or stress (*change fatigue*), any other change should wait until group resistance decreases. When work is in a constant state of flux, workers feel unsettled and unsure of themselves. The leader's role is to make sure that change does not happen for the sake of change alone (Huston, 2020).

For effective change to occur then, the change agent must make a thorough and accurate assessment of the extent of and interest in change, the nature and depth of motivation, and the environment in which the change will occur. In addition, because human beings have little control over many changes in their lives, the change agent must remember that people need a balance between stability and change in the workplace. Indeed, Sherman and Cohn (2021) note that the human brain loves predictability, and we feel safer when we know what to expect. As a result, over time, our work and personal lives often become a series of habits.

> Change should be implemented only for good reasons.

Initiating and coordinating change requires well-developed leadership and management skills. Leading organizational change always starts with a bit of mindset transformation because such changes often involve resource allocation. It also requires not only vision but expert planning skills because a vision is not the same as a plan. The failure to reassess goals proactively and to initiate these changes results in misdirected and poorly used fiscal and human resources. Leader-managers must be visionary in identifying where change is needed in the organization, and be flexible in adapting to change they directly initiated as well as change that has indirectly affected them. Display 8.2 delineates selected leadership roles and management functions necessary for leader-managers acting either in the change agent role or as a coordinator of the planned change team.

DISPLAY 8.2 LEADERSHIP ROLES AND MANAGEMENT FUNCTIONS IN PLANNED CHANGE

Leadership Roles

1. Is visionary in identifying areas of needed change in the organization and the health care system
2. Demonstrates risk taking in assuming the role of change agent
3. Demonstrates flexibility in goal setting in a rapidly changing health care system
4. Anticipates, recognizes, and creatively problem solves resistance to change
5. Serves as a role model to followers during planned change by viewing change as a challenge and opportunity for growth
6. Is a role model for high-level interpersonal communication skills in providing support for followers undergoing rapid or difficult change
7. Demonstrates creativity in identifying alternatives to problems
8. Demonstrates sensitivity to timing in proposing planned change
9. Takes steps to prevent aging in the organization and to keep current with the new realities of nursing practice
10. Supports and reinforces the individual adaptive efforts of those affected by change

Management Functions

1. Forecasts unit needs with an understanding of the organization's and unit's legal, political, economic, social, and legislative climate
2. Recognizes the need for planned change and identifies the options and resources available to implement that change
3. Appropriately assesses and responds to the driving and restraining forces when planning for change
4. Identifies and implements appropriate strategies to minimize or overcome resistance to change
5. Seeks subordinates' input in planned change and provides them with adequate information during the change process to give them some feeling of control
6. Supports and reinforces the individual efforts of subordinates during the change process
7. Identifies and uses appropriate change strategies to modify the behavior of subordinates as needed
8. Periodically assesses the unit/department for signs of organizational aging and plans renewal strategies
9. Continues to be actively involved in the refreezing process until the change becomes part of the new status quo

Lewin's Change Theory of Unfreezing, Movement, and Refreezing

Most of the current research on change builds on the classic change theories developed by Kurt Lewin in the mid-20th century. Lewin (1951) identified three phases through which the change agent must proceed before a planned change becomes part of the system: unfreezing, movement, and refreezing.

Unfreezing

Unfreezing occurs when the change agent convinces members of the group to change or when guilt, anxiety, or concern can be elicited. Thus, people become discontent and aware of a need to change. Carucci (2021) notes that leaders frequently underestimate the amount of work required for a change, overestimate the organization's capacity to make the change, and misjudge how the members of an organization view their connection to the change. Therefore, to make a change effort successful, the leader must clear away competing priorities and shine a spotlight on the need for a change to happen. Resistance should be expected, however, as most people cling to the status quo, even if they are not entirely pleased with it.

In addition, communication is critical during unfreezing so that those who will be most affected by the proposed change can examine it, provide input, and discover what, if any, benefits the change might have for them. Communicating change effectively then requires listening to the organization twice as much as telling the organization about the change (Carucci, 2021).

Movement

The second phase of planned change is *movement*. In movement, the change agent identifies, plans, and implements appropriate strategies, ensuring that driving forces exceed restraining forces. It is a manager's responsibility to maintain the excitement for a change by providing the required resources to their employees (Bhasin, 2020). However, because change is such a complex process, it requires a great deal of planning and intricate timing.

Simply put, most leaders want transformational change to be easier than it is. Transformational change starts with an honest acknowledgment of how hard the work will be, how much capacity and discipline the organization actually has, and the personal commitments of sponsoring executives to change first (Carucci, 2021).

Recognizing, addressing, and overcoming expected resistance may be a lengthy process, and whenever possible, change should be implemented gradually. Any change of human behavior, or the perceptions, attitudes, and values underlying that behavior, takes time. Indeed, addressing and responding appropriately to stress caused by change is a high-level leadership skill. Fear alone, however, is not a good reason for delaying or shunning change.

Refreezing

The last phase is *refreezing*. During the refreezing phase, the change agent assists in stabilizing the system change so that it becomes integrated into the status quo. If refreezing is incomplete, the change will be ineffective and prechange behaviors will resume. For refreezing to occur, the change agent must be supportive and reinforce the individual adaptive efforts of those affected by the change. Because change needs at least 3 to 6 months before it will be accepted as part of the system, the change agent must be sure to remain involved until the change is completed.

> Change agents must be patient and open to new opportunities during refreezing, as complex change takes time, and several different attempts may be needed before desired outcomes are achieved.

It is important to remember, though, that refreezing does not eliminate the possibility of further improvements to the change. Indeed, measuring the impact of change should always be a part of refreezing. Display 8.3 illustrates the change agent's responsibilities during the various stages of planned change.

Lewin's Change Theory of Driving and Restraining Forces

Lewin (1951) also theorized that people maintain a state of status quo or equilibrium by the simultaneous occurrence of both *driving forces* (facilitators) and *restraining forces* (barriers) operating within any field. Driving forces advance a system toward change; restraining forces impede change.

> The forces that push the system toward change are driving forces, whereas the forces that pull the system away from change are restraining forces.

DISPLAY 8.3 **STAGES OF CHANGE AND RESPONSIBILITIES OF THE CHANGE AGENT**

Stage 1—Unfreezing

1. Gather data.
2. Accurately diagnose the problem.
3. Decide if change is needed.
4. Make others aware of the need for change; often involves deliberate tactics to raise the group's discontent level; do not proceed to stage 2 until the status quo has been disrupted and the need for change is perceived by the others.

Stage 2—Movement

1. Develop a plan.
2. Set goals and objectives.
3. Identify areas of support and resistance.
4. Include everyone who will be affected by the change in its planning.
5. Set target dates.
6. Develop appropriate strategies.
7. Implement the change.
8. Be available to support others and offer encouragement through the change.
9. Use strategies for overcoming resistance to change.
10. Evaluate the change.
11. Modify the change, if necessary.

Stage 3—Refreezing

Support others so that the change continues.

Examples of driving forces might include a desire to please one's boss, to eliminate a problem, to get a pay raise, or to receive recognition. Restraining forces include conformity to norms, an unwillingness to take risks, and a fear of the unknown. Lewin's (1951) model suggested that people like feeling safe, comfortable, and in control of their environment. For change to occur then, driving forces must be increased or restraining forces decreased.

In Figure 8.1, the person wishing to return to school must reduce the restraining forces or increase the driving forces to alter the present state of equilibrium. There will be no change or action until this occurs. Therefore, creating an imbalance within the system by increasing the driving forces or decreasing the restraining forces is one of the tasks required of a change agent.

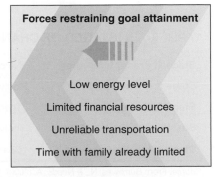

GOAL: RETURN TO SCHOOL

Forces driving to reach goal	Forces restraining goal attainment
Opportunity for advancement	Low energy level
Status—Social gratification	Limited financial resources
Enhanced self-esteem	Unreliable transportation
Family supportive of efforts	Time with family already limited

FIGURE 8.1 Driving and restraining forces.

LEARNING EXERCISE 8.1
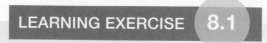

Making Change Possible

Identify a change that you would like to make in your personal life (such as losing weight, exercising daily, and stopping smoking). List the restraining forces keeping you from making this change. List the driving forces that make you want to change. Determine how you might be able to change the status quo and make the change possible.

A Contemporary Adaptation of Lewin's Model

Burrowes and Needs (2009) shared an adaptation of Lewin's model in their discussion of a five-step *stages of change model* (SCM). In this model, the first stage is *precontemplation*. During this stage, the individual "has no intention to change his or her behavior in the foreseeable future" (Burrowes & Needs, 2009, p. 41). Next comes the *contemplation* stage at which point the individual considers making a change but has not yet made a commitment to take action. This would be the phase in which unfreezing would occur according to Lewin.

A transition from unfreezing to movement begins in the *preparation* stage, as the individual intends to take action in the short-term future. The *action* stage then occurs (movement) in which the individual actively modifies their behavior. Finally, the process ends with the *maintenance* stage at which point the individual works to maintain changes made during the action stage and prevent relapse. This stage would be synonymous with refreezing. Table 8.1 illustrates the steps of the SCM.

Classic Change Strategies

In addition to being aware of the stages of change, the change agent must be highly skilled in the use of behavioral strategies to prompt change in others. Three such classic strategies for effecting change were described by Bennis et al. (1969), with the most appropriate strategy for any situation depending on the power of the change agent and the amount of resistance expected from the subordinates.

One of these strategies is to give current research as evidence to support the change. This group of strategies is often referred to as *rational–empirical* strategies. The change agent using this set of strategies assumes that resistance to change comes from a lack of knowledge and that humans are rational beings who will change when given information documenting the need for change. This type of strategy is used when there is little anticipated resistance to the change or when the change is perceived as reasonable.

TABLE 8.1 STAGES OF CHANGE MODEL

Stage 1: Precontemplation	No current intention to change.
Stage 2: Contemplation	Individual considers making a change.
Stage 3: Preparation	There is intent to make a change in the near future.
Stage 4: Action	Individual modifies behavior.
Stage 5: Maintenance	Change is maintained and relapse is avoided.

Source: From Burrowes, N., & Needs, A. (2009). Time to contemplate change? A framework for assessing readiness to change with offenders. *Aggression & Violent Behavior, 14*(1), 39–49.

In contrast, *normative–reeducative* strategies use group norms and peer pressure to socialize and influence people so that change will occur. The change agent assumes that humans are social creatures, more easily influenced by others than by facts. This strategy does not require the change agent to have a legitimate power base. Instead, they gain power by skill in interpersonal relationships, focusing on noncognitive determinants of behavior, such as people's roles and relationships, perceptual orientations, attitudes, and feelings, to increase acceptance of change.

LEARNING EXERCISE 8.2

Using Change Strategies to Increase Sam's Adherence

You are a staff nurse in a home health agency. One of your patients, Sam Little, is a 38-year-old man with type 1 diabetes. He has developed some loss of vision and had to have two toes amputated as consequences of his disease process. Sam's adherence to four-times-daily blood glucose monitoring and sliding-scale insulin administration has never been particularly good, but he has been worse than usual lately. Sam refuses to use an insulin pump; however, he has been willing to follow a prescribed diabetic diet and has kept his weight to a desired level.

Sam's wife called you at the agency yesterday and asked you to work with her in developing a plan to increase Sam's adherence with his blood glucose monitoring and insulin administration. She said that Sam, although believing it "probably won't help," has agreed to meet with you to discuss such a plan. He does not want, however, "to feel pressured into doing something he doesn't want to do."

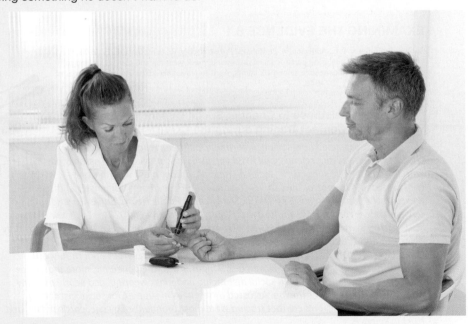

ASSIGNMENT:

What change strategy or combination thereof (rational–empirical, normative–reeducative, and power–coercive) do you believe has the greatest likelihood of increasing Sam's adherence? How could you use this strategy? Who would be involved in this change effort? What efforts might you undertake to increase the unfreezing so that Sam is more willing to actively participate in such a planned change effort?

The third group of strategies, *power–coercive* strategies, features the application of power by legitimate authority, economic sanctions, or the political clout of the change agent. These strategies include influencing the enactment of new laws and using group power for strikes or sit-ins. Using authority inherent in an individual position to effect change is another example of a power–coercive strategy. These strategies assume that people often are set in their ways and will change only when rewarded for the change or when they are forced by some other power–coercive method. Resistance is handled by authority measures; the individual must accept it or leave.

Often, the change agent uses strategies from each of these three groups. For example, imagine the change agent wants to convince someone to stop smoking. The change agent might present the person with the latest research on cancer and smoking (the rational–empirical approach), have friends and family encourage the person socially to quit (normative–reeducative approach), and refuse to ride in the person's car if the person smokes while driving (power–coercive approach). By selecting from each set of strategies, the change agent increases the chance of successful change.

Another example of a planned change that involved strategies from each of the three groups was described by Anderson et al. (2021) in their analysis of public resistance to the need for social distancing, mask wearing, and contact tracing to combat the COVID-19 pandemic. Factors such as beliefs about the trustworthiness of science (rational–empirical) played a role in the degree of resistance as did the normative–reeducative strategies associated with political partisanship. Finally, a generalized resistance to mandates (power–coercive) influenced some participants' choices to comply (see Examining the Evidence 8.1).

EXAMINING THE EVIDENCE 8.1

Source: From Barry, C. L., Anderson, K. E., Han, H., Presskreischer, R., & McGinty, E. E. (2021, May). Change over time in public support for social distancing, mask wearing, and contact tracing to combat the COVID-19 pandemic among US adults, April to November 2020. *American Journal of Public Health, 111*(5), 937–948.

Addressing Resistance to Change: Social Distancing, Indoor Mask Wearing, and Contact Tracing during the COVID-19 Pandemic

This research examined how sociodemographic, political, religious, and civic characteristics; trust in science; and fixed versus fluid worldview were associated with evolving public support for social distancing, indoor mask wearing, and contact tracing to control the COVID-19 pandemic. Researchers administered three waves of the Johns Hopkins COVID-19 Civic Life and Public Health Survey to a nationally representative cohort of US adults in April, July, and November 2020.

Over the 8-month study period, rhetoric on public health responses became increasingly polarized and "COVID fatigue" regarding the sustained effort needed to maintain social distancing set in. Support for social distancing dropped sharply from April to July, but then stabilized in November. By November, 9 months into the pandemic, more than three quarters of US adults supported social distancing and mask wearing, and nearly as many (73%) supported contact tracing. Adjusted differences in support for social distancing, indoor mask wearing, and contact tracing were most pronounced by age, partisanship, and trust in science.

Stark differences between adults trusting science and those with doubts about science persisted, however, in models controlling for political party affiliation. This suggests that trust in science crosscuts political partisanship. In adjusted models controlling for partisanship, having a fixed worldview was associated with lower support for contact tracing in November, but not mask wearing or social distancing.

The researchers concluded that to better mobilize support for the pandemic response, it is critical to understand the sources of people's skepticism and to develop broad and diverse strategies to attain the collective response needed for widespread immunity.

Resistance: The Expected Response to Change

Even though change is inevitable, it creates instability in our lives, and some conflict should always be expected. Indeed, Heathfield (2021) suggests that even the most cooperative, supportive employees often experience resistance because change alters the balance of a group. Proactive change is generally less emotional than mandated change; yet the lines often blur between the two because proactive change launched by one group may be perceived as mandated change by another.

The level of resistance also generally depends on the type of change proposed. Technologic changes encounter less resistance than changes that are perceived as socially driven or that are contrary to established customs or norms. For example, nursing staff may be more willing to accept a change in the type of intravenous (IV) pump to be used than a change regarding who is able to administer certain types of IV therapy.

Nursing leaders also must recognize that subordinates' values, educational levels, cultural and social backgrounds, and experiences with change (positive or negative) will have a tremendous impact on the degree of resistance. It is also much easier to change a person's behavior than it is to change an entire group's behavior. Likewise, it is easier to change knowledge levels than attitudes.

To eliminate resistance to change in the workplace, managers historically used an autocratic leadership style with specific guidelines for work, an excessive number of rules, and a coercive approach to discipline. The resistance, which occurred anyway, was both covert (such as delaying tactics and passive–aggressive behavior) and overt (openly refusing to follow a direct command). The result was wasted managerial energy and time and a high level of frustration.

> Because change disrupts the homeostasis or balance of the group, resistance should always be expected.

Currently, resistance is recognized as a natural and expected response to change, and leader-managers must resist the impulse to focus on blaming others when resistance to planned change occurs. Instead, they should immerse themselves in identifying and implementing strategies to minimize or manage this resistance to change. One such strategy is to encourage subordinates to speak openly so that options can be identified to overcome objections. In addition, it is the leader's role to envision what the future will be like after the change has taken place and to share that vision with their followers.

Likewise, workers should be encouraged to talk about their perceptions of the forces driving the planned change so that the leader can accurately assess change support and resources. It takes a strong leader to step up and engage when a change effort meets with pushback.

Still, there are individual variations in terms of risk taking and willingness to accept change. Temperament and personality play at least some role in this. Change agents then should be

LEARNING EXERCISE 8.3

What Is Your Attitude Toward Change?

How do you typically respond to change? Do you embrace it? Seek it out? Accept it reluctantly? Avoid it at all costs? Is this behavior like that of your friends and that of your family? Has your behavior always fit this pattern, or has the pattern changed throughout your life? If so, what life events have altered how you view and respond to change?

Try to remember a situation in your own life that involved unnecessary change. Why do you think that the change was unnecessary? What types of turmoil did it cause? Were there things a change agent could have done that would have increased unfreezing in this situation?

aware of life history variables as well as risk-taking propensity when assessing the likelihood of an individual or group being willing to change. Early in a planned change then, leader-managers should assess which workers are likely to promote or resist a specific change, by both observation and direct communication. Then, the manager can collaborate with change promoters on how best to convert those individuals more resistant to change.

Sherman and Cohn (2021) agree, noting how important it is for leaders to meet staff where they are in the change process. Not all staff accept change in the same way or on the same timeline. Some nurses are natural innovators or early adopters, whereas others will be slow to adopt change. Asking early adopters to serve as superusers will help others adapt.

Perhaps the greatest factor contributing to the resistance encountered with change, however, is a lack of trust between the employee and the manager or the employee and the organization. Workers want security and predictability. That is why trust erodes when the ground rules change, as the assumed "contract" between the worker and the organization is altered. Subordinates' confidence in the change agent's ability to manage change depends on whether they believe that they have adequate resources to cope with it.

In addition, the leader-manager must remember that subordinates in an organization will generally focus more on how a specific change will affect their personal lives and status than on how it will affect the organization. Heathfield (2021) advises leaders to always help employees identify what's in it for them to make the change. A good portion of the normal resistance to change disappears when employees are clear about the benefits the change brings to them as individuals.

> "True change in an organization often means that job positions and titles also change, which means that roles and responsibilities may shift as well. Resistance occurs when employees don't understand how they fit in with the new way of doing things" (Quain, 2019, para. 4).

Planned Change as a Collaborative Process

Often, the change process begins with a few people who meet to discuss their dissatisfaction with the status quo and an inadequate effort is made to talk with anyone else in the organization. This approach virtually guarantees that the change effort will fail. People abhor "information vacuums," and when there is no ongoing conversation about the change process, gossip usually fills the void. These rumors are generally much more negative than anything that is actually happening. McQuerrey (2019) suggests that leaders should quell this early discord by being as transparent as possible. "Call a meeting or issue a companywide memo that sets the record about imminent change. Even if the situation is still fluid, acknowledge that change is on the horizon and announce you will disseminate information as soon as it is available" (para. 3).

> "Resistance to change can gain its initial footing in unchecked gossip . . . People will speculate, make assumptions, and otherwise develop their thought patterns about what's going on" (McQuerrey, 2019, para 2).

In addition, generally, anyone who will be affected by a change should be included in planning it. When information and decision making are shared, subordinates feel that they have played a valuable role in the change. Change agents and the elements of the system—the people or groups within it—must openly develop goals and strategies together. All must have the opportunity to define their interest in the change, their expectation of its outcome, and their ideas on strategies for achieving change.

It is not always easy, however, to attain grassroots involvement in planning efforts. Even when managers communicate that change is needed and subordinate feedback is wanted, the message often goes unheeded. Some people in the organization may need to hear a message repeatedly before they listen, understand, and believe the message. If the message is one that they do not want to hear, it may take even longer for them to come to terms with the anticipated change.

When change agents fail to communicate with the rest of the organization, they prevent people from understanding the principles that guided the change, what has been learned from prior experience, and why compromises have been made. Likewise, subordinates affected by the change should thoroughly understand the change and the impacts that will likely result. Good, open communication throughout the process can reduce resistance. Leaders must ensure that group members share perceptions about what change is to be undertaken, who is to be involved and in what role, and how the change will directly and indirectly affect each person in the organization.

The Leader-Manager as a Role Model During Planned Change

Leader-managers must act as role models to subordinates during the change process. Heathfield (2021) suggests it is critical that leader-managers own the planned change, no matter where it originated. In addition, the leader-manager must attempt to view change positively and to impart this view to subordinates. Rather than viewing change as a threat, managers should embrace it as a challenge and the chance or opportunity to do something new and innovative. Indeed, the leader has two responsibilities in facilitating change in nursing practice. First, leader-managers must be actively engaged in change in their own work and model this behavior to staff. Second, leaders must be able to assist staff members in making the needed changes in their work.

Managers must also believe that they can make a difference. This feeling of control is probably the most important trait for thriving in a changing environment. Unfortunately, many leader-managers lack self-confidence in their ability to serve as an effective change agent. When this occurs, they can disengage from the change process and demonstrate to followers that the change may not be worth the time and energy necessary to bring it to fruition.

Organizational Change Associated with Nonlinear Dynamics

Most 21st-century organizations experience fairly brief periods of stability followed by intense transformation. In fact, some later organizational theorists feel that Lewin's (1951) refreezing to establish equilibrium should not be the focus of contemporary organizational change because change is unforeseeable and ever present. This is particularly true in health care organizations, where long-term outcomes are almost always unpredictable.

In the past, organizations looked at change and organizational dynamics as linear, occurring both in steps and sequentially. More contemporary theorists maintain that the world is so unpredictable that such dynamics are truly nonlinear. As a result, nonlinear change theories such as *complex adaptive systems (CAS) theory* and *chaos theory* now influence the thinking of many organizational leaders.

Complexity and Complex Adaptive Systems Change Theory

Complexity science has emerged from the exploration of the subatomic world and quantum physics and suggests that the world is complex as are the individuals who operate within it. Thus, control and order are emergent rather than predetermined, and mechanistic formulas do not provide the flexibility needed to predict what actions will result in what outcomes.

DISPLAY **8.4** **MAIN FEATURES OF OLSON AND EOYANG'S (2001) COMPLEX ADAPTIVE SYSTEMS APPROACH TO CHANGE**

- Change should be achieved through connections among change agents instead of from the top-down.
- There should be adaptation to uncertainty during the change instead of trying to predict stages of development.
- Goals, plans, and structures should be allowed to emerge instead of depending on clear, detailed plans and goals.
- Value differences should be amplified and explored instead of focusing on consensus in change efforts.
- Patterns in one part of the organization are often repeated in another part. Thus, change does not need to begin at the top of an organization to be successful. The goal instead is self-similarity rather than differences in how change is implemented in different parts of the organization.
- Successful change fits with the current organizational environment instead of with an ideal. This is what makes it sustainable.

CAS change theory, an outgrowth of complexity theory, suggests that the relationship between elements and agents within any system is nonlinear and that these elements are constantly in play to change the environment or outcome.

For example, although an individual may have behaved one way in the past, CAS theory suggests that future behavior may not always be the same (not always predictable). This is because that individual's prior experience and past learning may change their future choices. In addition, the rules or parameters of each situation are different, even if these differences are subtle; even small variations can dramatically alter choice of action. CAS theory also suggests that the actions of any agent within the system affect all other agents in the system; that is, that context and action are interconnected. Finally, CAS theory suggests that there are always hidden or unanticipated elements in systems that make linear thinking almost impossible.

In their classic work on CAS, Olson and Eoyang (2001) suggest that the self-organizing nature of human interactions in a complex organization leads to surprising effects. Rather than focusing on the macrolevel of the organization system, complexity theory suggests that most powerful change processes occur at the microlevel, where relationships, interactions, and simple rules shape emerging patterns. The main features of the CAS approach are shown in Display 8.4.

In applying CAS theory to planned change, it becomes clear that the multidimensionality of health care organizations, and the individuals who work within them, causes significant challenges for the change agent. Change agents then must carefully examine and focus on the relationships between the elements and avoid looking at one element in isolation from the others. They must give time and attention to trying to understand these relationships and interactions even before attempting unfreezing; continual monitoring and adaptation will likely be needed for movement and refreezing to be successful.

Chaos Theory

The roots of *chaos theory*, considered by some to be a subset of complexity science, likely emerged from the early work of meteorologist Edward Lorenz in the 1960s to improve weather forecasting techniques (MIT News, 2008). Lorenz discovered that even tiny changes in variables often dramatically affected outcomes. Lorenz also discovered that even though these chaotic changes appeared to be random, they were not. Instead, he found that there were deterministic sequences and physical laws, which prevail in nature, even if this does not appear to be the case.

> Chaos theory is really about finding the underlying order in apparently random data.

Determining this underlying order, however, is challenging, and the order itself is constantly changing. This chaos makes it difficult to predict the future. In addition, chaos theory suggests that even small changes in conditions can drastically alter a system's long-term behavior (commonly known as the *butterfly effect*). Thus, changes in outcomes are not proportional to the degree of change in the initial condition. Because of this sensitivity, the behavior of a system exhibiting chaos appears to be random, even though the system is deterministic, meaning it is well defined and contains no random parameters.

Chaos and complexity theories have great application within the health care arena. For example, despite having been created with much time and energy, many plans with sharply delivered strategies and targets are often not effective. This is because hidden variables are not explored, and general goals and boundaries are not developed. For example, a single individual or unit can undermine a planned organizational change, particularly if the actions of that individual or unit to undermine the change are covert. The change agent might inadvertently focus on the aftermath of the subversive action without ever realizing the root cause of the problem.

Because the use of nonlinear theories to explain organizational functioning and change is expected to increase in the 21st century, it is imperative that change agents understand complexity theory and chaos theory.

Organizational Aging: Change as a Means of Renewal

Organizations progress through developmental stages, just as people do—birth, youth, maturity, and aging. The young organization is characterized by high energy, movement, and virtually constant change and adaptation. As organizations age, structure increases to provide greater control and coordination. Aged organizations function in an orderly and predictable fashion and are focused on rules and regulations. Change is limited.

Organizations must find a balance between stagnation and chaos, between birth and death. During the process of maturing, workers within the organization can become prisoners of procedures, forget their original purposes, and allow means to become the ends. Without change, the organization may stagnate and die. Organizations need to keep foremost what they are going to do, not what they have done.

> "It is critical not to view change as a threat. When leaders look to the future, they help organizations stay young and ever-changing" (Huston, 2020, p. 119).

For example, Gordon (2012) and Owarish (2013) shared insights regarding Kodak. Founded in 1880 by George Eastman, and one of America's most notable companies, Kodak helped establish the market for camera film and then dominated the field. But it suffered from a variety of problems over the last four decades of its existence—almost all related to being an aged organization. Kodak's top management never fully grasped how the world around them was changing and they hung on to assumptions (such as the idea that digital prints will never replace film prints) long after they became obsolete.

In addition, Kodak followed a pattern seen by many aged organizations that face technologic change. First, they tried to ignore a new technology hoping it would go away by itself. Then they openly put it down by using various justifications such as it is too expensive, too slow, and too complicated. Then they tried to prolong the life of the existing technology by attempting to create synergies between the new technology and the old (such as photo CD). This further delayed any serious commitment to the new order of things.

In the end, Kodak failed to realize its limitations, ignored the data, and spent an additional 15 years in avoidance mode until it became virtually irrelevant in the market. With only 1 full

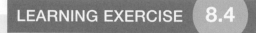

LEARNING EXERCISE   8.4

Young or Old Organization?

Reflect on the organization in which you work or the nursing school you attend. Do you believe that this organization has more characteristics of a young or aged organization? Diagram on a continuum from birth to death where you feel that this organization would fall. What actions has this organization taken to be dynamic and innovative? What further efforts could be made? Do you agree or disagree that most organizations change unpredictably? Can you support your conclusions with examples? If professions were classified the way organizations are, do you believe that the nursing profession would be classified as (a) an aging organization, (b) in constant motion and ever renewing, or (c) a closed system that does not respond well to change?

year of profit after 2004, Kodak ended up filing for bankruptcy in 2012, after 131 years of being the pioneer in the film industry.

Integrating Leadership Roles and Management Functions in Planned Change

Change and innovation are integral to organizational success. Leadership and management skills are necessary, however, for successful planned change to occur. The manager must understand the planning process and planning standards and be able to apply both to the work situation. The manager is also cognizant of the specific driving and restraining forces within a specific environment for change and can provide the tools or resources necessary to implement that change. The manager, then, is the mechanic who implements the planned change.

The leader, however, is the inventor or creator. Leaders today are forced to plan in a chaotic health care system that is changing at a frenetic pace. Out of this chaos, leaders must identify trends and changes that may affect their organizations and units and proactively prepare for these changes. Thus, the leader must retain a big-picture focus while dealing with each part of the system. In the inventor or creator role, the leader displays such traits as flexibility, confidence, tenacity, and the ability to articulate vision through insights and versatile thinking. The leader also must constantly look for and attempt to adapt to the changing and unpredictable interactions between agents and environmental factors as outlined by the complexity science theorists.

Both leadership and management skills are therefore necessary in planned change. The change agent fulfills a management function when identifying situations where change is necessary and appropriate and when assessing the driving and restraining forces affecting the plan for change. The leader is the role model in planned change. They are open and receptive to change, and view change as a challenge and an opportunity for growth. Other critical elements in successful planned change are the change agent's leadership skills—interpersonal communication, group management, and problem-solving abilities.

There is perhaps no greater need for the leader, though, than to be the catalyst for professional change as well as organizational change. Many people attracted to nursing now find that their values and traditional expectations no longer fit as they once did. It is the leader's role to help their followers confront the opportunities and challenges presented by the realities of emerging nursing practice; to create enthusiasm and passion for renewing the profession; to embrace the change of locus of control, which now belongs to the health care consumer; and to engage a new social context for nursing practice.

Key Concepts

- Change should not be viewed as a threat but as a challenge and a chance to do something new and innovative.
- Change, however, should be implemented only for good reason.
- Because change disrupts the homeostasis or balance of the group, resistance should be expected as a natural part of the change process.
- The level of resistance to change generally depends on the type of change proposed. Technologic changes encounter less resistance than changes that are perceived as social or that are contrary to established customs or norms.
- Perhaps the greatest factor contributing to the resistance encountered with change is a lack of trust between the employee and the manager or the employee and the organization.
- It is much easier to change a person's behavior than it is to change an entire group's behavior. It is also easier to change knowledge levels than attitudes.
- Change should be planned and thus implemented gradually, not sporadically or suddenly.
- Those who may be affected by a change should be involved in planning for it. Likewise, workers should thoroughly understand the change and its effect on them.

- The feeling of control is critical to thriving in a changing environment.
- Friends, family, and colleagues should be used as a network of support during change.
- The successful change agent has the leadership skills of problem solving and decision making as well as good interpersonal skills.
- In contrast to planned change, change by drift is unplanned or accidental.
- Historically, many of the changes that have occurred in nursing or have affected the profession are the results of change by drift.
- People maintain status quo or equilibrium when both driving and restraining forces operating within any field simultaneously occur. For change to happen, this balance of driving and restraining forces must be altered.
- Emerging theories such as complexity science suggest that change is unpredictable, occurs at random, and is dependent on rapidly changing relationships between agents and factors in the system and that even small changes can affect an entire organization.
- Organizations are preserved by change and constant renewal. Without change, they may stagnate and die.

Additional Learning Exercises and Applications

LEARNING EXERCISE 8.5

Implementing Planned Change in a Family Planning Clinic

You are a Hispanic registered nurse who has recently received a 2-year grant to establish a family planning clinic in a low-income area of a large city. This area has a primarily Hispanic population, which has been historically underserved in its access to health services. The project will be evaluated at the end of the grant to determine whether continued funding is warranted. As project director, you have the funds to choose and hire three health care workers. You will essentially be able to manage the clinic as you see fit.

The average age of your patients will be 14 years, and many come from single-parent homes. In addition, the population with which you will be working has high unemployment, high crime and truancy levels, and great suspicion and mistrust of authority figures due to experiences of discrimination. You are aware that many restraining forces exist that will challenge you, but you feel strongly committed to the cause. You believe that the high teenage pregnancy rate and maternal and infant morbidity can be reduced.

(continues on page 198)

LEARNING EXERCISE 8.5

Implementing Planned Change in a Family Planning Clinic (continued)

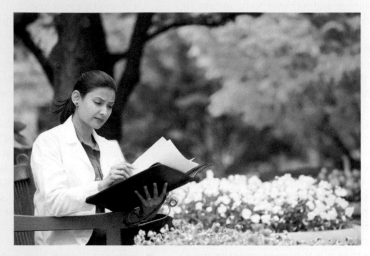

ASSIGNMENT:

1. Identify the restraining and driving forces in this situation.
2. Identify realistic short- and long-term goals for establishing the clinic. What can realistically be accomplished in 2 years?
3. How might the project director use hiring authority to increase the driving forces in this situation?
4. Is refreezing of the planned change possible so that changes will continue if the grant is not funded again in 2 years?

LEARNING EXERCISE 8.6

Retain the Status Quo or Implement Change?

Morale and productivity are low on the unit where you are the new manager. To identify the root of the problem, you have been meeting informally with staff to discuss their perceptions of unit functioning and to identify sources of unrest on the unit. You believe that one of the greatest factors leading to unrest is the limited advancement opportunity for your staff nurses. You have a fixed charge nurse on each shift. This is how the unit has been managed for as long as everyone can remember. You would like to rotate the charge nurse position but are unsure of your staff's feelings about the change.

ASSIGNMENT:

Using the phases of change identified by Lewin (1951), identify the actions you could take in unfreezing, movement, and refreezing. What are the greatest barriers to this change? What are the strongest driving forces?

LEARNING EXERCISE 8.7

How Would You Handle This Response to Change?

You are the unit manager of a cardiovascular surgical unit. The workstation on the unit is small, dated, and disorganized. The unit clerks have complained for some time that the chart racks on the counter above their desk are difficult to reach, that staff frequently impinge on the clerks' work space to discuss patients or to chart, that the call-light system is antiquated, and that supplies and forms need to be relocated. You ask all eight of your shift unit clerks to make a "wish list" of how they would like the workstation to be redesigned for optimum efficiency and effectiveness.

Construction is completed several months later. You are pleased that the new workstation incorporates what each unit clerk included in their top three priorities for change. There is a new revolving chart rack in the center of the workstation, with enhanced accessibility to both staff and unit clerks. A new, state-of-the-art call-light system has been installed. A small, quiet room has been created for nurses to chart and conference, and new cubbyholes and filing drawers now put forms within arm's reach of the charge nurse and unit clerk.

Almost immediately, you begin to be barraged with complaints about the changes. Several of the unit clerks find the new call-light system's computerized response system overwhelming and complain that patient lights are now going unanswered. Others complain that with the chart rack out of their immediate work area, charts can no longer be monitored and are being removed from the unit by physicians or left in the charting room by nurses. One unit clerk has filed a complaint that she was injured by a staff member who carelessly and rapidly turned the chart rack. She refuses to work again until the old chart racks are returned. The regular day-shift unit clerk complains that all the forms are filed backward for left-handed people and that after 20 years, she should have the right to put them the way that she likes it. Several of the nurses are complaining that the workstation is "now the domain of the unit clerk" and that access to the telephones and desk supplies is limited by the unit clerks. There have been some rumblings that several staff members believe that you favored the requests of some employees over others.

Today, when you make rounds at change of shift, you find the day-shift unit clerk and charge nurse involved in a heated conversation with the evening-shift unit clerk and charge nurse. Each evening, the charge nurse and unit clerk reorganize the workstation in the manner that they believe is most effective, and each morning, the charge nurse and unit clerk put things back the way they had been the prior day. Both believe that the other shift is undermining their efforts to "fix" the workstation organization and that their method of organization is the best. Both groups of workers turn to you and demand that you "make the other shift stop sabotaging our efforts to change things for the better."

ASSIGNMENT:

Despite your intent to include subordinate input into this planned change, resistance is high and worker morale is decreasing. Is the level of resistance a normal and anticipated response to planned change? If so, would you intervene in this conflict? How? Was it possible to have reduced the likelihood of such a high degree of resistance?

LEARNING EXERCISE   8.8

Overcoming Resistance to a Needed Change

You are the charge nurse of a medical/surgical unit. Recently, your hospital spent millions of dollars to implement a bedside medication verification (BMV) system to reduce medication errors and to promote a culture of patient safety. In this system, the nurse, using a handheld device, scans the drug they are planning to give against the patient's medication record to make sure that the right drug, at the right dose, is being given at the right time to the right patient. The nurse then scans the patient's name band/arm band to assure the right patient is receiving the drug and finally scans their own name badge to document who is administering the drug to the patient. If any of the codes do not match, a signal goes off, alerting the nurse of the discrepancy.

It has come to your attention, however, that some nurses are overriding the safety features built into the bar-coding system. For example, some nurses are reluctant to wake sleeping patients to scan their barcode before they administer an intravenous push medication and instead simply scan the chart label. Some nurses have overridden the bar code warning, assuming it was a technologic glitch. Some nurses have administered drugs to patients despite having name bands that have become smudged or torn and no longer scan well. Still other nurses are carrying multiple prescanned pills on one tray or charting that drugs have been given, even though they were left at the bedside. Finally, you learned that one nurse even affixed extra copies of her patient's bar codes to her clipboard, so that they could be scanned more quickly.

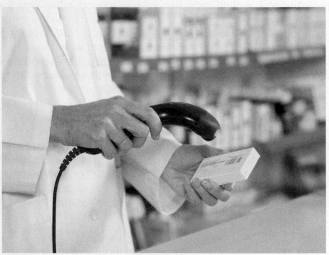

ASSIGNMENT:

Despite thorough orientation and training regarding BMV, some staff have developed "work-arounds" to the barcoding system, increasing the risk of medication errors and patient harm. Your staff suggests that although they understand BMV reduces risks to patients, the equipment does not always work and performing the additional safety checks often takes them more time than how they did it in the past, ultimately delaying medications to patients who need them. The staff states they will try to be more careful in implementing the BMV procedures, but you continue to sense resistance on their part. What strategies could you employ now to foster refreezing of the new system? Would rational–empirical, power–coercive, or normative–reeducative strategies be more effective? Provide a rationale for your choice.

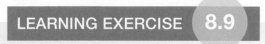

LEARNING EXERCISE 8.9

Promoting Evidence-Based Practice

In recent years, the implementation of evidence-based practice has been identified as a priority across nearly every nursing specialty. In addition, nurses are increasingly accepted as essential members, and often as leaders, of the interdisciplinary health care teams. To effectively participate and lead a health care team, nurses must have knowledge of the most effective and reliable evidence-based approaches to care, increase their expertise in critiquing research, and apply the evidence of their findings to select optimal interventions for their patients (Ford & Graves, 2023).

ASSIGNMENT:

Identify at least five things you might do to increase your knowledge and use of evidence in your practice. What are the most significant driving and restraining forces to make this change? Would you anticipate (overt or covert) resistance to your efforts? Will you need to enlist support from others or acquire additional resources for this planned change to occur? (Examples might be administrative support, access to scholarly journals, or mentoring.)

LEARNING EXERCISE 8.10

Implementing Change at the Unit Level

You are an oncology RN who has recently been selected chair of an oncology procedure committee. Your supervisor has suggested you guide the committee in creating a new procedure for shift report so that it is more efficient. Presently all team members of the oncoming shift gather in the break room and hear report for all the patients on the unit. The departing team leaders take turns coming into the break room to give report on their patients. Your supervisor feels that once team members hear report on all their assigned patients that they should begin their shift duties rather than listening to entire report, as this change would likely reduce overtime. She feels that if the procedure committee plans the change carefully it can be successful.

Your committee knows that there will be some resistance to the plan so in addition to developing a procedure for the new reporting system you feel you should plan for overcoming resistance to the change.

ASSIGNMENT:

1. Identify the restraining and driving forces in this situation.
2. Identify areas where your plan may be sabotaged.
3. How could you use research to increase the driving forces in this situation?
4. How long do you think it would take for refreezing of the planned change, so the unit does not go back to the old form of report?

REFERENCES

Bennis, W., Benne, K., & Chinn, R. (1969). *The planning of change* (2nd ed.). Holt, Rinehart, & Winston.

Bhasin, H. (2020, September 26). *Planned change: Definition, theories, effects and steps.* Retrieved June 24, 2022 from https://www.marketing91.com/planned-change/#:~:text=September%2026%2C%202020%20By%20Hitesh%20Bhasin%20Tagged%20With%3A,processes%2C%20or%20any%20other%20relevant%20and%20related%20aspect

Bligh, M. C., Kohles, J. C., & Yan, Q. (2018). Leading and learning to change: The role of leadership style and mindset in error learning and organizational change. *Journal of Change Management, 18*(2), 116–141.

Burrowes, N., & Needs, A. (2009). Time to contemplate change? A framework for assessing readiness to change with offenders. *Aggression & Violent Behavior, 14*(1), 39–49.

Carucci, R. (2021, April 30). How leaders get in the way of organizational change. *Harvard Business Review.* Retrieved June 24, 2022 from https://hbr.org/2021/04/how-leaders-get-in-the-way-of-organizational-change

Ford, C. D., & Graves, B. A. (2023). Evidence based practice (chapter 5). In Huston, C. (2023). *Professional issues in nursing: Challenges and opportunities* (6th ed., pp. 67–77). Wolters Kluwer.

Gordon, M. (2012, March 30). *The fall of Kodak: 5 Lessons for small business.* SCORE. Retrieved June 24, 2022 from https://nemassachusetts.score.org/resource/fall-kodak-5-lessons-small-business

Heathfield, S. M. (2021, February 4). *How to reduce employee resistance to change.* The Balance Careers. Retrieved June 24, 2022 from https://www.thebalancecareers.com/how-to-reduce-employee-resistance-to-change-1918992

Huston, C. (2020). *The road to positive work cultures.* Sigma Theta Tau International.

Lewin, K. (1951). *Field theory in social sciences: Selected theoretical papers.* Harper & Row.

McQuerrey, L. (2019, February 6). How to overcome resistance to change in an organization. *Chron.* Retrieved June 24, 2022 from https://smallbusiness.chron.com/overcome-resistance-change-organization-154.html

MIT News. (2008). *Edward Lorenz, father of chaos theory and butterfly effect, dies at 90.* Retrieved June 24, 2022 from http://web.mit.edu/newsoffice/2008/obit-lorenz-0416.html

Olson, E. E., & Eoyang, G. H. (2001). *Facilitating organization change: Lessons from complexity science.* Jossey-Bass/Pfeiffer.

Owarish, F. (2013). *Strategic leadership of technology: Lessons learned.* Retrieved June 24, 2022 from https://documents.pub/document/strategic-leadership-of-technology-lessons-learned.html

Quain, S. (2019, February 12). What causes resistance to change in an organization? *Chron.* Retrieved June 24, 2022 from https://smallbusiness.chron.com/causes-resistance-change-organization-347.html

Sherman, R. O., & Cohn, T. M. (2021, September 14). *Navigating an environment of continuous change.* American Nurse. Retrieved June 24, 2022 from https://www.myamericannurse.com/wp-content/uploads/2021/08/Leading-the-Way_Change_final-3.pdf

9

Time Management

… nothing is particularly hard if you divide it into small jobs.—**Henry Ford**

… things which matter most must never be at the mercy of things that matter least.—**Johann Wolfgang von Goethe**

… The bad news is time flies. The good news is you're the pilot.—**Michael Altshuler**

CROSSWALK

This chapter addresses:

- **AACN Essentials Domain 5:** Quality and safety
- **AACN Essentials Domain 7:** Systems-based practice
- **AACN Essentials Domain 8:** Information and health care technologies
- **AACN Essentials Domain 10:** Personal, professional, and leadership development
- **AONL Nurse Executive Competency 1:** Communication and relationship building
- **AONL Nurse Executive Competency 2:** A knowledge of the health care environment
- **ANA Standard of Professional Performance 10:** Communication
- **ANA Standard of Professional Performance 11:** Collaboration
- **ANA Standard of Professional Performance 12:** Leadership
- **ANA Standard of Professional Performance 15:** Quality of practice
- **ANA Standard of Professional Performance 17:** Resource stewardship
- **ANA Standard of Professional Performance 18:** Environmental health
- **QSEN Competency:** Safety
- **QSEN Competency:** Teamwork and collaboration

LEARNING OBJECTIVES

The learner will:

- analyze how time is managed both personally and at the unit level of the organization
- describe the importance of allowing adequate time for daily planning and priority setting
- describe factors that influence the perception of the time needed to complete a task
- complete tasks according to the priority level they have been assigned whenever possible
- build evaluation steps into planning so that reprioritization can occur
- identify common internal and external time wasters as well as interventions that can be taken to reduce their impact
- complete a time inventory to increase self-awareness regarding personal priority setting and time management
- identify how technology applications such as e-mail, the internet, telecommunications, and social networking can both facilitate and hinder personal time management
- involve subordinates and followers in maximizing time use and guiding work to its successful implementation and conclusion

Introduction

Another part of the planning process is short-term planning. This operational planning focuses on achieving specific tasks. Short-term plans involve a period of 1 hour to 3 years and are usually less complex than strategic or long-range plans. Short-term planning may be done annually, quarterly, monthly, weekly, daily, or even hourly.

Previous chapters examined the need for prudent planning of resources, such as money, equipment, supplies, and labor. Time is an equally important resource. It feels good to get things done in a timely manner. When we lack the time for this to occur, we feel overwhelmed, leading to increased errors, the omission of important tasks, and general feelings of stress and ineffectiveness.

If leaders are to empower others to achieve personal and shared goals, they need to become experts in the planning and implementation of goal attainment. If managers are to direct employees effectively and maximize other resources, they must first be able to find the time to do so. In other words, both must become experts at time management.

Time management can be defined as making optimal use of available time. Many people argue that there is not enough time in the day to do everything that must be done. Yet everyone has the same amount of time in a day, but some people consistently get much more done than others. The problem then may be how the time available is being used.

Optimizing time management must include priority setting, managing and controlling crises, and balancing work and personal time. All these activities require some degree of both leadership skills and management functions. Leadership roles and management functions needed for effective time management are listed in Display 9.1.

> Good time management skills allow an individual to spend time on things
> that matter.

DISPLAY 9.1 LEADERSHIP ROLES AND MANAGEMENT FUNCTIONS IN TIME MANAGEMENT

Leadership Roles

1. Is self-aware regarding personal blocks and barriers to efficient time management
2. Recognizes how one's own value system influences one's use of time and the expectations of followers
3. Functions as a role model, supporter, and resource person to others in setting priorities for goal attainment
4. Assists followers in working cooperatively to maximize time use
5. Prevents and/or filters interruptions that prevent effective time management
6. Role models flexibility in working cooperatively with other people whose primary time management style is different
7. Presents a calm and reassuring demeanor during periods of high unit activity
8. Prioritizes conflicting and overlapping requests for time
9. Appropriately determines the quality of work needed in tasks to be completed

Management Functions

1. Appropriately prioritizes day-to-day planning to meet short-term and long-term unit goals
2. Builds time for planning into the work schedule
3. Analyzes how time is managed on the unit level by using job analysis and time-and-motion studies
4. Eliminates environmental barriers to effective time management for workers
5. Handles paperwork promptly and efficiently and maintains a neat work area
6. Breaks down large tasks into smaller ones that can more easily be accomplished by unit members
7. Utilizes appropriate technology to facilitate timely communication and documentation
8. Discriminates between inadequate staffing and inefficient use of time when time resources are inadequate to complete assigned tasks

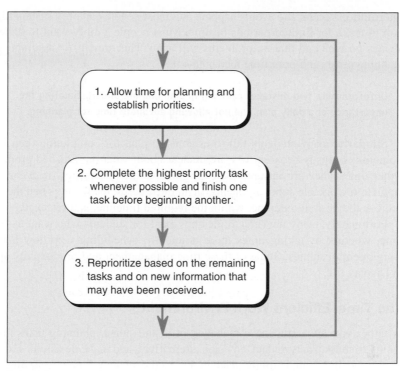

FIGURE 9.1 The three basic steps to time management.

Three Basic Steps to Time Management

There are three basic steps to time management (Fig. 9.1). The first step is setting aside time for planning and establishing priorities. The second step entails completing the highest priority task (as determined in Step 1) whenever possible and finishing one task before beginning another. In the final step, the person must reprioritize what tasks will be accomplished based on new information received. Because this is a cyclic process, all three steps must be accomplished sequentially.

Taking Time to Plan and Establishing Priorities

Planning is essential if an individual is to manage by efficiency rather than by crisis, and the adage "fail to plan—plan to fail" is timeless. Planning occurs first in the management process because the ability to be organized develops from good planning. During planning, there should be time to think about how plans will be translated into action. The planner must pause and decide how people, activities, and materials are going to be put together to carry out the objectives.

Many individuals believe that they are unproductive if they take time out early in their day to design a plan for action rather than immediately beginning work on tasks. Without adequate planning, however, the individual finds it difficult to get started and begins to manage by crisis. In addition, there can be no sense of achievement at day's end if the goals for the day are not clearly delineated. Managers who are new to time management may underestimate the importance of regular planning and fail to allot enough time for it.

In addition, many individuals repeatedly fail to complete planned tasks because they don't allow adequate resources (time, energy, human or physical resources, etc.) for task completion. For example, the student who carries home a full backpack every night with the expectation that every assignment or task will always be completed is likely to be disappointed.

Interruptions occur, life events happen, and most people can only sustain high levels of attention to tasks for limited periods of time. Most people simply want to believe that tasks will always go well and that no problems will arise. This unrealistic assumption leads to serious planning errors and poor time management.

> Unfortunately, two mistakes common in planning are underestimating the importance of a daily plan and not allowing adequate time for planning.

Similarly, many students fail to establish a plan for completing their learning activities. Sometimes, this is because they are unclear about what the finished product must look like. Other times, they are unsure when assignments are due or how to break large assignments down into workable subcomponents. In all these cases, the result is that the student's ability to achieve the desired outcome, within the required timeline, is threatened.

Fortunately, many new electronic apps exist for students who want to better manage their time, whether by taking notes more efficiently, scheduling workflow better, or sticking to assignment deadlines. Some of these time management and productivity apps are previewed in Display 9.2.

The Time-Efficient Work Environment

Whether you are a student, a manager, or a staff nurse, planning takes time; it requires the ability to think, analyze data, envision alternatives, and make decisions. Examples of the types of plans a charge nurse might make in day-to-day planning include staffing schedules, patient care assignments, coordination of lunch- and work-break schedules, and interdisciplinary coordination of patient care. Examples of an acute care staff nurse's day-to-day planning might include determining how handoff reports will be given and received; the timing and method used for initial patient assessments; the coordination of medication administration, treatments, and procedures; and organizing the documentation of the day's activities.

Some staff nurses, however, appear disorganized in their efforts to care for patients, which may result in *unfinished nursing care* (UNC) (any task that is omitted or significantly delayed). Indeed, nurses report leaving at least one patient care task incomplete up to 98% of the time. Commonly reported UNC include providing patients with comfort and emotional support, documenting care plans, and providing patient education (Bryant & Yoder, 2021). This may be the result of poor planning, or it may be a symptom of a work environment that is not conducive to efficient time management.

The following suggestions, based on industrial engineering principles, may assist the staff nurse in planning work activities, especially when the environment poses obstacles to time efficiency:

- *Gather all the supplies and equipment that will be needed before starting an activity.* Breaking a job down mentally into parts before beginning the activity may help the staff nurse identify what supplies and equipment will be needed to complete the activity.

LEARNING EXERCISE 9.1

Making Big Projects Manageable

Think of the last major paper you wrote for a class. Did you set short-term and intermediate deadlines? Did you break the task down into smaller tasks to prevent a last-minute crisis? What short-term and intermediate deadlines have you set to accomplish major projects that have been assigned to you this quarter or semester? Are you realistic about the time that will be required to complete the task or are you likely to experience planning fallacies?

DISPLAY 9.2 SAMPLE TIME MANAGEMENT AND COMMUNICATION PRODUCTIVITY APPS

- **Time Doctor:** tracks other people's schedules and offers screen monitoring software, a tool to monitor internet usage, website application monitoring, and more.
- **Calendar:** offers multiple ways to gauge how you are spending your own time and offers insights about your team's productivity.
- **Roadmap:** tracking app for remote employees. Balances the schedules of multiple people and provides insights as to how project goals are lining up with the realities of available resources so that adjustments can be made accordingly.
- **Click Up:** cloud-based project management software that coordinates an organization's projects and tasks on a single platform.
- **Basecamp:** organizes all important tasks into three categories and displays them on one convenient dashboard. In addition, there is a "project" section where members of different teams can work together to finish a project. Here people can share tasks and see every step of the project from start to completion.
- **Asana:** a project management app that breaks down tasks into either a list or a calendar. This allows users to see when they have something due on a calendar, and to address tasks in an orderly fashion. This app also emails notifications about upcoming due dates.
- **Float:** a project management task software with a click and drop scheduler that helps users visualize teamwork load, assign tasks, and make updates. Also helps make task assignments, mark milestones, group projects, and add tasks notes.
- **ProofHub:** project management software that helps to plan what needs to be done, discusses ideas, organizes documents, and delivers projects of all sizes.
- **Hive:** all-in-one project management tool that includes action templates, proofing and approvals, time-tracking, and forms.
- **Google Hangouts:** video meeting software that allows meetings and chat through a voice or video call.
- **Skype:** communication platform that allows easy messaging, voice calls, screen sharing, and video conference calls across all desktop, iOS, and Android devices.
- **Join.me:** communication system to organize meetings. Includes free conference calling capabilities, video conferencing, screen sharing, and chat (through Slack), but also offers additional benefits like webinar training services and a mobile whiteboard.
- **Slack:** chat tool for quick group or one-on-one communications.
- **Workplace by Facebook:** functions as a joint Facebook account for team members. This allows members to hold group discussions, post updates about projects, comment and offer suggestions on posts, and also participate in voice and video calling.
- **Troop Messenger:** business collaboration tool which offers secure and seamless team collaboration.
- **I Done This:** productivity app that is essentially a to-do list. When tasks are accomplished, an incomplete red "x" turns to a green completed check mark.
- **Todoist:** productivity app to list tasks to be accomplished. Tasks are labeled, assigned a due date, and then filtered by priority.
- **Dropbox:** cloud storage app for file sharing.
- **Google Drive:** cloud storage app for file sharing, collaboration, editing, commenting on documents, and more.
- **Shift:** streamlines workflows to get things done more efficiently.
- **Evernote:** note taking app to jot down thoughts and ideas.

Source: Adapted from *21 Best time management apps to be more productive in 2021*. (2021). Time Doctor. https://biz30. timedoctor.com/best-time-management-apps/

- *Get organized.* Rampton (2018) notes that the average American spends 2.5 days each year looking for misplaced items. Have a home for everything and make sure that items are put back where they belong. Rampton also suggests single tasking because most people cite multitasking as the main culprit for misplacing items.
- *Group activities that are in the same location.* If you have walked a long distance down a hallway, attempt to do several things there before going back to the nurses' station. If you

are a home health nurse, group patient visits geographically when possible, to minimize travel time and maximize time with patients.

- *Use time estimates.* For example, if you know an intermittent intravenous medication (IV piggyback) will take 30 minutes to complete, then use that time estimate for planning some other activity that can be completed in that 30-minute window of time.
- *Document your nursing interventions as soon as possible after an activity is completed.* Waiting until the end of the workday to complete necessary documentation increases the risk of inaccuracies and incomplete documentation.
- *Always strive to end the workday on time.* Although this is not always possible, delegating appropriately to others and making sure that the workload goal for any given day is reasonable are two strategies that will accomplish this goal.

Like staff nurses, unit managers need to coordinate how their duties will be carried out and devise methods to make work simpler and more efficient. Often, this includes simple tasks such as organizing how supplies are stored or determining the most efficient lunch and break schedules for staff. In addition, it is the manager's responsibility to see that units are appropriately stocked with the equipment nurses need to do their work. This reduces the time spent in trying to locate needed supplies.

Daily planning actions that may help the unit manager identify and utilize time as a resource most efficiently might include the following:

- At the start of each workday, identify key priorities to be accomplished that day. Identify what specific actions need to be taken to accomplish those priorities and in what order they should be done. Also, identify specific actions that should be taken to meet ongoing, long-term goals.
- Determine the level of achievement that you expect for each prioritized task. Is a maximizing or "satisficing" approach more appropriate or more reasonable for each of the goals you have identified?
- Assess the staff assigned to work with you. Assign work that must be delegated to staff members who are both capable and willing to accomplish the priority task that you have identified. Be sure that you have clearly expressed any expectations you may have about how and when a delegated task must be completed. (Delegation is discussed further in Chapter 20.)
- Review the short- and long-term plans of the unit regularly. Include colleagues and subordinates in identifying unit problems or concerns so that they can be fully involved in planning for needed change.
- Plan ahead for meetings. Prepare and distribute agendas in advance.
- Allow time at several points throughout the day and at the end of the day to assess progress in meeting established daily goals and to determine if unanticipated events have occurred or if new information has been received that may have altered your original plan. Ongoing realities for the unit manager include work situations that are constantly changing, and with them, setting new priorities and adjusting older ones.
- Take regularly scheduled breaks. Planning for periodic breaks from work during the workday is an integral part of time and task management. These work breaks allow both managers and staff to refresh physically and mentally.
- Using an electronic calendar to organize your day can help make a day feel less chaotic. It can also help you identify pockets of spare time that you could use for breaks.

> Setting new priorities or adjusting priorities to reflect ever-changing work situations is an ongoing reality for the manager.

LEARNING EXERCISE   9.2

Setting Daily Priorities

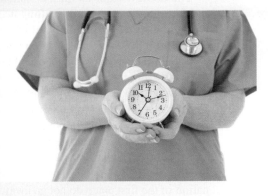

You are the registered nurse-leader of a team with one licensed vocational nurse and one nursing assistant on the 7 AM to 3 PM shift at an acute care hospital. The three of you are responsible for providing total care to 10 patients. Prioritize the following list of 10 things that you need to accomplish this morning. Use a "1" for the first thing you will do and a "10" for the last. Be prepared to provide rationale for your priorities.

_____ Check medication sheet against the patient medication record.
_____ Listen to night shift handoff.
_____ Take brief walking rounds to assess the night shift report and to introduce yourself to patients.
_____ Hang four 9:00 AM intravenous medications.
_____ Set up the schedule for breaks and lunch among your team members.
_____ Give 8:45 AM preoperative medications on patient going to surgery at 9:00 AM.
_____ Pass 8:30 AM breakfast trays.
_____ Meet with team members to plan the schedule for the day and to clarify roles.
_____ Read charts of patients who are new to you.
_____ Check 6:00 AM blood glucose laboratory results for 7:30 AM insulin administration.

Priority Setting and Procrastination

Because most individuals are inundated with requests for their time and energy, the next step in time management is prioritizing, which may well be the key to good time management. Unfortunately, some individuals lack self-awareness about what is important and therefore how to spend their time.

> Priority setting is perhaps the most critical skill in good time management because all actions we take have some type of relative importance.

One simple means of prioritizing what needs to be accomplished is to divide all requests into three categories: "don't do," "do later," and "do now" (Display 9.3). The don't do items probably reflect problems that will take care of themselves, are already outdated, or are better accomplished by someone else. The individual either throws away the unnecessary information or passes it on to the appropriate person in a timely fashion. In either case, the individual removes unneeded clutter from the work area.

Before setting "do later" items aside, the leader-manager must be sure that large projects have been broken down into smaller projects and that a specific timeline and plan for implementation are in place. The plan should include short-term, intermediate, and final deadlines.

DISPLAY 9.3   THREE CATEGORIES OF PRIORITIZATION

1. "Don't do"
2. "Do later"
3. "Do now"

Likewise, one cannot ignore items without immediate time limits forever and must make a definite time commitment soon to address these requests.

The do now requests most commonly reflect a unit's day-to-day operational needs. These requests may include daily staffing needs, dealing with equipment shortages, meeting schedules, conducting hiring interviews, and giving performance appraisals. Do now requests also may represent items that had been put off earlier.

Some do later items reflect trivial problems or those that do not have immediate deadlines; thus, they may be procrastinated. To *procrastinate* means to put off something until a future time, to postpone, or to delay needlessly. Wang et al. (2021, para 1) go so far as to say that procrastination is the "quintessence of self-regulatory failure"; however, procrastination can be justified if it is more important to do something of higher priority now, but it should not be used to avoid a task because it is overwhelming or unpleasant.

More often, however, procrastination is a barrier to effective time management. This occurs because typically, the task is just delayed in its completion and the things that led to procrastination in the first place do not go away. In addition, people who procrastinate often feel guilty later and regret having put off the task at hand.

Procrastination, however, is a difficult problem to solve because it rarely results from a single cause and can involve a combination of dysfunctional attitudes, rationalizations, and resentment. For example, sometimes, procrastination is caused by perfectionism. It can also occur when someone feels too overwhelmed to even begin.

New research even suggests that procrastination may have neurobiologic causes. The tendency to procrastinate seems to run in families. Indeed, one landmark study examining identical twins argued that 46% of a person's tendency to procrastinate was due to genetic factors, making the problem "moderately heritable" and a second study found compelling evidence linking procrastination to a gene involved in the production enzyme tyrosine hydroxylase (associated with the regulation of neurotransmitter dopamine) (Ling, 2021).

In addition, new research has found a relationship between the gray matter volume of the amygdala in the brain and difficulties in initiating action. Theoretically, this is known as *decision-related action orientation*. Those who have greater gray matter volume in the amygdala are more likely to procrastinate (Davis, 2021). This neural signature of action suggests that procrastination may reflect a problem with emotion regulation.

Whether procrastination has a neurobiologic cause or not, it can and does interfere with productivity. Individuals who frequently procrastinate should establish clear goals and attempt to understand why it is that they are procrastinating. They should also focus on increasing self-control and developing an action plan for the completion of tasks. The key to successful procrastination is to use it appropriately and selectively.

LEARNING EXERCISE   9.3

Targeting Personal Procrastination

Spend a few moments reflecting on the last 2 weeks of your life. What are the things you put off doing? Do these things form a pattern? For instance, do you always put off writing a school paper until the last minute? Do you wait to do certain tasks at work until you cannot avoid the task any longer? What things do you do when you really do not want to do something? Do you eat? Play video games? Watch TV? Read?

ASSIGNMENT:

Write a one-page essay on at least two things that you procrastinate and then develop two strategies for breaking each of these habits.

Making Lists

In prioritizing the do now items, the leader-manager may find preparing a written list helpful. Remember, however, that a list is a plan, not a product, and that the creation of the list is not the final goal. The list is a planning tool.

Although the individual may use monthly or weekly lists, a list also can assist in coordinating daily operations. This daily list, however, should not be longer than what can be realistically accomplished in 1 day; otherwise, it demotivates instead of assists.

In addition, although the leader-manager must be cognizant of and plan for routine tasks, it is not always necessary to place them on the list because they may only distract attention from other priority tasks. Lists should allow adequate time for each task and have blocks of time built in for the unexpected. In addition, individuals who use lists to help them organize their day must be careful not to confuse importance and urgency.

> Not all important things are urgent, and not all urgent things are important. This is especially true when the urgency is coming from an external source.

In addition, the individual should periodically review lists from previous days to see what was not accomplished or completed. If a task appears on a list for several successive days, the manager must reexamine it and assess why it was not accomplished. Sometimes, tasks just need to be removed from the list. This occurs when a task has low priority or when it is better done by someone else. Other times, undone tasks on the list should be discarded because they are duplicative or unimportant.

Sometimes, however, items on the list remain unaccomplished because they are not divided into steps or tasks that can be completed. Breaking a big job down into smaller parts can make the task seem more manageable. For example, many well-meaning people begin thinking about completing their tax returns in early January but feel overwhelmed by a project that cannot be accomplished in a day or two. If preparing a tax return is not broken down into several smaller tasks with intermediate deadlines, it may be almost perpetually procrastinated.

> Some projects are not accomplished because they are not broken down into manageable tasks.

Reprioritizing

The last step in time management is reprioritizing. Often, one's priorities or list will change during a day, week, or longer because new information is received. If the individual does not take time to reprioritize after each major task is accomplished, other priorities set earlier may no longer be accurate. In addition, despite outstanding planning, an occasional crisis may erupt.

> No amount of planning can prevent an occasional crisis.

If a crisis does occur, the individual may need to set aside the original priorities for the day and reorganize, communicate, and delegate a new plan reflecting the new priorities associated with the unexpected event causing the crisis.

Dealing with Interruptions

All managers experience interruptions, but lower-level managers typically experience the most. This occurs in part because first- and middle-level managers are more involved in daily planning than higher-level managers and thus directly interact with a greater number of subordinates. In addition, many lower-level managers do not have a quiet workspace or clerical help to filter interruptions.

LEARNING EXERCISE 9.4

Creating Planning Lists

Do you make a daily plan to organize what needs to be done? Mentally or on paper, develop a list of five items that must be accomplished today. Prioritize that list. Now make a list of five items that must be done this week. Prioritize that list as well.

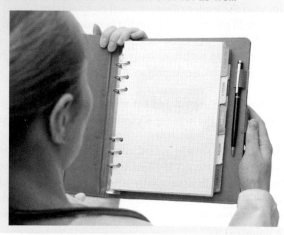

Interruptions can cause a great deal of time wasting because attention is continually diverted from the task at hand. All managers need protected time to respond to time-sensitive phone calls or e-mails, and it is important not to be disturbed during these times unless there is an urgent request for an answer or guidance on dealing with an emergency.

Frequent work interruptions also cause situational stress and lowered job satisfaction. That's because interruptions cause us to split our attention between what we should be doing and addressing the new demands. James Clear suggests the result of this divided attention is "*half–work*," work that takes twice as long to accomplish half as much (Rampton, 2018). Managers then need to develop skill in preventing interruptions that threaten effective time management.

> Lower–level managers experience more interruptions than higher–level managers.

Dealing with interruptions also requires leadership skills. Leaders role model flexibility and the ability to regroup when new information or tasks emerge as priorities. Followers often observe how their leaders are coping with change and even crisis, and their reactions often mirror those of their leaders. That is often why a staff nurse who feels harried or out of control typically finds these same feelings reflected in the individuals they are assigned to work with.

Time Wasters

There are many time wasters, and the time wasters that are used most often vary by the individual. Four time wasters warrant special attention here (Display 9.4). The first of these surprisingly is technology, which generally has been promoted as a time saver for most people. Indeed, technology can and does save time. E-mail now makes instantaneous, asynchronous communication to multiple parties possible simultaneously, and the internet provides virtually

DISPLAY 9.4   TIME WASTERS

1. Technology (internet, gaming, e-mail, and social media sites)
2. Socializing
3. Paperwork overload
4. A poor filing system
5. Interruptions

unlimited access to emerging, state of the science knowledge globally. In addition, social networks such as Facebook, Pinterest, and Twitter have created new opportunities for communicating in real time to vast networks of users.

Yet, this same technology increasingly consumes more and more of our time. Many individuals find themselves randomly searching the internet or playing online games to distract themselves from the tasks at hand. In addition, the need to check and respond to so many different communication mediums is time consuming in itself.

Finally, all this technology can make it difficult to find an appropriate balance between the need for virtual and face-to-face interaction and between work and personal life. Staying plugged in and checking e-mails nonstop throughout the day can waste time and use significant energy. This causes boundaries between work and personal life to blur.

A second time waster is socializing. Socializing with colleagues during the workday can waste significant amounts of time in a workday. Although socializing can help workers meet relationship needs or build power, it can tremendously deter productivity. This is especially true for managers with an open-door policy. Subordinates can be discouraged from taking up a manager's time with idle chatter in several ways:

- *Do not make yourself overly accessible.* Make it easy for people to ignore you. Try not to "work" at the nursing station, if this is possible. If charting is to be done, sit with your back to others. If you have an office, close the door. Have people make appointments to see you. All these behaviors will discourage casual socializers.
- *Interrupt.* When someone is rambling on without getting to the point, break in and say gently, "Excuse me. I'm not getting your message. What exactly are you saying?"
- *Avoid promoting socialization.* Having several comfortable chairs in your office, a full candy dish, and posters on your walls that invite comments encourage socializing in your office.
- *Be brief.* Watch your own long-winded comments and stand up when you are finished. This will signal an end to the conversation.
- *Schedule time for people who tend to ramble or like to talk.* If someone has a pattern of lengthy chatter and manages to corner you on rounds or at the nurse's station, say, "I can't speak with you now, but I'm going to have some free time at 11 AM. Why don't you see me then?" Unless the meeting is important, the person who just wishes to chat will not bother to make a formal appointment. If you would like to chat and have the time to do so, use breaks and lunch hours for socializing.

Other external time wasters that a manager must conquer are paperwork overload and a poor filing system. Managers are generally inundated with paper clutter, including organizational memos, staffing requests, quality assurance reports, incident reports, and patient evaluations. Because paperwork is often redundant or unnecessary, the manager needs to become an expert at handling it. Whenever possible, incoming correspondence should be handled the day it arrives; it should either be thrown away or filed according to the date to be completed. Try to address each piece of correspondence only once.

An adequate filing system also is invaluable to handling paper overload. Keeping correspondence organized in easily retrievable files rather than disorganized stacks saves time when the manager needs to find specific information. The manager also may want to consider increased use of computerization and e-mail to reduce the paper use and to increase response time in time-sensitive communication.

Personal Time Management

Personal time management refers in part to self-knowledge. Self-awareness is a leadership skill. For people who are not certain of their own short- and long-term goals, time management, in general, poses difficulties. These goals give structure to what should be accomplished today, tomorrow, and in the future. However, goals alone are not enough; a concrete plan with timelines is needed. Plans outlined in manageable steps are clearer, more realistic, and attainable. By being self-aware and setting goals accordingly, people determine how their time will be spent. If goals are not set, others often end up deciding how a person should spend their time.

Indeed, many college students often report feeling time challenged and overwhelmed by their numerous academic, work, and personal commitments. This may reflect a lack of priority or goal setting, or it may simply reflect too many things to be reasonably accomplished in the time frame given. In addition, perceived content relevance, technology usability, and innate learner conscientiousness may influence learners' ability to complete coursework on time (see Examining the Evidence 9.1). Research by Cheng and Xie (2021) suggests, however, that instructor engagement is not a predictor of academic procrastination, suggesting even highly engaged instructors may not be able to help some students avoid procrastination.

EXAMINING THE EVIDENCE 9.1

Source: From Cheng, S.-L., & Xie, K. (2021, June). Why college students procrastinate in online courses: A self-regulated learning perspective. *Internet & Higher Education, 50.* https://www.sciencedirect.com/science/article/abs/pii/S1096751621000166?via%3Dihub

Why Students Procrastinate in Online Courses

The purpose of this research was to examine why college students procrastinated in online courses from a self-regulated learning perspective. A sample of 207 college students enrolled in six two-credit, 7-week online undergraduate courses in animal sciences, anthropology, educational psychology, entomology, history, and nursing at a mid-western university in the United States during the spring 2019 semester, completed surveys for the study.

The study found that on average, students in the sample experienced a moderate level of procrastination and that this procrastination stemmed from the interrelationships between students' perceptions of learning context, personality traits, and motivational beliefs. Perceptions of instructor engagement, peer interaction, and content relevance were positively associated with one another as were perceptions of technology usability and content relevance. Conscientious students were, however, less likely to procrastinate in online courses.

When students perceived that course materials were intellectually stimulating and comprehensible, they were more likely to see the value of engaging in learning activities and procrastinated less frequently. Similarly, when they perceived that technology and multimedia implemented in a course were not disruptive, they were less likely to experience emotional distress and had a greater tendency to complete academic tasks on time.

The researchers concluded that procrastination by college students in online courses was indirectly related to external factors, including perceived content relevance and technology usability, and directly related to internal factors, including conscientiousness, task value, and emotional cost. To help students avoid procrastination, making course materials relevant and technology components well implemented should be a top priority for instructors. However, instructor engagement did not predict academic procrastination, suggesting even highly engaged instructors may not be able to help some students avoid procrastination.

Think for a moment about last week. Did you accomplish all that you wanted to accomplish? How much time did you or others waste? In your clinical practice, did you spend your time hunting for supplies and medicines instead of teaching your patient about their condition?

Too often, irrelevant decisions and insignificant activities take priority over real purposes. Work redesign, clarification of job descriptions, or a change in the type of care delivery system may alleviate some of these problems. However, the same general principle holds: Individuals who are self-aware and have clearly identified personal goals and priorities have greater control over how they expend their energy and what they accomplish.

When individuals lack this self-awareness, they may find it difficult to find a balance between time spent on personal and professional priorities. Indeed, a study of more than 50,000 employees from a variety of manufacturing and service organizations found that 2 out of every 5 employees were dissatisfied with the balance between their work and their personal lives (Hansen, 2022). Effective time management then is an essential part of finding that balance between work life and personal life.

In addition to being self-aware regarding the values that influence how people prioritize the use of their time, people must be self-aware regarding their general tendency to complete tasks in isolation or in combination. Some people prefer to do one thing at a time, whereas others typically do two or more things simultaneously. Some individuals begin and finish projects on time, have clean and organized desks by handling each piece of paperwork only once, and are highly structured. Others tend to change plans, borrow and lend things frequently, and emphasize relationships rather than tasks. It is important to recognize one's own preferred time management style and to be self-aware about how this orientation may affect one's interaction with others in the workplace. A significant part of personal time management depends on self-awareness about how and when a person is most productive.

> Everyone avoids certain types of work or has methods of wasting time.

Likewise, each person works better at certain times of the day or for certain lengths of time. Rampton (2018) suggests the biggest and most challenging tasks should be addressed in the morning because most people have the greatest amount of energy in the morning. Accomplishing the most important tasks in the morning also provides a sense of accomplishment the rest of the day. Mornings may not be the most productive time, however, for everyone. Self-aware people schedule complex or difficult tasks during the periods they are most productive and simpler or routine tasks during less productive times.

Finally, each individual should be cognizant of how they value others' time. For example, being punctual goes beyond common courtesy. Tardiness reflects some disregard for the value of other people's time.

> A lack of punctuality suggests that you do not value other people's time.

A list of tips for optimum personal time management is shown in Display 9.5. All 25 tips (McBeth, 2020) involve self-awareness of what is important to accomplish in one's life, staying focused on the things that matter, taking care of oneself, and following through in a timely and consistent manner.

Using a Time Inventory

Because most people have an inaccurate perception of the time they spend on a specific task or the total amount of time they are productive during the day, a time inventory (Display 9.6) may provide insight. A time inventory allows you to compare what you planned to do, as outlined by your appointments and "to-do" entries, with what you actually did. Electronic time

DISPLAY **9.5**   **TIPS FOR PERSONAL TIME MANAGEMENT**

1. Create a daily task list.
2. Prioritize your tasks.
3. Do the most critical tasks in the morning.
4. Track your time.
5. Minimize distractions.
6. Avoid multitasking.
7. Use time management apps and tools.
8. Perform audits of your time weekly.
9. Create meeting agendas.
10. Don't wait for inspiration to start working.
11. Schedule your breaks.
12. Keep a list of backup tasks.
13. Organize your desk, task list, inbox, etc.
14. Use your calendar.
15. Skip ahead when you feel stuck.
16. Communicate your workload with your team.
17. Delegate nonessential tasks if you can.
18. Check your email once a day.
19. Learn to say no.
20. Group similar tasks together.
21. Find your flow state (the ability to "get in the zone" and be engaged mentally).
22. Focus on your work-life balance.
23. Practice removing bad habits.
24. Make another to-do list for tomorrow.
25. Seek a mentor for more guidance.

Source: Adapted from McBeth, K. (2020, June 26). 25 Time management tips for work. *Quickbooks Blog*. https://quickbooks. intuit.com/r/manage-employees/time-management-tips/

inventory apps such as *RescueTime*, *Toggl*, or *my app Calendar* can track everything you do for a week (Rampton, 2018).

Because the greatest benefit from a time inventory is being able to objectively identify patterns of behavior, it may be necessary to maintain the time inventory for several days or even several weeks. It may also be helpful to repeat the time inventory annually to see if long-term behavior changes have been noted. Remember, there is no way to beg, borrow, or steal more hours in the day. If time is habitually used ineffectively, managing time will be stressful.

Integrating Leadership Roles and Management Functions in Time Management

There is a close relationship between time management and stress. Managing time appropriately reduces stress and increases productivity. The current status of health care, health care professional shortages, and decreasing reimbursements have resulted in many health care organizations trying to do more with less. The effective use of time management tools, therefore, becomes even more important to enable leader-managers to meet personal and professional goals.

The leadership skills needed to manage time resources draw heavily on interpersonal communication skills. The leader is a resource and role model to subordinates in how to manage time. As has been stressed in other phases of the management process, the leadership skill of self-awareness is also necessary in time management. Leaders must understand their own value system, which influences how they use time and how they expect subordinates to use time.

DISPLAY **9.6** **TIME INVENTORY**

5:00 AM _____
6:00 AM _____
6:30 AM _____
7:00 AM _____
7:30 AM _____
8:00 AM _____
8:30 AM _____
9:00 AM _____
9:30 AM _____
10:00 AM _____
10:30 AM _____
11:00 AM _____
11:30 AM _____
12:00 PM _____
12:30 PM _____
1:00 PM _____
1:30 PM _____
2:00 PM _____
2:30 PM _____
3:00 PM _____
3:30 PM _____
4:00 PM _____
4:30 PM _____
5:00 PM _____
5:30 PM _____
6:00 PM _____
6:30 PM _____
7:00 PM _____
7:30 PM _____
8:00 PM _____
8:30 PM _____
9:00 PM _____
9:30 PM _____
10:00 PM _____
11:00 PM _____
12:00 PM _____
1:00 AM _____
2:00 AM _____
3:00 AM _____
4:00 AM _____

LEARNING EXERCISE **9.5**

Writing a Personal Time Inventory

ASSIGNMENT:

Use the time inventory shown in Display 9.6 to identify your activities for a 24-hour period. Record your activities on the time inventory on a regular basis. Be specific. Do not trust your memory. Star the periods of time when you were most productive. Circle periods of time when you were least productive. Do not include sleep time. Was this a typical day for you? Could you have modified your activity during your least productive time periods? If so, how?

The management functions inherent in using time resources wisely are more related to productivity. The manager must be able to prioritize activities of unit functioning to meet short- and long-term unit needs. To do this, the leader-manager must initiate an analysis of time management on the unit level, involve team members and gain their cooperation in maximizing time use, and guide work to its conclusion and successful implementation.

Successful leader-managers integrate leadership skills and management functions; they accomplish unit goals in a timely and efficient manner in a concerted effort with subordinates. They also recognize time as a valuable unit resource and share responsibility for the use of that resource with subordinates. Perhaps most importantly, the integrated leader-manager with well-developed time management skills can maintain greater control over time and energy constraints in their personal and professional life.

 Key Concepts

- Because time is a finite and valuable resource, learning to use it wisely is essential for effective management.
- Time management can be reduced to three cyclic steps: (a) allow time for planning and establish priorities; (b) complete the highest priority task, and whenever possible, finish one task before beginning another; and (c) reprioritize based on remaining tasks and any new information.
- Setting aside time at the beginning of each day to plan the day allows the manager to spend appropriate time on high-priority tasks.
- Many individuals fall prey to planning fallacies, where they are overly optimistic about the time it will take to complete a task.
- Making lists is an appropriate tool to manage daily tasks. This list should not be any longer than what can realistically be accomplished in a day and must include adequate time to accomplish each item on the list and time for the unexpected.
- A common cause of procrastination is failure to break large tasks down into smaller ones so that the manager can set short-term, intermediate, and long-term goals.

- Lower-level managers have more interruptions in their work than do higher-level managers. This results in situational stress and lowered job satisfaction.
- Managers must learn strategies to cope with interruptions from socializing.
- Because so much paperwork is redundant or unnecessary, the manager needs to develop expertise at prioritizing it and eliminating unnecessary clutter at the work site.
- An efficient filing system is invaluable to handling paper overload.
- Personal time management refers to "the knowing of self." Managing time is difficult if a person is unsure of their priorities, including personal short-term, intermediate, and long-term goals.
- Being punctual implies that you value other people's time and creates an imperative for them to value your time as well.
- Effective time management is an essential part of finding that balance between work life and personal life.
- Using a time inventory is one way to gain insight into how and when a person is most productive. It also assists in identifying internal time wasters.

LEARNING EXERCISE   9.8

Creating a Shift Time Inventory

You are a 3 PM to 11 PM shift coordinator for a skilled nursing facility. You are the only registered nurse on your unit this shift. All the other personnel assigned to work with you this evening are unlicensed. The unit census is 21. As the shift coordinator, your responsibility is to make shift assignments, provide needed patient treatments, administer medications, and coordinate the work of team members. This evening, you will need to administer treatments and/or medications to the following patients:

Room 101 A	Gina Adams	88 years old. Senile dementia. Resident for 6 years. Confused—strikes out at staff. Insulin dependent diabetic. Has small grade 2 pressure injury on coccyx, which requires evaluation and dressing change each shift.
Room 102 B	Gus Taylor	64 years old. Diabetes. New resident. Bilateral above-knee amputee. Right amputation 2 weeks ago. Left amputation performed 8 years ago. Needs stump dressing on right amputation site this shift. Has developed methicillin-resistant *Staphylococcus aureus* in wound site. Wound isolation ordered. IV antibiotics due at 4:00 PM and 10:00 PM tonight. Blood glucose monitoring due at 4:30 PM and 9:00 PM with sliding-scale coverage.
Room 106 A	Marvin Young	26 years old. Closed head injury 5 years ago. Resident since that time. Decerebrate posturing only. Does not follow commands. Percutaneous endoscopic gastrostomy feeding tube site red and inflamed; medical doctor has not yet been notified. Needs feeding solution bag change this PM.
Room 107 A	Sheila Abood	93 years old. Functional decline. Refusing to eat. Physician has written an order not to resuscitate in the event of cardiac or respiratory failure but wants an IV line begun this PM to minimize patient dehydration. Family will also be here this PM and wants to talk about their mother's status.
Room 109 C	Tina Crowden	89 years old. Admit from local hospital, 2 weeks postoperative left hip replacement. Anticipated length of stay—2 weeks. Arrives by ambulance at 3:30 PM. Needs to have admission assessment and paperwork completed and care plan started.

Oral Medications Schedule

Room 101 A—4 PM, 8 PM
Room 101 B—4 PM, 8 PM
Room 102 A—5 PM, 9 PM
Room 103 B—4 PM, 10 PM
Room 104 C—5 PM, 6 PM, 9 PM
Room 106 B—6 PM, 9 PM
Room 108 C—9 PM
Room 109 C—5 PM, 6 PM, 8 PM, 9 PM

ASSIGNMENT:

Create a time inventory from 3:00 PM to 11:30 PM using 1-hour blocks of time. Plan what activities you will do during each 1-hour block. Be sure that you start with the activities you have prioritized for the shift. Also, remember that you will be in shift report from 3:00 PM to 3:30 PM and from 11:00 PM to 11:30 PM and that you need to schedule a dinner break for yourself. Allow adequate time for planning and dealing with the unexpected. Compare the inventory that you created with other students in your class. Did you identify the same priorities? Were you more focused on professional, technical, or amenity care? Will your plan require multitasking? Was the time inventory that you created realistic? Is this a workload that you believe you could handle?

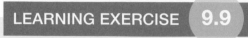

LEARNING EXERCISE   9.9

Plan Your Day

It is October of your second year as nursing coordinator for the surgical department. A copy of your appointment calendar for Monday, October 27, follows.

Appointment Calendar for Monday, October 27

8:00 AM	Arrive at work
8:15 AM	Daily rounds with each head nurse in your area
8:30 AM	Continuation of daily rounds with head nurses
9:00 AM	Open
9:30 AM	Open
10:00 AM	Department head meeting
10:30 AM	United Givers committee
11:00 AM	United Givers committee continued
11:30 AM	Open
Noon	Lunch
12:30 PM	Lunch
1:00 PM	Weekly meeting with administrator—budget and annual report due
1:30 PM	Open
2:00 PM	Infection control meeting
2:30 PM	Infection control meeting continued
3:00 PM	Fire drill and critique of drill
3:30 PM	Fire drill and critique of drill continued
4:00 PM	Open
4:30 PM	Open
5:00 PM	Off duty

You will review your unfinished business from the preceding Friday and look at the new items of business that have arrived on your desk this morning. (The new items follow the appointment calendar.) The unit ward clerk is usually free in the afternoon to provide you with 1 hour of clerical assistance, and you have a charge nurse on each shift to whom you may delegate.

1. Assign a priority to each item, with 1 being the most important and 5 being the least important.
2. Decide when you will deal with each item, being careful not to use more time than you have open on your calendar.
3. If the problem is to be handled immediately, explain how you will do this (e.g., delegated, phone call).
4. Explain the rationale for your decisions.

Correspondence

Item 1

From the desk of M. Jones, personnel manager
October 24
Dear Joan:

I am sending you the names of two new graduate nurses who are interested in working in your area. I have processed their applications; they seem well qualified. Could you manage to see them as early as possible in the week? I would hate to lose these prospective employees, and they are anxious to obtain definite confirmation of employment.

Item 2

From the desk of John Brown, purchasing agent
October 23
Joan:

We really must get together this week and devise a method to control supplies. Your area has used three times the amount of isolation gowns than you did this same time period last year. Are there that many more patients in isolation? This is just one of the supplies your area uses excessively. I'm open to suggestions.

Item 3

Roger Johnson, MD, chief of surgical department
October 24
Ms. Kerr:

I know you have your budget ready to submit, but I just remembered this week that I forgot to include an arterial pressure monitor. Is there another item that we can leave out? I'll drop by Monday morning, and we'll figure something out.

Item 4

October 23
Ms. Kerr:

The following personnel are due for merit raises, and I must have their completed and signed evaluations by Tuesday afternoon: Mary Rocas, Jim Newman, Marge Newfield.
M. Jones, personnel manager

Item 5

Roger Johnson, MD, chief of surgical department
October 23
Ms. Kerr:

The physicians are complaining about the availability of nurses to accompany them on rounds. I believe you and I need to sit down with the doctors and head nurses to discuss this recurring problem. I have some free time Monday afternoon.

Item 6

5 AM
Joan:

Sally Knight (your regular night registered nurse) requested a leave of absence due to her mother's illness. I told her it would be OK to take the next three nights off. She is flying out of town on the 9 AM commuter flight to San Francisco, so phone her right away if you don't want her to go. I felt I had no choice but to say yes.
Nancy Peters, night supervisor
P.S. You'll need to find a replacement for her for the next three nights.

(continues on page 224)

LEARNING EXERCISE 9.9

Plan Your Day (continued)

Item 7

To: Ms. Kerr
From: Administrator
Re: Patient complaint
Date: October 23

Please investigate the following patient complaint. I would like a report on this matter this afternoon.

Dear Sir:

My mother, Gertrude Boswich, was a patient in your hospital, and I just want to tell you that no member of my family will ever go there again.

She had an operation on Monday, and no one gave her a bath for 3 days. Besides that, she didn't get anything to eat for 2 days, not even water. What kind of a hospital do you run anyway?

Elmo Boswich

Item 8

To: Joan Kerr
From: Nancy Newton, RN, head nurse
Re: Problems with X-ray department
Date: October 23

We have been having problems getting diagnostic x-ray procedures scheduled for patients. Many times, patients have had to stay an extra day to get x-ray tests done. I have talked to the radiology chief several times, but the situation hasn't improved. Can you do something about this?

Item 9

To: All department heads
From: Storeroom
Re: Supplies
Date: October 23

The storeroom is out of the following items: toilet paper, paper clips, disposable diapers, and pencils. We are expecting a shipment next week.

Telephone Messages

Item 10

Sam Surefoot, Superior Surgical Supplies, Inc., returned your call at 7:50 AM on October 27. He will be at the hospital this afternoon to talk about problems with defective equipment received.

Item 11

Donald Drinkley, Channel 32-TV, called at 8:10 AM on October 27 to say he will be here at 11:30 AM to do a feature story on the open-heart surgery unit.

Item 12

Lila Green, director of nurses at St. Joan's Hospital, called at 8:05 AM on October 24 about a phone reference on Jane Jones, RN. Ms. Jones has applied for a job there. Isn't that the one we fired last year?

Item 13

Betty Brownie, Bluebird Troop 35, called at 8 AM on October 27 about the Bluebird Troop visit to patients on Halloween with trick-or-treat candy. She will call again.

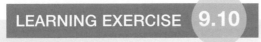

LEARNING EXERCISE 9.10

Avoiding Crises

The following scenarios depict situations that likely could have been avoided with better planning. Write down what could have been done to prevent the crisis. Then outline at least three alternatives to deal with the problem, as it already exists.

- It is the end of your 8-hour shift. Your team members are ready to go home. You have not yet begun to chart on any of your six patients. You have neither completed your intake/output totals nor given patients the medications that were due 1 hour ago. The arriving shift asks you to give your handoff report now.
- You need to use the home computer to write your midterm essay, which is due tomorrow, but your mother is online doing the family's taxes, which must be mailed by midnight. The taxes will likely take several additional hours.
- Your computer hard drive crashes when you try to print your term paper, which is due tomorrow.
- An older adult, frail patient pulls out her intravenous line. You make six attempts, over a 1-hour period, to restart the line but are unsuccessful. You have missed your lunch break and now must choose between taking time for lunch and finishing your shift on time.

LEARNING EXERCISE 9.11

The Need to Reprioritize

You have just arrived home from a long day at school (it's 4 PM on Wednesday) and sit down to look at your to-do list for the week. You have several major deadlines looming and are aware that you have procrastinated their completion far too long. Items on your list that must be completed by week's end include the following:

1. You have a 15-page term paper due in your leadership class on Friday (9 AM), which you have not begun. This will require 3 to 4 hours of literature review before you can begin and likely 4 to 6 hours to write the paper. There is a 10% loss of points for every day the paper is late, including weekends.
2. You have to create clinical preparation sheets tonight for the four medical/surgical patients you will be caring for tomorrow (Thursday) at the hospital (7:00 AM to 3:30 PM). Each of these preparation sheets will take approximately 30 minutes to complete. These preparation sheets will be used to provide patient care tomorrow and will be discussed at the postclinical conference from 3:30 PM to 4:30 PM.
3. You have a test tomorrow night (Thursday) in your political science class, which begins at 7 PM. You have read the materials but want to review them one last time because the test counts for 25% of your grade.
4. You need to finish writing your reflective journal analysis, a weekly assignment for your clinical course. The analysis is typically four to six pages and reflects what you learned in your clinical experiences each week. It is due by noon on Friday.
5. You are the maid of honor for your best friend's wedding and as such are responsible for hosting her bridal shower on Saturday afternoon. You have not yet purchased the food or bought the materials you need for the activities you have planned. You also realize that your apartment is a mess and that it needs to be cleaned before guests arrive.
6. Your car is critically low on oil. The oil light has been on for the last week, and you know that you are likely to burn up the engine if you keep driving it. You must take it in for an oil change immediately because the campus and hospital are too far away to take your bike and there is no public transportation system.

(continues on page 226)

LEARNING EXERCISE 9.11

The Need to Reprioritize (continued)

As you create your time inventory for the next 4 days, you realize just how tight your schedule is. If you work until at least midnight each night and get up just in time to make it to clinical and class (6:00 AM), you should be able to get everything done.

At 6 PM, the phone rings. It is one of your peers from school. She has just broken up with her fiancé and is in a crisis state. She asks that you come over right away and stay with her as she does not want to be alone. In addition, shortly after you hang up the phone, your roommate knocks on your door and says she needs to have a conversation with you about the "house rules" the two of you set. She says the rules are not working and that she has grown increasingly frustrated the last week. She wants to resolve the conflict right now and is threatening to move out. Finally, there is a knock at the door. One of your neighbors tells you that he just saw your dog running down the street. The gate must have been left open when your roommate returned home.

ASSIGNMENT:

How will you reprioritize your plans for this evening as well as the rest of the week? Can any items be eliminated from your list? Can any items be further procrastinated? What "satisficing" choices will you make regarding the items you will accomplish from your to-do list for the week?

REFERENCES

Bryant, S., & Yoder, L. (2021, May–June). Implementing the Lean Management System to influence unfinished nursing care. *MEDSURG Nursing, 30*(3), 181–217.

Cheng, S.-L., & Xie, K. (2021, June). Why college students procrastinate in online courses: A self-regulated learning perspective. *Internet & Higher Education, 50.* https://www.sciencedirect.com/science/article/abs/pii/S1096751621000166?via%3Dihub

Davis, M. (2021, May 10). Procrastination: Why people wait before doing a task and how to break this pattern. *The Science Times.* https://www.sciencetimes.com/articles/31098/20210510/procrastination-why-people-wait-before-doing-task-break-pattern.htm

Hansen, R. S. (2022). *Is your life in balance? Work/life balance quiz. A quintessential careers quiz.* Live Career. https://www.livecareer.com/resources/jobs/search/work-life-balance-quiz

Ling, T. (2021, July 7). Can't break the procrastination cycle? Blame your parents. *Science Focus.* https://www.sciencefocus.com/the-human-body/is-procrastination-genetic/

McBeth, K. (2020, June 26). 25 Time management tips for work. *QuickBooks Blog.* https://quickbooks.intuit.com/r/manage-employees/time-management-tips/

Rampton, J. (2018, May 1). Manipulate time with these powerful 20 time management tips. *Forbes.* https://www.forbes.com/sites/johnrampton/2018/05/01/manipulate-time-with-these-powerful-20-time-management-tips/?sh=7ef0a3be57ab

Wang, Y., Gao, H., Sun, C., Liu, J., & Fan, X. (2021). Academic procrastination in college students: The role of self-leadership. *Personality & Individual Differences, 178.* https://www.sciencedirect.com/science/article/abs/pii/S0191886921002415

Fiscal Planning and Health Care Reimbursement

… nurses are practicing caring in an environment where the economics and costs of health care permeate discussions and impact decisions.—Marian C. Turkel

… the trouble with a budget is that it's hard to fill up one hole without digging another.—Dan Bennett

… Don't tell me what you value, show me your budget, and I'll tell you what you value.—Joe Biden

CROSSWALK

This chapter addresses:

- **AACN Essentials Domain 5:** Quality and safety
- **AACN Essentials Domain 6:** Interprofessional partnerships
- **AACN Essentials Domain 7:** Systems-based practice
- **AACN Essentials Domain 8:** Information and health care technologies
- **AACN Essentials Domain 10:** Personal, professional, and leadership development
- **AONL Nurse Executive Competency 2:** A knowledge of the health care environment
- **AONL Nurse Executive Competency 5:** Business skills
- **ANA Standard of Professional Performance 8:** Advocacy
- **ANA Standard of Professional Performance 9:** Respectful and equitable practice
- **ANA Standard of Professional Performance 11:** Collaboration
- **ANA Standard of Professional Performance 12:** Leadership
- **ANA Standard of Professional Performance 15:** Quality of practice
- **ANA Standard of Professional Performance 17:** Resource stewardship
- **QSEN Competency:** Quality improvement
- **QSEN Competency:** Safety

LEARNING OBJECTIVES

The learner will:

- define basic fiscal terminology
- differentiate among the three major types of budgets (personnel, operating, and capital) and the four most common budgeting methods (incremental, zero-based, flexible, and new performance budgeting)
- identify the strengths and weaknesses of flexible budgets
- recognize the need to involve subordinates and followers in fiscal planning whenever possible
- design a decision package to aid in fiscal priority setting
- anticipate, recognize, and creatively problem solve budgetary constraints
- accurately compute the standard formula for calculating nursing care hours per patient-day

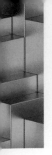

- describe the impetus for the development of diagnosis-related groups, the prospective payment system, and other managed care initiatives
- describe the resulting impact on cost and quality when health care reimbursement shifted from a health care system dominated by third-party, fee-for-service plans to capitated, managed care programs
- describe the impact of the increasing shift in government and private insurer reimbursement from volume to value based
- recognize that rapidly changing federal and state reimbursement policies make long-range budgeting and planning very difficult for health care organizations
- discuss how spiraling health care costs that had little relationship to health care outcomes led to comprehensive health care reform in the United States in 2010
- describe key components of the *Patient Protection and Affordable Care Act* (PPACA or ACA) as well as its implementation plan between 2010 and 2014
- consider how ongoing legislative efforts to repeal the ACA and the 2019 elimination of the "individual mandate" to have health insurance, may affect health care in the future
- describe why nurses need to understand and actively be involved in fiscal planning and health care reform

Introduction

For at least 40 years, health care organizations have faced financial challenges because of shrinking reimbursement and rising costs. Regulatory controls have tightened, quality expectations have risen, and the public is increasingly demanding more and higher-quality services at little to no out-of-pocket cost.

In addition, costs for health care have soared, posing a financial burden to many Americans. The Kaiser Family Foundation (2020) noted that annual premiums for employer-sponsored family health coverage reached $21,342 in 2020, up 4% from 2019, with workers on average paying $5,588 toward the cost of their coverage.

In addition, as we entered the second decade of the 21st century, 44 million people in the United States lacked any type of health insurance and an even greater number were underinsured (Huston, 2023). Of the millions of people whose incomes were too low to afford health insurance, many did not qualify for federally provided health insurance. In addition, small businesses, in tough economic times, lacked the resources to provide health insurance benefits to all employees. All these factors suggested a need for health care reform that provided universal health care insurance coverage.

Comprehensive, systematic efforts to reform this clearly broken health care system achieved no real momentum, however, until late in the first decade of the 21st century. Even then, convergence on proposals for reform was limited, so the relatively swift passage of controversial national health care reform in the United States in March 2010 came as a surprise to many. This legislation, the *Patient Protection and Affordable Care Act* (PPACA), hereafter called the *Affordable Care Act* (ACA), promised significant reductions in numbers of uninsured people, greater access to coverage for those with preexisting conditions, and mandated health care insurance provision by employers. Provisions of the ACA are discussed later in this chapter.

In addition, health care reform accelerated a shift in reimbursement from *volume* to *value* to remove incentives for redundant and inappropriate care. Unlike volume, which simply considers how much of a product is purchased, *value* considers quality, efficiency, safety, and cost. The ACA's payment reform provisions included *value-based purchasing* (VBP), *accountable care organizations* (ACOs), *bundled payments*, the *medical home*, and the *health insurance* marketplace, all of which are based on value and discussed later in this chapter.

Great change also occurred in fiscal planning at the organizational level over the past four decades in terms of scope of responsibility and accountability for cost and outcomes. Nurse leader-managers in the 21st century are expected to be fiscally knowledgeable because nursing budgets generally account for the greatest share of health care institutional expenses. Yet, shrinking resources and increasing demands increasingly pose challenges for nursing managers.

Unfortunately, many nurses perceive fiscal planning to be the most difficult type of planning. This is often the result of inadequate formal education or training on budget preparation as well as *forecasting* (making an educated budget estimate by using historical data). It is important to remember that fiscal planning is an acquired skill that improves with use; that's because it requires vision; creativity; and a thorough knowledge of the political, social, and economic forces that shape health care. Fiscal planning, then, must be included in nursing program curricula and in management preparation programs.

> Fiscal planning is not intuitive; it is a learned skill that improves with practice.

This chapter discusses the leader-manager's role in fiscal planning, identifies types of budgets, and delineates the budgetary process. Learners will also examine health care reimbursement concepts with specific attention given to the recent change from volume-based reimbursement to value-based reimbursement. The leadership roles and management functions involved in fiscal planning are outlined in Display 10.1.

DISPLAY 10.1 LEADERSHIP ROLES AND MANAGEMENT FUNCTIONS IN FISCAL PLANNING

Leadership Roles

1. Is visionary in identifying or forecasting short- and long-term unit needs, thus inspiring proactive rather than reactive fiscal planning
2. Is knowledgeable about political, social, and economic factors that shape fiscal planning and reimbursement in health care today
3. Demonstrates flexibility in fiscal goal setting in a rapidly changing system
4. Anticipates, recognizes, and creatively solves budgetary constraints
5. Influences and inspires group members to become active in short- and long-range fiscal planning
6. Recognizes when fiscal constraints have resulted in an inability to meet organizational or unit goals and communicates this insight effectively, following the chain of command
7. Ensures that patient safety is not jeopardized by cost containment
8. Role models leadership in needed health care reform efforts
9. Proactively prepares followers for the plethora of changes in health care associated with health care reform and implementation of the *Patient Protection and Affordable Care Act*

Management Functions

1. Identifies the importance of and develops short- and long-range fiscal plans that reflect unit needs
2. Articulates and documents unit needs effectively to higher administrative levels
3. Assesses the internal and external environment of the organization in forecasting to identify driving forces and barriers to fiscal planning
4. Demonstrates knowledge of budgeting and uses appropriate techniques to budget effectively
5. Provides opportunities for subordinates to participate in relevant fiscal planning
6. Coordinates unit-level fiscal planning to be congruent with organizational goals and objectives
7. Accurately assesses personnel needs by using predetermined standards or an established patient classification system
8. Coordinates the monitoring aspects of budget control
9. Ensures that documentation of patients' need for services and services rendered is clear and complete to facilitate organizational reimbursement
10. Collaborates with other health care administrators to proactively determine how health care reform initiatives such as value-based purchasing, accountable care organizations, bundled payments, the medical home, and the health insurance marketplace may impact organizational viability and the provision of services

Balancing Cost and Quality

Complicating fiscal planning in health care organizations today are the dual goals of cost containment and quality care. *Cost containment* refers to the effective and efficient delivery of services while generating needed revenues for operations. Cost containment is the responsibility of every health care provider, and the viability of most health care organizations today depends on their ability to use their fiscal resources wisely.

Being *cost-effective*, however, is not the same as being inexpensive; *cost-effective* means producing good results for the money spent; in other words, the product is worth the price (YourDictionary, 2021). Expensive items can be cost-effective, and inexpensive items may not. Cost-effectiveness then must consider factors such as anticipated length of service, need for such a service, and availability of other alternatives.

In addition, cost and quality do not necessarily have a linear relationship in health care. Sometimes, high spending represents a duplication of services, an overutilization of services, and the use of technology that exceeds a specific patient's needs. In fact, numerous studies over the past decade have examined the relationship between higher spending and the quality and outcomes of care and found that higher spending does not necessarily result in better-quality care.

> Spending more does not always equate to better-quality health outcomes.

These findings are true on the macrolevel as well. The US health care system is the most expensive in the world, spending almost twice as much on health care, as a percentage of its economy, in 2019, as other advanced industrialized countries—totaling $3.6 trillion, or 16.8% of gross domestic product (GDP) (Congressional Research Service, 2021).Yet, our outcomes in terms of teenage pregnancy rates, lifespan, low–birth-weight infants, and access to care are worse than many countries that spend significantly less.

In addition, health care costs are simply higher in the United States. For example, the average cost of a magnetic resonance imaging (MRI) in the United States in 2017 was US$1,430, compared to US$190 in the Netherlands (Stewart, 2020). Similarly, prescription drug prices in the United States are 2.56 times those in other 32 countries (Mulcahy, 2021). The gap between prices in the United States and other countries is even larger for brand-named drugs, with US prices averaging 3.44 times those in comparison nations (Mulcahy, 2021). This occurs because of government protected "monopoly" rights for drug manufacturers. The problem then is not a scarcity of resources. The problem is that we do not use the resources we have available in a cost-effective manner.

Responsibility Accounting

An essential feature of fiscal planning is *responsibility accounting*, which means that each of an organization's revenues, expenses, assets, and liabilities is someone's responsibility. The leader-manager at the unit level then should be an active participant in unit budgeting, have a high degree of control over what is included in the unit budget, receive regular data reports that compare actual expenses with budgeted expenses, and be held accountable for the financial results of the operating unit.

The unit manager also can best monitor and evaluate all aspects of a unit's budget control. Like other types of planning, the unit manager has a responsibility to communicate budgetary planning goals to the staff. The more the staff understands the budgetary goals and the plans to carry out those goals, the more likely the goal attainment is. Sadly, many nurses have little knowledge of the nursing budget model used by their hospital system.

Budget Basics

A *budget* is a financial plan that includes estimated expenses as well as income for a set period of time. The more accurate the budget blueprint, the better the institution can plan the most efficient use of its resources.

> The budget's value is directly related to its accuracy.

Because a budget is at best a prediction, a plan, and not a rule, however, fiscal planning requires flexibility, ongoing evaluation, and revision. In the budget, expenses are classified as fixed or variable and either controllable or noncontrollable. *Fixed* expenses do not vary with volume, whereas *variable* expenses do. Examples of fixed expenses might be a building's mortgage payment or a manager's salary; variable expenses might include the payroll of hourly wage employees and the cost of supplies.

Controllable expenses can be controlled or varied by the manager, whereas *noncontrollable* expenses cannot. For example, the unit manager can control the number of personnel working on a certain shift and the staffing mix; they cannot, however, control equipment depreciation, the number and type of supplies needed by patients, or overtime that occurs in response to an emergency. A list of the fiscal terminology that a manager needs to know is shown in Display 10.2.

DISPLAY 10.2 FISCAL TERMINOLOGY

Accountable care organizations—groups of providers and suppliers of service who work together to better coordinate care for Medicare patients (does not include Medicare Advantage) across care settings

Acuity index—weighted statistical measurement that refers to severity of illness of patients for a given time. Patients are classified according to acuity of illness, usually in one of four categories. The acuity index is determined by taking a total of acuities and then dividing by the number of patients.

Affordable Care Act—officially known as the *Patient Protection and Affordable Care Act*, this act passed in March 2010 to provide more Americans access to affordable health insurance

Assets—financial resources that a health care organization receives, such as accounts receivable

Baseline data—historical information on dollars spent, acuity level, patient census, resources needed, hours of care, and so forth. This information is used as the basis for projecting future needs.

Break-even point—point at which revenue covers costs

Bundled payment—a payment structure in which different health care providers who are treating a patient for the same or related conditions are paid an overall sum for taking care of that condition rather than being paid for each individual treatment, test, or procedure. In doing so, providers are rewarded for coordinating care, preventing complications and errors, and reducing unnecessary or duplicative tests and treatments (HealthCare.gov, n.d., para 1).

Capitation—a prospective payment system (PPS) that pays health plans or providers a fixed amount per enrollee per month for a defined set of health services, regardless of how many (if any) services are used

Case mix—type of patients served by an institution. A hospital's case mix is usually defined in such patient-related variables as type of insurance, acuity levels, diagnosis, personal characteristics, and patterns of treatment.

Cash flow—rate at which dollars are received and dispersed

continues on page 232

DISPLAY 10.2 (CONTINUED)

Controllable costs—costs that can be controlled or that vary. An example would be the number of personnel employed, the level of skill required, wage levels, and quality of materials.

Cost–benefit ratio—numerical relationship between the value of an activity or procedure in terms of benefits and the value of the activity's or procedure's cost. The cost–benefit ratio is expressed as a fraction.

Cost center—smallest functional unit for which cost control and accountability can be assigned. A nursing unit is usually considered a cost center, but there may be other cost centers within a unit (orthopedics is a cost center, but often, the cast room is considered a separate cost center within orthopedics).

Diagnosis-related groups (DRGs)—rate-setting PPS used by Medicare to determine payment rates for an inpatient hospital stay based on admission diagnosis. Each DRG represents a case type for which Medicare provides a flat dollar amount of reimbursement. This set rate may be higher or lower than the cost of treating the patient in a particular hospital.

Direct costs—costs that can be attributed to a specific source, such as medications and treatments; costs that are clearly identifiable with goods or service

Fee-for-service (FFS) system—a reimbursement system whereby insurance companies reimburse health care providers a billed amount for services after the services are delivered

Fixed budget—style of budgeting that is based on a fixed, annual level of volume, such as number of patient-days or tests performed, to arrive at an annual budget total. These totals are then divided by 12 to arrive at the monthly average. The fixed budget does not make provisions for monthly or seasonal variations.

Fixed costs—costs that do not vary according to volume. Examples of fixed costs are fixed rate or loan payments.

For-profit organization—organization in which the providers of funds have an ownership interest in the organization. These providers own stocks in the for-profit organization and earn dividends based on what is left when the cost of goods and of carrying on the business is subtracted from the amount of money taken in.

Full costs—total of all direct and indirect costs

Full-time equivalent (FTE)—number of hours of work for which a full-time employee is scheduled for a weekly period. For example, 1.0 FTE = five 8-hour days of staffing, which equals 40 hours of staffing per week. One FTE can be divided in different ways. For example, two part-time employees, each working 20 hours per week, would equal 1 FTE. If a position requires coverage for more than 5 days or 40 hours per week, the FTE will be greater than 1.0 for that position. Assume a position requires 7-day coverage, or 56 hours, then the position requires 1.4 FTE coverage (56/40 = 1.4). This means that more than one person is needed to fill the FTE positions for a 7-day period.

Health maintenance organization—historically, a prepaid organization that provided health care to voluntarily enrolled members in return for a preset amount of money on a per-person, per-month basis; often referred to as a *managed care organization*

Hours per patient-day (HPPD)—hours of nursing care provided per patient per day by various levels of nursing personnel. HPPD are determined by dividing total production hours by the number of patients.

Indirect costs—costs that cannot be directly attributed to a specific area. These are hidden costs and are usually spread among different departments. Housekeeping services are considered indirect costs.

International Classification of Disease (ICD) codes—coding used to report the severity and treatment of patient diseases, illnesses, and injuries to determine appropriate reimbursement; currently in its 10th revision (ICD-10)

Managed care—term used to describe a variety of health care plans designed to contain the cost of health care services delivered to members while maintaining the quality of care

Medicaid—federally assisted and state-administered program to pay for medical services on behalf of certain groups of low-income individuals. In general, these individuals are not covered by Social Security. Certain groups of people (e.g., older adults, those who are blind, people with disabilities, members of families with dependent children, and certain other children and pregnant people) also qualify for coverage if their incomes and resources are sufficiently low.

DISPLAY 10.2 (CONTINUED)

Medicare—nationwide health insurance program authorized under Title 18 of the Social Security Act that provides benefits to people aged 65 years or older. Medicare coverage also is available to certain groups of people with catastrophic or chronic illness, such as patients with renal failure requiring hemodialysis, regardless of age.

Noncontrollable costs—indirect expenses that cannot usually be controlled or varied. Examples might be rent, lighting, and depreciation of equipment.

Not-for-profit organization—this type of organization is financed by funds that come from several sources, but the providers of these funds do not have an ownership interest. Profits generated in the not-for-profit organization are frequently funneled back into the organization for expansion or capital acquisition.

Operating expenses—daily costs required to maintain a hospital or health care institution

Patient classification system—method of classifying patients. Different criteria are used for different systems. In nursing, patients are usually classified according to acuity of illness.

Pay for performance (also known as P4P) programs—incentives are paid to providers to achieve a targeted threshold of clinical performance, typically a process or outcome measure associated with a specified patient population

Pay for value programs—incentive payments that are linked to both quality and efficiency improvements

Preferred provider organization (PPO)—health care financing and delivery program with a group of providers, such as physicians and hospitals, who contract to give services on an FFS basis. This provides financial incentives to consumers to use a select group of preferred providers and pay less for services. Insurance companies usually promise the PPO a certain volume of patients and prompt payment in exchange for fee discounts.

Production hours—total amount of regular time, overtime, and temporary time. This also may be referred to as *actual hours*.

Prospective payment system—a hospital payment system with predetermined reimbursement ratio for services given

Revenue—source of income or the reward for providing a service to a patient

Staffing mix—ratio of registered nurses (RNs), licensed vocational nurses (LVNs)/licensed practical nurses (LPNs), and unlicensed workers (e.g., a shift on one unit might have 40% RNs, 40% LPNs/LVNs, and 20% others). Hospitals vary on their staffing mix policies.

Third-party payment system—a system of health care financing in which providers deliver services to patients, and a third party, or intermediary, usually an insurance company or a government agency, pays the bill

Turnover ratio—rate at which employees leave their jobs for reasons other than death or retirement. The rate is calculated by dividing the number of employees leaving by the number of workers employed in the unit during the year and then multiplying by 100.

Value-based purchasing—a payment methodology that rewards quality of care through payment incentives

Variable costs—costs that vary with the volume. Payroll costs are an example.

Workload units—in nursing, workloads are usually the same as patient-days. For some areas, however, workload units might refer to the number of procedures, tests, patient visits, injections, and so forth.

Steps in the Budgetary Process

The nursing process provides a model for the steps in budget planning:

1. The first step is to *assess* what needs to be covered in the budget. In general, this determination should reflect input from all levels of the organizational hierarchy because budgeting is most effective when all personnel using the resources are involved in the process.

2. The second step is *diagnosis*. In the case of budget planning, the diagnosis would be the goal or what needs to be accomplished, which is to create a cost-effective budget that maximizes the use of available resources. Unfortunately, some managers artificially inflate their department budgets as a cushion against budget cuts. If several departments partake in this unsound practice, the entire institutional budget may be ineffective. If a major change in the budget is indicated, the entire budgeting process must be repeated. Top-level managers must watch for and correct unrealistic budget projections before they are implemented.

3. The third step is to develop a *plan*. The budget plan may be developed in many ways. A budgeting cycle that is set for 12 months is called a *fiscal-year budget*. This fiscal year, which may or may not coincide with the calendar year, is then usually broken down into quarters or subdivided into monthly or semiannual periods.

   Most budgets are developed for a 1-year period, but a *perpetual budget* may be done on a continual basis each month so that 12 months of future budget data are always available. Selecting the optimal time frame for budgeting is also important. Errors are more likely if the budget is projected too far in advance. Conversely, if the budget is shortsighted, compensating for unexpected major expenses or purchasing capital equipment may be difficult.

4. The fourth step is *implementation*. In this step, ongoing monitoring and analysis occur to avoid inadequate or excess funds at the end of the fiscal year. In most health care institutions, monthly statements outline each department's projected budget and deviations from that budget.

5. The last step is *evaluation*. The budget must be reviewed periodically and modified as needed throughout the fiscal year. Each unit manager is accountable for budget deviations in their unit. Most units can expect some change from the anticipated budget, but large deviations must be examined for possible causes and remedial action taken if necessary.

A budget that is predicted too far in advance has greater probability for error.

LEARNING EXERCISE 10.1

Would You Accept This Gift?

You are the director of the education department in a 40-bed, rural, critical access hospital. A simulation vendor has offered to give you a 5-year-old, used, high-fidelity manikin for staff development training purposes (cardiopulmonary resuscitation, advanced cardiac life support, pediatric advanced life support, annual skills updates). His only request is that all supplies used with the manikin and the maintenance contract be purchased through his company. The chief nursing officer is very excited about the offer and has asked all the unit directors to consider how the manikin might be used for their staff training needs. The hospital currently does not have the funds available to purchase a new manikin.

ASSIGNMENT:

1. Justify acceptance or rejection of the gift. What influenced your choice?
2. What are the fixed and variable costs?
3. What are the controllable and noncontrollable costs?
4. What factors determine whether this gift is cost-effective?
5. Who will have control over how and when the manikin is used?

Types of Budgets

The nurse-manager may be directly involved in the fiscal planning of three major types of budgets: personnel, operating, and capital budgets.

The Personnel Budget

The largest of the budget expenditures is the *workforce* or *personnel budget* because health care is *labor-intensive*. To handle fluctuating patient census and acuity, managers need to use historical data about unit census fluctuations in forecasting short- and long-term personnel needs. Likewise, a manager must monitor the personnel budget closely to prevent understaffing or overstaffing. As patient-days or volume decreases, managers must decrease personnel costs in relation to the decrease in volume.

> The largest of the budget expenditures is the workforce or personnel budget because health care is labor-intensive.

In addition to numbers of staff, the manager must be cognizant of the *staffing mix*. Staffing mix refers to the mix (percentages) of licensed (registered nurse [RN] and licensed vocational nurse [LVN]) and unlicensed assistive personnel (certified nursing assistant [CNA]/nursing assistive personnel) working at a given time. The manager must also be aware of the patient acuity so that the most economical level of nursing care that will meet patient needs can be provided.

Most staffing is based on a predetermined *standard*. This standard may be addressed in hours per patient-day (HPPD) (medical units), visits per month (home health agencies), or minutes per case (the operating room). Because the patient census, number of visits, or cases per day never remains constant, the manager must be ready to alter staffing when volume increases or decreases.

The standard formula for calculating *nursing care hours per patient-day (NCH/PPD)* is shown in Figure 10.1.

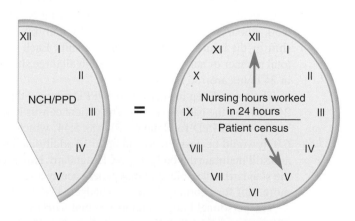

FIGURE 10.1 Standard formula for calculating nursing care hours per patient-day (NCH/PPD).

$$\text{NCH/PPD} = \frac{\text{Nursing hours worked in 24 hours}}{\text{Patient census}}$$

A unit manager in an acute care facility might use this formula to calculate daily staffing needs. For example, assume that your budgeted NCH are 6 NCH/PPD. You are calculating the NCH/PPD for today, January 31; at midnight, it will be February 1. The patient census at midnight is 25 patients. In checking staffing, you find the following information:

Shift	Staff on Duty	Hours Worked
11:00 PM (1/30) to 7:00 AM (1/31)	2 RNs	8 h each
	1 LVN	8 h
	1 CNA	8 h
7:00 AM to 3:00 PM (1/31)	3 RNs	8 h each
	2 LVNs	8 h each
	1 CNA	8 h
	1 ward clerk	8 h
3:00 PM to 11:00 PM (1/31)	2 RNs	8 h each
	2 LVNs	8 h each
	1 CNA	8 h
	1 ward clerk	8 h
11:00 PM (1/31) to 7:00 AM (2/1)	2 RNs	8 h each
	2 LVNs	8 h each
	1 CNA	8 h

RNs, registered nurses; LVNs, licensed vocational nurses; CNA, certified nursing assistant.

Ideally, you would use 12 midnight to compute the NCH/PPD for January 31, but most staffing calculations based on traditional 8-hour shifts are made beginning at 11:00 PM and ending at 11:00 PM the following night. Therefore, in this case, it would be acceptable to figure the NCH/PPD for January 31 by using numerical data from the 11:00 PM to 7:00 AM shift last night and the 7:00 AM to 3:00 PM and 3:00 PM to 11:00 PM shifts today. The first step in this calculation requires a computation of total NCH worked in 24 hours (including the ward clerk's hours). This can be calculated by multiplying the total number of staff on duty each shift by the hours each worked in their shift. Each shift total then is added together to get the total number of nursing hours worked in all three shifts or 24 hours: The nursing hours worked in 24 hours are 136 hours.

The second step in solving NCH/PPD requires that you divide the nursing hours worked in 24 hours by the patient census. The patient census in this case is 25. Therefore, 136/25 = 5.44.

The NCH/PPD for January 31 was 5.44, which is less than your budgeted NCH/PPD of 6.0. It would be possible to add up to 14 additional hours of nursing care in the next 24 hours and still maintain the budgeted NCH standard. However, the unit manager must remember that the standard is flexible, and that patient acuity and staffing mix may suggest the need for even more staff for February 1 than the budgeted NCH/PPD.

The personnel budget includes actual *worked time* (also called *productive time* or *salary expense*) and time that the organization pays the employee for not working (*nonproductive* or *benefit time*). Nonproductive time includes the cost of benefits, new employee orientation, employee turnover, sick and holiday time, and education time. For example, the average 8.5-hour shift includes a 30-minute lunch break and two 15-minute breaks. Thus, this employee would work 7.5 productive hours and have 1.0 hours of nonproductive time.

For a more detailed discussion of staffing, see Unit V.

LEARNING EXERCISE　10.2

Calculating Nursing Care Hours per Patient-Day

Calculate the nursing care hours per patient-day (NCH/PPD) if the midnight census is 25, but use the following as the number of hours worked:

12 midnight to 12 noon	2 RNs	12 h each
	2 LVNs	12 h each
	1 CNA	12 h
	1 ward clerk	5 h
12 noon to 12 midnight	3 RNs	12 h each
	2 LVNs	12 h each
	1 CNA	12 h
	1 ward clerk	12 h

Now, calculate the NCH/PPD if the following staff were working:

12 midnight to 12 noon	3 RNs	12 h each
	1 LVN	12 h
12 noon to 12 midnight	2 RNs	12 h each
	1 LVN	12 h
	1 ward clerk	4 h

RNs, registered nurses; LVNs, licensed vocational nurses; CNA, certified nursing assistant.

The Operating Budget

The *operating budget* is the second area of expenditure that involves all managers. The operating budget reflects expenses that change in response to the volume of service, such as the cost of electricity, repairs and maintenance, and supplies. Although personnel costs lead the hospital budget, the cost of supplies typically runs a close second.

> Next to personnel costs, supplies are typically the second most significant component in the hospital budget.

Effective unit managers should be alert to the types and quantities of supplies used in their unit. They should also understand the relationship between supply use and patient mix, occupancy rate, technology requirements, and types of procedures performed on the unit. Saving unused supplies from packs or trays, reducing obsolete and slow-moving inventory, eliminating pilferage, and monitoring the uncontrolled usage of supplies and giveaways all represent potential cost savings. Other ways to cut supply costs might be in rental versus facility-owned equipment, stocking products on consignment, and just-in-time stockless inventory. *Just-in-time ordering* is a process whereby inventory is delivered to the organization by suppliers only when it is needed and immediately before it is to be used.

The Capital Budget

The third type of budget used by managers is the *capital budget*. Capital budgets plan for the purchase of buildings or major equipment, which include equipment that has a long life (usually greater than 5 to 7 years), is not used in daily operations, and is more expensive than operating supplies. Examples of these types of capital expenditures might include the acquisition of a positron emission tomography imager or the renovation of a major wing in a hospital. The short-term component of the capital budget includes equipment purchases within the annual budget cycle, such as call-light systems, hospital beds, and medication carts.

Often, the designation of capital equipment requires that the value of the equipment exceed a certain dollar amount. That dollar amount will vary from institution to institution, but $5,000 is common. Managers are usually required to complete specific capital equipment request forms to justify their request.

Budgeting Methods

Budgeting is frequently classified according to how often it occurs and the base on which budgeting takes place. Four of the most common budgeting methods are incremental budgeting (also called *flat-percentage increase budgeting*), zero-based budgeting, flexible budgeting, and performance budgeting.

Incremental Budgeting

Incremental or the *flat-percentage increase method* is the simplest method for budgeting. By multiplying current-year expenses by a certain figure, usually the inflation rate or consumer price index, the budget for the coming year may be projected. Although this method is simple and quick and requires little budgeting expertise on the part of the manager, it is generally inefficient fiscally because there is no motivation to contain costs and no need to prioritize programs and services. Hospitals historically used incremental budgeting in fiscal planning.

LEARNING EXERCISE   10.3

Missing Supplies

You are a unit manager in an acute care hospital. You are aware that staff occasionally leave at the end of the shift with forgotten hospital supplies in their pockets. You remember how often as a staff nurse you would unintentionally take home rolls of adhesive tape, syringes, penlights, and bottles of lotion. Usually, you remembered to return the items, but other times, you did not.

Recently, however, your budget has shown a dramatic and unprecedented increase in missing supplies, including gauze wraps, blood pressure cuffs, stethoscopes, surgical instruments, and personal hygiene kits. Although this increase represents only a fraction of your total operating budget, you believe that it is necessary to identify the source of their use. An audit of patient charts and charges reveals that these items were not used in patient care.

When you ask your charge nurses for an explanation, they reveal that a few employees have openly expressed that taking a few small supplies is, in effect, an expected and minor fringe benefit of employment. Your charge nurses do not believe that the problem is widespread, and they cannot objectively document which employees are involved in pilfering supplies. The charge nurses suggest that you ask all employees to document in writing when they see other employees taking supplies and then turn in the information to you anonymously for follow-up.

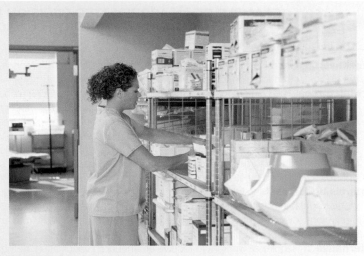

ASSIGNMENT:

Because supplies are such a major part of the operating budget, you believe that some action is indicated. You must determine what that action should be. Analyze your actions in terms of the desirable and undesirable effects on the employees involved in taking the supplies and those who are not. Is the amount of the fiscal debit in this situation a critical factor? Is it worth the time and energy that would be required to truly eliminate this problem?

Zero-Based Budgeting

In comparison, managers who use *zero-based budgeting* must rejustify their program or needs every budgeting cycle. This method does not automatically assume that because a program has been funded in the past, it should continue to be funded. Thus, this budgeting process is labor-intensive for nurse-managers. The use of a *decision package* to set funding priorities is a key feature of zero-based budgeting. Key components of decision packages are shown in Display 10.3. Display 10.4 presents an example of an abbreviated decision package.

Decision packages and zero-based budgeting are advantageous because they force managers to set priorities and to use resources most efficiently. Though it is complex and time-consuming, this method encourages participative management because information from peers and subordinates is needed to analyze adequately and prioritize the activities of each unit.

Flexible Budgeting

Flexible budgets are budgets that flex up and down over the year depending on volume. A flexible budget automatically calculates what the expenses should be, given the volume that is

---

DISPLAY 10.3 KEY COMPONENTS OF DECISION PACKAGES IN ZERO-BASED BUDGETING

1. Listing of all current and proposed objectives or activities in the department
2. Alternative plans for carrying out these activities
3. Costs for each alternative
4. Advantages and disadvantages of continuing or discontinuing an activity

DISPLAY 10.4 **EXAMPLE OF AN ABBREVIATED DECISION PACKAGE FOR IMPLEMENTING MANDATORY FLU VACCINATIONS FOR HOSPITAL EMPLOYEES**

Objective: To determine if annual mandatory flu vaccination is an appropriate strategy for reducing the risk of flu transmission to and from hospital employees

Driving forces: The Centers for Disease Control and Prevention (CDC) recommend that all health care workers receive an annual flu vaccine, arguing it is one of the most important ways to prevent transmission of influenza, not only in the hospital but also in other health care settings. Flu vaccines typically protect against the three or four viruses (depending on vaccine) that research suggests will be most common that year (CDC, 2019). Individual hospitals and health systems have some latitude to devise and implement policies based on their own strategies within the bounds established by state laws.

Restraining forces: Mandatory flu vaccine policies may fail to include safeguards to protect worker rights. In addition, it is not possible to predict what any flu season will be like because the timing, severity, and length of the season varies from one season to another as does the efficacy of the vaccine.

Alternative 1: Require all workers to receive an annual flu vaccination, at the hospital's expense.

Advantage: There is no out-of-pocket expense to employees for the vaccination. There is greater likelihood that employees will be protected against the flu while working in a high-risk clinical setting.

Disadvantage: The effectiveness of the vaccine varies from year to year. Some employees may believe that requiring the vaccine infringes on their right to control choices about their bodies. In addition, mandatory vaccination policies may violate certain employee's religious beliefs or pose health risks. Employee lawsuits arguing a violation of their rights are likely.

Alternative 2: Require all workers to be vaccinated, at the hospital's expense, unless an employee can show evidence that the vaccination poses a health risk or violates religious beliefs. Require workers who cannot have the flu vaccine, and are approved for an exemption, to wear masks during the flu season. Educate employees about the importance of immunization.

Advantage: There is no out-of-pocket expense to employees for the vaccination. Employees can refuse the vaccine for documented medical or religious reasons.

Disadvantage: The effectiveness of the vaccine varies from year to year. Resources will be needed to process requests for religious and medical exemption as well as appeals. Some employees may have less protection against the flu while working in a high-risk clinical setting. Employee lawsuits arguing a violation of their rights may occur.

Alternative 3: Encourage, but do not require, employees to have annual flu vaccinations. Provide education about the value of flu vaccination and provide incentives to workers who do agree to be vaccinated. Require workers who choose not to have the flu vaccine wear masks during the flu season.

Advantage: There is no out-of-pocket expense to employees for the vaccination. Employees have a choice regarding whether to have the vaccinations and assume the responsibility of protecting their health themselves.

Disadvantage: The effectiveness of the vaccine varies from year to year. Some employees may have less protection against the flu while working in a high-risk clinical setting.

occurring. This works well in many health care organizations because of changing census and manpower needs that are difficult to predict despite historical forecasting tools.

Performance Budgeting

The fourth method of budgeting, *performance budgeting*, emphasizes outcomes and results instead of activities or outputs. Thus, the manager would budget as needed to achieve specific outcomes and would evaluate budgetary success accordingly. For example, a home health agency would set and then measure a specific outcome in a group, such as patients with diabetes, as a means of establishing and justifying a budget.

LEARNING EXERCISE 10.4

Developing a Decision Package

Given the following objective, develop a decision package to aid you in fiscal priority setting.

Objective: To have reliable, economic, and convenient transportation when you enter nursing school in 3 months

Additional information: You currently have no car and rely on public transportation, which is inexpensive and reliable but not very convenient. Your current financial resources are limited, although you could probably qualify for a car loan if your parents were willing to cosign the loan. Your nursing school's policy states that you must have a car available to commute to clinical agencies outside the immediate area. You know that this policy is not enforced and that some students do carpool to clinical assignments.

ASSIGNMENT:

Identify at least three alternatives that will meet your objective. Choose the best alternative based on the advantages and disadvantages that you identify. You may embellish information presented in the case to help your problem solving.

Critical Pathways and Variance Analysis

Critical pathways (also called *clinical pathways* and *care pathways*) are a strategy for assessing, implementing, and evaluating the cost-effectiveness of patient care. These pathways reflect relatively standardized predictions of patients' progress for a specific diagnosis or procedure. For example, a critical pathway for a specific diagnosis might suggest an average length of stay of 4 days, with certain interventions completed by certain points on the pathway (much like a program evaluation and review technique flow diagram; see Fig. 1.5 in Chapter 1). Patient progress that differs from the critical pathway prompts a *variance analysis*.

> Critical pathways are predetermined courses of progress that patients should make after admission for a specific diagnosis or after a specific surgery.

The advantage of critical pathways is that they do provide some means of standardizing care for patients with similar diagnoses. Their weakness, however, is the difficulties they pose in accounting for and accepting what are often justifiable differentiations between unique patients who have deviated from their pathway. They also pose yet another paperwork and utilization review function in a system already burdened with administrative costs. Despite these challenges, research suggests that critical pathways can standardize care according to evidence-based best practices, leading to improved patient outcomes and lower costs.

Health Care Reimbursement

Historically, health care institutions used incremental budgeting and placed little or no emphasis on budgeting. Because insurance carriers reimbursed fully on virtually a limitless basis, there was little motivation to save costs, and organizations found it unnecessary to justify charges. Reimbursement was based on costs incurred to provide the service plus profit (fee-for-service [FFS]), with no ceiling placed on the total amount that could be charged. Indeed, under FFS, the more services provided, the greater the amount that could be billed, encouraging the overtreatment of clients. The result of uncontrolled FFS reimbursement was skyrocketing health care costs with health care increasingly assuming a greater percentage of GDP each year. Few efforts to shift from FFS to more cost-effective reimbursement models began before the late-1970s.

Medicare and Medicaid

The US federal government became a major insurer of health care with the advent of Medicare and Medicaid in the mid-1960s. Both Medicare and Medicaid are coordinated by the *Centers for Medicare & Medicaid Services* (CMS). *Medicare* is a federally sponsored health insurance program for individuals older than 65 years and for certain groups of people with catastrophic or chronic illness regardless of age. Medicare currently provides coverage for items and services for more than 62 million beneficiaries, approximately 18% of the US population (Kaiser Family Foundation, 2022b). Approximately 86% of enrollees are older adults, 14% are disabled, and less than 1% have end-stage renal disease (Kaiser Family Foundation, 2022a). Medicare enrollments are expected to increase dramatically in the coming years as the result of the aging population.

Medicare Part A is the hospital insurance program. *Medicare Part B* is the supplementary medical insurance program that pays for outpatient care (including laboratory and x-ray services) and physician (or other primary care provider) services. *Medicare Part C* (now called *Medicare Advantage*) allows Medicare eligible patients to participate in managed care plans and *Medicare Part D* allows Medicare patients to purchase at least limited prescription drug coverage, either through standalone prescription drug plans or Medicare Advantage prescription drug (MA-PD) plans. Approximately 22 million beneficiaries (34%) participated in Medicare Advantage in 2019 (Kaiser Family Foundation, 2019). Out-of-pocket costs for Medicare beneficiaries in 2022 are shown in Table 10.1.

TABLE **10.1** **MEDICARE COSTS PER BENEFICIARY FOR 2022**

Medicare Insurance Plan	Cost
Part B premium	$170.10 each month (or higher depending on your income)
Part B deductible and coinsurance	$233 per year. After the deductible is met, patients typically pay 20% of the Medicare-approved amount for most doctor services (including most doctor services while a hospital inpatient), outpatient therapy, and durable medical equipment.
Part A premium	Most people do not pay a monthly premium for Part A. (About 99% of Medicare beneficiaries do not have a Part A premium since they had at least 40 quarters of Medicare-covered employment.) If you must buy Part A, the cost is up to $499 each month.
Part A hospital inpatient deductible and coinsurance	Beneficiaries pay: • $1556 deductible for each benefit period • Days 1–60: $0 coinsurance for each benefit period • Days 61–90: $389 coinsurance per day • Days 91 and beyond: $778 coinsurance per each "lifetime reserve day" after day 90 for each benefit period (up to 60 days over your lifetime) • Beyond lifetime reserve days: all costs
Part C	Monthly premium varies by plan.
Part D	Monthly premium varies by plan (higher-income consumers may pay more).

Source: From Centers for Medicare & Medicaid Services. (2021, November 12). *2022 Medicare Parts A & B Premiums and Deductibles/2022 Medicare Part D Income-Related Monthly Adjustment Amounts.* https://www.cms.gov/news-room/fact-sheets/2022-medicare-parts-b-premiums-and-deductibles2022-medicare-part-d-income-related-monthly-adjustment

Medicaid is a federal-state cooperative health insurance plan created primarily for low-income children and adults, although it also provides medical and long-term care coverage for people with disabilities and assistance with health and long-term care expenses for low-income seniors. Over the past 30 years, Medicaid enrollment increased substantially during two major recessions and again in 2015 with implementation of the ACA. As a result, Medicaid provided coverage to about one in five Americans, or just over 84 million people as of March 2021 (Medicaid.gov, 2021). During economic downturns, when individuals lose their jobs and incomes decline, more people qualify and enroll in Medicaid, which in turn drives increases in total Medicaid spending.

The Prospective Payment System

With the advent of Medicare, Medicaid, and FFS reimbursement, health care costs skyrocketed as large segments of the population that previously had no health insurance or inadequate coverage began accessing services. In addition, health care providers saw the government as having "deep pockets," which suggested almost limitless reimbursement, and began providing services accordingly. Because of rapidly escalating costs, the government began establishing regulations requiring organizations to justify the need for services and to monitor the quality of services. Health care providers were forced for the first time to submit budgets and justify costs. This new surveillance and existence of external controls had a tremendous effect on the health care industry.

The advent of *diagnosis-related groups* (DRGs) in the early 1980s added to the need for monitoring cost containment. DRGs were predetermined payment schedules that reflected historical costs for the treatment of specific patient conditions. *Medicare Severity* DRGs were implemented in 2007 and have been updated annually since.

With DRGs, hospitals joined the prospective payment system (PPS), whereby they receive a specified amount for each Medicare patient's admission regardless of the actual cost of care. Exceptions to this occur when providers can demonstrate that a patient's case is an *outlier*, meaning that the cost of providing care for that patient justifies extra payment. PPS and consequent cost-containment efforts lead to decreased length of stays for most patients.

> Because of the PPS and the need to contain costs, the length of stay for most hospital admissions has decreased greatly.

Many argue that quality standards have been lowered because of the PPS and that patients are being discharged before they are ready. It is the nurse-leader's responsibility to recognize when cost containment is impinging on patient safety and to take appropriate action to guarantee at least a minimum standard of care.

In addition, hospitals must use the International Classification of Diseases (ICD) to code diseases, signs and symptoms, and abnormal findings. Currently in its 10th revision, *ICD-10* provides significantly more coding options for treatment, reporting, and payment processes, including more than 78,000 clinical modification codes as compared with 15,000 in ICD-9 (CMS, 2021).

The government again deeply affected health care administration in the United States in 1997 with the passage of the *Balanced Budget Act* (BBA). This act contained numerous cost-containment measures, including reductions in provider payments for traditional FFS Medicare program participants. The bulk of the savings resulted from limiting the growth rates for hospital and physician payments. A second major source of savings derived from restructuring the payment methods for rehabilitation hospitals, home health agencies, skilled nursing facilities, and outpatient services. The BBA also, for the first time, authorized payments to nurse practitioners for Medicare-provided services at 85% of the physician-fee schedule.

The ever-increasing impact of the federal government on how health care is delivered in the United States must be recognized. Accompanying this funding is an increase in regulations for facilities treating these patients and a system that rewards cost containment. Health care providers are encountering financial crises as they attempt to meet unlimited health care needs and services with limited fiscal reimbursement. Competition has intensified, reimbursement levels have declined, and utilization controls have increased. In addition, rapidly changing federal and state reimbursement policies make long-range budgeting and planning very difficult for health care facilities.

Managed Care

Managed care has also been a significant factor affecting health care delivery and reimbursement since the early 1990s. Broadly defined, *managed care* is a system that attempts to integrate efficiency of care, access, and cost of care. Common denominators in managed care include the use of primary care providers as "gatekeepers," a focus on prevention, a decreased emphasis on inpatient hospital care, the use of clinical practice guidelines for providers, and *selective contracting* (whereby providers agree to lower reimbursement levels in exchange for patient population contracts). In addition, managed care typically uses formularies to manage pharmacy care and focuses on continuous quality monitoring and improvement.

Utilization review is another common component of managed care. Utilization review is a process used by insurance companies to assess the need for medical care and to assure that payment will be provided for the care. Utilization review typically includes precertification or preauthorization for elective treatments, concurrent review, and, if necessary, retrospective review for emergency cases.

Another frequent hallmark of managed care is *capitation*, whereby providers receive a fixed monthly payment regardless of services used by that patient during the month. If the cost to provide care to someone is less than the capitated amount, the provider profits. If the cost is greater than the capitated amount, the provider suffers a loss. The goal, then, for capitated providers is to see that patients receive the essential services to stay healthy or to keep from becoming ill but to eliminate unnecessary use of health care services. Critics of capitation argue that this reimbursement strategy leads to undertreatment of patients.

A summary of managed care characteristics is found in Display 10.5.

Types of Managed Care Organizations

One of the most common types of managed care organizations (MCOs) is the health maintenance organization (HMO). An HMO is a network of providers funded by insurance premiums. The HMO's physicians and other professionals practice medicine within certain financial, geographic, and professional limits to individuals and families who have enrolled in the HMO. Although HMOs originated as an alternative to traditional health insurance plans, some of the largest private insurers, including Blue Cross and Blue Shield and Aetna, have created HMOs within their organization while maintaining their traditional indemnity plans.

It is important to remember that there are different types of HMOs as well as different types of plans within HMOs to which members may subscribe. Several types of HMOs include (a) *staff*, (b) *independent practice association* (IPA), (c) *group*, and (d) *network*. In *staff HMOs*, physician providers are salaried by the HMO and under direct control of the HMO. In *IPA HMOs*, the HMO contracts with a group of physicians through an intermediary to provide services for members of the HMO. In a *group HMO*, the HMO contracts directly with one independent physician group. In *network HMOs*, the HMO contracts with multiple independent physician group practices.

DISPLAY 10.5 MANAGED CARE AT A GLANCE

- Represents a wide range of financing alternatives that focus on managing the cost and quality of health care by:
  - Using panels of selectively contracted providers
  - Limiting benefits to subscribers who use noncontracted providers
  - Implementing some type of authorization system
  - Focusing on primary care rather than specialists and inpatient services
  - Emphasizing preventive health care
  - Relying on clinical practice guidelines for providers
  - Regularly reviewing the use of health care resources
  - Continuously monitoring and improving the quality of health services
- Patients have less choice about the providers they can see and services they can access, in exchange for small copayments and no deductibles.
- Managed care organizations often use primary care gatekeepers to:
  - Be sure that the provider-ordered services are needed and appropriate
  - See that patients are cared for in outpatient settings whenever possible
  - Ration care by queuing and wait times for authorizations
  - Encourage providers to follow more standardized care pathways and clinical guidelines for treatment
- Managed care is based on the concept of capitation, whereby providers prospectively receive a fixed monthly payment, regardless of what services are used by that patient during the month. This encourages providers to treat less because their potential profits decline as treatment increases.

The types of plans available within HMOs typically vary according to the degree of provider choice available to enrollees. Two such plans include *point-of-service* (POS) and *exclusive provider organization* (EPO) options. In POS plans, the patient has the option, at the time of service, to select a provider outside the network but pays a higher premium as well as a *copayment* (amount of money enrollees pay out of their pocket at the time a service is provided) for the flexibility to do so. In the EPO option, enrollees must seek care from the designated HMO provider or pay all the costs out of pocket.

Another common type of MCO is the *preferred provider organization* (PPO). PPOs render services on an FFS basis but provide financial incentives to consumers (they pay less) when the preferred provider is used. Providers are motivated to become part of a PPO because it ensures them an adequate population of patients.

Medicare and Medicaid Managed Care

Although Medicare and Medicaid patients historically were excluded from managed care under the *free choice of physician rule*, these patients can now participate in private HMOs and other types of managed care programs through *Medicare Part C* (formerly the Medicare + Choice program and now known as *Medicare Advantage*). To join a Medicare Advantage plan, patients must have both Medicare Parts A and Part B. The payment system for these programs (effective 1982) was to be prospective, and the HMO was at risk for providing all benefits in return for the capitated payment.

MCOs receive reimbursement for Medicare-eligible patients based on a formula established by the CMS, which looks at age, gender, geographic region, and the average cost per patient at a given age. Then, the government gives itself a small discount and gives the rest to the MCO. The *BBA of 1997* expanded the role of private plans under Medicare + Choice to include PPOs, *provider-sponsored organizations*, *private FFS plans*, and *medical savings accounts*, coupled with high-deductible insurance plans.

The CMS is now the largest purchaser of managed care in the United States.

Proponents and Critics of Managed Care Speak Up

Proponents of managed care argue that prepaid health care plans, such as those offered by HMOs, decrease health care costs, provide broader benefits for patients than under the traditional FFS model, appropriately shift care from inpatient to outpatient settings, result in higher provider productivity, and have high enrollee satisfaction levels. Managed care plans have also rapidly expanded their use of telehealth options to maximize provider efficiency and to save costs. A recent study by Zakaria and colleagues (2021) found that the implementation of a teledermatology triage system in a managed care setting was associated with significant cost savings, suggesting this mode of care can effectively triage and manage patients (see Examining the Evidence 10.1).

Critics, however, suggest that participation in MCOs may result in a loss of existing physician–patient relationships, a limited choice of physicians for consumers, a lower level of continuity of care, reduced physician autonomy, longer wait times for care, and consumer confusion about the many rules to be followed. A common complaint heard from managed care subscribers is that services must be preapproved or preauthorized by a gatekeeper or that second opinions must be obtained before surgery. Although this loss of autonomy is difficult for consumers accustomed to an FFS system with few limits on choice and access, such utilization constraints are necessary due to *moral hazard*, which is the risk that the insured will overuse services just because the insurance will pay the costs. Because the copayment is typically small for patients in managed care programs, the risk of moral hazard rises.

> Moral hazard refers to the propensity of insured patients to use more medical services than necessary because their insurance covers so much of the cost.

EXAMINING THE EVIDENCE 10.1

Source: From Zakaria, A., Miclau, T. A., Maurer, T., Leslie, K. S., & Amerson, E. (2021). Cost minimization analysis of a teledermatology triage system in a managed care setting. *JAMA Dermatology, 157*(1), 52–58.

● ● ● ● ● ● ● ● ● ●

Cost Savings in a Managed Care Teledermatology Model

Teledermatology (TD) enables remote triage and management of dermatology patients. It also reduces societal costs by enabling patients to attend fewer in-person appointments and by providing more timely dermatology diagnosis and treatment. Previous analyses of TD systems, however, have demonstrated improved access to care but an inconsistent fiscal impact.

A retrospective cost minimization analysis was conducted of 2,098 patients referred to a dermatology department in a managed care setting to determine mean cost to manage newly referred patients with or without TD triage. To estimate costs, decision-tree models were constructed to characterize possible care paths with TD triage and within a conventional dermatology care model.

In the decision-tree model with TD triage, the mean (SD) cost per patient to the health care organization was $559.84. In the decision-tree model for conventional dermatology care, the mean (SD) cost per patient was $699.96. Therefore, the TD model demonstrated a statistically significant mean (SE) cost savings of $140.12 per patient. Given an annual dermatology referral volume of 3,150 patients, the analysis estimated an annual savings of $441,378. Study findings also suggested that TD produced these cost savings despite implementation costs (purchase of equipment and the training of personnel). Thus, the cost savings are lowest at the outset and should steadily increase over time.

The researchers concluded that the implementation of a TD triage system within this dermatology department was associated with cost savings, suggesting that managed health care settings may experience significant cost savings from using TD to triage and manage patients.

LEARNING EXERCISE 10.5

Providing Care with Limited Reimbursement

You are the manager at a home health agency. One of your older adult patients has insulin-dependent diabetes. He has no family support. He speaks limited English and has little understanding of his disease. He lives alone in a rural community, which requires significant time to be spent commuting to his home. Your reimbursement from a government agency pays $100 per visit. Because this gentleman needs so much care and because of the travel time and costs, you find that the actual cost to your agency is $135 for each visit to him. What will be the impact to your agency if this patient is seen twice a week for 3 months? How can you recover the lost revenue? How can you make each visit less costly and still meet the needs of the patient?

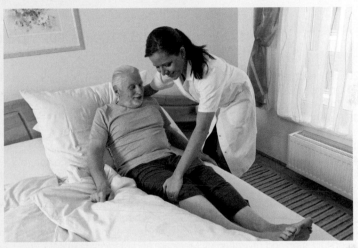

Another aspect complicating health care reimbursement through the PPS, an HMO, or a PPO is that clear and comprehensive documentation of the need for services and actual services provided is mandatory. Provision of service no longer guarantees reimbursement. Thus, the fiscal accountability of nurses goes beyond planning and implementing; it includes responsible recording and communication of activities.

> Provision of service no longer guarantees reimbursement. Documentation must be complete.

Perhaps the most serious concern about the advancement of managed care in this country is the change in relationships among insurers, physicians, nurses, and patients. The full impact on clinical judgment of tying physician and nursing salaries to bonuses, incentives, and penalties designed to reduce utilization of services and resources and increase profit is unknown. As a result, a need for self-awareness regarding the values that guide individual professional nursing practice has never been greater.

The Future of Managed Care

Managed care continues to change the face of health care in the United States. The contractual complexity and the use of prospective payment in managed care make it much more difficult for providers to anticipate potential revenues and then to bill for and collect reimbursement for services provided. Indeed, some critics of managed care suggest that health care practitioners and institutions now bear more of the financial risk for the cost of care than insurers.

Some declines in managed care participation have occurred in part because these plans are no longer significantly less expensive for consumers to purchase or for insurers to provide. In addition, providers have grown increasingly frustrated with limited and delayed reimbursement for services provided as well as the need to justify need for services ordered. Indeed, some providers have filed lawsuits against managed care insurers for delay of payment or nonpayment for services provided. Even with this discontent, managed care is not going to go away—at least not any time soon. It will, however, continue to change. Certainly, in reviewing the health care reimbursement milestones of the past 90 years (Display 10.6), one can see that health care reimbursement has changed dramatically in a relatively short time and that managed care is just one more reimbursement schema that has changed the face of health care in the United States.

DISPLAY 10.6 **US HEALTH CARE MILESTONES: 90+ YEARS OF REIMBURSEMENT**

1929 First health maintenance organization (HMO), the Ross-Loos Clinic, is established in Los Angeles.

1929 Origins of Blue Cross, when Baylor University Hospital agreed to provide 1,500 schoolteachers up to 21 days of hospital care for $6.00 per year.

1935 Passage of Social Security Act. This act originally included compulsory health insurance for states that voluntarily chose to participate, but the American Medical Association fought it and the health insurance provisions were omitted from the act.

1942 First nationwide hospital insurance bill introduced into Congress, but it failed to pass.

1946 Hill–Burton Act promoted hospital development and renovation after World War II. Authorized $75 million yearly for 5 years to aid in hospital construction.

1965 Passage of Medicare and Medicaid as part of Lyndon B. Johnson's Great Society. Resulted in 50% increase in the number of medical schools in the United States.

1972 Professional standards review organizations established by Congress to prevent excess hospitalization and utilization by Medicare and Medicaid patients.

1973 The Health Maintenance Act authorized the spending of $375 million over 5 years to set up and evaluate HMOs in communities across the country.

1974 The National Planning Act created a system of state and local health planning agencies largely supported by federal funds. This created health systems agencies to inventory each community's health care resources and to issue Certificates of Need.

1974 The Employment Retirement Income Security Act (ERISA) passed, generally preempting state regulation of self-insuring employee benefit plans.

1983 Diagnosis-related groups established, which changed the structure of Medicare payments from a retrospectively adjusted cost-reimbursement system to a prospective, risk-based one.

1986 Consolidated Omnibus Budget Reconciliation Act (COBRA) of 1986 passed. Allowed terminated employees or those who lose coverage because of reduced work hours to buy group coverage for themselves and their families for limited periods of time (up to 60 days to decide).

1988 Medicare Catastrophic Coverage Act (MCCA) enacted, which expanded Medicare benefits greatly to include a portion of out-of-pocket drug and physician expenses.

1989 Medicare system of paying physician charges changed to a resource-based relative value scale to be phased in starting in 1992.

1993 Former President William J. Clinton introduced the Health Security Act, legislation assuring universal access to all Americans. The act failed to pass.

1996 Health Insurance Portability and Accountability Act passed. Created medical savings accounts and required the U.S. Department of Health and Human Services to establish national standards for electronic health care transactions and national identifiers for providers, health plans, and employers. It also addressed the security and privacy of health data.

1997 Approximately one quarter of Americans enrolled in HMOs. Almost 6 million Medicare beneficiaries enrolled in HMOs. Balanced Budget Act gives states the authority to implement managed care programs without federal waivers.

DISPLAY 10.6 (CONTINUED)

1999 Health care spending comprised approximately 15% of the gross domestic product of the United States, exceeding $1 trillion in annual health care expenditures for the first time. Approximately 37 million Americans were uninsured, and between 50 and 70 million were inadequately insured.

2001 More than 1.5 million older adult Medicare HMO patients forced to find new insurance arrangements as their HMOs pulled out of the Medicare program after losing money on Medicare enrollees. Increasing disenchantment noted with managed care.

2003 The Medicare Prescription Drug, Improvement, and Modernization Act of 2003 passed, providing a voluntary program for prescription drug coverage under the Medicare program. It also commissioned the Institute of Medicine to prioritize options to align performance and payment in Medicare, supporting a "pay for performance" (P4P) approach.

2009 Congressional committees began active debate of a comprehensive health care reform package. Former President Barack Obama announced the release of nearly $600 million in funding to strengthen community health centers that would serve 500,000 additional patients and use health information technology.

2010 Former President Barack Obama's Health Care Reform bill *Patient Protection and Affordable Care Act* (PPACA) passed, resulting in sweeping overhauls of the US health care system and the introduction of a new Patient's Bill of Rights related to insurance coverage. Provisions related to eliminating lifetime limits on insurance coverage, extending coverage to young adults, and providing new coverage to individuals who have been uninsured for at least 6 months due to a preexisting condition were implemented.

2011 PPACA provisions related to providing free preventive care to seniors, the establishment of a Community-Based Care Transitions Program, and the creation of a new Center for Medicare & Medicaid Innovation were put into place.

2012 The PPACA established hospital value-based purchasing programs in traditional Medicare to provide incentives for health care providers to work together to form accountable care organizations as well as new, voluntary options for long-term care insurance.

2013 The PPACA provided new funding to state Medicaid programs that chose to cover preventive services for patients at little or no cost, expanded the authority to bundle payments, increased medical payments for primary care doctors, and began open enrollment in the *Healthcare Insurance Marketplace*.

2014 The final provisions of the PPACA were phased in, including the implementation of the Healthcare Insurance Marketplace, prohibition of discrimination due to preexisting conditions or gender, the elimination of annual limits on insurance coverage, and ensuring coverage for individuals participating in clinical trials.

2015 The tax penalty for being uninsured increased. The 2015 penalty was the larger of 2% of income or $325 per person ($162.50 per child younger than 18 years). Businesses with 100 or more full-time equivalent (FTE) employees were required to offer affordable coverage to full-time staff that offered the essential benefits required under the Affordable Care Act (ACA). In addition, these policies were required to cover full-time employees' dependent children up through age 26 years. If businesses of this size chose not to offer insurance, they had to pay a tax penalty to the government. This provision applied to businesses with 50 or more full-time employees in 2016.

2016 Under the PPACA, all businesses with 100 or fewer FTE employees were able to purchase insurance through the state SHOP Exchange. A new program also began, allowing states to form health care choice compacts and allowing insurers to sell policies in any state participating in the compact.

2017 Under the PPACA, a state's ability to allow large employers (with 100+ employees) to provide coverage through a SHOP Exchange took effect.

2017 Multiple bills to repeal and replace the ACA were introduced into either the House or the Senate in fall 2017, although legislative consensus was not achieved. Although the bills were different in some respects, the common theme was a reduction in mandates for individuals and businesses to buy or provide health insurance and a reduction of government subsidies for vulnerable populations like older adults and those with incomes below the federal poverty threshold.

continues on page 250

2017 The Tax Cuts and Jobs Act (passed by Congress and signed into law by former President Donald Trump in late December 2017). This made significant changes to the ACA, including eliminating the penalty of the "individual mandate" to purchase health insurance in 2018 and repealing the individual mandate effective January 2019.

2018 Former President Donald Trump revealed the *American Patients First* plan. This plan sought to reform the rebates drug companies pay to pharmacy benefit managers (PBMs), who negotiate prices between drug manufacturers, pharmacies, and health insurance companies. The rebates create incentives for PBMs to suggest higher cost drugs. In addition, PBMs can charge insurers more than they're charging pharmacies. As a result, everyone pays different prices for drugs. Although a number of actions were taken in the first 100 days to enable the plan, full implementation of the blueprint required Congress to amend the act that established Medicare Part D because it prohibited Medicare from negotiating (Huston, 2023). This had not occurred as of mid-2022.

2019 The Department of Justice (DOJ) asked the U.S. Court of Appeals for the Fifth Circuit to invalidate the entire ACA. On January 10, 2020, the DOJ, however, urged the Supreme Court to delay consideration of the lawsuit in which the Administration and 18 states asked the courts to strike down the entire ACA.

2021 In November 2020, The Supreme Court began its debate of the constitutionality of the individual mandate to buy insurance under the ACA and to determine if the entire ACA should be discarded if a portion of the law was found unconstitutional. The court's final decision was rendered in June 2021, concluding that the plaintiffs did not have standing to challenge the constitutionality of the now penalty-less individual mandate (Keith, 2021).

Health Care Reform Efforts: The Patient Protection and Affordable Care Act. What Comes Next?

In March 2010, former President Barack Obama signed the ACA that put in place comprehensive insurance reforms to be phased in over a 4-year period. The act included a new *Patient's Bill of Rights* implemented in 2010, a provision for Medicare beneficiaries to get preventive services for free, and discounts on brand name drugs for some patients using Medicare Part D beginning in 2011. It also introduced "bundled payments," the addition of ACOs and other programs to help doctors and health care providers work together to deliver better care in 2012, hospital VBP and open enrollment in the *Health Insurance Marketplace* beginning in October 2013, and greater access for most Americans to affordable health insurance options in 2014 (Assistant Secretary for Public Affairs, 2021).

Bundled Payments

Passed in October 2011 and implemented in 2013, the *Bundled Payments for Care Improvement Initiative* gave providers flexibility to work together to coordinate care for patients over the course of a single episode of an illness. There are four broadly defined models of *bundled care*: Three of these models involve retrospective payment, and one is prospective. In the retrospective payment models, CMS and providers set a target payment amount for a defined episode of care. This target amount would reflect a discount to total costs for a similar episode of care as determined from historical data. Participants then would be paid for their services under the original Medicare FFS system but at a negotiated discount (CMS, 2022a).

The prospective payment model differs in that CMS makes a single, prospectively determined bundled payment to a hospital that would encompass all services furnished during the inpatient stay by the hospital, physicians, and other practitioners. Physicians and other practitioners would be paid by the hospital out of the bundled payment.

Accountable Care Organizations

ACOs are groups of providers and suppliers of service who work together to better coordinate care for Medicare patients (does not include Medicare Advantage) across care settings. The goal of an ACO is to deliver seamless, high-quality care in an environment that is truly patient centered and where patients and providers are partners in decision making.

Although patient and provider participation in ACOs is voluntary, the *Medicare Shared Savings Program* rewards ACOs that lower growth in health care costs while meeting performance standards of quality of care and putting patients first (Medicare & Medicaid Services, 2022b). ACOs are entitled to these shared savings when savings exceed the minimum sharing rate and if the ACO meets or exceeds the quality performance standards. Additional shared savings can be earned by ACOs that include beneficiaries who receive services from a federally qualified health center or rural health clinic during the performance year (Medicare & Medicaid Services, 2022b).

Hospital Value-Based Purchasing

Beginning in 2013, for the first time, the hospital VBP program paid inpatient acute care services partially on care quality, not just on the quantity of the services they provide. In VBP, providers are held accountable for the quality and cost of the health care services they provide by a system of rewards and consequences. This requires the reporting of standardized, comparable patient outcomes.

The Patient-Centered Medical Home

The *patient-centered medical home* (PCMH), also known as the *medical home*, is a coordinated effort to meet patient needs through the better coordination of quality care. The medical home uses a team of providers—such as physicians, nurses, nutritionists, pharmacists, and social workers—to integrate all aspects of health care, including physical health, behavioral health, access to community-based social services, and the management of chronic conditions. Communication occurs through well-developed health information technology including electronic health records.

Payment reform is also a critical part of the medical home initiative as financial incentives are offered to providers to focus on the quality of patient outcomes rather than the volume of services they provide. Although the model is still evolving, national and state medical home accreditation is available, facilitating payment from both public and private payers.

Health Insurance Marketplaces

As of October 2013, new *health insurance marketplaces*, also called *exchanges*, were created for individuals without access to health insurance through a job, for implementation in January 2014. Small businesses were also eligible to buy affordable and qualified health benefit plans in this competitive insurance marketplace. Every health insurance plan in the marketplace offered comprehensive coverage (10 essential health benefits). From doctors to medications to hospital visits, options could be compared based on price, benefits, and quality. Prospective clients could not be turned down because of preexisting conditions. Tax credits were also provided to lower insurance costs for individuals and families earning below certain levels.

Outcomes of the Affordable Care Act

The outcomes of the ACA included successes and failures (Huston, 2023). With the passage of ACA, approximately 20 million uninsured working-aged adults (aged 18 to 64 years) gained health insurance coverage (How Many Americans Are Uninsured, 2021). The program was especially successful for Black Americans, children, and small business owners.

Despite this progress, major opportunities to improve the health care system remained. The ACA itself was shrouded in confusion and misinformation, starting well before it was signed into law. This was due partly to partisan politics and poor communication about the law to the public. Some of this discontent came about because of the broken promise that people who were satisfied with their previous coverage could remain on their plan. It quickly became apparent this would not be the case. Other consumers found the rollout of the ACA and the marketplace confusing. They felt enrollment periods were too limited and the website was too complicated.

In addition, costs were prohibitive for both the government and consumers and the cost of health care insurance continued to be beyond reach for many Americans. Individuals found it difficult to find affordable plans in the Health Insurance Marketplace, often choosing lower cost plans with high deductibles or copayments that, ultimately, they could not pay. In addition, choice was limited in the Health Insurance Marketplace, existing coverage was disrupted, and bureaucracy created even more rules and regulations. Of even greater concern were the staggering costs of the federal subsidies to insurers as well as what many perceived to be uneven allocation of their use.

With the election of Donald Trump as president in 2017, the vision for comprehensive health care changed and repeal of the ACA became a priority. Legislative efforts during his 4-year presidential term to repeal the ACA failed, but executive orders, including elimination of the individual mandate to have health insurance or face financial penalty (effective January 2019), undermined many of its key elements. In addition, the Trump administration cut subsidies to insurers that were in place to encourage them to stay in the ACA insurance exchanges and to help keep premiums down. As a result, many health insurance companies left the ACA marketplaces (Huston, 2023).

The final attempt to dismantle the ACA under the Trump administration was a hearing brought to the U.S. Supreme Court in November 2020, challenging whether the ACA could be thrown out entirely, if one section of the act was deemed unconstitutional (Huston, 2023). The case before the court—*California v. Texas* (known as Texas v. United States in the lower courts)—disputed the constitutionality of the individual mandate to purchase health insurance. The court's final decision was rendered in June 2021, concluding that the plaintiffs did not have standing to challenge the constitutionality of the now penalty-less individual mandate (Keith, 2021).

In contrast, Simmons-Duffin (2019) notes that while Trump's presidency was marked by scaled-back federal investment and involvement in health care, President Joe Biden, elected in November 2020, has pledged to reverse that trend. Indeed, Biden states that he intends to expand eligibility for the Medicare and Medicaid programs and to double-down and invest in the changes the ACA made to the country's health care system.

President Biden's campaign promises also included pouring trillions into a unified coronavirus strategy, and to work with Congress to create a Medicare-like public insurance plan that anyone could buy into—what he called the "public option" (Simmons-Duffin, 2019, para 3). As of mid 2022, however, the "public option" had fallen off the national radar and will be difficult to revive without a major push by the White House (Sarlin & Kapur, 2021).

Warner et al. (2020) suggest, however, that future reform efforts will bring us closer to meaningful health coverage for all people living in the United States. These initiatives must promote a strong, stable health system; adequate provider networks; consumer-focused transparency of costs and coverage benefits; and a health system that is navigable for patients and consumers. In addition, this coverage must facilitate access to the services and treatments needed by patients, including those with unique or complex medical needs, and the patient protections currently in place, including prohibitions on preexisting condition exclusions, annual and lifetime limits, insurance policy rescission, gender pricing, and excessive premiums for older adults (Warner et al., 2020).

Integrating Leadership Roles and Management Functions in Fiscal Planning

Managers must understand fiscal planning and health care reimbursement, be aware of their budgetary responsibilities, and be cost-effective in meeting organizational goals. The ability to forecast unit fiscal needs with sensitivity to the organization's political, economic, social, and legislative climate is a high-level management function. Managers also must be able to articulate unit needs through budgeting to ensure adequate nursing staff, supplies, and equipment. Finally, managers must be skillful in the monitoring aspects of budget control.

Leadership skills allow the manager to involve all appropriate stakeholders in developing the budget and implementing needed reforms. This has likely never been as important as it is now, given the current climate of health care reform with almost countless initiatives and phased-in implementation. Other leadership skills required in fiscal planning include flexibility, creativity, and vision regarding future needs. The skilled leader can anticipate budget constraints and act proactively. In contrast, many managers allow budget constraints to dictate alternatives. In an age of inadequate fiscal resources, the leader must creatively identify alternatives to meet patient needs.

The skilled leader, however, also ensures that cost containment does not jeopardize patient safety. Leaders are assertive, articulate people who ensure that their department's budgeting receives a fair hearing. Because leaders can delineate unit budgetary needs in an assertive, professional, and proactive manner, they generally obtain a fair distribution of resources for their unit.

To provide care and appropriately advocate for patients in the 21st century, all nurses need at least a basic understanding of health care costs. They also need to know how reimbursement strategies directly and indirectly impact patients and affect their practice. Only then can nurses be active participants in the proactive and visionary fiscal planning required to survive in the current health care marketplace and to reform a broken health care system.

Key Concepts

- Fiscal planning, as in all types of planning, is a learned skill that improves with practice.
- Historically, nursing management played a limited role in determining resource allocation in health care institutions.
- The personnel–workforce budget often accounts for the majority of a health care organization's expenses because health care is labor intensive.
- Personnel budgets include actual worked time (productive time or salary expense) and time that the organization pays the employee for not working (nonproductive or benefit time).

- A budget is at best a forecast or prediction; it is a plan and not a rule. Therefore, a budget must be flexible and open to ongoing evaluation and revision.
- A budget that is predicted too far in advance is open to greater error. If the budget is short-sighted, compensating for unexpected major expenses or capital equipment purchases may be difficult.
- The desired outcome of budgeting is maximal use of resources to meet organizational short- and long-term needs. Its value to the institution is directly related to its accuracy.

- The operating budget reflects expenses that flex up or down in a predetermined manner to reflect variation in volume of service provided.
- Capital budgets plan for the purchase of buildings or major equipment. This includes equipment that has a long life (usually greater than 5 years), is not used daily, and is more expensive than operating supplies.
- Managers must rejustify their program or needs every budgeting cycle in zero-based budgeting. Using a decision package to set funding priorities is a key feature of zero-based budgeting.
- With the advent of state and federal reimbursement for health care in the 1960s, providers were forced to submit budgets and costs to payers that more accurately reflected their actual cost to provide these services.
- With DRGs, hospitals join the PPS, whereby they receive a specified amount for each Medicare patient's admission, regardless of the actual cost of care. Exceptions occur when the provider can demonstrate that a patient's case is an outlier, meaning that the cost of providing care for that patient justifies extra payment.
- Key principles of managed care include the use of primary care providers as gatekeepers, a focus on prevention, a decreased emphasis on inpatient hospital care, the use of clinical practice guidelines for providers, selective contracting, capitation, utilization review, the use of formularies to manage pharmacy care, and continuous quality monitoring and improvement.
- The types of plans available within HMOs typically vary according to the degree of provider choice available to enrollees.
- Managed care has altered the relationships among insurers, physicians, nurses, and patients, with providers today often having to assume a role as an agent for the patient as well as an agent of resource allocation for an insurance carrier, hospital, or particular practice plan.
- Provision of service no longer guarantees reimbursement. Clear and comprehensive

documentation of the need for services and actual services provided is needed for reimbursement.
- The 2010 PPACA (often shortened as ACA) put in place comprehensive insurance reforms, which were phased in over a 4-year period.
- With bundled payments, providers agree to accept a discounted payment either retrospectively or prospectively, which represents a coordinated plan of care for patients over the course of a single episode of an illness.
- ACOs are groups of providers and suppliers of service who work together to better coordinate care for Medicare patients (does not include Medicare Advantage) across care settings with the expectation that efficiency as well as quality of care will result in shared savings.
- In VBP, providers are held accountable for the quality and cost of the health care services they provide by a system of rewards and consequences, conditional upon achieving prespecified performance measures.
- The medical home, or PCMH, relies on a team of providers to integrate all aspects of health care through well-developed health information technology, including electronic health records.
- Health insurance marketplaces, also called exchanges, are online insurance supermalls created for individuals without access to health insurance through a job or for small businesses who wish to buy affordable and qualified health benefit plans in a competitive insurance marketplace.
- The ACA experienced successes and failures. Legislative efforts to repeal the ACA failed, but executive orders, including elimination of the individual mandate, undermined many of its key elements.
- While Trump's presidency was marked by scaled-back federal investment and involvement in health care, his successor, President Joe Biden, has pledged to reverse that trend, by expanding eligibility for the Medicare and Medicaid programs and reinvesting in the ACA.

Additional Learning Exercises and Applications

LEARNING EXERCISE 10.6

How Does Policy Influence Your Decision?

You are the evening house supervisor of a small, private, rural hospital. In your role as house supervisor, you are responsible for staffing the upcoming shift and for troubleshooting all problems that cannot be handled at the unit level.

Tonight, you receive a call to come to the emergency department (ED) to handle a "patient complaint." When you arrive, you find a woman arguing vehemently with the ED charge nurse and physician. When you intercede, the woman introduces herself as Teresa Garcia and states, "There is something wrong with my father, and they won't help him because we only have Medicaid insurance. If we had private insurance, you would be willing to do something." The charge nurse intercedes by saying, "Teresa's father began vomiting about 2 hours ago and blacked out approximately 45 minutes ago, following a 14-hour drinking binge." The ED physician adds, "Mr. Garcia's blood alcohol level is 0.25 [2.5 times the level required to be declared legally intoxicated], and my baseline physical examination would indicate nothing other than he is drunk and needs to sleep it off. Besides, I have seen Mr. Garcia in the ED before, and it's always for the same thing. He does not need further treatment."

Teresa persists in her pleas to you that "there is something different this time" and that she believes this hospital should evaluate her father further. She intuitively feels that something terrible will happen to her father if he is not cared for immediately. The ED physician becomes even angrier after this comment and states to you, "I am not going to waste my time and energy on someone who is just drunk, and I refuse to order any more expensive lab tests or x-rays on this patient. I've met the legal requirements for care. If you want something else done, you will have to find someone else to order it." With that, he walks off and returns to the examination room, where other patients are waiting to be seen. The ED nurse turns to look at you and is waiting for further directions.

ASSIGNMENT:

How will you handle this situation? Would your decision be any easier if there were no limitations in resource allocation? Are your values to act as an agent for the patient or for the agency more strongly developed?

LEARNING EXERCISE 10.7

Weighing Choices in Budget Spending

One of your goals as the unit manager of a critical care unit is to prepare all your nurses to be certified in advanced cardiac life support. You currently have five staff nurses who need this certification. You can hire someone to teach this class locally and rent a facility for $1,000; however, the cost will be taken out of the travel and education budget for the unit, and this will leave you short for the rest of the fiscal year. It also will be a time-consuming effort because you must coordinate the preparation and reproduction of educational materials needed for the course and make arrangements for the rental facility. A certification class also will be provided soon in a large city approximately 150 miles from the hospital. The cost per participant will be $300. In addition, there would be travel and lodging expenses.

(continues on page 256)

> ## LEARNING EXERCISE 10.7
>
> ### Weighing Choices in Budget Spending (continued)
>
> **ASSIGNMENT:**
>
> You have several decisions to make. Should the class be held locally? If so, how will you organize it? Are you going to require your staff to have this certification or merely highly recommend that they do so? If it is required, will the unit pay the costs of the certification? Will you pay the staff nurses their regular hourly wage for attending the class on regularly scheduled work hours? Can this certification be cost-effective? Use group process in some way to make your decision.

> ## LEARNING EXERCISE 10.8
>
> ### How Will You Meet New Budget Restrictions?
>
> You are the director of the local agency that cares for ill and well older adult patients. You are funded by a private corporation grant, which requires matching of city and state funds. You received a letter in the mail today from the state that says state funding will be cut by $40,000, effective in 2 weeks, when the state's budget year begins. This means that your private funding also will be cut $40,000, for a total revenue loss of $80,000. It is impossible at this time to seek alternative funding sources.
>
> In reviewing your agency budget, you note that, as in many health care agencies, your budget is labor-intensive. More than 80% of your budget is attributable to personnel costs, and you believe that the cuts must come from within the personnel budget. You may reduce the patient population that you serve, although you do not really want to do so. You briefly discuss this communication with your staff; no one is willing to reduce their hours voluntarily, and no one is planning to terminate their employment at any time in the near future.
>
> **ASSIGNMENT:**
>
> Given the following brief description of your position and each of your five employees, decide how you will meet the new budget restrictions. What is the rationale for your choice? Which decision do you believe will result in the least disruption of the agency and of the employees in the agency? Should group decision making be involved in fiscal decisions such as this one? Can fiscal decisions such as this be made without value judgments?
>
> Your position is project director. As the project director, you coordinate the day-to-day activities in the agency. You also are involved in long-term planning, and a major portion of your time is allotted to securing future funding for the agency to continue. As the project director, you have the authority to hire and fire employees. You are in your early 30s and have a master's degree in nursing and health administration. You enjoy your job and believe that you have done well in this position since you started 4 years ago. Your yearly salary as a full-time employee is $80,000.
>
> Employee 1 is Mrs. Potter. Mrs. Potter has worked at the agency since it started 7 years ago. She is a registered nurse (RN) with 30 years of experience working with the geriatric population in public health nursing, care facilities, and private duty. She plans to retire in 7 years and travel with her independently wealthy husband. Mrs. Potter has a great deal of expertise that she can share with your staff, although at times, you believe she overshadows your authority because of her experience and your young age. Her yearly salary as a full-time employee is $65,000.

Employee 2 is Mr. Boone. Mr. Boone has Bachelor of Science degrees in both nursing and dietetics and food management. As an RN and registered dietitian, he brings a unique expertise to your staff, which is vital when dealing with a chronically ill and improperly nourished older adult population. In the 6 months since he joined your agency, he has proven to be a dependable, well-liked, and highly respected member of your staff. His yearly salary as a full-time employee is $60,000.

Employee 3 is Ms. Barns. Ms. Barns is the receptionist-secretary in the agency. In addition to all the traditional secretarial duties, such as typing, filing, and transcription of dictation, she screens incoming telephone calls and directs people who come to the agency for information. Her efficiency is a tremendous attribute to the agency. Her full-time yearly salary is $28,000.

Employee 4 is Ms. Lake. Ms. Lake is a licensed practical nurse/licensed vocational nurse with 15 years of work experience in a variety of health care agencies. She is especially attuned to patient needs. Although her technical nursing skills are also good, her caseload frequently is more focused around older adult patients who need companionship and emotional support. She does well at patient teaching because of her outstanding listening and communication skills. Many of your patients request her by name. She is a single mother, supporting six children, and you are aware that she has great difficulty in meeting her personal financial obligations. Her full-time yearly salary is $48,000.

Employee 5 is Mrs. Long. Mrs. Long is an "elderly help aide." She has completed nurse aide training, although her primary role in the agency is to assist well older adults with bathing, meal preparation, driving, and shopping. The time that Mrs. Long spends in performing basic care has decreased the average visit time for each member of your staff by 30%. She is widowed and uses this job to meet her social and self-esteem needs. Financially, her resources are adequate, and the money she earns is not a motivator for working. Mrs. Long works 3 days a week, and her yearly salary is $22,000.

LEARNING EXERCISE 10.9

Identifying, Prioritizing, and Choosing Program Goals

Jane is the supervisor of a small cardiac rehabilitation program. The program includes inpatient cardiac teaching and an outpatient exercise rehabilitation program. Because of limited reimbursement by third-party insurance payers for patient education, there has been no direct charge for inpatient education. Outpatient program participants pay $240 per month to attend three 1-hour sessions per week, although the revenue generated from the outpatient program still leaves an overall budget deficit for the program of approximately $6,800 per month.

Today, Jane is summoned to the associate administrator's office to discuss her budget for the upcoming year. At this meeting, the administrator states that the hospital is experiencing extreme financial difficulties due to declining reimbursements. He states that the program must become self-supporting in the next fiscal year; otherwise, services must be cut. On returning to her office, Jane decides to make a list of several alternatives for problem solving and to analyze each for driving and restraining factors. These alternatives include the following:

1. *Implement a charge for inpatient education.* This would eliminate the budget deficit, but the cost would probably have to be borne by the patient. (*Implication*: Only patients with adequate fiscal resources would elect to receive vital education.)
2. *Reduce department staffing.* There are currently three staff members in the department, and it would be impossible to maintain the same level or quality of services if staffing were reduced.
3. *Reduce or limit services.* The inpatient education program or educational programs associated with the outpatient program could be eliminated. These are both considered to be valuable aspects of the program.

(continues on page 258)

LEARNING EXERCISE 10.9

Identifying, Prioritizing, and Choosing Program Goals (continued)

4. *The fee for the outpatient program could be increased.* This could easily result in a decrease in program participation because many outpatient program participants do not have insurance coverage for their participation.

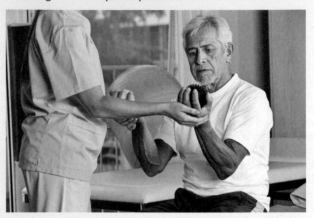

ASSIGNMENT:
• • • • • • • •

Identify at least five program goals and prioritize them as you would if you were Jane. Based on the priorities that you have established, which alternative would you select? Explain your choice.

LEARNING EXERCISE 10.10

Addressing Conflicting Values

You are a single parent of two children younger than 5 years and are currently employed as a pediatric office nurse. You enjoy your job, but your long-term career goal is to become a pediatric nurse practitioner, and you have been taking courses part-time preparing to enter graduate school in the fall. Your application for admission has been accepted, and the next cycle for admissions will not be for another 3 years. Your recent divorce and assignment of sole custody of the children have resulted in a need for you to reconsider your plan.

Restraining Forces

You had originally planned to reduce your work hours to part-time to allow time for classes and studying, but this will be fiscally impossible now. You also recognize that tuition and educational expenses will place a strain on your budget even if you continue to work full-time. You have not investigated the availability of scholarships or loans and have missed the deadline for the upcoming fall. In addition, you have not yet overcome your anxiety and guilt about leaving your small children for even more time than you do now.

Driving Forces

You also recognize, however, that gaining certification as a pediatric nurse practitioner should result in a large salary increase over what you are able to make as an office nurse and that it would allow you to provide resources for your children in the future that you otherwise may be unable to do. Furthermore, you recognize that although you are not dissatisfied with your current job, you have a great deal of ability that has gone untapped and that your potential for long-term job satisfaction is low.

ASSIGNMENT:

Fiscal planning always requires priority setting, and often, this priority setting is determined by personal values. Priority setting is made even more difficult when there are conflicting values. Identify the values involved in this case. Develop a plan that addresses these value conflicts and has the most desirable outcomes.

REFERENCES

Assistant Secretary for Public Affairs. (2021, March 23). *About the Affordable Care Act*. U.S. Department of Health and Human Services. Retrieved August 23, 2021, from http://www.hhs.gov/healthcare/facts-and-features/key-features-of-aca/index.html

Centers for Disease Control and Prevention. (2019, January 10). *Frequently asked flu questions 2018–2019 influenza season*. https://www.cdc.gov/flu/about/season/flu-season-2018-2019.htm

Centers for Medicare & Medicaid Services. (2021, December 10). *ICD-10*. http://www.cms.gov/Medicare/Coding/ICD10/index.html?redirect=/icd10

Centers for Medicare & Medicaid Services. (2022a). *Bundled payments for care improvement (BPCI) initiative: General information*. https://innovation.cms.gov/initiatives/bundled-payments/

Centers for Medicare & Medicaid Services. (2022b). *Shared savings program*. https://www.cms.gov/Medicare/Medicare-Fee-for-Service-Payment/sharedsavingsprogram

Congressional Research Service (2021, January 26). *U.S. health care coverage and spending*. United States Congress. https://fas.org/sgp/crs/misc/IF10830.pdf

HealthCare.gov. (n.d.). *Payment bundling*. Retrieved August 23, 2021, from https://www.healthcare.gov/glossary/payment-bundling/

How many Americans are uninsured? (2021, May 6). *Balancing Everything*. https://balancingeverything.com/how-many-americans-are-uninsured/

Huston, C. J. (2023). Health care reform: Is the Affordable Care Act the answer? In C. J. Huston (Ed.), *Professional issues in nursing: Challenges and opportunities* (6th ed., pp. 319–336). Wolters Kluwer.

Kaiser Family Foundation. (2019, June 6). *Medicare Advantage*. https://kff.org/medicare/fact-sheet/medicare-advantage/

Kaiser Family Foundation. (2020). *2020 Employer health benefits survey*. https://www.kff.org/health-costs/report/2020-employer-health-benefits-survey/

Kaiser Family Foundation. (2022a). *Distribution of Medicare beneficiaries by eligibility category. Timeframe: 2019*. https://www.kff.org/medicare/state-indicator/distribution-of-medicare-beneficiaries-by-eligibility-category-2/?currentTimeframe=0&sortModel=%7B%22colId%22:%22Location%22,%22sort%22:%22asc%22%7D

Kaiser Family Foundation. (2022b). *Medicare beneficiaries as a percent of total population. Timeframe: 2018*. https://www.kff.org/medicare/state-indicator/medicare-beneficiaries-as-of-total-pop/?currentTimeframe=0&sortModel=%7B%22colId%22:%22Location%22,%22sort%22:%22asc%22%7D

Keith, K. (2021, June 17). Supreme Court rejects ACA challenge; Law remains fully intact. *Health Affairs*. https://www.healthaffairs.org/do/10.1377/hblog20210617.665248/full/

Medicaid.gov. (2021). *March 2021 Medicaid & CHIP enrollment data highlights*. https://www.medicaid.gov/medicaid/program-information/medicaid-and-chip-enrollment-data/report-highlights/index.html

Mulcahy, A. W. (2021, January 28). *Prescription drug prices in the United States are 2.56 times those in other countries*. Rand Corporation. https://www.rand.org/news/press/2021/01/28.html

Sarlin, B., & Kapur, S. (2021). *The health insurance public option might be fizzling. The left is OK with that*. NBC News. https://www.nbcnews.com/politics/joe-biden/health-insurance-public-option-might-be-fizzling-left-ok-n1269571

Simmons-Duffin, S. (2019, October 14). *Trump is trying hard to thwart Obamacare. How's that going?* NPR. https://www.npr.org/sections/health-shots/2019/10/14/768731628/trump-is-trying-hard-to-thwart-obamacare-hows-that-going

Stewart, C. (2020, January 7). *Average prices of a magnetic resonance imaging (MRI) in selected countries in 2017 (in U.S. dollars)*. Statista. https://www.statista.com/statistics/312020/price-of-mri-diagnostics-by-country/

Warner, J. J., Benjamin, I. J., Churchwell, K., Firestone, G., Gardner, T. J., Janay, C., Johnson, J. C., Ng-Osorio, J., Rodriguez, C. J., Todman, L., Yaffe, K., Yancy, C. W., Harrington, R. A.; American Heart Association Advocacy Coordinating Committee. (2020, February 3). Advancing healthcare reform: The American Heart Association's 2020 statement of principles for adequate, accessible, and affordable health care: A presidential advisory from the American Heart Association. *Circulation, 141*(10), e601–e614. https://doi.org/10.1161/CIR.0000000000000759

YourDictionary. (2021). Cost effective. Retrieved August 23, 2021, from http://www.yourdictionary.com/cost-effective

11

Career Planning and Development in Nursing

… every individual you hire for a leadership role should have the capability to grow into that role.—**Carolyn Hope Smeltzer**

… career plans are about where you are today and, more importantly, where you're going tomorrow.—**Phil McPeck**

… The number one role of any leader is to identify and prepare their successor.—**Bill Bliss**

CROSSWALK

This chapter addresses:

- **AACN Essentials Domain 1:** Knowledge for nursing practice
- **AACN Essentials Domain 4:** Scholarship for nursing practice
- **AACN Essentials Domain 8:** Information and health care technologies
- **AACN Essentials Domain 9:** Professionalism
- **AACN Essentials Domain 10:** Personal, professional, and leadership development
- **AONL Nurse Executive Competency 3:** Leadership
- **AONL Nurse Executive Competency 4:** Professionalism
- **AONL Nurse Executive Competency 5:** Business skills
- **ANA Standard of Professional Performance 8:** Advocacy
- **ANA Standard of Professional Performance 12:** Leadership
- **ANA Standard of Professional Performance 13:** Education
- **ANA Standard of Professional Performance 14:** Scholarly inquiry
- **ANA Standard of Professional Performance 15:** Quality of practice
- **ANA Standard of Professional Performance 16:** Professional practice evaluation

LEARNING OBJECTIVES

The learner will:

- describe the impact a career development program has on employee attrition, future employment opportunities, quality of work life, and competitiveness of the organization
- differentiate among the promise, momentum, and harvest stages of a career as identified by Shirey (2009)
- discuss changes in practical knowledge based on clinical experience that occurs in the transition from novice to expert nurse (Benner, 1982)
- differentiate between the employer's and the employee's responsibilities for career development
- describe three phases of long-term coaching for career development

- identify support by top management, systematic planning and implementation, and inclusion of social learning activities as integral components of management development programs
- identify the organization's responsibility for effective promotions
- recognize lifelong learning as a professional expectation and responsibility
- define continued competency and identify strategies for assuring and measuring it
- identify driving and restraining forces for specialty certification in professional nursing
- identify factors creating the current, pressing need for transition-to-practice programs to retain new graduate nurses and prepare them for successful employment
- develop a personal career plan
- create and/or critique a resumé for content, format, grammar, punctuation, sentence structure, and appropriate use of language

Introduction

To be a fully engaged professional requires commitment to career development. *Career development* is intentional career planning and should be viewed as a critical and deliberate life process involving both the individual and the employer. It provides individuals with choices about career outcomes rather than leaving them to chance.

Currently, subordinate career development is recognized as essential to organizational success, and most organizations accept at least some responsibility for helping employees with this function. For the most part, however, organizational career development efforts have historically centered on management development rather than activities that promote growth in nonmanagement employees. Indeed, a survey by Infopro Learning found that only 83% of organizations felt it was important to develop leaders at all levels (Velasquez, 2020). Given that more than 80% of an organization's employees are typically nonmanagement, this is often a neglected part of career development.

> Career development in an organization must include more than management employees.

This chapter examines organizational justifications for employee career development, suggests the existence of career stages, and emphasizes the need for career coaching. The use of competency assessment, professional certification, and transition-to-practice programs (TPPs) are identified as strategies for career management with the goal of lifelong learning. Finally, professional resumés, reflection, and portfolios are discussed as career planning tools. The leadership roles and management functions inherent in career planning and development in nursing are shown in Display 11.1.

Career Stages

Before individuals can plan a successful career development program, they need to understand the typical career stages. Shirey (2009) suggests that there are three different career phases or stages among nurses: promise, momentum, and harvest. *Promise* is the earliest of the career phases and typically reflects the first 10 years of nursing employment. Individuals in this stage are less experienced and tend to experience reality overload as a result. Making wise early career choices is critical in this phase. Milestones to be attained include socialization to the nursing role (becoming an insider); building knowledge, skills, abilities, credentials, and an education base; gaining exposure to a variety of experiences; identifying strengths and building confidence; and positioning for the future.

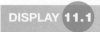

DISPLAY 11.1   LEADERSHIP ROLES AND MANAGEMENT FUNCTIONS IN CAREER PLANNING AND DEVELOPMENT IN NURSING

Leadership Roles

1. Is self-aware regarding personal values influencing career development
2. Encourages employees to take responsibility for their own career planning
3. Identifies, encourages, and develops future leaders
4. Shows a genuine interest in the career planning and career development of all employees
5. Encourages and supports the development of career paths within and outside the organization
6. Supports employees' personal career decisions based on each employee's needs and values
7. Is a role model for continued professional development via specialty certification, continuing education, and portfolio development
8. Emphasizes the need for employees to develop the skill set necessary for evidence-based practice
9. Supports new graduate nurses in their transition to practice through positive role modeling as well as the creation of nurse residencies, internships, and externships
10. Role models lifelong learning as a professional expectation and responsibility
11. Encourages others to continue their formal education as part of their career ladder and professional journey

Management Functions

1. Develops fair policies related to career development opportunities and communicates them clearly to subordinates
2. Provides fiscal resources and release time for subordinate training and education
3. Uses a planned system of short- and long-term coaching for career development and documents all coaching efforts
4. Disseminates career and job information
5. Works with employees to establish career goals that meet both employee and organizational needs
6. Works cooperatively with other departments in arranging for the release of employees to take other positions within the organization
7. Views transition-to-practice programs as an investment strategy to mitigate nurse turnover and promote employee satisfaction
8. Coaches employees to create professional portfolios that demonstrate reflection as well as the maintenance of continued competence
9. Attempts to match position openings with capable employees who seek new learning opportunities
10. Creates possibilities for career progression
11. Provides opportunities for "legacy" clinicians to "reinvent" themselves to renew their potential value to the organization and their coworkers

Benner (1982) describes this early phase as a transition from *novice* to *expert*, arguing that nurses develop skills and understanding of patient care over time through a sound educational base as well as a multitude of experiences. As nurses progress from novice to advanced beginner, to competent, to proficient, and finally to expert, they extend their practical knowledge ("know how") through research and the understanding of the "know how" of clinical experience (Benner, 1982). In other words, the new nurse moves from reliance on past abstract principles to the use of past concrete experience as paradigms and changes their perception of situations to whole parts rather than separate pieces (Display 11.2).

Shirey (2009) identifies *momentum* as the middle career phase, which typically reflects the nurse with 11 to 29 years of experience. Nurses in this phase are experienced clinicians with expert knowledge, skills, abilities, credentials, and education base. This is a time of accomplishment, challenge, and a sense of purpose, and the individual often achieves enough expertise to be a role model to others. Milestones include further building confidence in one's

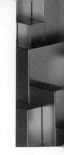

DISPLAY 11.2 BENNER'S LEVELS OF NURSING EXPERIENCE

Novice

- Beginner with no experience
- Taught general rules to help perform tasks
- Rules are context-free, independent of specific cases, and applied universally
- However, rules cannot express which tasks are most relevant in real life or when exceptions are needed

Advanced Beginner

- Demonstrates acceptable performance
- Has gained prior experience in actual situations to recognize recurring meaningful components
- Principles, based on experiences, begin to be formulated to guide actions

Competent

- Typically, 2 to 3 years' work experience in the same area or in similar day-to-day situations
- More aware of long-term goals
- Gains perspective from planning own actions based on conscious, abstract, and analytical thinking and helps to achieve greater efficiency and organization

Proficient

- Perceives and understands situations as whole parts
- More holistic understanding improves decision making
- Learns from experiences what to expect in certain situations and how to modify plans

Expert

- No longer relies on principles, rules, or guidelines to connect situations and determine actions
- Much greater background of experience
- Has intuitive grasp of clinical situations
- Performance is now fluid, flexible, and highly proficient

Source: From Benner, P. (1982). From novice to expert. *American Journal of Nursing, 82*(3), 402–407.

competence; developing experience, gaining mastery, and establishing a professional track record; and finding a voice through aligning strengths with passion. One of the most significant challenges to nurses in this phase, however, is creating possibilities for career progression rather than stagnation. A commitment to lifelong learning and being willing to seize unexpected opportunities that may present themselves over time are often key to career divergence at this point in life.

Shirey (2009) notes that the last stage, *harvest*, commences in late career. Shirey labels nurses with 30 to 40 years as having "prime" experience and nurses with more than 40 years of experience as being "legacy" clinicians. Although viewed as expert clinicians, the experiential value of nurses in the harvest phase may begin to decline if others perceive them as obsolescent. These prime or legacy nurse-leaders then must actively strive for ongoing "reinvention" to renew their potential value to their coworkers. Success then is defined not only by being knowledgeable but also by being savvy and adaptable. The potential for career divergence in this phase is mixed, depending on choices made in the momentum phase. Milestones to be conquered include elevating their mastery to sage practice for advancing the profession and positioning as a professional statesperson and establishing a legacy.

Finally, an argument might be made that another career stage exists in nursing—that of *reentry*. Concurrent with nursing shortages, many nurses who were no longer working in the profession but who possess the necessary training and experience to do so may reenter the work setting.

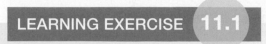

LEARNING EXERCISE 11.1

Exploring Career Stages

In a group, discuss the job stages described by Shirey (2009). What stage most closely reflects your present situation? Think about the nurses that you work with or those you aspire to be like. What career stage are they currently in? Do you believe that male and female nurses have similar or dissimilar career stages?

Justifications for Career Development

The following, summarized in Display 11.3, is a list of justifications for career development programs:

- *Reduced employee attrition*. Career development can reduce the turnover of ambitious employees who might otherwise seek other jobs because of a lack of job advancement.
- *Equal employment opportunity*. Underrepresented minorities and other underserved groups have more opportunities to move up in an organization if they are identified and developed early in their careers.
- *Increased opportunities for employee growth*. When employees are kept in jobs that they have outgrown, their productivity is often reduced.
- *Improved quality of work life*. Nurses increasingly desire to control their own careers. They want greater job satisfaction and more career options.
- *Improved competitiveness of the organization*. Highly educated professionals often prefer organizations that have a good track record of career development. During nursing shortages, a recognized program of career development can be the deciding factor for professionals selecting a position.
- *Obsolescence can be avoided and new skills acquired*. Because of the rapid changes in health care, especially in the areas of consumer demands and technology, employees may find that their skills have become obsolete. A successful career development program begins to retrain employees proactively, providing them with the necessary skills to remain current in their field and, therefore, valuable to the organization.
- *Evidence-based practice promoted*. Evidence-based practice is now the gold standard for nursing practice; yet, many nurses still lack both skill and confidence in knowing how to use research and best practices to inform their practice. The astute leader-manager recognizes this knowledge deficit and uses career planning and goal setting to give these nurses the time and resources needed to acquire these skills.

DISPLAY 11.3 JUSTIFICATIONS FOR CAREER DEVELOPMENT

- Reduces employee attrition
- Provides equal employment opportunity
- Increases opportunities for employee growth
- Improves quality of work life
- Improves competitiveness of the organization
- Avoids obsolescence and builds new skills
- Promotes evidence-based practice

Individual Responsibility for Career Development

Despite the many obvious benefits of career development programs, some nurses never create a personal career plan or set goals they wish to accomplish during their career. Instead, nursing becomes just a job. This viewpoint limits the opportunities for professional advancement and personal growth because what cannot be imagined rarely becomes a reality. The impact of positive role modeling by nurse-leaders in influencing this perception cannot be overstated.

Career development should begin with an assessment of self as well as work environment, job analysis, education, training, job search and acquisition, and work experience. This is known as *career planning*. Career planning includes evaluating one's strengths and weaknesses, setting goals, examining career opportunities, preparing for potential opportunities, and using appropriate developmental activities.

Career planning in nursing should begin with an individual's decision about educational entry level for practice and quickly expand to developing advanced skills in an area of nursing practice. Even for the entry-level nurse, career planning should include, at minimum, a commitment to the use of evidence-based practice, learning new skills or bettering practice with the assistance of role models and mentors, staying aware of and being involved in professional issues, and furthering one's education. It should also include long-term career goals as well as a specific plan to achieve lifelong learning.

> Every nurse should proactively develop a career plan that provides opportunities for new learning, challenges, and opportunities for career divergence.

The Organization's Role in Employee Career Development

Organizations also have some responsibility to assist employees with their career development. One such responsibility is the creation of career paths and *advancement/career ladders* (the progression from entry level positions to higher levels of pay, skill, responsibility, or authority; frequently used to denote upward mobility within a stratified promotion mode) (STANDS4 LLC, 2022). It must also attempt to match position openings with appropriate people. This includes accurately assessing employees' performance and potential to offer the most appropriate career guidance, education, and training. Other organizational responsibilities include:

- *Integrating needs.* The human resources department, nursing division, nursing units, and education department must work together to match job openings with the skills and talents of present employees.
- *Establishing career paths.* Career paths must be developed, communicated to the staff, and implemented consistently. When designing career paths, each successive job in each path should contain additional responsibilities and duties that are greater than the previous jobs in that path. Each successive job also must be related to and use previous skills.
- Once career paths are established, they must be communicated effectively to all staff. What employees must do to advance in a path should be very clear.
- *Disseminating career information.* The education department, human resources department, and unit manager are all responsible for sharing career information; however, employees should not be encouraged to pursue unrealistic goals.
- *Posting job openings.* Although this is usually the responsibility of the human resources department, the manager should communicate this information, even when it means staff may transfer to another area. Effective managers know who should be encouraged to apply for openings and who is ready for more responsibility and challenges.

TABLE **ROLES AND RESPONSIBILITIES FOR CAREER DEVELOPMENT**

Career Planning (Individual)	Career Management (Organizational)
• Self-assess interests, skills, strengths, weaknesses, and values • Determine goals • Assess the organization for opportunities • Assess opportunities outside the organization • Develop strategies • Implement plans • Evaluate plans • Reassess and make new plans as necessary, at least biannually	• Integrate individual employee needs and organizational needs • Establish, design, communicate, and implement career paths • Disseminate career information • Post and communicate all job openings within the organization • Assess employees' career needs • Provide work experiences to further employee development • Give support and encouragement • Develop new personnel policies as necessary, at least biannually • Provide training and education

- *Assessing employees.* One of the benefits of a good appraisal system is the important information that it gives the manager on the performance, potential, and abilities of all staff members. The use of short- and long-term coaching will give managers insight into their employees' needs and wants so that appropriate career counseling can proceed.
- *Providing challenging assignments.* Planned work experience is one of the most powerful career development tools. This includes jobs that temporarily stretch employees to their maximum skill, temporary projects, assignment to committees, shift rotation, assignment to different units, and shift charge duties.
- *Giving support and encouragement.* Because excellent subordinates make managers' jobs easier, managers are often reluctant to encourage these subordinates to move up the corporate ladder or to seek more challenging experiences outside the manager's span of control. Thus, many managers hoard their talent. A leadership role requires that managers look beyond their immediate unit or department and consider the needs of the entire organization. Leaders recognize and share talent.
- *Developing personnel policies.* An active career development program often reveals certain personnel policies and procedures that are impeding the success of the program. When this occurs, the organization should reexamine these policies and make necessary changes.
- *Providing education and training.* The impact of education and training on career development and retention of subordinate staff is discussed more fully in Chapter 16. The need for organizations to develop leaders and managers is presented later in this chapter.

A comparison of roles and responsibilities individuals and organizations have for employee career development is shown in Table 11.1.

LEARNING EXERCISE 11.2

Encouragement and Coaching for Goal Achievement

In your employment, has someone ever coached you, either formally or informally, to develop your career? For example, has an employer told you about career or educational opportunities? Have they offered tuition reimbursement? If so, how did you find out about such policies? Have you ever coached (something more than just encouraging) someone to pursue educational or career goals? Share the answers to these questions in class.

Career Coaching

Organizations also have some responsibility to assist employees with career coaching. Unit managers sometimes take on this role, but it may also be provided by informal organization leaders who are willing to act in a mentoring capacity.

Career coaching involves helping others to identify professional goals and career options and then designing a career plan to achieve those goals. Handrick (2022) defines a career coach as an individual whose role is to assist leaders in identifying their leadership strengths, building their organizations and careers whether as corporate executives or business owners.

Career coaching typically has three steps:

1. *Gathering data.* When managers spend time observing employees, they can determine who has good communication skills, who is well organized, who uses effective negotiating skills, and who works collaboratively. Managers also should seek information about the employee's past work experience, performance appraisals, and educational experiences. Data also should include academic qualifications and credentials. Most of this information is retrievable in the employee's personnel file. Finally, employees themselves are an excellent source of information about career needs and wants.

2. *Asking what is possible.* As part of career planning, the manager should assess the department for possible changes in the future, openings or transfers, and potential challenges and opportunities. The manager should anticipate what needs lie ahead, what projects are planned, and what staffing and budget changes will occur. After carefully assessing the employee's profile and future opportunities, managers should consider each staff member and ask the following questions: How can this employee be helped so that they are better prepared to take advantage of the future? Who needs to be encouraged to return to school, to become credentialed, or to take a special course? Which employees need to be encouraged to transfer to a more challenging position, given more responsibility on their present unit, or moved to another shift? Managers can create a stimulating environment for career development by being aware of the uniqueness of their employees.

3. *Conducting the coaching session.* The goals of career coaching include helping employees increase their effectiveness; identifying potential opportunities in the organization; and advancing knowledge, skills, and experience. It is important not to intimidate employees when questioning them about their future and their goals. Although there is no standard procedure for career coaching, the main emphasis should be on employee's growth and future development.

Career coaching, then, can be either short- or long-term. In *short-term career coaching*, the manager regularly asks the employees questions to develop and motivate them. Thus, short-term coaching is a spontaneous part of the experienced manager's repertoire.

Long-term career coaching, on the other hand, is a planned management action that occurs over the duration of employment. Because this type of coaching may cover a long time, it is frequently neglected unless the manager uses a systematic scheduling plan and a form for documentation. Because employees and managers move frequently within an organization, documentation of career coaching is crucial. Figure 11.1 is an example of a long-term coaching form.

The effective manager should have at least one coaching session with each employee annually, in addition to any coaching that may occur during the appraisal interview. Although some coaching should occur during the performance appraisal interview, additional coaching should be planned at a less stressful time.

Name of employee: _____

Name of supervisor: _____

Date: _____ Date of last coaching interview: _____

1. What new challenges and responsibilities could be given to this employee that would utilize their special talents? _____
   _____

2. What events happening in the organization do you foresee affecting this employee? *(Examples would be plans to go to an all-RN staff, changing the mode of patient care delivery, increasing emphasis on credentialing by new CEO of the nursing division, changing medication system, or changing the ratio of nonprofessionals to professionals for nurse staffing.)* _____
   _____

3. How should the employee be preparing to meet new or changing expectations?_____
   _____
   _____

4. What specific suggestions and guidance for the future can you give this employee? *(Examples would be taking specific courses to prepare for change, urging employee to pursue an advanced degree or seek challenges outside of the unit, considering changing shifts, or suggesting that they apply for the next management opening.)*_____
   _____
   _____

5. What specific organizational resources can you offer the employee?_____
   _____
   _____

6. What new information regarding this employee's long-term plans, aspirations, and potential have your review of the personnel record, your observations, and this interview given?
   _____
   _____

7. Do the organizational and professional career plans held by the individual match your vision of their future? If not, how do they differ?_____
   _____

8. What developmental and professional growth has taken place since the last coaching?_____
   _____
   _____

9. Date of next coaching interview: _____

FIGURE 11.1 Sample long-term coaching form.

Management Development

Management development is a planned system of training and developing people so that they acquire the skills, insights, and attitudes needed to manage people and their work effectively within the organization.

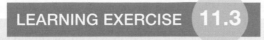

LEARNING EXERCISE   11.3

Career Coaching a Bored Employee

You are the registered nurse (RN) team leader on a busy step-down critical care unit. One of the certified nursing assistants (CNAs) assigned to your team is technically very competent and always completes her work on time but frequently appears to be bored. The only time she seems to be excited about work is when she is assisting you or the other RNs with more complex skills such as central line dressing changes, peripherally inserted central catheters, and complex wound packings. She has shared at times that her long-term career goal is to become an RN but has never verbalized any specific plan to achieve this. Although she is highly capable, her formal education to date is limited to a high school diploma she earned 3 years ago. She currently provides full-time financial support for herself and her 3-year-old daughter.

ASSIGNMENT:

1. Identify questions you might ask the CNA that could be a part of both short- and long-term career coaching for this employee.
2. What resources might be explored to support this employee in attaining higher education?
3. What leadership role modeling could be made available to this employee to encourage her in furthering her career goals?

Management development is often referred to as *succession planning*. Many nurses feel uncertain that they have the skills needed to be effective managers, and they lack confidence that the decision making, interpersonal, and organizational skills they learned as staff nurses can translate to the management role.

> Many nurses feel that they lack the knowledge and experience necessary to become a manager.

Although many of these skills do transfer, becoming an effective manager is generally not intuitive. New leader-managers will likely need the formal education and training that are a part of a management development program. The program must include a means of developing appropriate attitudes through social learning theory as well as adequate content on management theory.

Support for such management development programs by the organization should occur in two ways. First, top-level management must do more than bear the cost of management development classes. They must create an organizational structure that allows managers to apply their new knowledge.

Second, training outcomes improve if nursing executives are active in planning and developing a systematic and integrated program. Whenever possible, nursing administrators should teach some of the classes and, at the very least, make sure that the program supports top management philosophy. Just as nurses are required to be certified in critical care before they accept a position in a critical care unit, nurses should be required to take part in a management development program before their appointment to a management position. This requires early identification and grooming of potential management candidates.

The first step in the process would be an appraisal of the present management team and an analysis of possible future needs. The second step would be the establishment of a training and development program. This would require decisions such as the following: How often should the formal management course be offered? Should outside educators be involved, or should in-house staff teach it? Who should be involved in teaching the didactic portion? Should there be two levels of classes, one for first-level and one for middle-level managers? Should the management development courses be open to all, or should people be recommended by someone from management? In addition to formal course content, what other methods should be used to develop managers? Should other methods be used, such as job rotation through an understudy system of pairing selected people with a manager and management coaching?

The inclusion of *social learning activities* also is a valuable part of management development. Management development will not be successful unless learners have ample chance to try out new skills. Providing potential managers with didactic management theory alone does not prepare them for the attitudes, skills, and insights necessary for effective management. Case studies, management games, transactional analysis, and sensitivity training are also effective in changing attitudes and increasing self-awareness. All these techniques appropriately use social learning theory strategies.

Promotion: A Career Management Tool

Promotions are reassignments to positions of higher rank. It is normal for promotions to include a pay raise. Most promotions include increased status, title changes, more authority, and greater responsibility; therefore, they can be used as significant motivational tools.

Because of the importance that US society places on promotions, certain guidelines must accompany promotion selection to ensure that the process is fair, equitable, and motivating. When position openings occur, they are often posted and filled quickly with little thought of long-term organizational or employee goals. This frequently results in negative personnel outcomes. To avoid this, the following elements should be determined in advance:

- *Whether recruitment will be internal or external.* There are obvious advantages and disadvantages to recruiting for promotions from both inside and outside the organization. Recruiting from within can help to develop employees to fill higher-level positions as they become vacant. It can also serve as a powerful motivation and recognition tool because all employees know that opportunities for advancement are possible, and this encourages them to perform at a higher level.

   There are advantages to recruiting from outside the organization, however. When promotions are filled with people outside the organization, the organization is infused with people with new ideas. External candidates, however, often cost more in terms of salary than internal ones. This is because external candidates generally need a financial incentive to leave their current positions for something else.

   Regardless of what the organization decides, the policy should be consistently followed and communicated to all employees. Some companies recruit from within first and recruit from outside the organization only if they are unable to find qualified people from among their own employees.

- *What the promotion and selection criteria will be.* Employees should know in advance what the criteria for *promotion* are and what selection method is to be used. Some organizations use an interview panel as a selection method to promote all employees beyond the level of charge nurse. Decisions regarding the selection method and promotion criteria should be justified with rationale. In addition, employees need to know what place seniority will have in the selection criteria.

- *The pool of candidates that exists.* When promotions are planned, as in succession management, the leader-manager's role is to identify and prepare an adequate pool of candidates to seek higher-level positions. It is not their role to urge employees to seek a position in a manner that would lead the employee to think that they were guaranteed the job or to unduly influence them in the decision to seek such a job.

When employees actively seek promotions, they are making a commitment to do well in the new position. When they are pushed into such positions, the commitment to expend the energy to do the job well may be lacking. In addition, for many reasons, the employee may not feel ready, either due to personal commitments or because they feel inadequately educated or experienced. Indeed, it is possible to promote an individual beyond their level of capability (known as the *Peter Principle*). In this case, promotions demotivate that individual as well as everyone in the organization.

> The Peter Principle suggests that individuals often rise "to the level of their incompetence."

- *Handling rejected candidates.* All promotion candidates who are rejected should be notified before or at the same time the selected candidate is notified. This is common courtesy. They should be thanked for applying and, when appropriate, encouraged to apply for future position openings. Sometimes, managers should tell employees what prevented them from getting the position. For instance, employees should be told if they lack some educational component or work experience that would make them a stronger competitor for future promotions. This can be an effective way of encouraging career development.
- *How employee releases are to be handled.* Knowledge that the best candidate for the position currently holds a critical job or difficult position to fill should not influence decisions regarding promotions. Managers frequently find it difficult to release employees to another position within the organization. Policies regarding the length of time that a manager can delay releasing an employee should be written and communicated. On the other hand, some managers are so good at developing their employees that they frequently become frustrated because their success at career development results in constantly losing their staff to other departments. In such cases, higher-level management should reward such leaders and set release policies that are workable and realistic.

Continued Competency as Part of Career Development

Continued competency is also a part of career management. Merriam-Webster Dictionary (2022) defines a *professional* as one that engages in a pursuit or activity professionally or a person who does a job that requires special education or skill. Being professional then is characterized by conforming to the technical or ethical standards of a profession, in other words, being competent.

Competency assessment, however, continues to pose challenges in nursing. Huston (2023) agrees, noting that unfortunately, in many states, a practitioner is determined to be competent when initially licensed and thereafter, unless proven otherwise. However, passing a licensing exam and continuing to work as a clinician does not assure competence throughout a career. Competence requires continual updates to knowledge and practice, and this is difficult in a health care environment characterized by rapidly emerging new technologies, chaotic change, and perpetual clinical advancements.

The National Academy of Science publication entitled *Future of Nursing 2020–2030* notes that by the year 2030, the nursing profession will look vastly different and will be caring for a changing America. "Nursing school curricula need to be strengthened so that nurses are prepared to help promote health equity, reduce health disparities, and improve the health and well-being of everyone. Nursing schools will need to ensure that nurses are prepared to understand and identify the social determinants of health, have expanded learning experiences in the community so they can work with different people with varied life experiences and cultural values, have the competencies to care for an aging and more diverse population, can engage in new professional roles, are nimble enough to adapt continually to new technologies, and can lead and collaborate with other professions and sectors" (National Academies Press, 2021, p. 189). One must at least question how many nurses currently in practice would be able to demonstrate competency in all these areas.

Assessing, maintaining, and supporting *continued competence* then is a challenge in professional nursing. For example, Huston (2023) notes that some nurses develop high levels of competence in specific areas of nursing practice because of work experience and specialization, at the expense of staying current in other areas of practice. In addition, employers often ask nurses to provide care in areas of practice outside their area of expertise because a nursing shortage encourages them to do so. In addition, many current competence assessments focus more on skills than they do on knowledge (Huston, 2023). The issue is also complicated by the fact that there are no national standards for defining, measuring, or requiring continuing competence in nursing.

Managers should appraise each employee's competency level not only as part of performance appraisal but also as part of career development. This appraisal should lead to the development of a plan that outlines what the employee must do to achieve desired competencies in both current and future positions. Often, however, competency assessment focuses only on whether the employee has achieved required minimal competency levels to meet current federal, state, or organizational standards and not on how to exceed these competency levels. Thus, competency assessment and goal setting in career planning is proactive, with the employee identifying areas of potential future growth and the manager assisting in identifying strategies that can help the employee achieve that goal.

> Competency assessment and goal setting in career planning should help the employee identify how to exceed minimum levels of competency.

Some individual responsibility for maintaining competence and pursuing lifelong learning is suggested by the American Nurses Association (ANA, 2015) *Code of Ethics for Nurses with Interpretive Statements* in its assertion that nurses are obligated to provide adequate and competent nursing care. State Nurse Practice Acts also hold nurses accountable for being reasonable and prudent in their practice. Both standards require the nurse to have at least some personal responsibility for continually assessing their professional competence through reflective practice (Huston, 2023). In addition, the Institute of Medicine (IOM, 2010) report *The Future of Nursing* calls for nursing schools and nurses to pursue lifelong learning.

> The individual registered nurse (RN) has a professional obligation to seek lifelong learning and maintain competence.

Mandatory Continuing Education to Promote Continued Competence

Many professional associations and states have mandated continuing education (CE) for RN license renewal to promote continued competence. Most states in the United States require CE for RN license renewal with requirements varying from a few hours to 30 hours, every 2 years. There is no requirement for CE for RNs (nonadvanced practice), however, in Arizona, Colorado, Connecticut, Indiana, Maine, Maryland, Mississippi (unless RN has been out of practice for more than 5 years), Missouri, South Dakota, Vermont, and Wisconsin. Every other state has some sort of requirement for RNs (AAACEUs, 2022).

Does Mandatory Continuing Education Assure Competence in Nursing?

Most states in the United States have mandatory requirements for continuing education (CE) for professional nurse license renewal even though there is limited research demonstrating correlation among CE, continuing competence, and improved patient outcomes. In addition, CE taken is not required to relate to the area a registered nurse (RN) practices in, nor is there agreement on the optimal number of annual credits needed to ensure competence.

ASSIGNMENT:

Determine the CE requirements for RN license renewal in the state in which you live or practice. In small groups, debate the use of CE as a valid and reliable measure of continuing competence in nursing.

The CE approach to continuing competence continues to be very controversial because there is limited research demonstrating correlation among CE, continuing competence, and improved patient outcomes. In addition, many professional organizations have expressed concern about the quality of mandated CE courses and the lack of courses for experts and specialists. Likewise, there is no agreement on the optimal number of annual credits needed to ensure competence, and the type of CE needed to assure continued competence can vary significantly. Until consensus can be reached regarding how CE should be provided, what and how much is needed, and until research findings show an empirical link between CE and provider competence, it is difficult to tout CE as a valid and reliable measure of continuing competence.

Professional Specialty Certification

Professional specialty certification is one way an employee can demonstrate advanced achievement of competencies. Specialty certification achieves multiple purposes such as validating specialized knowledge, skills, and abilities; clarifying roles and responsibilities; providing professional support; and shaping future practice (Halm, 2021). For organizations, certification can improve processes of care, enhance work culture, improve job satisfaction and recruitment/retention, and advance the safety and quality of care. It can also reduce vacancy and turnover rates (see Examining the Evidence 11.1).

To achieve professional certification, nurses must meet eligibility criteria that may include years and types of work experience as well as minimum educational levels, active nursing licenses, and successful completion of a nationally administered examination (Huston, 2023). Certifications normally last 5 years.

Professional associations grant specialty certification as a formal but voluntary process of demonstrating expertise in a specific area of nursing. For example, the ANA established the ANA Certification Program in 1973 to provide tangible recognition of professional achievement in a defined functional or clinical area of nursing. The American Nurses Credentialing Center, a subsidiary of ANA, became its own corporation in 1991 and since then has certified hundreds of thousands of nurses throughout the United States and its territories in more than 40 specialty and advanced practice areas of nursing. A few of the other organizations offering specialty certifications for nurses are the American Association of Critical-Care Nurses, the American Association of Nurse Anesthetists, the American College of Nurse-Midwives, the Board of Certification for Emergency Nursing, and the Rehabilitation Nursing Certification Board.

EXAMINING THE EVIDENCE 11.1

Source: From Halm, M. A. (2021, March). Specialty certification: A path to improving outcomes. *American Journal of Critical Care, 30*(2), 156–160.

Specialty Certification Outcomes

This synthesis of the literature examined the impact of specialty certification on numerous patient, nurse, and organizational outcomes. For patients, certification was associated with lower rates of complications, failure to rescue (i.e., inpatient deaths following complications), and intensive care unit mortality and 30-day mortality.

For nurses, certification was positively associated with improved knowledge and skills. Certified critical care nurses reported increased competence with 20 skills. Recognizing one's own abilities and professional competence was the skill with the largest increase after certification.

Organizationally, certification affected intent to leave and, subsequently, turnover and vacancy rates. In two studies, certified nurses reported lower intent to leave their current positions.

The researchers noted, however, that because patient outcomes are measured at the unit level, a certain proportion of certified nurses may be needed to improve outcomes. The proportion of certified nurses reported in this synthesis ranged from 11.7% to 63%. Such wide variation leads to challenges in interpreting links between certification and outcomes. This should be a key focus for future work.

Huston (2023) notes that middle- and top-level nurse-managers play the most significant role in creating work environments that value and reward certification. For example, nurse-managers can grant tuition reimbursement or salary incentives to workers who seek certification. Managers can also show their support for professional certification by giving employees paid time off to take the certification exam and by publicly recognizing employees who have achieved specialty certification.

The certified nurse often finds many personal benefits related to the attainment of such status, including more rapid promotions on career ladders, advancement opportunities, and feelings of accomplishment. Certified nurses also often earn more than their noncertified counterparts. In addition, research in the past decade suggests that certification leads to both improved patient outcomes and the creation of a positive work environment. A summary of the benefits associated with professional certification is shown in Display 11.4.

DISPLAY 11.4 BENEFITS OF PROFESSIONAL CERTIFICATION

- Provides a sense of accomplishment and achievement
- Validation of specialty knowledge and competence to peers and patients
- Increased credibility
- Increased self-confidence
- Promotes greater autonomy of practice
- Provides for increased career opportunities and greater competitiveness in the job market
- May result in salary incentives
- Improved patient outcomes
- Increased levels of perceived empowerment creating more positive work cultures
- Demonstrates commitment to the profession
- Promotes lifelong learning and professional development

Sources: From American Association of Colleges of Nursing. (2021). *CNL certification*. http://www.aacnnursing.org/CNL-Certification; Halm, M. A. (2021, March). Specialty certification: A path to improving outcomes. *American Journal of Critical Care, 30*(2), 156–160; Huston, C. J. (2023). Assuring provider competence through licensure, continuing education, and certification (chapter 20). In C. J. Huston (Ed.), *Professional issues in nursing: Challenges and opportunities* (6th ed., pp. 288–301). Wolters Kluwer.

DISPLAY 11.5	WATKINS'S SEVEN STEPS OF REFLECTION

R—RECALL the event.
E—EXAMINE your responses.
F—Acknowledge FEELINGS.
L—LEARN from the experience.
E—EXPLORE options.
C—CREATE a plan of action.
T—Set TIMESCALE.

Source: From Watkins, A. (2018). *Reflective practice as a tool for growth.* Ausmed. https://www.ausmed.com/articles/reflective-practice/

Reflective Practice and the Professional Portfolio

Reflective practice has also been suggested as a strategy for promoting personal growth and continued competence in nursing. Reflective practice is defined by the North Carolina Board of Nursing (NCBN, 2022) as a process for the assessment of one's own practice to identify and seek learning opportunities to promote continuing competence. Inherent in the process is the evaluation and incorporation of this learning into one's practice. Such self-assessment is gaining popularity as a tool to promote professional practice and maintain competence.

Watkins (2018) notes that in its simplest form, reflective practice is the ability to reflect on your actions and engage in a process of continuous learning. Steps in the reflective process, as represented by the mnemonic REFLECT, are shown in Display 11.5. Inherent in the process is the evaluation and incorporation of this learning into one's practice. Such self-assessment is gaining popularity as a means to promote professional practice and maintain competence. Often, this is done using professional portfolios for competence assessment.

For example, North Carolina now requires RNs to use a reflective practice approach to carry out self-assessments of their practice and develop plans for maintaining competence. Each assessment is individualized to the licensed nurse's area of practice. RNs seeking license renewal or reinstatement must attest to having completed the learning activities required for continuing competence and be prepared to submit evidence of completion if requested by the board on random audit (NCBN, 2022). This is typically collated in some type of professional portfolio.

A *professional portfolio* is as a collection of materials that document a nurse's competencies and illustrate the expertise of the nurse. The professional portfolio typically contains core components, such as biographical information; educational background; certifications achieved; employment history; a resumé; a competence record or checklist; personal and professional goals; professional development experiences, presentations, consultations, and publications; professional and community activities; honors and awards; and letters of thanks from patients, families, peers, organizations, and others.

> All nurses should maintain a portfolio to reflect their professional growth throughout their career.

Maintaining a professional portfolio prevents the loss of important documentation that professional nurses should always have readily available to pursue a promotion, to consider a new position, or to apply for another position in their present employment.

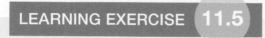

LEARNING EXERCISE 11.5

Creating a Professional Portfolio

ASSIGNMENT:

1. Identify the categories of evidence you would use to organize a professional portfolio if you were to create one today.
2. Identify specific evidence you could include in each of these categories. What evidence currently exists and what would need to be created?
3. How would you incorporate reflection in creating a personal professional portfolio?

Career Planning and the New Graduate Nurse

During the economic downturn at the start of the second decade in 20th century, some new graduates rushed to find a "job"—any job—in nursing, forgetting that even early employment decisions are critical to the achievement of their long-term career plans. New graduates must select their first employment wisely and seek work in a facility with a strong reputation for shared governance, positive work cultures, and a reputation of excellence in multiple arenas.

Finding work in a facility with orientation programs, internships, residencies, and fellowships is also important to the new graduate because it takes time to gain the expertise and self-confidence that is a part of being an expert nurse. Mentors and preceptors should also be available to support the new graduate nurse and to role model high-quality, evidence-based decision making and clinical practice. If the new graduate has a positive, nurturing first employment experience, they are much more likely to take future career risks, to pursue lifelong learning, and to have the energy and commitment to become involved in the bigger issues of their profession.

New graduates also have responsibility during the crucial first few years of employment to gain the expertise they need to have more opportunities for career divergence in the future. This includes becoming an expert in one or more areas of practice, gaining professional certifications, and being well informed about professional nursing and health care issues. This is also a time where participation in professional associations has great value because of opportunities for mentoring and networking. Finally, all new graduates should consider at what point continued formal education will be a part of their career ladder and professional journey.

Transition-to-Practice Programs/Residencies for New Graduate and Experienced Nurses in New Roles

Arguments have grown the last decade regarding the need for TPPs (also known as residences, externships, or internships) for new graduates of nursing programs and for nurses taking on new clinical roles in acute care settings. While TPPs are more common for new graduates, when the COVID-19 pandemic occurred, many health care organizations faced the challenge of transitioning nurses from the academic setting to clinical practice as well as transitioning other practice-based nurses to critical care settings (ANA, 2021). Nurse residency program have been used successfully to transition both these groups into practice.

Wallace et al. (2023) suggest the ever-changing health care delivery care system, with its increasing complexity of patient care, evolving technology, and focus on patient safety, has raised the bar in terms of expectations for new graduate nurses. New graduate nurses must now hit the ground running with well-developed critical thinking and problem-solving skills, the ability to exercise clinical judgment with know-how to practice from an evidence-based and outcome-driven perspective, and the ability to develop effectively from a novice to an expert in competency. Unfortunately, many new nurses begin working with little more than a few weeks of orientation, in contrast to most other professions, which require formal and often standardized internships or residencies. This is largely a residual outcome of the traditional nursing educational system that was grounded in apprenticeship and hospital-based training programs.

Such high expectations accompanied by inadequate advanced apprenticeship training often lead to high turnover rates for new graduate nurses. In addition, patient safety and quality of care are at risk if new graduates do not have the critical thinking skills or competencies needed to apply critical judgments to patient situations. Wallace et al. (2023) suggest that TPPs bridge the gap by providing the new graduate opportunities to take the learning from nursing school and apply it in an expanded, intensive, and integrated clinical learning situation while providing direct patient care—much in the same way that the internship of physicians is based on applying academic learning to actual care of patients and transition into the professional role.

The IOM in its landmark 2010 report *The Future of Nursing* called for the implementation and evaluation of nursing residency programs. Recent compelling evidence suggests that TPPs can improve outcomes for new nurses in their first year of practice including improved quality and safety practices, reduced work stress, and increased job satisfaction. In addition, health care institutions with transition programs report marked drops in attrition (NCBN, 2022).

Wallace et al. (2023) also suggest that employers and academe share the obligation to provide bridges from student to practicing nurse and that the inclusion of TPP is increasingly considered an expectation of the nursing education process and career development. Indeed, the IOM (2010) report *The Future of Nursing* identified TPPs/residencies as one of the eight key recommendations to actualize nursing contributions to the demands of health care reform. The IOM suggests "state Boards of Nursing, accrediting bodies, the federal government, and health care organizations should take action to support nurses' completion of a transition-to-practice program (nurse residency) after they have completed a prelicensure or advanced practice degree program or when they are transitioning into new clinical practice areas" (p. 280).

Multiple types of TPP exist (Wallace et al., 2023). There are programs that begin in the final year of nursing school and continue through licensure, although these programs are generally not intended to take the place of employer-based residencies, which often extend to 1 year and have a planned structured, mentored experience. Most TPPs are employer-based "new graduate classes" within a hospital- or employer- (hospital) based programs that take up to a year to complete. Still others are for new graduates who have yet to be hired, so they may gain skills to become more employable.

Traditional TPPs (residencies) are typically funded and provided by employers (usually hospitals). The hospital hires a group of new graduate RNs and provides a curriculum over the first 6 months to 1 year of their employment. The new graduate hires may receive partial to full pay, although they do not have a full patient load for some time into their residency. TPPs are also found, however, in nonacute settings, such as primary care clinics, behavior health clinics, long-term care, home health, corrections, schools of nursing, and public health, and they provide exposure to career paths that new graduates may not have previously considered. They also provide an opportunity for nonacute employers to consider hiring new graduate nurses (Wallace et al., 2023).

Resumé Preparation

Despite the best efforts of organizations to help subordinates identify career needs, wants, and opportunities, it is how employees represent themselves that often determines whether desired career opportunities become a reality. Creating a positive image often depends on having well-developed interviewing skills (see Chapter 15) and a well-prepared resumé.

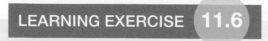

LEARNING EXERCISE 11.6

Addressing Nurse Residency Concerns

Wallace et al. (2023) note that although many groups are actively working to assure that nurse residences exist to provide a solid foundation for successful career development in nursing, many questions continue to exist about resource allocation (human and fiscal).

ASSIGNMENT:

Select any two of the following four questions and write a one-page essay defending your answers.

1. Schools have voiced concerns that transition-to-practice programs (TPPs) are taking preceptorship slots that have been historically allocated to prelicensure students. Do you support this reallocation of resources?
2. Should TPPs/residencies be a requirement for the completion of entry-level nursing education?
3. Residencies have historically been a cost hospitals or employers have assumed. Should this cost be shared and why?
4. Would you participate in a school-based TPP without an associated stipend if it could help you gain experience? Would you pay to participate?

Resumé Format

Various acceptable styles and formats of resumés exist. However, because the resumé represents the professionalism of the applicant and recruiters use it to summarize an applicant's qualifications, it must be professionally prepared, make an impression, and quickly capture the reader's attention. General guidelines for resumé preparation are shown in Display 11.6. A sample resumé is shown in Figure 11.2.

DISPLAY 11.6 GENERAL GUIDELINES FOR RESUMÉ PREPARATION

- Keep the resumé one to two pages long (*5 Ways*, 2022).
- Keep your writing concise and clear.
- Target the job you desire and your qualifications with what you write. The average resumé receives only a few seconds of attention from recruiters, so make important points stand out.
- Type the document in a single-font format that is easy to read (12-point font or larger is recommended).
- Use bulleted points or sentences.
- Add your LinkedIn address next to your name and contact information and make sure your LinkedIn profile is current and robust.
- Include educational background, work history, awards or honors received, scholarly achievements such as publications and presentations, and community service activities.
- Do not include personal information such as marital status, age, whether you have children, ethnicity, or religious affiliations.
- Maximize your strong points and minimize your weaknesses.
- Do not overstate your accomplishments because doing so places your credibility at great risk.
- Use good grammar, correct punctuation, and proper sentence structure. Typographic errors suggest you may not be serious about the job application or that the quality of your work will be substandard.
- Try to avoid overuse of "confidence inspiring" words like passionate, driven, or results-oriented as those words have little meaning without context. Instead, keep your resumé direct and to the point and show, do not tell, how you accomplish things (*5 Ways*, 2022).

DISPLAY 11.6 (CONTINUED)

- Choose words carefully. Use keywords applicable to the job you're applying for.
- Use high-quality, heavy white, or off-white paper to print the resumé.
- Consider adding a splash of color to your black-and-white resumé to make it "pop" out from your competition but do not go overboard (5 Ways, 2022). Black and another color is good enough. Use the color on your headings and keep your bullet points black.
- Include a cover letter (whether by mail or e-mail), addressed to a specific individual when possible, to introduce yourself, briefly highlight key points of the resumé, and make a positive first impression.
- Objective statements are considered old-fashioned; consider adding a summary statement instead.
- Make sure only to list references who know you well. You should inform the referees that you have listed them in your resumé so that when they are contacted, they are prepared to answer questions about the person who has applied for the job.

SUSAN ELAINE TINCHELL
628 Normal Road
Chico, CA 95928
Home phone: (530) 555-3718
stinchell@emailaccount.com
www.linkedin.com/in/susan-tinchell-5529362

CAREER GOAL: To practice professional nursing within a progressive environment that provides challenges and opportunities for professional and personal growth.

EDUCATION
- Bachelor of Science in Nursing, California State University, Chico (CSUC), May 2022. California Public Health Certificate. Cumulative GPA 3.88; Nursing GPA 3.74.

HONORS
- Sigma Theta Tau International Society of Nursing, Kappa Omicron Chapter.
- CSUC School of Nursing Scholarship Award 2020 and 2021.
- Publication of "An Expression of Nursing, A Journal of Student Writing" in The CSUC School of Nursing Alumni newsletter, spring 2021.

WORK EXPERIENCE
- June 2019–Present
  Per Diem Certified Nurses Aide. Memorial Hospital, Chico, CA. Performed direct patient care under the supervision and guidance of a registered nurse. (Job description available on request.)

- July 2017–May 2019
  Per Diem Home Health Aide/Respite Worker. Sommers Elder Services, Chico, CA. Performed custodial care and light housekeeping duties for home-bound older adults and patients with disabilities.

REFERENCES: Available on request.

FIGURE 11.2 Sample nursing resumé.

Integrating Leadership Roles and Management Functions in Career Planning and Development

Appropriate career management should foster positive career planning and development, alleviate burnout, reduce attrition, and promote productivity. Management functions in career planning and development include disseminating career information and posting job openings. The manager should have a well-developed, planned system for career development for all employees; this system should include long-term coaching, the appropriate use of transfers, and a plan for how promotions are to be handled. These policies should be fair and communicated effectively to all employees.

With the integration of leadership, managers become more aware of how their own values shape personal career decisions. In addition, the leader-manager shows genuine interest in the career development of all employees. Career planning is encouraged, and potential leaders are identified and developed. Present leaders are rewarded when they see those whom they have helped to develop advance in their careers and in turn develop leadership and management skills in others.

Effective managers recognize that in all career decisions, the employee must decide when they are ready to pursue promotions, return to school, or take on greater responsibility. Leaders are aware that every person perceives success differently. Although career development programs benefit all employees and the organization, there is a bonus for the professional nurse. When professional nurses can experience a well-planned career development program, a greater viability for and increased commitment to the profession are often evident.

Key Concepts

- There are many outcomes of a career development program that justify its implementation.
- Career job sequencing should assist the manager in career management.
- Career development programs consist of a set of personal responsibilities called career planning and a set of management responsibilities called career management.
- Employees often need to be encouraged to make more formalized long-term career plans.
- Career planning should include, at minimum, a commitment to the use of evidence-based practice, learning new skills or bettering practice through the use of role models and mentors, staying aware of and being involved in professional issues, and furthering one's education.
- Designing career paths is an important part of organizational career management.
- Managers should plan specific interventions that promote growth and development in each of their subordinates.
- Most individuals progress through normal and predictable career stages. Shirey (2009) describes these stages as promise, momentum, and harvest.
- Benner (1982) suggests that in the transition from novice to expert, nurses develop skills and an understanding of patient care over time through a sound educational base as well as a multitude of experiences. Thus, the new nurse moves from reliance on past abstract principles to the use of past concrete experience and changes their perception of situations to whole parts rather than separate pieces.
- Career coaching involves helping others to identify professional goals and career options and designing a career plan to achieve those goals. This coaching should be both short and long term.
- Because of the importance that American society places on promotions, certain guidelines must accompany promotion selection to ensure that the process is fair, equitable, and motivating.
- It is possible to promote individuals beyond their level of capability. The Peter Principle, as it is known, suggests that individuals may rise "to the level of their incompetence."
- Competency assessment and goal setting in career planning should help the employee identify how to exceed the minimum levels of competency required by federal, state, or organizational standards.
- Professional specialty certification is one way that an employee can demonstrate advanced achievement of competencies.
- To be successful, management development must be planned and supported by top-level management. This type of planned program is called succession planning.
- If appropriate management attitudes and insight are goals of a management development program, social learning techniques need to be part of the teaching strategies used.
- Multiple types of transition-to-practice programs exist, but all are focused on helping nursing students bridge from school into employment.
- All nurses should maintain a professional portfolio (a collection of materials that document a nurse's competencies and illustrate the expertise of the nurse) to reflect their professional growth over their career.
- Maintaining a current, professional resumé is a career-planning necessity for the health care professional and should not be undertaken lightly.
- Cover letters (whether by mail or e-mail) should always be used when submitting a resumé. Their purpose is to introduce the applicant, briefly highlight key points of the resumé, and make a positive first impression.

Additional Learning Exercises and Applications

Developing a 20-Year Career Plan Using a Career Map

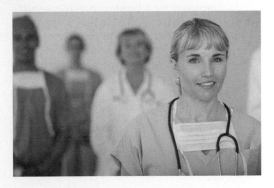

Develop a 20-year career plan, considering the constraints of family responsibilities such as marriage, children, and aging parents. Have your career plan critiqued to determine whether it is feasible and whether the timelines and goals are realistic.

In addition, career planning is often made easier when a career map is created to assist in developing a long-term master plan. Use the career guide shown in Figure 11.3, along with the individual responsibilities for career development outlined in Table 11.1, to assist with developing your 20-year career plan.

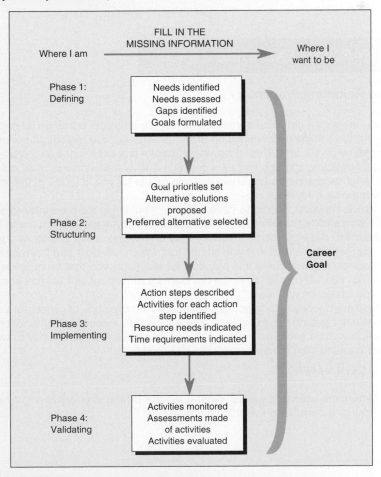

FIGURE 11.3 A career planning guide for a professional nurse.

LEARNING EXERCISE 11.8

Preparing a Resumé

The medical center where you have applied for a position has requested that you submit a resumé along with your application. Prepare a professional resumé using your actual experience and education. You may use any style and format that you desire. The resumé will be critiqued on its professional appearance and appropriateness of included content.

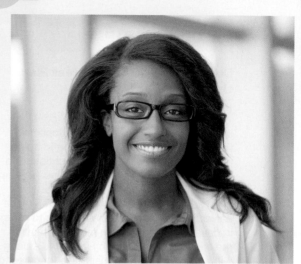

LEARNING EXERCISE 11.9

The Reluctant Preceptor

You are a new graduate nurse in your first job as a staff nurse on an oncology unit. You have been assigned to orient with Steve, an experienced registered nurse (RN) and longtime employee on the unit. This is, however, Steve's first experience as a preceptor. Steve is an expert clinician, and you marvel at his high-quality assessments and how intuitive his nursing diagnoses seem to be. Steve is a role model for you in terms of the level of clinical skills you hope to achieve.

Steve, however, seems to have difficulty teaching in the preceptor role. He accomplishes his work quickly and often, without explanation—even though you are at his side. He also is resistant to allowing you to practice many of the basic skills and tasks you are qualified to do, suggesting instead that you should just watch him do it and learn by shadowing. When you question Steve about this practice, he reassures you that he believes you are competent and that you will be a good nurse but states that he does not yet feel comfortable in "letting you do things on your own."

You are becoming increasingly frustrated with this style of preceptorship and worry that you are not getting the experience you will need to autonomously function as an RN when your orientation ends in 4 weeks. Yet, you also value the opportunity to work so closely with such a skilled clinician and wonderful role model.

ASSIGNMENT:

Determine what you will do. What goals are driving your decision? What are the potential risks and benefits inherent in your plan?

REFERENCES

AAACEUs. (2022). *Nursing continuing education requirements by state.* Retrieved April 30, 2022, from https://www.aaaceus.com/state_nursing_requirements.asp

American Nurses Association. (2015). *Code of ethics for nurses with interpretive statements.*

American Nurses Association. (2021, July 7). Nurse residency program helps successfully transition new nurses in pandemic. *Nurse.com by Relias Blog.* https://www.nurse.com/blog/2021/07/07/nurse-residency-program-helps-successfully-transition-new-nurses-in-pandemic/?utm_source=newsletter&utm_medium=email&utm_campaign=hc+weekly+newsletter&utm_content=091221

Benner, P. (1982). From novice to expert. *The American Journal of Nursing, 82*(3), 402–407.

5 ways to spruce up your resume right now. (2022). *Undercover Recruiter.* https://theundercoverrecruiter.com/spruce-up-resume-new-year/

Halm, M. A. (2021, March). Specialty certification: A path to improving outcomes. *American Journal of Critical Care, 30*(2), 156–160.

Handrick, L. (2022, March). *Best executive coaching certification programs.* The Balance Careers. Retrieved April 30, 2022, from https://www.thebalancecareers.com/best-executive-coaching-certification-programs-5111891#:~:text=Updated%20May%2025%2C%202021%20An%20executive%20coach%20is,whether%20as%20a%20corporate%20executive%20or%20business%20owner

Huston, C. J. (2023). Assuring provider competence through licensure, continuing education, and certification (chapter 20). In C. J. Huston (Ed.), *Professional issues in nursing: Challenges and opportunities* (6th ed., pp. 288–301). Wolters Kluwer.

Institute of Medicine. (2010). *The future of nursing: Leading change, advancing health.* National Academies Press.

Merriam-Webster Dictionary. (2022). Professional. In *Merriam-Webster.com.* Retrieved April 30, 2022, from https://www.merriam-webster.com/dictionary/professional

National Academies of Sciences, Engineering, and Medicine. (2021). *The future of nursing 2020–2030: Charting a path to achieve health equity.* The National Academies Press. https://doi.org/10.17226/25982

North Carolina Board of Nursing. (2022). *Continuing competence requirements.* https://www.ncbon.com/licensure-listing-continuing-competence

Shirey, M. (2009). Building an extraordinary career in nursing: Promise, momentum, and harvest. *Journal of Continuing Education in Nursing, 40*(9), 394–402.

STANDS4LLC. (2022). Career ladder. *Definitions.net.* Retrieved April 30, 2022, from https://www.definitions.net/definition/CAREER%20LADDER

Velasquez, R. (2020, July 13). 13 Shocking leadership development statistics (infographic). *Infopro Learning.* https://www.infoprolearning.com/blog/13-shocking-leadership-development-statistics-infopro-learning/

Wallace, J., Hooper-Arana, E., & West, N. (2023). Bridging the academic–practice gap in nursing (chapter 2). In C. J. Huston (Ed.), *Professional issues in nursing: Challenges and opportunities* (6th ed., pp. 16–31). Wolters Kluwer.

Watkins, A. (2018). *Reflective practice as a tool for growth.* Ausmed. https://www.ausmed.com/articles/reflective-practice/

Roles and Functions in Organizing

12

Organizational Structure

*… The days of the traditional pyramid shaped corporate hierarchy as a viable business model are coming to an end.—**Michael Hugos***

*… Basic philosophy, spirit and drive of an organization have far more to do with its relative achievements than do technological or economic resources, organizational structure, innovation, and timing.—**Marvin Bower***

*… Every company has two organizational structures: The formal one is written on the charts; the other is the everyday relationship of the men and women in the organization.—**Harold Geneen***

CROSSWALK

This chapter addresses:

- **AACN Essentials Domain 2**: Person-centered care
- **AACN Essentials Domain 5:** Quality and safety
- **AACN Essentials Domain 6:** Interprofessional partnerships
- **AACN Essentials Domain 7:** Systems-based practice
- **AACN Essentials Domain 8:** Information and health care technologies
- **AONL Nurse Executive Competency 1:** Communication and relationship building
- **AONL Nurse Executive Competency 2:** A knowledge of the health care environment
- **AONL Nurse Executive Competency 4:** Professionalism
- **AONL Nurse Executive Competency 5:** Business skills
- **ANA Standard of Professional Performance 10:** Communication
- **ANA Standard of Professional Performance 11:** Collaboration
- **ANA Standard of Professional Performance 12:** Leadership
- **ANA Standard of Professional Performance 15:** Quality of practice
- **ANA Standard of Professional Performance 17:** Resource stewardship
- **ANA Standard of Professional Performance 18:** Environmental health
- **QSEN Competency:** Teamwork and collaboration
- **QSEN Competency:** Quality improvement
- **QSEN Competency:** Safety

LEARNING OBJECTIVES

The learner will:

- describe how the structure of an organization facilitates or impedes communication, flexibility, and job satisfaction
- identify characteristics of a bureaucracy as defined by Max Weber
- identify line-and-staff relationships, span of control, unity of command, and scalar chains on the organization chart
- describe components of the informal organization structure including employee interpersonal relationships, the formation of primary and secondary groups, and group leaders without formal authority

- differentiate between first, middle, and top levels of management
- contrast centralized and decentralized decision making
- analyze how position on the organization chart is related to centrality
- describe common components of shared governance models and differentiate shared governance from participatory decision making
- contrast individual authority, responsibility, and accountability in given scenarios
- identify appropriate strategies the leader-manager may take to create a constructive organizational culture
- describe characteristics of effective committees and committee members
- define "groupthink" and discuss the impact of groupthink on organizational decision making and risk taking
- identify symptoms of poorly designed organizations
- describe the five model components of Magnet-designated health care organizations as well as the 14 foundational forces required to achieve Magnet status
- provide examples of an organization's potential stakeholders

Introduction

Unit III provided a background in planning, the first phase of the management process. *Organizing* follows planning as the second phase of the management process and is explored in this unit. In the organizing phase, relationships are defined, procedures are outlined, equipment is readied, and tasks are assigned. Organizing also involves establishing a formal structure that provides the best possible coordination or use of resources to accomplish objectives. This chapter looks at how the structure of an organization facilitates or impedes communication, flexibility, productivity, and job satisfaction. Chapter 13 examines the role of authority and power in organizations and how power may be used to meet individual, unit, and organizational goals. Chapter 14 looks at how human resources can be organized to accomplish patient care.

Formal and Informal Organizational Structure

Because people spend most of their lives in social, personal, and professional organizations, they need to understand how organizations are structured—their formation, methods of communication, channels of authority, and decision-making processes. Each organization has both a formal and an informal structure. In the *formal structure*, the emphasis is on organizational positions and formal power. Thus, it provides a framework for defining managerial authority, responsibility, and accountability. Formal structure is generally highly planned and visible, roles and functions are defined and systematically arranged, different people have differing roles, and rank and hierarchy are evident.

> Organizational structure refers to the way in which a group is formed, its lines of communication, and its means for channeling authority and making decisions.

In contrast, in the *informal structure,* the focus is on employees, their relationships, and the informal power that is inherent within those naturally forming social relationships (Hartzell, 2012). Thus, it is generally unplanned. Hartzell (2012) argues that informal structure allows employees to network with one another to get work done. Because informal structures are typically based on camaraderie, they often result in a more immediate response from individuals, saving people's time and effort. People also rely on informal structure if the formal structure has stopped being effective, which often happens as an organization grows or changes but does not reevaluate its hierarchy or work groups (Quain, 2019).

The informal structure even has its own communication network, known as the *grapevine*. According to Hartzell (2012), grapevine communication is at the heart of the informal organization; it is the conversations that occur in the break room, down the halls, during the carpool, and in between work that allows the relationships of informal groups to develop. In addition, social media sites (Facebook, Instagram, Snapchat, Twitter, etc.) and electronic communication such as e-mail and text messages are also used to facilitate communication among informal group members.

Although grapevine communication is fast and can facilitate information upward, downward, and horizontally, it is difficult to control or to stop. With little accountability for the message, grapevine communication often becomes a source for rumor or gossip.

> The informal structure also has its own leaders. In addition, it also has its own communication channels, often referred to as the grapevine.

Informal authority and lines of communication exist in every group, even when they are never formally acknowledged. The primary emphasis of this chapter, however, is the identification of components of organizational structure, the leadership roles and management functions associated with formal organizational structure (Display 12.1), and the proper utilization of work groups or committees to accomplish organizational objectives.

Organizational Theory and Bureaucracy

Max Weber, a German social scientist, is known as the father of organizational theory. Generally acknowledged to have developed the most comprehensive classic formulation on the characteristics of *bureaucracy*, Weber wrote from the vantage point of a manager instead of that of a scholar. During the 1920s, Weber saw the growth of the large-scale organization and correctly predicted that this growth required a more formalized set of procedures for administrators. His statement on bureaucracy, published after his death, is still the most influential statement on the subject.

Weber postulated three "ideal types" of authority or reasons why people throughout history have obeyed their rulers. One of these, *legal-rational authority*, was based on a belief in the legitimacy of rules and the rights of those elevated to authority under such rules to issue commands. Obedience, then, was owed to the legally established impersonal set of rules rather than to a personal ruler. It is this type of authority that is the basis for Weber's concept of bureaucracy.

Weber argued that the great virtue of bureaucracy—indeed, perhaps its defining characteristic—was that it was an institutional method for applying general rules to specific cases, thereby making the actions of management fair and predictable. Other characteristics of bureaucracies as identified by Weber include the following:

- There must be a clear *division of labor* (i.e., all work must be divided into units that can be undertaken by individuals or groups of individuals competent to perform those tasks).
- A well-defined *hierarchy of authority* must exist in which superiors are separated from subordinates; based on this hierarchy, remuneration for work is dispensed, authority is recognized, privileges are allotted, and promotions are awarded.
- There must be impersonal rules and *impersonality of interpersonal relationships*. In other words, bureaucrats are not free to act in any way they please. Bureaucratic rules provide superiors systematic control over subordinates, thus limiting the opportunities for arbitrary behavior and personal favoritism.

DISPLAY 12.1   LEADERSHIP ROLES AND MANAGEMENT FUNCTIONS ASSOCIATED WITH ORGANIZATIONAL STRUCTURE

Leadership Roles

1. Evaluates the organizational structure frequently to determine if management positions should be eliminated to shorten the chain of command
2. Encourages and guides employees to follow the chain of command and counsels employees who do not do so
3. Supports personnel in advisory (staff) positions
4. Models responsibility and accountability for subordinates
5. Assists staff to see how their roles are congruent with and complement the organization's mission, vision, and goals
6. Facilitates constructive informal group structure
7. Encourages upward communication
8. Fosters a positive organizational culture between work groups and subcultures that facilitates shared values and goals
9. Promotes participatory decision making and shared governance to empower subordinates
10. Uses committees to facilitate group goals, not to delay decisions

Management Functions

1. Is knowledgeable about the organization's internal structure, including personal and department authority and responsibilities within that structure
2. Facilitates constructive formal group structure
3. Provides the staff with an accurate unit organization chart and assists with interpretation
4. When possible, maintains unity of command
5. Clarifies unity of command when there is confusion
6. Follows appropriate subordinate complaints upward through the chain of command
7. Establishes an appropriate span of control
8. Strives to create a constructive organizational culture and positive organizational climate
9. Uses the informal organization to meet organizational goals
10. Uses committee structure to increase the quality and quantity of work accomplished
11. Works, as appropriate, to achieve a level of operational excellence befitting an organization such as Magnet status or some other recognition of excellence
12. Continually identifies, analyzes, and promotes stakeholder interests in the organization

- A system of procedures for dealing with work situations (i.e., regular activities to get a job done) must exist.
- A system of rules covering the rights and duties of each position must be in place.
- Selection for employment and promotion is based on technical competence.

Bureaucracy was the ideal tool to harness and routinize the energy and prolific production of the Industrial Revolution. Weber's work did not, however, consider the complexity of managing organizations in the 21st century. Weber wrote during an era when worker motivation was taken for granted, and his simplification of management and employee roles did not examine the bilateral relationships between employee and management prevalent in most organizations today.

Since Weber's research, management theorists have learned much about human behavior, and most organizations have modified their structures and created alternative organizational designs that reduce rigidity and impersonality. Yet, more than 100 years after Weber's findings, components of bureaucratic structure continue to be found in the design of most large organizations.

Current research suggests that changing an organization's structure in a manner that increases autonomy and work empowerment for health care employees will lead to more effective patient care.

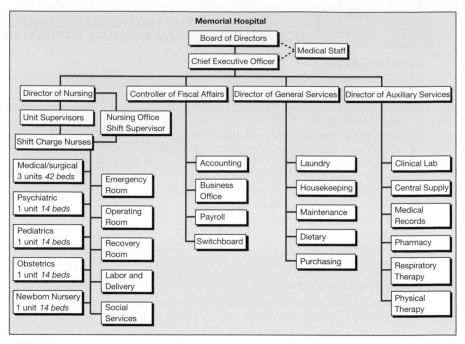

FIGURE 12.1 Sample organizational chart.

Components of Organizational Structure

Weber is also credited with the development of the organization chart to depict an organization's structure. Because the organization chart (Fig. 12.1) is a picture of an organization, the knowledgeable manager can derive much information from reading the chart. For example, an organization chart can help identify roles and their expectations.

In addition, by observing elements, such as which departments report directly to the chief executive officer (CEO), inferences can be drawn about the organization. For instance, reporting to a middle-level manager rather than a chief executive officer suggests that person has less status and influence than someone who reports to an individual higher on the organization chart. Leader-managers who understand an organization's structure and relationships will be able to expedite decisions and have a greater understanding of the organizational environment.

Relationships and Chain of Command

The organization chart defines formal relationships within the institution. Formal relationships, lines of communication, and authority are depicted on a chart by unbroken (solid) horizontal or vertical lines. Solid horizontal lines represent communication between people with similar spheres of responsibility and power but different functions. Solid vertical lines between positions denote the official *chain of command*, the formal paths of communication and authority. Those having the greatest decision-making authority are located at the top; those with the least are at the bottom. The level of position on the chart also signifies status and power.

Dotted or broken lines on the organization chart represent *staff* positions. Individuals in these positions are advisory, providing information or assistance to their manager. Staff positions increase a manager's sphere of influence, enabling them to handle more activities and interactions than would otherwise be possible. These positions also provide for specialization

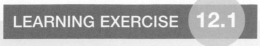

LEARNING EXERCISE 12.1

Who Is the Boss?

In groups or individually, analyze the following and give an oral or written report.

1. Have you ever worked in an organization in which the lines of authority were unclear? Have you been a member of a social organization in which this happened? How did this interfere with the organization's functioning?
2. Do you believe that the "one boss/one person" rule is a good idea? Do hospital clerical workers frequently have many bosses? If you have worked in a situation in which you had more than one boss, what was the result?

that would be impossible for a manager to achieve alone. Although staff positions can make line personnel more effective, organizations can function without them.

Advisory (staff) positions, however, do not have inherent legitimate authority. Accomplishing the role expectations in a staff position may therefore be more difficult. For example, clinical specialists and education directors in staff positions often lack the authority that accompanies a line relationship. Staff positions then may result in an ineffective use of support services unless job descriptions and responsibilities for these positions can be clearly spelled out.

Unity of command is indicated by the vertical solid line between positions on the organizational chart. This concept is best described as "one person/one boss," in which employees have one manager to whom they report and to whom they are responsible. This greatly simplifies the manager–employee relationship because the employee needs to maintain only a minimum number of relationships and accept the influence of only one person as an immediate supervisor.

> Unity of command is difficult to maintain in some large health care organizations because the nature of health care requires an interprofessional approach.

Nurses sometimes feel as though they have many individuals to account to including their immediate supervisor, the patient, the patient's family, central administration, and the physician. All have some input in directing a nurse's work. Weber was correct when he determined that a lack of unity of command results in some conflict and lost productivity. This is demonstrated when health care workers become confused about unity of command.

Span of Control

Span of control also can be determined from the organization chart. The number of people directly reporting to any one manager represents that manager's span of control. Thus, there is an inverse relation between the span of control and the number of levels in hierarchy in an organization, that is, the narrower the span, the greater the number of levels in an organization (Juneja, 1996–2022).

Theorists are divided regarding the optimal span of control for any one manager. Quantitative formulas for determining the optimal span of control have been attempted, with suggested ranges from 3 to 50 employees. The ideal span of control, however, depends on various factors, such as the nature of the job, the manager's abilities, the employees' maturity, the task complexity, and the level in the organization at which the work occurs. The number of people directly reporting to any one supervisor should be the number that maximizes productivity and worker satisfaction.

> Too many people reporting to a single manager delays decision making, whereas too few results in an inefficient, top-heavy organization.

Until early this century, narrow spans of control at top levels of management, with slightly wider spans at other levels, was widely accepted. Indeed, Juneja (1996–2022) explains that most modern management theorists would suggest an ideal span of control as 15 to 20 subordinates per manager, as compared with the 6 subordinates per manager touted in the past. With increased financial pressures on health care organizations to remain fiscally solvent and electronic communication technology advances, many have increased their spans of control and reduced the number of administrative levels in the organization. This is often termed *flattening the organization*.

One of the leadership responsibilities of organizing is to periodically examine the number of people in the chain of command and the span of control each person has. Organizations frequently add levels until there are too many managers. Therefore, the leader-manager should carefully weigh the advantages and disadvantages of adding a management level.

Managerial Levels

In large organizations, several levels of managers often exist. *Top-level managers* look at the entire organization, coordinating internal and external influences, and generally make decisions with few guidelines or structures. Examples of top-level managers include the organization's CEO and the highest-level nursing administrator. Current nomenclature for top-level nurse-managers includes vice president of nursing, nurse administrator, director of nursing, chief nurse, or chief nurse officer (CNO). It is necessary to remember only that the CEO is the organization's highest-ranking person, and the top-level nurse-manager is its highest-ranking nurse. Responsibilities common to top-level managers include determining the organizational philosophy, setting policy, and creating goals and priorities for resource allocation. Top-level managers have a greater need for leadership skills and are not as involved in routine daily operations as are lower-level managers.

Middle-level managers coordinate the efforts of lower levels of the hierarchy and are the conduit between lower- and top-level managers. Middle-level managers carry out day-to-day operations but are still involved in some long-term planning and in establishing unit policies. Examples of middle-level managers include nursing supervisors, department heads, coordinators, directors, and unit managers.

Currently, there are many health facility mergers and acquisitions, and reduced levels of administration are frequently apparent within these consolidated organizations. Consequently, many health care facilities have expanded the scope of responsibility for middle-level managers and given them the title of "director" to indicate new roles. The proliferation of titles among health care administrators has made it imperative that individuals understand what roles and responsibilities go with each position.

First-level managers are concerned with their specific unit's workflow. They deal with immediate problems in the unit's daily operations, with organizational needs, and with personal needs of employees. First-level managers need good management skills. Because they work so closely with patients and health care teams, first-level managers also have an excellent opportunity to practice leadership roles that will greatly influence productivity and subordinates' satisfaction. Examples of first-level managers include primary care nurses, team leaders, case managers, and charge nurses. In many organizations, every registered nurse (RN) is considered a first-level manager. A composite look at top-, middle-, and first-level managers is shown in Table 12.1.

TABLE **12.1** **LEVELS OF MANAGERS**

	Top Level	Middle Level	First Level
Examples	Chief nursing officer Chief executive officer Chief financial officer	Unit supervisor Department head Director	Charge nurse Team leader Primary nurse
Scope of responsibility	Look at organization as a whole as well as external influences	Focus is on integrating unit-level day-to-day needs with organizational needs	Focus primarily on day-to-day needs at unit level
Primary planning focus	Strategic planning	Combination of long- and short-range planning	Short-range, operational planning
Communication flow	More often top-down but receives subordinate feedback both directly and via middle-level managers	Upward and downward with great centrality	More often upward; generally relies on middle-level managers to transmit communication to top-level managers

Centrality

Centrality, the extent to which an employee communicates or interacts with others, is determined by distance on the organization chart. Employees with relatively small organizational distance can receive more information than those who are more peripherally located. Therefore, the middle manager often has a broader view of the organization than other levels of management. A middle manager has a large degree of centrality because this manager receives information upward, downward, and horizontally.

> Centrality refers to the location of a position on an organization chart where frequent and various types of communication occur, creating a network of interpersonal relationships.

Because all communication involves a sender and a receiver, messages may not be received clearly because of the sender's hierarchical position. Similarly, status and power often influence the receiver's ability to hear information accurately. An example of the effect of status on communication is found in the "principal syndrome." Most people can recall panic, when they were school age, at being summoned to the principal's office. Thoughts of "What did I do?" travel through one's mind. Even adults find discomfort in communicating with certain people who hold high status. This may be fear or awe, but both interfere with clear communication. The difficulties with upward and downward communication are discussed in more detail in Chapter 19. It is important, then, to be aware of how the formal structure affects overall relationships and communication. This is especially true because organizations change their structures frequently, resulting in new communication lines and reporting relationships. Unless one understands how to interpret a formal organization chart, confusion and anxiety will result when organizations are restructured.

Is it ever appropriate to go outside the chain of command? Of course, there are isolated circumstances when the chain of command must be breached. However, those rare conditions usually involve a question of ethics. In most instances, those being bypassed in a chain of command should be forewarned. Remember that unity of command provides the organization with a workable system for procedural directives and orders so that productivity is increased, and conflict is minimized.

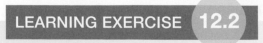

LEARNING EXERCISE 12.2

Change Is Coming

This Learning Exercise refers to the organization chart in Figure 12.1. Because Memorial Hospital is expanding, the board of directors has made several changes that require modification of the organization chart. The directors have just announced the following changes:

- The name of the hospital has been changed from Memorial Hospital to Memorial Medical Center.
- State approval has been granted for open-heart surgery.
- One of the existing medical-surgical units will be remodeled and will become two critical care units (one six-bed coronary and open-heart unit and one six-bed trauma and surgical unit).
- A part-time medical director will be responsible for medical care on each critical care unit.
- The hospital chief executive officer's title has been changed to executive director.
- An associate hospital administrator has been hired.
- A new hospital-wide educational department has been created.
- The old pediatric unit will be remodeled into a seven-bed pediatric wing and a seven-bed rehabilitation unit.
- The director of nursing's new title is vice president of patient care services.

ASSIGNMENT:

If the hospital is viewed as a large, open system, it is possible to visualize areas where problems might occur. In particular, it is necessary to identify changes anticipated in the nursing department and how these changes will affect the organization as a whole. Depict all of these changes on the old organization chart, delineating both staff and line positions. Give the rationale for your decisions. Why did you place the education department where you did? What was the reasoning in your division of authority? Where do you believe there might be potential conflict in the new organization chart? Why?

Limitations of Organization Charts

Because organization charts show only formal relationships, what they can reveal about an institution is limited. The chart does not show the informal structure of the organization, which is powerful and dynamic. Knowledgeable leaders never underestimate the importance of this informal structure because it includes employees' interpersonal relationships, the formation of primary and secondary groups, and the identification of group leaders without formal authority. These groups provide workers with a feeling of belonging and can either facilitate or sabotage planned change. Their ability to determine a unit's norms and acceptable behavior also has a great deal to do with the socialization of new employees. Informal leaders are frequently found among long-term employees or people in select *gatekeeping positions*, such as the CNO's secretary. Frequently, the informal organization evolves from social activities or from relationships that develop outside the work environment.

Organization charts are also limited in their ability to depict each line position's degree of authority. *Authority* is defined as the official power to act. It is power given by the organization to direct the work of others. A manager may have the authority to hire, fire, or discipline others.

Equating status with authority, however, frequently causes confusion. The distance from the top of the organizational hierarchy usually determines the degree of status: the closer to the top, the higher the status. Status also is influenced by skill, education, specialization, level of

DISPLAY 12.2   ADVANTAGES AND LIMITATIONS OF THE ORGANIZATION CHART

Advantages

1. Maps lines of decision-making authority
2. Helps people understand their assignments and those of their coworkers
3. Reveals to managers and new personnel how they fit into the organization
4. Contributes to sound organizational structure
5. Shows formal lines of communication

Limitations

1. Shows only formal relationships
2. Does not indicate degree of authority
3. Is difficult to keep current
4. May show things as they are supposed to be or used to be rather than as they are
5. May define roles too narrowly
6. Possibility of confusing authority with status exists

responsibility, autonomy, and salary accorded a position. People sometimes have status with little accompanying authority.

Another limitation of the organization chart is currency. Because organizations are so dynamic, an organization chart becomes obsolete very quickly, so trying to keep an organization chart current is almost impossible. It is also possible that the organization chart may depict how things are supposed to be, when the organization is still functioning under an old structure because employees have not yet accepted new lines of authority.

Another limitation of the organization chart is that although it defines authority, it does not define responsibility and accountability. A *responsibility* is a duty or an assignment. It is the implementation of a job. For example, a responsibility common to many charge nurses is establishing the unit's daily patient care assignment. Individuals should always be assigned responsibilities with concomitant authority. If authority is not commensurate to the responsibility, role confusion occurs for everyone involved. For example, supervisors may have the responsibility of maintaining high professional care standards among their staff. If the manager is not given the authority to discipline employees as needed, however, this responsibility is virtually impossible to implement.

Accountability is like responsibility, but it is internalized. Thus, to be accountable means that individuals agree to be morally responsible for the consequences of their actions. One individual cannot be accountable for another. Society holds us accountable for our assigned responsibilities, and people are expected to accept the consequences of their actions. A nurse who reports a medication error is being accountable for the responsibilities inherent in the position.

The leader-manager should understand the interrelationships and differences among these three terms. Display 12.2 discusses the advantages and limitations of an organization chart. Because the use of authority, power building, and political awareness are so important to functioning effectively in any structure, Chapter 13 discusses these organizational components in depth.

Types of Organizational Structures

Traditionally, organizations have used one of the following structural patterns: bureaucratic, ad hoc, matrix, flat, or various combinations of these. The type of structure used in any health care facility affects communication patterns, relationships, and authority.

Line Structures

Bureaucratic organizational designs are commonly called *line structures* or *line organizations*. Those with staff authority may be referred to as *staff organizations*. Both types of organizational structures are found frequently in large health care facilities and usually resemble Weber's original design for effective organizations. Because of most people's familiarity with these structures, there is little stress associated with orienting people to these organizations. In these structures, authority and responsibility are clearly defined, which leads to efficiency and simplicity of relationships. The organization chart in Figure 12.1 is a line-and-staff structure.

These formal designs, however, have some disadvantages. They often produce monotony, alienate workers, and make adjusting rapidly to altered circumstances difficult. Another problem is their adherence to chain of command communication, which restricts upward communication. Good leaders encourage upward communication to compensate for this disadvantage. However, when line positions are clearly defined, going outside the chain of command for upward communication is usually inappropriate.

Ad Hoc Design

The *ad hoc design* is a modification of the bureaucratic structure and is sometimes used on a temporary basis to facilitate completion of a project within a formal line organization. The ad hoc structure is a means of overcoming the inflexibility of line structure and serves as a way for professionals to handle the increasingly large amounts of available information. Ad hoc structures use a project team or task approach and are usually disbanded after a project is completed. This structure's disadvantages are decreased strength in the formal chain of command and decreased employee loyalty to the parent organization.

Matrix Structure

A *matrix organization* structure is designed to focus on both product and function. Function is described as all the tasks required to produce the product, and the product is the end result of the function. For example, good patient outcomes are the product, and staff education and adequate staffing may be the functions necessary to produce the outcome.

The matrix organization structure has a formal vertical and horizontal chain of command. Figure 12.2 depicts a matrix organizational structure and shows that the manager of Nursing Women's Services care could report both to a vice president for Maternal and Women's Services (product manager) and a vice president for Nursing Services (functional manager). Although there are fewer formal rules and fewer levels in the hierarchy, a matrix structure is not without disadvantages. For example, in this structure, decision making can be slow because of the necessity of information sharing, and it can produce confusion and frustration for workers because of its dual-authority hierarchical design. The primary advantage of centralizing expertise is frequently outweighed by the complexity of the communication required in the design.

Service Line Organization

Like the matrix design, a service line organization can be used in some large institutions to address the shortcomings that are endemic to traditional large bureaucratic organizations. *Service lines*, sometimes called *care-centered organizations*, are smaller in scale than a large bureaucratic system. For example, in this organizational design, the overall goals would be determined by the larger organization, but the service line would decide on the processes to be used to achieve the goals.

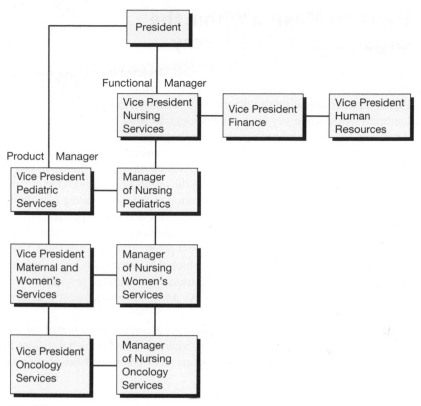

FIGURE 12.2 Matrix organizational structure.

Flat Designs

Flat organizational designs attempt to remove hierarchical layers by flattening the chain of command and decentralizing the organization. Thus, a single manager or supervisor would oversee many subordinates and have a wide span of control (Juneja, 1996–2022). In strong economic times, it is easy to add layers to the organization in order to get the work done, but when the organization begins to feel a financial strain, they often look at their hierarchy to see where they can cut positions.

In *flattened organizations*, there continues to be line authority, but because the organizational structure is flattened, more authority and decision making can occur where the work is being carried out. Figure 12.3 shows a flattened organizational structure. Many managers have difficulty letting go of control, and even very flattened types of structure organizations often retain many characteristics of a bureaucracy.

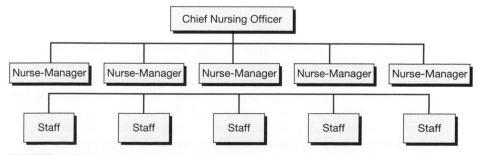

FIGURE 12.3 Flattened organizational structure.

Decision Making Within the Organizational Hierarchy

The decision-making hierarchy, or pyramid, depicted by a chain from the top management positions to the lowest rank, is called a *scalar chain*. By reviewing the organization chart in Figure 12.1, it is possible to determine where decisions are made within the organizational hierarchy. Although every manager has some decision-making authority, its type and level are determined by the manager's position on the chart.

In organizations with *centralized decision making*, a few managers at the top of the hierarchy make the decisions and the emphasis is on top-down control. In other words, the vision or thinking of one or a few individuals in the organization guides the organization's goals and how those goals are accomplished. Execution of decision making in centralized organizations is fairly rapid because role conflict is minimized, and role expectations are clarified.

Decentralized decision making diffuses decision making throughout the organization and allows problems to be solved by the lowest practical managerial level. Often, this means that problems can be solved at the level at which they occur, although some delays may occur in decision making if the problem must be transmitted through several levels to reach the appropriate individual to solve the problem. As a rule, however, larger organizations benefit from decentralized decision making.

This occurs because the complex questions that must be answered can best be addressed by a variety of people with distinct areas of expertise. Leaving such decisions in a large organization to a few managers burdens those managers tremendously and could result in devastating delays in decision making.

> In general, the larger the organization, the greater the need to decentralize decision making.

Stakeholders

Stakeholders are those entities that play a role in an organization's health and performance or that are affected by the organization. Stakeholders may be both internal and external, they may include individuals and large groups, and they may have shared goals or diverse goals. *Internal stakeholders*, for example, may include the nurse in a hospital or the dietitian in a nursing home. Examples of *external stakeholders* for an acute care hospital might be the local school of nursing, home health agencies, and managed care providers who contract with consumers in the area. Even the Chamber of Commerce in a city could be considered a stakeholder for a health care organization.

> Every organization should be viewed as being part of a greater community of stakeholders.

Stakeholders have interests in what the organization does but may or may not have the power to influence the organization to protect their interests. Stakeholders' interests are varied, however, and their interests may coincide on some issues and not others. For example, research by Tyler et al. (2021) found significant differences between five different stakeholder groups regarding perceptions of safety in mental health discharge (see Examining the Evidence 12.1). This suggests that engaging in critical conversations with stakeholders about organizational strategic initiatives whenever possible may offer viewpoints or perceptions that might otherwise not be considered.

EXAMINING THE EVIDENCE 12.1

Source: From Tyler, N., Wright, N., Panagioti, M., Grundy, A., & Waring, J. (2021). What does safety in mental healthcare transitions mean for service users and other stakeholder groups: An open-ended questionnaire study. *Health Expectations, 24,* 185–194.

A Significant Variance in Stakeholder Perceptions

The purpose of this international cross-sectional study, using an online survey investigated perceptions of safety in mental health transitions (hospital to community) among five stakeholder groups; individuals with lived experience/ service users; families and carers; mental health care professionals (HCPs); researchers; and end users of research (the people who will use research to make decisions—i.e., policy makers, service managers, charity workers, and commissioners). Ninety-three participants from 12 different countries responded.

Study findings noted that safety in mental health discharge was perceived differently by service users and families compared to HCPs and researchers. Traditional safety indicators such as suicide, self-harm, risk, or adverse drug events were raised as important safety outcomes and priorities, particularly by HCPs. However, service users and families in particular had a much wider perception of safety outcomes and priorities in mental health discharge, which incorporated human, behavioral and social and system-level factors. Contrastingly, service users/families considered safety largely nonclinically, focusing instead on human elements of communication, emotions, and relationships.

This work highlighted the differences between the scientific-technical cultures and the lived experience cultures of risk. Because perspectives about its critical components and priorities differed across different groups, there is a critical need to engage a broad variety of stakeholders in the design, conduct, and analysis of quality and safety research.

Therefore, *stakeholder analysis* is an important aspect of the management process. Such an analysis should be performed when there is a need to clarify the consequences of decisions and changes. In addition to identifying which stakeholders will be impacted by a change, it is necessary to prioritize them and determine their influence. Astute leaders are always cognizant as to who their stakeholders are and the impact they may have on an organization. A depiction of possible stakeholders for a local community hospital appears in Table 12.2.

Organizations, however, do not generally choose their own stakeholders; rather, the stakeholders choose to have a stake in the organizations' decisions. Stakeholders may have a supportive or threatening influence on organizational decision making. For many decisions an organization makes, it may face a diverse set of stakeholders with varied and conflicting interest and goals.

TABLE 12.2 EXAMPLES OF STAKEHOLDERS IN A COMMUNITY HOSPITAL

External Stakeholders	Internal Stakeholders
Local businesses	Hospital employees
Area colleges and universities	Physicians
Insurance companies and HMOs	Patients
Community leaders	Patients' families
Unions	Union shop stewards
Professional organizations	Board of directors
Philanthropic donors	

HMO, health maintenance organization.

Organizational Culture

Organizational culture is the total of an organization's values, language, traditions, and customs, as well as those things present in an institution that are not open to discussion or change. For example, the hospital logo that had been designed by the original board of trustees is an item that may not be considered for updating or change.

Similarly, Cancialosi (2017) defines *organizational culture* as the underlying beliefs, assumptions, values and ways of interacting that contribute to the unique social and psychological environment of an organization. The organizational culture includes an organization's expectations, experiences, philosophy, and values that hold it together and is expressed in its self-image, inner workings, interactions with the outside world, and future expectations. It is based on shared attitudes, beliefs, customs, and written and unwritten rules that have been developed over time and are considered valid.

Huston (2020, p. 4) agrees, noting that culture provides the "feel" of an organization and determines what is right or wrong, important or unimportant, and workable or unworkable. In other words, culture is everywhere and affects everything. All these definitions impart a sense of the complexity and importance of organizational culture.

> Organizational culture is a system of symbols and interactions unique to each organization. It is the ways of thinking, behaving, and believing that members of a unit have in common.

Although assessing unit culture is a management function, building a constructive culture, particularly if a negative culture is in place, requires the interpersonal and communication skills of a leader. The leader must take an active role in creating the kind of organizational culture that will ensure success. Groysberg et al. (2018) agree, noting that although most leaders understand the fundamentals of strategy as a lever in their quest to maintain organizational viability and effectiveness, culture is more elusive because much of it is anchored in unspoken behaviors, mindsets, and social patterns. Groysberg et al. argue, however, that for better or for worse, culture and leadership are inextricably linked: "Founders and influential leaders often set new cultures in motion and imprint values and assumptions that persist for decades. Over time an organization's leaders can also shape culture, through both conscious and unconscious actions (sometimes with unintended consequences). The best leaders we have observed are fully aware of the multiple cultures within which they are embedded, can sense when change is required, and can deftly influence the process" (Groysberg et al., 2018, para. 3).

It should be noted, however, that the more entrenched the culture and pattern of actions, the more challenging the change process is for the leader. Given such entrenchment of culture, success in building a new culture sometimes requires new leadership or the assistance of outside leadership.

Organizations, if large enough, also have many different and competing value systems that create *subcultures*. These subcultures shape perceptions, attitudes, and beliefs and influence how their members approach and execute their roles and responsibilities. A critical challenge then for the nurse-leader is to recognize these subcultures and to do whatever is necessary to create shared norms and priorities. Such transformation requires both management assessment and leadership direction.

In addition, much of an organization's culture is not available to staff in a retrievable source and must be related by others. For example, feelings about collective bargaining, nursing education levels, nursing autonomy, and nurse–physician relationships differ from one organization to another. These beliefs and values, however, are rarely written down or appear in a philosophy. Therefore, in addition to creating a constructive culture, a major leadership role is to assist subordinates in understanding the organization's culture. Display 12.3 identifies questions that leaders and followers should ask when assessing organizational culture.

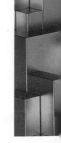

DISPLAY 12.3 ASSESSING THE ORGANIZATIONAL CULTURE

What Is the Organization's Physical Environment?

1. Is the environment attractive?
2. Does it appear that there is adequate maintenance?
3. Are nursing stations crowded or noisy?
4. Is there an appropriate-sized lobby? Are there quiet areas?
5. Is there sufficient seating for families in the dining room?
6. Are there enough conference rooms? A library? A chapel or place of worship?

What Is the Organization's Social Environment?

1. Are many friendships maintained beyond the workplace?
2. Is there an annual picnic or holiday party that is well attended by the employees?
3. Do employees seem to generally like each other?
4. Do all shifts and all departments cooperate and work together collaboratively?
5. Are certain departments disliked or resented?
6. Are employees on a first-name basis with coworkers, doctors, charge nurses, and supervisors?
7. How do employees treat patients and visitors?

How Supportive Is the Organization?

1. Is tuition reimbursement available?
2. Are good, low-cost meals available to employees?
3. Are there adequate employee lounges?
4. Are funds available to send employees to workshops or classes for professional development?
5. Are employees recognized for extra effort?
6. Does the organization help pay for the holiday party or other social functions?

What Is the Organizational Power Structure?

1. Who holds the most power in the organization?
2. Which departments are viewed as powerful? Which are viewed as powerless?
3. Who gets free meals? Who gets special parking places?
4. Who wears laboratory coats? Who has overhead pages?
5. Who has the biggest office?
6. Who is never called by their first name?

How Safe Is the Organization?

1. Is there a well-lighted parking place for employees arriving or departing when it is dark?
2. Is there an active and involved safety committee?
3. Are security guards needed and visible?

What Is the Communication Environment?

1. Is upward communication usually written or verbal?
2. Is there much informal communication?
3. Is there an active grapevine? Is it reliable?
4. Where is important information exchanged—in the parking lot, the doctors' surgical dressing room, the nurses' station, the coffee shop, or during surgery or during the delivery room?

What Are the Organizational Taboos? Who Are the Heroes?

1. Are there special rules and policies that can never be broken?
2. Are certain subjects or ideas forbidden?
3. Are there relationships that cannot be threatened?

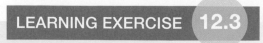

Cultures and Hierarchies

Having been with the county health department for 6 months, you are very impressed with the physician who is the county health administrator. She seems to have a genuine concern for patient welfare. She has a tea for new employees each month to discuss the department's philosophy and her own management style. She says that she has an open-door policy, so employees are always welcome to visit her.

Because you have been assigned to the evening immunization clinic as charge nurse, you have become concerned with a persistent problem. The housekeeping staff often spend part of the evening sleeping on duty or socializing for long periods. You have reported your concerns to your health department supervisor twice. Last evening, you found the housekeeping staff having another get-together. This mainly upsets you because the clinic is chronically in need of cleaning. Sometimes, the public bathrooms get so untidy that they embarrass you and your staff. You frequently remind the housekeepers to empty overflowing wastepaper baskets. You believe that this environment is demeaning to patients. This also upsets you because you and your staff work hard all evening and rarely have a chance to sit down. You believe it is unfair to everyone that the housekeeping staff is not doing their share.

ASSIGNMENT:

Note: Attempt to solve this problem before referring to a possible solution posted in the Appendix.

On your way to the parking lot this evening, the health administrator stops to chat and asks you how things are going. Should you tell her about the problem with the house-keeping staff? Is this following an appropriate chain of command? Do you believe that there is a conflict between the housekeeping unit's culture and the nursing unit's culture? What should you do? List choices and alternatives. Decide what you should do and explain your rationale.

Finally, organizational culture should not be confused with *organizational climate*—how employees perceive an organization. For example, an employee might perceive an organization as fair, friendly, and informal or as formal and very structured. The perception may be accurate or inaccurate, and people in the same organization may have different perceptions about the same organization. Therefore, because the organizational climate is the view of the organization by individuals, the organization's climate and its culture may differ.

> In terms of importance, more people rank "workplace well-being" over monetary or "material benefits"—and that well-being is created through a positive organizational culture (Thiefels, 2020, para 2).

Shared Governance: Organizational Design for the 21st Century

Shared governance, one of the most innovative and empowering organization structures, was developed in the mid-1980s as an alternative to the traditional bureaucratic organizational

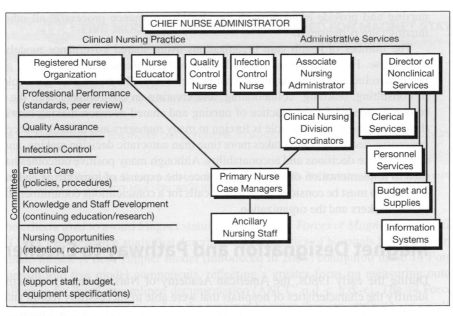

FIGURE 12.4 Shared governance model.

structure. A flat type of organizational structure is often used to describe shared governance but differs somewhat, as shown in Figure 12.4. In shared governance, the organization's governance is shared among board members, nurses, physicians, and management. Thus, decision making and communication channels are altered. Group structures, in the form of *joint practice committees*, are developed to assume the power and accountability for decision making, and professional communication takes on an egalitarian structure.

In health care organizations, shared governance empowers decision makers, and this empowerment is directed at increasing nurses' authority and control over nursing practice. Shared governance thus gives nurses more control over their nursing practice by being an accountability-based governance system for professional workers. In addition, shared governance can be used to improve communication and joint decision making between nursing and other members of the interprofessional health care team.

> The stated aim of shared governance is the empowerment of employees within the decision-making system.

Although participatory management lays the foundation for shared governance, they are not the same. *Participatory management* implies that others can participate in decision making over which someone has control. Thus, the act of "allowing" participation identifies the real and final authority for the participant.

There is no single model of shared governance, although all models emphasize the empowerment of staff nurses. In general, issues related to nursing practice are the responsibility of nurses, not managers, and nursing councils are used to organize governance. These *nursing councils*, elected at the organization and unit levels, use a congressional format organized like a representative form of government, with a president and cabinet.

Typical governance councils include a nursing practice council, a research council, professional development or education council, a nursing performance improvement or quality council, and a leadership council. Sometimes, organizations will have a retention council as well. The councils participate in decision making and coordination of the department of

LEARNING EXERCISE **12.4**

Why Work for Them?

A list of current Magnet-recognized organizations and their contact information can be found at the ANCC (n.d.-b) website: https://www.nursingworld.org/organizational-programs/magnet/find-a-magnet-facility/

ASSIGNMENT:

Select one of the current organizations and prepare a one-page written report about how that organization demonstrates the excellence exemplified by Magnet status. Speak to at least five of the "forces of magnetism." Would you want to work for this particular organization?

Committee Structure in an Organization

Managers are also responsible for designing and implementing appropriate work group or committee structures. Poorly structured committees can be nonproductive for the organization and frustrating for committee members. However, there are many benefits to and justifications for well-structured committees. For example, committees can facilitate upward communication and assist with management functions. In addition, as organizations seek new ways to revamp old bureaucratic structures, committees may pave the road to increased staff participation in organization governance. Committees may be advisory or may have a coordinating or informal function. They generate ideas and creative thinking to solve operational problems or improve services and often improve the quality and quantity of work accomplished. Committees also can pool specific skills and expertise and help reduce resistance to change.

> Because committees communicate upward and downward and encourage the participation of interested or affected employees, they assist the organization in receiving valuable feedback and important information.

However, these positive benefits can be achieved only if committees are appropriately organized and led. If not properly used, the committee becomes a liability to the organizing process because it wastes energy, time, and money and can defer decisions and action. One of the leadership roles inherent in organizing work is to ensure that committees are not used to avoid or delay decisions but to facilitate organizational goals. Display 12.6 lists factors to consider when organizing committees.

Responsibilities and Opportunities of Committee Work

Committees present the leader-manager with many opportunities and responsibilities; however, managers need to be well grounded in group dynamics to assure the committee uses its time wisely and is productive. The manager should use appropriate power strategies, such as coming to meetings well prepared and skillfully guiding group process to generate influence and gain power at meetings.

Another responsibility is to create an environment at committee meetings that leads to shared decision making. Encouraging an interaction free of status and power is important. Likewise, an appropriate seating arrangement, such as a circle, will increase motivation for

DISPLAY 12.6 **FACTORS TO CONSIDER WHEN ORGANIZING COMMITTEES**

- The committee should be composed of people who want to contribute in terms of commitment, energy, and time.
- The members should have a variety of work experience and educational backgrounds. Composition should, however, ensure expertise sufficient to complete the task.
- Committees should have enough members to accomplish assigned tasks but not so many that discussion cannot occur. Six to eight members in a committee are usually ideal.
- The tasks and responsibilities, including reporting mechanisms, should be clearly outlined.
- Assignments should be given ahead of time, with clear expectations that assigned work will be discussed at the next meeting.
- All committees should have written agendas and effective committee chairpersons.

committee members to speak up. The responsible manager is also aware that staff from different cultures may have different needs in groups, which is why multicultural committees should be the norm. In addition, because gender differences are increasingly being recognized as playing a role in problem solving, communication, and power, efforts should be made to include all genders on committees.

> When assigning members to committees, diversity should always be a goal.

The manager must not rely too heavily on committees or use them as a method to delay decision making. Numerous committee assignments exhaust staff, and committees then become poor tools for accomplishing work. An alternative that will decrease the time commitment for committee work is to make individual assignments and gather the entire committee only to report progress.

In addition, it is important for the manager to be aware of the possibility for groupthink to occur in any group or committee structure. *Groupthink* occurs when group members fail to take adequate risks by disagreeing, being challenged, or assessing discussion carefully. If the manager is actively involved in the work group or on the committee, groupthink is less likely to occur. The leadership role includes teaching members to avoid groupthink by demonstrating critical thinking and being a role model who allows their own ideas to be challenged.

Committees may be chaired by an elected member of the group, appointed by the manager, or led by the department or unit manager. Informal leaders may also emerge from the group process. There is an opportunity for leaders to have significant influence on committee and group effectiveness because leaders keep group work on course. Dynamic leaders also inspire people to work toward shared goals, and this demonstrates their commitment to participatory management. Finally, leaders should be sure to celebrate committee successes and goal completion.

Integrating Leadership Roles and Management Functions Associated with Organizational Structure

Despite the known difficulties, it has been difficult for some organizations to move away from a bureaucratic model of organization. However, efforts to redesign and restructure organizations to make them more flexible and decentralized continue.

There is no one "best" way to structure an organization. Variables such as the size of the organization, the capability of its human resources, and the commitment level of its workers should always be considered. Regardless of what type of organizational structure is used, certain minimal requirements can be identified:

- The structure should be clearly defined so that employees know where they belong and where to go for assistance.
- The goal should be to build the fewest possible management levels and have the shortest possible chain of command. This eliminates friction, stress, and inertia.
- The unit staff need to be able to see where their tasks fit into common tasks of the organization.
- The organizational structure should enhance, not impede, communication.
- The organizational structure should facilitate decision making that results in the greatest work performance.
- Staff should be organized in a manner that encourages informal groups to develop a sense of community and belonging.
- Nursing services should be organized to facilitate the development of future leaders.

Integrated leader-managers need to look at organizational structure as the road map that tells them how organizations operate. Without organizational structure, people would work in a chaotic environment. Structure becomes an important tool, then, to facilitate order and enhance productivity.

Astute leader-managers understand both the structure of the organization in which they work and external stakeholders. The integrated leader-manager, however, goes beyond personal understanding of the larger organizational design. The leader-manager takes responsibility for ensuring that subordinates also understand the overall organizational structure and the structure at the unit level. This can be done by being a resource and role model to subordinates. The role modeling includes demonstrating accountability and the appropriate use of authority.

The effective manager recognizes the difficulties inherent in advisory positions and uses leadership skills to support staff in these positions. This is accomplished by granting enough authority to enable advisory staff to carry out the functions of their role.

Leadership requires that problems are pursued through appropriate channels, that upward communication is encouraged, and that unit structure is periodically evaluated to determine if it can be redesigned to enable increased lower-level decision making. The integrated leader-manager also facilitates constructive informal group structure. It is important for the manager to be knowledgeable about the organization's culture and subcultures. It is just as important for the leader to promote the development of a shared constructive culture with subordinates.

It is a management role to evaluate the types of organizational structure and governance and to implement those that will have the most positive impact in the department. It is a leadership skill to role model the shared authority necessary to make newer models of organizational structure and governance possible.

When serving on committees, leaders look for opportunities to gain influence to meet the needs of patients and staff appropriately. In addition, the integrated leader-manager comes to meetings well prepared and contributes thoughtful comments and ideas. The leader's critical thinking and role-modeling behavior discourages groupthink among work groups or in committees.

Integrated leader-managers also refrain from judging and encourage all members of a committee to participate and contribute. An important management function is to see that appropriate work is accomplished in committees, that they remain productive, and that they are not used to delay decision making. A leadership role is the involvement of staff in organizational decision making, either informally or through more formal models of organizational design, such as shared governance. The integrated leader-manager understands the organization and recognizes what can be molded or shaped and what is constant. Thus, the interaction between the manager and the organization is dynamic.

Key Concepts

- Many modern health care organizations continue to be organized around a line or line-and-staff design and have attributes of a bureaucracy; however, there is a movement toward less bureaucratic designs, such as ad hoc, matrix, and care-centered systems.

- A bureaucracy, as proposed by Max Weber, is characterized by a clear chain of command, rules and regulations, specialization of work, division of labor, and impersonality of relationships.

- An organization chart depicts formal relationships, channels of communication, and authority through line-and-staff positions, scalar chains, and span of control.

- Unity of command means that each person should have only one boss so that there is less confusion and greater productivity.

- Centrality refers to the degree of communication of a management position.

- In centralized decision making, decisions are made by a few managers at the top of the hierarchy. In decentralized decision making, decision making is diffused throughout the organization, and problems are solved at the lowest practical managerial level.

- Organizational structure affects how people perceive their roles and the status given to them by other people in the organization.

- Organizational structure is effective when the design is clearly communicated, there are as few managers as possible to accomplish goals, communication is facilitated, decisions are made at the lowest possible level, informal groups are encouraged, and future leaders are developed.

- The entities in an organization's environment that play a role in the organization's health and performance, or which are affected by the organization, are called stakeholders.

- Authority, responsibility, and accountability differ in terms of official sanctions, self-directedness, and moral integration.

- Organizational culture is the total of an organization's beliefs, history, taboos, formal and informal relationships, and communication patterns.

- Much of an organization's culture is not available to staff in a retrievable source and must be related by others.

- Subunits of large organizations may also have a culture. These subcultures may support or conflict with other cultures in the organization.

- Informal groups are present in every organization. They are often powerful, although they have no formal authority. Informal groups determine norms and assist members in the socialization process.

- Shared governance refers to an organizational design that empowers staff nurses by making them an integral part of patient care decision making and providing accountability and responsibility in nursing practice.

- Magnet designation is conferred by the ANCC to health care organizations that exemplify five model components: transformational leadership; structural empowerment; exemplary professional practice; new knowledge, innovation, and improvements; and empirical quality results.

- Magnet-designated organizations demonstrate improved patient outcomes and higher staff nurse satisfaction than organizations that do not have Magnet status.

- The Pathway to Excellence designation, also conferred by the ANCC, recognizes health care organizations and long-term care institutions with foundational quality initiatives in creating a positive work environment, as defined by nurses and supported by research.

- The existence of too many committees in an organization is a sign of a poorly designed organizational structure.

- Committees should have an appropriate number of members, prepared agendas, clearly outlined tasks, and effective leadership if they are to be productive.

- Groupthink occurs when there is too much conformity to group norms.

Additional Learning Exercises and Applications

LEARNING EXERCISE 12.5

Restructuring—In Depth

You are the supervisor at a home health agency. There are 22 registered nurses in your span of control. In a meeting today, John Dao, the chief nurse officer (CNO), tells you that your span of control needs adjustment to be effective. Therefore, the CNO has decided to flatten the organization and decentralize the department. To accomplish this, he plans to designate three of your staff as shift coordinators. These shift coordinators will "schedule patient visits for all the staff on their shift and be accountable for the staff that they super-vise." The CNO believes that this restructuring will give you more time for implementing a continuous quality improvement program and promoting staff development.

Although you are glad to have the opportunity to begin these new projects, you are somewhat unclear about the role expectations of the new shift coordinators and how this will change your job description. In fact, you worry that this is just a precursor to the elimina-tion of your position. Will these shift coordinators report to you? If so, will you have direct line authority or staff authority? Who should be responsible for evaluating the performance of the staff nurses now? Who will handle employee disciplinary problems? How involved should the shift coordinators be in strategic planning or determining next year's budget? What types of management training will be needed by the shift coordinators to prepare for their new role? Are you the most appropriate person to train them?

ASSIGNMENT:

There is great potential for conflict here. In small groups, make a list of 10 questions (not including the ones listed in the Learning Exercise) that you would want to ask the CNO at your next meeting to clarify role expectations. Discuss tools and skills that you have learned in the preceding units that could make this role change less traumatic for all involved.

LEARNING EXERCISE 12.6

Problem Solving: Working Toward Shared Governance

You are the supervisor of a surgical services department in a nonunion hospital. The staff on your unit have become increasingly frustrated with hospital policies regarding staffing ratios, on-call pay, and verbal medical orders but feel that they have limited opportunities for providing feedback to change the current system. You would like to explore the possibility of moving toward a shared governance model of decision making to resolve this issue and others like it but are not quite sure where to start.

ASSIGNMENT:

Assume that you are the supervisor in this case. Answer the following questions:
1. Who do I need to involve in this discussion and at what point?
2. How might I determine if the overarching organizational structure supports shared governance? How would I determine if external stakeholders would be impacted? How would I determine if organizational culture and subculture would support a shared governance model?

3. What types of nursing councils might be created to provide a framework for operation?
4. Who would be the members on these nursing councils?
5. What support mechanisms would need to be in place to ensure success of this project?
6. What would be my role as a supervisor in identifying and resolving employee concerns in a shared governance model?

LEARNING EXERCISE 12.7

Finding Direction

You are a new graduate working on the 3:00 PM to 11:00 PM shift in a large, metropolitan hospital on the pediatrics unit. You feel frustrated because you had many preceptors while you were being oriented, and each told you slightly different variations of the unit routine. In addition, the regular charge nurse has just been promoted and moved to another unit, and the charge nurse position on your unit is being filled by two part-time nurses.

You feel inadequately prepared for the job and do not know where to turn or to whom you should direct your questions. If your organization chart resembles the one in Figure 12.1, outline a plan of action that would be appropriate to take. Share your plan with a larger group.

LEARNING EXERCISE 12.8

Thinking About Committee Work

As a writing exercise, choose one of the following to examine in depth:

1. What has contributed to the productivity of the committees on which you have served? What practices have led committees you have served on to be ineffective?
2. Have you ever served on a committee that made recommendations on which higher authority never acted? What was the effect on the group?

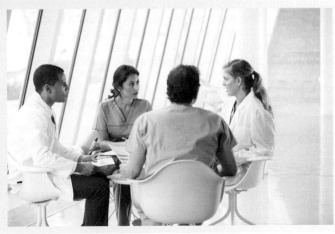

LEARNING EXERCISE 12.9

Participation and Productivity

You are a 3:00 PM to 11:00 PM charge nurse on a surgical unit. You have been selected to chair the unit's safety committee. Each month, you have a short committee meeting with the other committee members. Your committee's main responsibility is to report upward any safety issues that have been identified. Lately, you have found an increase in needle-stick incidents, and the committee has been addressing this problem.

The committee is made up of two nursing assistants, one unit clerk, two staff registered nurses, and two licensed practical nurses/licensed vocational nurses. All shifts and staff cultures are represented. Lately, you have found that the meetings are not going well because one member of the group, Mary, has begun to monopolize the meeting time. She is especially outspoken about the danger of blood borne infections and seems more interested in pointing blame regarding the needle sticks than in finding a solution to the problem.

You have privately spoken to Mary about her frequent disruption of the committee business; although she apologized, the behavior has continued. You feel that some members of the committee are becoming bored and restless, and you believe that the committee is making little progress.

ASSIGNMENT:

Using your knowledge of committee structure and effectiveness, outline steps that you would take to facilitate more group participation and make the committee more productive. Be specific and explain exactly what you would do at the next meeting to prevent Mary from taking over the meeting.

LEARNING EXERCISE 12.10

Finding an Organizational Culture That Fits

Joanie Smith is a 32-year-old single mother of two who will graduate in 3 months from a local associate degree nursing program. Joanie has accrued some debts in completing her nursing education. She has been offered two jobs upon graduation: one is at a local medium-sized hospital (Community Center Hospital) and one is in a larger city some distance away (Metropolitan City Hospital). Both job offers are in the obstetrical unit, which is Joanie's desired place of work because some day, she hopes to return to school to become a nurse midwife.

Research on the two hospitals shows that both are accredited and have good medical staffs, and Joanie has received positive feedback on both from people whose judgment she trusts.

ASSIGNMENT:

Pretend you are this nurse. What additional type of information should you gather to be able to decide which of these organizations is a better fit? What particular assessment of organizational culture can you do that would help you make a better decision? Are there particular organization culture characteristics that are a better fit for you than others?

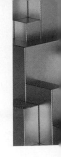

REFERENCES

American Nurses Credentialing Center. (n.d.-a). Eligibility criteria. *ANCC Magnet Recognition Program®*. Retrieved September 14, 2021, from https://www.nursingworld.org/organizational-programs/magnet/apply/eligibility-criteria/

American Nurses Credentialing Center. (n.d.-b). *Find a Magnet facility*. Retrieved September 14, 2021, from https://www.nursingworld.org/organizational-programs/magnet/find-a-magnet-facility/

American Nurses Credentialing Center. (n.d.-c). *Forces of magnetism*. Retrieved September 10, 2018, from https://www.nursingworld.org/organizational-programs/magnet/history/forces-of-magnetism/

American Nurses Credentialing Center. (n.d.-d). *ANCC Magnet Recognition Program®*. Retrieved September 14, 2021, from https://www.nursingworld.org/organizational-programs/magnet/

American Nurses Credentialing Center. (n.d.-e). *Magnet model. Creating a magnet culture*. Retrieved September 14, 2021, from https://www.nursingworld.org/organizational-programs/magnet/magnet-model/

American Nurses Credentialing Center. (n.d.-f). *ANCC Pathway to Excellence® program*. Retrieved August 25, 2019, from https://www.nursingworld.org/organizational-programs/pathway/

American Nurses Credentialing Center. (n,d.-g). *Pathway program overview*. Retrieved September 14, 2021, from https://www.nursingworld.org/organizational-programs/pathway/overview/

American Nurses Credentialing Center. (n.d.-h). *Why become Magnet?* Retrieved December 14, 2021, from https://www.nursingworld.org/organizational-programs/magnet/about-magnet/why-become-magnet/

Cancialosi, C. (2017). *What is Organizational Culture?* Gotham Culture. https://gothamculture.com/what-is-organizational-culture-definition/

Groysberg, B., Lee, J., Price, J., & Cheng, J. Y.-J. (2018). The leader's guide to corporate culture. *Harvard Business Review.* https://hbr.org/2018/01/the-culture-factor

Hartzell, S. (2012). *Characteristics of informal organizations: The grapevine & informal groups*. Study.com. http://education-portal.com/academy/lesson/characteristics-of-informal-organizations-the-grapevine-informal-groups.html

Huston, C. J. (2020). *The road to positive work cultures*. Sigma Theta Tau International.

Juneja, H. (1996–2022). *Span of control in an organization*. SelfGrowth.com. http://www.selfgrowth.com/articles/Span_of_Control_in_an_Organization.html

Pabico, C., & Graystone, R. (2018). Comparing Pathway to Excellence® and Magnet Recognition® programs. *American Nurse Today, 13*(3). https://www.americannursetoday.com/comparing-pathway-excellence-magnet-recognition-programs/

Quain, S. (2019). *Basic types of organizational structure: Formal & informal*. Chron. http://smallbusiness.chron.com/basic-types-organizational-structure-formal-informal-982.html

Thiefels, J. (2020). 5 Simple ways to assess company culture. *Achievers.* https://www.achievers.com/blog/2018/04/5-simple-ways-assess-company-culture/

Tyler, N., Wright, N., Panagioti, M., Grundy, A., & Waring, J. (2021). What does safety in mental healthcare transitions mean for service users and other stakeholder groups: An open-ended questionnaire study. *Health Expectations, 24,* 185–194.

13

Organizational, Political, and Personal Power

*… nearly all men can stand adversity, but if you want to test a man's character, give him power.—**Abraham Lincoln***

*… Being powerful is like being a lady. If you have to tell people you are, you aren't.—**M. Thatcher***

*… Power should not be concentrated in the hands of so few, and powerlessness in the hands of so many.—**Maggie Kuhn***

LEARNING OBJECTIVES

The learner will:

- assess how one's experience of power dynamics in the family unit as a child may affect one's perception of power as an adult as well as the ability to use it appropriately
- explore the influence of gender in how an individual may view power and politics
- differentiate among legitimate, reward, coercive, expert, referent, charismatic, self, and information power

- recognize the need to create and maintain a small authority–power gap
- identify and use appropriate strategies to increase one's personal power base
- use power on behalf of other people rather than over them
- empower subordinates and followers by providing them with opportunities for success
- describe how to access and build political alliances and coalitions through networking
- use appropriate political strategies in resolving unit problems
- use cooperation rather than competition and avoid overt displays of power and authority whenever possible
- explore factors that historically led to nursing's limited power as a profession
- identify driving forces in place as well as specific strategies to increase the nursing profession's power base
- identify political strategies the novice manager could use to minimize the negative effects of organizational politics
- serve as a role model of an empowered nurse

Introduction

Chapter 12 reviewed organizational structure and introduced the concepts of status, authority, and responsibility at different levels of the organizational hierarchy. In this chapter, the organization is examined further, with emphasis on the management functions and leadership roles inherent in effective use of authority, establishment of a personal power base, empowerment of others, and the impact of organizational politics on power. In addition, factors that have historically contributed to nursing's limited power as a profession are presented as well as the driving forces in place to change this phenomenon. Finally, this chapter introduces strategies the individual and the nursing profession could use to increase their power base.

The word *power* is derived from the Latin verb *potere* (to be able); thus, power may be appropriately defined as that which enables one to accomplish goals. Power can also be defined as the capacity to act or the strength and potency to accomplish something. It is almost impossible to achieve organizational or personal goals without an adequate power base. It is even more difficult to help subordinates, patients, or clients achieve their goals when powerless because having access to and control over resources is often related to the degree of power one holds.

> Having power gives one the potential to change the attitudes and behaviors of individual people and groups, and to bestow resources to accomplish goals.

Authority, or the right to command, accompanies any management position and is a source of legitimate power, although components of management, authority, and power are also necessary, to a degree, for successful leadership. The manager who is knowledgeable about the wise use of authority, power, and political strategy is more effective at meeting personal, unit, and organizational goals. Likewise, powerful leaders can raise morale because they delegate more and build with a team effort. Thus, their followers become part of the growth and excitement of the organization as their own status is enhanced. The leadership roles and management functions inherent in the use of authority and power are shown in Display 13.1.

DISPLAY 13.1   LEADERSHIP ROLES AND MANAGEMENT FUNCTIONS ASSOCIATED WITH ORGANIZATIONAL, POLITICAL, AND PERSONAL POWER

Leadership Roles

1. Creates a climate that promotes followership in response to authority
2. Recognizes the impact of power on relationships that exist within an organization
3. Uses a powerful persona and referent power to increase respect and decrease fear in subordinates
4. Recognizes when it is appropriate to have authority questioned or to question authority
5. Is personally comfortable with power in the political arena
6. Empowers others whenever possible
7. Assists others in using appropriate political strategies
8. Serves as a role model of the empowered nurse
9. Strives to eliminate a perception of powerlessness among others
10. Uses power judiciously and mindfully
11. Role models political skill in developing consensus, inclusion, and follower involvement
12. Builds alliances and coalitions inside and outside of nursing

Management Functions

1. Uses authority to ensure that organizational goals are met
2. Uses political strategies that are complementary to the unit and organization's functioning
3. Builds a power base appropriate for the assigned management role
4. Creates and maintains a small authority–power gap
5. Is knowledgeable about the essence and appropriate use of power
6. Maintains personal credibility with subordinates
7. Avoids using power over others rather than on behalf of others whenever possible
8. Demonstrates reasoned risk taking in decision making with political implications
9. Uses reward power, coercive power, legitimate power, and expert power when appropriate to positively influence the achievement of organizational goals
10. Limits visible displays of legitimate power and avoids overusing commands
11. Understands the organizational structure in which they work, functions effectively within that structure, and deals effectively with the institution's inherent politics
12. Promotes subordinate identification and recognition

Understanding Power

How individuals view power varies greatly. Indeed, power may be feared, worshipped, or mistrusted, and it is frequently misunderstood. Our first experience with power usually occurs in the family unit. Because children's roles are likened to later subordinate roles and the parental power position is like management, adult views of the management–subordinate relationship are often influenced by how power was used in the family unit and the often-unacknowledged impact of gender on power in family dynamics. A positive or negative familial power experience may greatly affect a person's ability to deal with power in adulthood.

Gender and Power

Successful leaders are attentive to the influence of gender on power as well. Many women (and thus nurses) have historically demonstrated ambivalence toward the concept of power, and some have even eschewed the pursuit of power. This likely occurred because of the way some women have been socialized to view power, believing that women do not inherently possess power (formal or informal) or authority (Huston, 2023). In addition, rather than feeling capable of achieving and managing power, some women feel that power manages them.

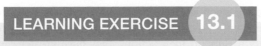

LEARNING EXERCISE 13.1

Is Power Different for Men and Women?

Research studies suggest differences in how men and women view power and how others view men and women in positions of authority. Do you think that there are gender differences in how power is perceived? Who did you feel was most powerful in your family while growing up? Why do you think that person was powerful? If you are using group work, how many in your group named powerful male figures; how many named powerful female figures? Discuss this in a group and then go to the library or use internet sources to see if you can find recent studies that support your views.

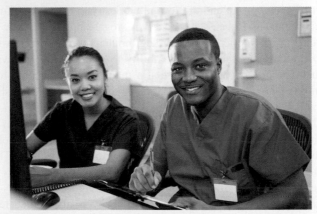

These gender-based perceptions are changing; yet, many women still need to learn how to use power as a tool for personal and professional success. In contemporary society, people are finding new ways for leaders, regardless of gender, to acquire and manage power. These changes are taking place within women, in women's view of other women holding power, in organizational hierarchies, and among male subordinates and male colleagues (Huston, 2023). Indeed, skills that have often been linked to female characteristics such as political skill in developing consensus, inclusion, and involvement are now viewed as strengths in the corporate world. These attributes are certainly not limited to women, but it is notable that the same attributes that once closed corporate doors and created the barrier popularly called the *glass ceiling* are now generally welcomed in the boardroom.

Power and Powerlessness

In determining what degree of power is desirable, it may be helpful to look at its opposite: *powerlessness*. Most people agree that they dislike being powerless. Everyone needs to have some control in life, and when that is not the case, the result is typically a bossy and rules-oriented individual, desperate to have some degree of power or control. Leader-managers who feel powerless often create an ineffective, petty, dictatorial, and rule-minded management style. They may become oppressive leaders, punitive and rigid in decision making, or withhold information from others, and they become difficult to work with. This suggests that although the adage that power corrupts might be true for some, it is also likely correct to say that powerlessness holds at least as much potential for corruption.

> Power is likely to bring more power in an ascending cycle, whereas powerlessness will only generate more powerlessness.

In contrast, truly powerful individuals know they are powerful and do not need to display this overtly. Instead, their power is evident in the respect and cooperation of their followers. Because the powerful have credibility to support their actions, they have greater capacity to get things accomplished and can enhance their base.

Apparently, then, power has a negative and a positive face. The negative face of power is the "I win, you lose" aspect of dominance versus submission. The positive face of power occurs when someone exerts influence on behalf of—rather than over—someone or something. Power, therefore, is not good or evil; it is how it is used and for what purpose that matters.

Types of Power

For leadership to be effective, some measure of power must often support it. This is true for the informal social group and the formal work group. The Mind Tools Content Team (2022) describes French and Raven's classical work regarding the bases or sources of power: reward power, punishment or coercive power, legitimate power, expert power, and referent power.

Reward power is obtained by the ability to grant favors or reward others with whatever they value. The arsenal of rewards that a manager can dispense to get employees to work toward meeting organizational goals is very broad. Positive leadership through rewards tends to develop a great deal of loyalty and devotion toward leaders.

Punishment or *coercive power*, the opposite of reward power, is based on fear of punishment if the manager's expectations are not met. The manager may obtain compliance through threats (often implied) of transfer, layoff, demotion, or dismissal. The manager who shuns or ignores an employee is exercising power through punishment, as is the manager who berates or belittles an employee.

Legitimate power is position power. Authority is also called legitimate power. It is the power gained by a title or official position within an organization. Legitimate power has inherent in it the ability to create feelings of obligation or responsibility. The socialization and culture of subordinate employees will influence to some degree how much power a manager has due to their position.

Expert power is gained through knowledge, expertise, or experience. Having critical knowledge allows a manager to gain power over others who need that knowledge. This type of power is limited to a specialized area. For example, someone with vast expertise in music would be powerful only in that area, not in another specialization. When Florence Nightingale used research to quantify the need for nurses in the Crimea (by showing that when nurses were present, fewer soldiers died), she was using her research to demonstrate expertise in the health needs of the wounded.

Referent power is power that a person has because others identify with that leader or with what that leader symbolizes. Referent power also occurs when one gives another person feelings of personal acceptance or approval. It may be obtained through association with the powerful. People may also develop referent power because others perceive them as powerful. This perception could be based on personal charisma, the way the leader talks or acts, the organizations to which they belong, or the people with whom they associate. People who others accept as role models or leaders enjoy referent power. Physicians use referent power very effectively; society, as a whole, views physicians as powerful, and physicians carefully maintain this image.

Although correlated with referent power, *charismatic power* is distinguished by some from referent power. Referent power is gained only through association with powerful others, whereas charisma is a more personal type of power.

Another type of power, which is often added to French and Raven's list of power sources, is *informational power*. This source of power is obtained when people have information that others must have to accomplish their goals. The various sources of power are summarized in Table 13.1.

TABLE **13.1** SOURCES OF POWER

Type	Source
Referent	Association with powerful others
Legitimate	Position
Coercive	Fear
Reward	Ability to grant favors
Expert	Knowledge and skill
Charismatic	Personal
Informational	The need for information

The Authority–Power Gap

If authority is the right to command, then a logical question is "Why do workers sometimes not follow orders?" Sometimes, it is because they believe management does not understand their point of view or that they are insensitive to worker needs. When followers feel that their needs and wants don't matter and that the person in charge does not care, their innate motivation to be a good follower declines.

Clearly then, the right to command does not ensure that employees will follow orders. The gap that sometimes exists between a position of authority and subordinate response is called the *authority–power gap*. The more power subordinates perceive a manager to have, the smaller the gap between the right to expect certain things and the resulting fulfillment of those expectations by others.

The negative effect of a wide authority–power gap is that organizational chaos may develop. There would be little productivity if every order was questioned. The organization should rightfully expect that its goals will be accomplished. One of the core dynamics of civilization is that there will always be a few authority figures pushing the many for a certain standard of performance.

People in the United States are socialized very early to respond to authority figures. In many cases, children are conditioned to accept the directives of their parents, teachers, and community leaders. This early conditioning informs how adults respond to authority figures, an example of which can be seen in the relationship between nursing students and nurse educators. Some nurse educators present themselves as authoritarians who demand unconditional obedience. Indeed, educators who maintain a very narrow authority–power gap reinforce dependency and obedience by emphasizing extreme consequences, including the death of the patient. Thus, nursing students may be socialized to be overly cautious and to hesitate when making independent nursing judgments. Because of these types of early socialization, the gap between the manager's authority and the worker's response to that authority tends to be relatively small; however, it has grown in the last 50 years.

At times, however, authority should be questioned by either the leader or the subordinates. This is demonstrated in health care by the increased questioning of the authority of physicians—many of whom feel they have the authority to command—by nurses and consumers. Figure 13.1 shows the dynamics of the relationships in the organizational authority–power response.

Bridging the Authority–Power Gap

For an organization to be successful, mutual trust must be present between managers and employees. This means that managers need to trust their employees, employees need to trust their managers, and employees need to trust each other.

Empowering Subordinates

The empowerment of staff is a hallmark of transformational leadership. To empower means to enable, develop, or allow. *Empowerment*, as discussed in Chapter 2, can be defined as decentralization of power. Empowerment occurs when leaders communicate their vision; employees are given the opportunity to make the most of their talents; and learning, creativity, and exploration are encouraged.

Empowerment is not the relinquishing of rightful power inherent in a position. Nor is it a delegation of authority or its commensurate responsibility and accountability. Instead, the actions of empowered staff are freely chosen, owned, and committed to on behalf of the organization without any requests or requirements to do so. Empowerment plants seeds of leadership, collegiality, self-respect, and professionalism.

Empowerment can also be as simple as assuring that all individuals in the organization are treated with dignity. Empowerment, however, is not an easy one-step process. Instead, it is a complex process that consists of responsibility for the individual desiring empowerment as well as the organization and its leadership.

One way that leaders empower subordinates is when they delegate assignments to provide learning opportunities and allow employees to share in the satisfaction derived from achievement. Delegation can motivate employees and fuel creativity, but it can also create work overload and cause stress that may hurt performance. Managers then must understand that empowering leadership has its limits and that factors like trust and experience affect how their behaviors are perceived.

> Empowerment creates and sustains a work environment that speaks to values, such as facilitating the employee's choice to invest in and own personal actions and behaviors that result in positive contributions to the organization's mission.

Not being committed to empowerment, though, is a barrier to creating an environment for empowerment in an organization. Other barriers would include a rigid organizational belief about authority and status. A manager's personal feelings regarding empowerment's potential effect on the manager's own power can also impede the empowering process.

Once organizational barriers have been minimized or eliminated, the leader should develop strategies at the unit level to empower staff. The easiest strategy is to be a role model of an empowered nurse. Another strategy would be to assist staff in building their own personal power base. This can be accomplished by showing subordinates how their personal, expert, and referent power can be expanded. Empowerment also occurs when workers are involved in planning and implementing change and when workers believe that they have some input in what is about to happen to them and some control over the environment in which they will work in the future.

Mobilizing the Power of the Nursing Profession

Until the nursing profession has a seat at all health care policy-making tables, individual nurses and leader-managers will be limited in how much personal power they will hold. Huston (2023) argues that nursing has not been the force it could be in the policy arena, stating that nurses have often been reactive rather than proactive in addressing policy decisions and legislation after the fact rather than taking part in drafting and sponsoring legislation. However, she cites several driving forces that should increase nursing's power base (Display 13.2):

> **DISPLAY 13.2 SIX DRIVING FORCES TO INCREASE NURSING'S POWER BASE**
>
> 1. The timing is right
> 2. The size of the nursing profession
> 3. Nursing's referent power
> 4. Increasing knowledge base and education for nurses
> 5. Nursing's unique perspective
> 6. Desire of consumers and providers for change

Source: From Huston, C. (2023). The nursing profession's historic struggle to increase its power base. In C. Huston (Ed.), *Professional issues in nursing: Challenges and opportunities* (6th ed., pp. 338–352). Wolters Kluwer.

- *The timing is right.* The errors reported in our medical system, the numbers of uninsured, and the shortcomings of our current health care system are all reasons that consumers and legislators are willing to listen to nurses as an attempt is made to fix the health care crisis. Clearly, the public wants a better health care system, and nurses want to be able to provide high-quality nursing care. Both are powerful elements for change, and new nurses are entering the profession at a time when their energy and expertise will be more valued than ever.

  The passage and implementation of the *Patient Protection and Affordable Care Act* only escalated public awareness and debate about flaws in publicly funded or subsidized health care in the United States. Furthermore, because of publications such as the Institute of Medicine's (IOM's) *To Err Is Human*, consumers, health care providers, and legislators are more aware than ever of the shortcomings of the current health care system, and the clamor for action has never been louder.

- *Size of the nursing profession.* Numbers are very important in politics, and the nursing profession's size is its greatest asset. The United States had 3,047,530 employed RNs as of May 2021 (U.S. Department of Labor, 2022), which represents an impressive potential voting bloc.

- *Nursing's referent power.* The nursing profession has a great deal of referent power because of the high degree of trust and credibility the public places in them.

- *Increasing knowledge base and education for nurses.* There are more nurses being awarded master's and doctoral degrees than ever before. One of the greatest areas of growth is in the number of Doctor of Nursing Practice (DNP) students. As of 2021, DNP programs were available in all 50 states plus the District of Columbia, and from 2018 to 2019, the number of students enrolled in DNP programs increased from 32,678 to 36,069. During that same period, the number of DNP graduates increased from 7,039 to 7,944 (American Association of Colleges of Nursing, 2022). In addition, more nurses are stepping into advanced practice roles as nurse practitioners, clinical nurse specialists, certified nurse midwives, RN anesthetists, or clinical nurse-leaders. If knowledge is power, then those having knowledge can influence others, gain credibility, and gain power.

LEARNING EXERCISE 13.4

Cultural Diversity and Empowerment

Do you think that cultural diversity might be a challenge when empowering nurses? Think of ways that various cultures may view power and empowerment differently. If you know people from other cultures, ask them how powerful people or those in authority positions are viewed in their culture and compare that with your own culture.

Furthermore, leadership, management, and political theory are increasingly a part of baccalaureate nursing education, although many nurses still do not hold baccalaureate degrees. These are learned skills, and collectively, the nursing profession's knowledge of leadership, politics, negotiation, and finance is increasing. This can only strengthen the nursing profession's influence outside the field (Huston, 2023).

- *Nursing's unique perspective*. Professionals have power over the practice of their discipline. This is referred to as *professional autonomy*. Nursing has long been recognized as having a strong caring component. The combination of caring with nursing's recent surge in scientific knowledge and critical thinking creates a blend of art and science that brings a unique perspective to the health care arena.
- *Desire of consumers and providers for change*. Limited consumer choice, hospital restructuring, inadequate RN staffing, and the IOM medical error reports were sparks needed to mobilize nurses, as well as consumers, to act. Nurses began speaking out about how downsizing and restructuring were affecting the care they were providing, and the public began demanding accountability. The public does care who is caring for them and how that affects the quality of their care. The flaws of the health care system are no longer secret, and nursing can use its expertise and influence to help create a better health care system for the future.

An Action Plan for Increasing Professional Power in Nursing

Huston (2023) also developed an action plan for the nursing profession to build its power base (Display 13.3 shows a summary of these actions). This action plan includes the following strategies:

- *Place more nurses in positions of influence*. The National Academy of Sciences report *The Future of Nursing 2020–2030* suggests that nurses must lead and participate in multisectoral collaborations, serve in professional associations and organizations as well as on boards and expert panels, hold C-suite positions, and pursue political office. Fulfillment of this goal will require support, encouragement, mentorship, and advancement opportunities, with nurses operating to the full scope of their education, training, and expertise (National Academies Press, 2021). Progress to achieve this goal is being made through the work of groups such as the Nurses on Boards Coalition (NBC), a coalition founded by the ANA, the American Academy of Nursing, and the American Nurses Foundation (ANF), the charitable and philanthropic arm of ANA. The coalition, which first convened in 2014, set a goal to ensure that nurses filled at least 10,000 board seats by 2020. As of December 30, 2021, 10,353 nurses held board seats (NBC, 2022).

DISPLAY 13.3 ACTION PLAN FOR INCREASING THE POWER OF THE NURSING PROFESSION

1. Place more nurses in positions of influence.
2. Recognize and highlight the potential nurses have to make a difference.
3. Nurses must become better informed about all health care policy efforts.
4. Coalition building must occur within and outside of nursing.
5. More research must be done to strengthen evidence-based practice.
6. Nursing leaders must be supported.
7. Attention must be paid to mentoring future nurse-leaders and leadership succession.

Source: From Huston, C. J. (2023). The nursing profession's historic struggle to increase its power base. In C. J. Huston (Ed.), *Professional issues in nursing: Challenges and opportunities* (6th ed., pp. 338–352). Wolters Kluwer.

EXAMINING THE EVIDENCE 13.1

Source: From Millenbach, L., Niyirora, J., Sellers, K., & DeChance, C. (2021, August). Nursing expertise in the boardroom: NYONEL survey shows progress. *Nurse Leader, 19*(4), 341–347.

Characteristics and Roles of Nurses on Boards

The New York Organization of Nurse Executives and Leaders (NYONEL) conducted a survey of members regarding board membership, including examining board types and characteristics and the roles of nurses on boards. The study also looked at factors contributing to nurses obtaining positions on boards. A total of 84 of 518 potential participants completed the survey for a 16% return rate.

The data showed board members to be highly educated, with 48% (n = 30) having a doctorate degree, 47% (n = 29) had a master's degree, and the remainder 5% (n = 3) had a bachelor's degree. A majority of the respondents (n = 37) had some type of nursing executive certification. More than 85% of the respondents (n = 52) had been in their nursing careers for more than 20 years—a percentage that aligned with the respondents' age distribution and the vast majority (85%) were working full-time. Fifty-five percent (n = 32) were practicing nursing administrators.

Concerning their roles on the boards on which they served, 34 respondents (55%) were voting members with no other role. The remainder of the respondents held various positions, including chair and co-chair of the board.

Most respondents suggested that power structures on boards have become more equal, interprofessional, and collaborative over the past generation and the majority believed that boards work toward consensus as a decision-making model. In addition, most respondents believed that board members valued nursing's worldview and expertise. All respondents stressed that nursing perspective, experience, and leadership on various health care matters and community needs were invaluable.

The researchers concluded that although the results showed some encouraging results, there is a need for nursing associations at the state and national levels to continue their efforts, assisting nurses and nurse leaders to become prepared for board membership.

Research by Millenbach et al. (2021) noted that the most successful means of gaining a board seat was through expertise and networking (see Examining the Evidence 13.1). This suggests that increased education (graduate and doctoral level), the achievement of specialty nurse executive certification, coaching, and broad interprofessional networking may be helpful for younger nurses and those from underrepresented groups in gaining board seats.

Running for and holding elected office is, however, the ultimate in political activism and involvement. Only three nurses were serving in Congress as of May 2022 (American Nurses Association, 2022). Many more nurses hold elected office in state legislatures. Huston (2023) argues that nurses are uniquely qualified to hold public office because they have the greatest firsthand experience of problems faced by patients in today's health care system as well as an uncanny ability to translate the health care experience to the public. As a result, more nurses need to seek out this role. In addition, because the public respects and trusts nurses, nurses who choose to run for public office are often elected. The problem then is not that nurses are not elected; the problem is that not enough nurses are running for office.

- *Recognize and highlight the potential nurses have to make a difference.* Huston (2023) suggests it is critical that nurses never lose sight of their potential to make a difference. The bottom line is that the profession will only be as smart, as motivated, and as directed as its weakest link. If the nursing profession is to be the powerful force it can be, it needs to be filled with bright, highly motivated people who want to make a difference in the lives of the clients with whom they work as well as in the health care system itself.

"Some legislators and employers have argued that 'a nurse is a nurse, is a nurse.' This is wrong. Nurses can be whatever they want to be in nursing and they can achieve that goal at whatever level of quality they choose" (Huston, 2023).

- *Become better informed about all health care policy efforts.* This means becoming involved with grassroots knowledge building and becoming better informed consumers and providers of health care with a commitment to collective strength. This is difficult because no one can do this but nurses. Cardillo (2022) argues that every nurse can and should learn the ABCs of politics and power as a first step to personal and professional empowerment. She suggests that nurses should develop relationships with their legislators and contact their assemblypersons, congresspersons, and senators by phone or e-mail. These nurses should also introduce themselves as constituents in their district and offer to be a resource on nursing and health care issues. Cardillo (2022) goes on to suggest that every step an RN takes toward political awareness and activism benefits the entire profession. It is also one more way to impact the greater good and advocate for better health care for all.

- *Build coalitions inside and outside of nursing.* Health policy takes place in a virtual network of participants, professions, and organizations, both locally and nationally. Nurses have not always done well in building political coalitions with other interdisciplinary professionals who face similar challenges. In addition to belonging to nursing professional organizations, nurses need to reach out to other non-nursing groups with the same concerns and goals. This interdependence and strength in numbers is what will ultimately help the profession achieve its goals.

- *Conduct more research to strengthen evidence-based practice.* Great strides have been made in researching what it is that nurses do that makes a difference in patient outcomes (research on *nursing sensitivity*), but more needs to be done. Nurses must use research to present the case that nursing skills are vital to competent health care. In addition, building and sustaining evidence-based practice in nursing will require far greater numbers of master's- and doctorally prepared nurses as well as entry into practice at an educational level similar to other professions (Huston, 2023).

- *Support nursing leaders.* Rather than supporting their leaders' efforts to lead, nurses have sometimes viewed their leaders as deviants, and this has occurred at a high personal cost to the innovator. In addition, nurses often resist change from their leaders and instead look to leaders in medicine or other health-related disciplines. Thus, the division in nursing often comes from within the profession itself (Huston, 2023).

- *Mentor future nurse-leaders and plan for leadership succession.* Female-dominated professions such as nursing often exemplify the *queen bee syndrome*. The "queen bee" is a woman who has struggled to become successful, but once successful, she refuses to help other women reach the same success. This leads to inadequate empowering of new leaders by the older, more established leaders. Increased and adequate empowering of others, mentoring the young, and ensuring leadership succession are clearly needed to advance nursing leadership. Remember that the profession is responsible for ensuring leadership succession and is morally bound to do it with the brightest, most highly qualified individuals (Huston, 2023).

> Changing nurse's view of both power and politics is perhaps the most significant key to proactive rather than reactive participation in policy setting.

Strategies for Building a Personal Power Base

In addition to assisting with empowering the profession, nurse-leaders and nurse-managers must build a personal power base to further organizational goals, fulfill the leadership role, carry out management functions, and meet personal goals. Even a novice manager or newly graduated nurse can begin to build a power base in many ways. Habitual behaviors resulting from early lessons, passivity, and focusing on wrong targets can be replaced with new power-gaining behaviors. The following are suggested strategies for enhancing power.

Maintain Personal Energy

Power and energy go hand in hand. To take care of others, you must first take care of yourself. Effective leaders take enough time to unwind, reflect, rest, and have fun when they feel tired. Leader-managers who do not take care of themselves begin to make mistakes in judgment that may result in terrible political consequences.

> You must take care of yourself before you can take care of others.

Present a Powerful Picture to Others

How people look, act, and talk influence whether others view them as powerful or powerless. The nurse who stands tall and is poised, assertive, articulate, and well groomed presents a picture of personal control and power. The manager who looks like a victim will undoubtedly become one. When individuals take the time for self-care, they exude confidence. This is apparent in not only how they dress and act but also how they interact with others.

Work Hard and Be a Team Player

Newcomers who stand out and appear powerful are those who do more, work harder, and contribute to the organization. A power base is not achieved by slick, easy, or quick maneuvers but through hard work. It is important to be a team player. Showing a genuine interest in others, being considerate of other people's needs and wants, and offering others support whenever possible are all part of a successful team building. These interpersonal skills are part of emotional intelligence.

Determine the Powerful in the Organization

Understanding and working successfully within both formal and informal power structures are important strategies for building a personal power base. Individuals must be cognizant of their limitations and seek counsel appropriately. One should know the names and faces of those with both formal power and informal power. The powerful people in the informal structure are often more difficult to identify than those in the formal structure. When working with powerful people, look for similarities and shared values and avoid focusing on differences.

Learn the Language and Symbols of the Organization

Each organization has its own culture and value system. New members must understand this culture and be socialized into the organization if they are to build a power base. Being unaware of institutional taboos often results in embarrassment for the newcomer.

Learn How to Use the Organization's Priorities

Every group has its own goals and priorities for achieving those goals. Those seeking to build a power base must be cognizant of organizational goals and use those priorities and goals to meet management needs. For example, a need for a new manager in a community health service might be to develop educational programs on chemotherapy because some of the new patient caseload includes this nursing function. If fiscal management is a high priority, the manager needs to show superiors how the cost of these educational programs will be offset by additional revenues or improved quality of care.

Increase Professional Skills and Knowledge

Because employees are expected to perform their jobs well, one's performance must be extraordinary to enhance power. One method of being extraordinary is to increase professional skills and knowledge to an expert level. Having knowledge and skill that others lack greatly augments a person's power base. Excellence that reflects knowledge and demonstrates skill enhances a nurse's credibility and determines how others view them.

> Individuals may be born average, but staying average is a choice.

Maintain a Broad Vision

Vision is one of the most powerful tools that a leader has in their toolbox. Because workers are assigned to a unit or department, they often develop a narrow view of the total organization. Power builders always look upward and outward. The successful leader recognizes not only how the individual unit fits within the larger organization but also how the institution as a whole fits into the scheme of the total community. People without vision rarely become very powerful.

Use Experts and Seek Counsel

Newcomers should seek out role models. *Role models* are experienced, competent individuals an individual wants to emulate. Even though there may be no significant interpersonal relationship, one can learn a great deal about successful leadership, management, and decision making by observing and imitating positive role models. Aligning oneself with appropriate veterans in the organization is excellent for building power.

Be Flexible

Great leaders understand the power of flexibility. Anyone wishing to acquire power should develop a reputation as someone who can compromise. The rigid, uncompromising newcomer is viewed as being insensitive to the organization's needs.

Develop Visibility and a Voice in the Organization

Newcomers to an organization must become active in committees or groups that are recognized by the organization as having clout. When working in groups, the newcomer must not monopolize committee time. In addition, novice leaders and managers must develop observational, listening, and verbal skills. Their spoken contributions to the committee should be valuable and articulated well.

Experienced leader-managers must strive for visibility and voice as well. Managers who are too far removed from workers in the organization hierarchy can have a view that is cloudy or distorted. If workers do not know their managers, they will not trust them.

Learn to Accept Compliments

Accepting compliments is an art. One should be gracious but certainly not passive when praised for extraordinary effort. In addition, one should let others know when one has achieved some special professional recognition. This should be done in a manner that is not bragging but reflects the self-respect of one who is talented and unique.

TABLE **13.2** **LEADERSHIP STRATEGIES: DEVELOPING POWER AND POLITICAL SAVVY**

Power-Building Strategies	Political Strategies
Maintain personal energy	Develop information acquisition skills
Present a powerful persona	Communicate astutely
Work hard	Become a proactive decision maker
Be a team player	Assume authority
Determine the powerful	Engage in networking
Learn the organizational culture	Expand personal resources
Use organizational priorities	Maintain maneuverability
Increase skills and knowledge	Develop political alliances and coalitions
Have a broad vision	Remain sensitive to people, timing, and situations
Use experts and seek counsel	Promote subordinate identification
Be flexible	Meet organizational needs
Be visible and have a voice	Minimize ego-driven reactions
Accept compliments graciously	
Maintain a sense of humor	
Empower others	

Maintain a Sense of Humor

Appropriate humor is very effective. The ability to laugh at oneself and not take oneself too seriously is a most important power builder. Humor allows the leader to relax so that they can step away from the challenge and look at the circumstance in a different perspective.

Empower Others

Leaders need to empower others, and followers must empower their leaders. When nurses empower each other, they gain referent power. Nurses can empower other nurses by sharing knowledge, maintaining cohesiveness, valuing the profession, and supporting each other. Power-building and political strategies are summarized in Table 13.2.

LEARNING EXERCISE 13.5

Building Power as the New Nurse

You have been a registered nurse for 3 years. Six months ago, you left your position as a day charge nurse at one of the local hospitals to accept a position at the public health agency. You really miss your friends at the hospital and find most of the public health nurses older and aloof. However, you love working with your patients and have decided that this is where you want to build a lifetime career. Although you believe that you have some good ideas, you are aware that because you are new, your ability to act as a change agent will be limited. Eventually, you would like to be promoted to agency supervisor and become a powerful force for stimulating growth within the agency. You decide that you can do a few things to build a power base. You spend a weekend designing a personal power-building plan.

(continues on page 330)

LEARNING EXERCISE **13.5**

Building Power as the New Nurse (continued)

ASSIGNMENT:

Create a power-building plan. Give 6 to 10 specific examples of things you would do to build a power base in the new organization. Provide rationale for each selection. (Do not merely select from the general lists in the text. Outline specific actions that you would take.) It might be helpful to consider your own community and personal strengths when solving this learning exercise.

The Politics of Power

Politics is the art of using legitimate power wisely. It requires clear decision making, assertiveness, accountability, and the willingness to express one's own views. It also requires being proactive rather than reactive and demands decisiveness. Leader-managers in powerful positions in today's health care settings are more likely to recognize their innate abilities that support the effective use of power.

It is useless to argue the ethics or value of politics in an organization because politics exists in every organization. Thus, nurses waste energy and remain powerless when they refuse to learn the art and skill of political maneuvers. It is important then for managers to understand politics within the context of their employing organization and to function effectively within that structure.

After the employee has built a power base through hard work, increased personal power, and knowledge of the organization, developing skills in the politics of power is necessary. After all, power may not be gained indefinitely; it may be fleeting. For example, people often lose hard-earned power in an organization because they make political mistakes. Even seasoned leaders occasionally blunder in this arena.

> Although power is a universally available resource, it does not have a finite quality and can be lost as well as gained.

Understanding one's own power, however, can be frightening, especially when one considers that "attacks" (or opposition) from various fronts may reduce that power. When these attacks occur, people who hold powerful positions may undermine themselves by regressing rather than progressing and by being reactive rather than proactive. The following political strategies will help the novice manager to negate the negative effects of organizational politics:

- *Become an expert handler of information and communication.* Beware that facts can be presented seductively and out of context since information is often changed to fit others' needs. Managers must become artful at acquiring information and questioning others. Delay decisions until adequate and accurate information has been gathered and reviewed. Failing to do the necessary homework may lead to decisions with damaging political consequences.

  In addition, managers must not trap themselves by discussing something about which they know very little. The politically astute manager says, "I don't know" when adequate information is unavailable. Grave consequences can result from sharing the wrong information with the wrong people at the wrong time. Determining who should know, how much they should know, and when they should know requires great finesse.

One of the most politically serious errors that one can make is lying to others within the organization. Unlike withholding and refusing to divulge information, which may be good political strategies, lying destroys trust, and leaders must never underestimate the power of trust.

- *Be a proactive decision maker.* Proactive leaders prepare for the future instead of waiting for it. Seeing changes approaching in the health care system, they prepare to meet them, not fight them.

  Assuming authority is one way that nurses can become proactive. Instead of asking, "May I?", some leaders assume that they may. When people ask permission, they are really asking someone to take responsibility for them. If something is not expressly prohibited in an organization or a job description, the powerful leader assumes that it may be done. Politically astute nurses have been known to create new positions or new roles within a position simply by gradually assuming that they could do things that no one else was doing. In other words, they saw a need in the organization and started meeting it. The organization, by default, allowed expansion of the role. People need to be aware, however, that if they assume authority and something goes wrong, they will be held accountable, so this strategy is not without risk. Do not, however, ask for permission if "no" is not an option.

- *Expand personal resources.* Because organizations are dynamic and the future is impossible to predict, the proactive nurse prepares for the future by expanding personal resources. Personal resources include economic stability, higher education, and a broadened skill base. Some call this the political strategy of "having maneuverability." People with "money in the bank and gas in the tank" have a political freedom of maneuverability that others do not. People lose power if others within the organization know that they cannot afford to make a job change or lack the necessary skills to do so. Likewise, the nurse who has not developed additional skills or sought further education loses the political strength that comes from being able to find quality employment elsewhere.

- *Develop political alliances and coalitions.* Nurses often can increase their power and influence by forming coalitions and alliances (networking) with other groups, be they peers, sponsors, or subordinates, especially when these alliances are with peers outside the organization. In this manner, the manager keeps abreast of current happenings and consults others for advice and counsel. More power and political clout result from working together rather than alone. When a person faces political opposition from others in the organization, group power is very useful.

> Nurses must be represented in mass, in some way, before they will be able to significantly impact the decisions that directly influence their own profession.

- *Be sensitive to timing.* Successful leaders are sensitive to the appropriateness and timing of their actions. The person who presents a request to attend an expensive nursing conference on the same afternoon that their supervisor just had extensive dental work typifies someone who is insensitive to timing. Besides being able to choose the right moment, the effective manager should develop skill in other areas of timing, such as knowing when it is appropriate to do nothing. The sensitive manager also learns when to stop requesting something. That time is before your boss issues a firm "no," at which point continuing to press the issue is politically unwise.

- *Promote subordinate identification.* Rewarding excellence is an effective political strategy. A manager can promote the identification of subordinates in many ways. A simple "thank you" for a job well done works well when spoken in front of someone else. Calling attention to the extra efforts of subordinates says in effect, "Look what a good job we are capable of doing." Sending subordinates sincere notes of appreciation is another way of praising and promoting.

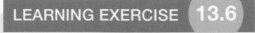

LEARNING EXERCISE 13.6

A Shifting of Power

The following is based on a real event. The cast includes Sally Jones, the chief nursing officer; Jane Smith, the hospital administrator and chief executive officer; and Bob Black, the assistant hospital administrator. Sally has been in her position at Memorial Hospital for 2 years. She has made many improvements in the nursing department and is generally respected by the hospital administrator, the nursing staff, and the physicians.

The present situation involves the newly hired Bob Black. Previously too small to have an assistant administrator, the hospital has grown, and this position was created. One of the departments assigned to Bob is the personnel and payroll department. Until now, nursing, which comprises 45% of all personnel, has done its own recruiting, interviewing, and selecting. Since Bob has been hired, he has shown obvious signs that he would like to increase his power and authority. Now, Bob has proposed that he hire an additional clerk who will do much of the personnel work for the nursing department, although nursing administration will be able to make the final selections in hiring. Bob proposes that his department should do the initial screening of applicants, seeking references, and so on. Sally has grown increasingly frustrated in dealing with the encroachment of Bob. Having just received Bob's latest proposal, she has requested to meet with Jane Smith and Bob to discuss the plan.

ASSIGNMENT:

What danger, if any, is there for Sally Jones in Bob Black's proposal? Explain two political strategies that you believe Sally could use in the upcoming meeting. Is it possible to facilitate a win–win solution to this conflict? If so, how? If there is not a win–win solution, how much can Sally win?
Note: Attempt to solve this case before reading the solution presented in the Appendix.

- *View personal and unit goals in terms of the organization.* Even extraordinary and visible activities will not result in desired power unless those activities are used to meet organizational goals. Frequently, novice managers think only in terms of their needs and their problems rather than seeing the large picture. Moreover, people often look upward for solutions rather than attempting to find answers themselves. When problems are identified, it is more politically astute to take the problem and a proposed solution upward rather than just presenting the problem to the superior. Although the superior may not accept the solution, the effort to problem solve will be appreciated.
- *Minimize ego-driven reactions.* Although political actions can be negative, you should try not to take political attacks personally. Likewise, be careful about accepting credit for political successes because you may just have been in the right place at the right time. Be prepared as a manager to make political errors. The key to success is how quickly you rebound.

Integrating Leadership Roles and Management Functions When Using Authority and Power in Organizations

A manager's ability to gain and wisely use power is critical to their success. Nurses will never be assured of adequate resources until they gain the power to manipulate the needed resources legitimately. To do this, managers must be able to bridge the authority–power gap, build a personal power base, and minimize the negative politics of the organization.

One of the most critical leadership roles in the use of power and authority is the empowerment of subordinates. The leader recognizes that some degree of power is held by all in the organization, including subordinates, peers, and higher administrators.

The key then to establishing and keeping authority and power in an organization is for the leader-manager to be able to accomplish four separate tasks:

- Maintain a small authority–power gap.
- Empower subordinates whenever possible.
- Use authority in such a manner that subordinates view what happens in the organization as necessary.
- When needed, implement political strategies to maintain power and authority.

Integrating the leadership roles and the functions of management reduces the risk that power will be misused. Power and authority will be used to increase respect for the position and for nursing as a whole. The leader comfortable with power ensures that the goal of political maneuvers is cooperation, not personal gain. The successful manager who has integrated the role of leadership will not seek to have power over others but instead will empower others. It is imperative for leader-managers to become skillful in the art of politics and the use of political strategy if they are to survive in the corporate world of the health care industry. It is with the use of such strategies that organizational resources are obtained and goals are achieved.

 Key Concepts

- Power and authority are necessary components of leadership and management.
- A person's response to authority is influenced early through authority figures, experiences in the family unit, and gender role identification.
- The gap that sometimes exists between a position of authority and subordinate response is called the authority–power gap.
- The empowerment of staff is a hallmark of transformational leadership. Empowerment means to enable, develop, or allow.
- Power has both a positive and a negative face.
- Traditionally, women have been socialized to view power differently than men do. However, recent studies show that gender differences regarding power are changing.
- Reward power is obtained by the ability to grant rewards to others.
- Coercive power is based on fear and punishment.
- Legitimate power is the power inherent in one's position.
- Expert power is gained through knowledge or skill.
- Referent power is obtained through association with others.
- Charismatic power results from a dynamic and powerful persona.

- Information power is gained when someone has information that another needs.
- Female-dominated professions such as nursing often exemplify the *queen bee syndrome*. The "queen bee" is a woman who has struggled to become successful, but once successful, she refuses to help other women reach the same success.
- Even a novice manager or newly graduated nurse can begin to build a power base by using appropriate power-building tactics.
- Power gained may be lost because one is politically naive or fails to use appropriate political strategies.
- Politics exist in every organization, and leader-managers must learn the art and skills of politics.
- The nursing profession has not been the political force it could be because historically, it has been more reactive than proactive in addressing needed policy decisions and legislation.
- Numerous driving forces are in place to increase the nursing profession's power base, including timing, the size of the profession, nursing's referent power, the increasing educational levels of nurses, nursing's unique perspective, and the desire of consumers and providers for change.

Additional Learning Exercises and Applications

LEARNING EXERCISE 13.7

Empowering Your Staff

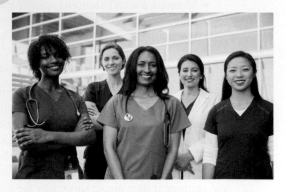

After 5 years as a public health nurse, you have just been appointed as supervisor of the Western region of the county health department. There is one supervisor for each region, a nursing director, and an assistant director. You have eight nurses who report directly to you. Your organization seems to have few barriers to prevent staff empowerment, but in talking with the staff who report to you, they frequently express feelings of powerlessness in their ability to effect lasting change in their patients or in changing policies within the organization. Your first planned change, therefore, is to develop strategies to empower them.

ASSIGNMENT:

Devise a political strategy for successfully empowering the staff who report directly to you. Consider the three elements necessary in the empowerment process: professional traits of the staff, a supportive environment, and effective leadership. Of these things, what is in your sphere of control? Where is the danger of your plan being sabotaged? What change tactics can you use to increase the likelihood of success?

LEARNING EXERCISE 13.8

Friendships and Truth

You are a middle-level manager in a public health department. One of your closest friends, Janie, is a registered nurse under your span of control. Today, Janie calls and tells you that she injured her back yesterday during a home visit after she slipped on a wet front porch. She said that the homeowners were unaware that she fell and that no one witnessed the accident. She has just returned from visiting her doctor who advises 6 weeks of bed rest. She requests that you initiate the paperwork for workers' compensation and disability because she has no sick days left.

Shortly after your telephone conversation with Janie, you take a brief coffee break in the lounge. You overhear a conversation between Jon and Lacey, two additional staff members in your department. Jon says that he and Janie were water skiing last night, and she took a terrible fall and hurt her back. He planned to call her to see how she was feeling.

You initially feel hurt and betrayed by Janie because you believe that she has lied to you. You want to call Janie and confront her. You want to deny her request for workers' compensation and disability. You are angry that she has placed you in this position. You are also aware that proving Janie's injury is not work related may be difficult.

ASSIGNMENT:

How should you proceed? What are the political ramifications if this incident is not handled properly? How should you use your power and authority when dealing with this problem?

LEARNING EXERCISE 13.9

Decision Making: Conflict and Dilemma

You are the director of a small Native American health clinic. Other than yourself and a part-time physician, your only professional staff members are two registered nurses (RNs). The remaining staff members are Native Americans and have been trained by you.

Because Nurse Bennett, a 26-year-old female Bachelor of Science in Nursing graduate, has had several years of experience working at a large southwestern community health agency, she is familiar with many of the patients' problems. She is hard working and extremely knowledgeable. Occasionally, her assertiveness is mistaken for bossiness among the Native American workers. However, everyone respects her judgment.

The other RN, Nurse Mikiou, is a 34-year-old male Native American. He started as a medic in the Persian Gulf War and attended several career-ladder external degree programs until he was able to take the RN examination. He does not have a baccalaureate degree. His nursing knowledge is occasionally limited, and he tends to be very casual about performing his duties. However, he is competent and has never shown unsafe judgment. His humor and good nature often reduce tension in the clinic. The Native American population is very proud of him, and he has a special relationship with them. However, he is not a particularly good role model because his health habits leave much to be desired, and he is frequently absent from work.

Nurse Bennett has come to find Nurse Mikiou intolerable. She believes that she has tried working with him, but this is difficult because she does not respect him. As the director of the clinic, you have tried many ways to solve this problem. You feel especially fortunate to have Nurse Bennett on your staff. It is difficult to find many nurses of her quality willing to come and live on a Native American reservation. On the other hand, if the care is to be as culturally relevant as possible, the Native Americans themselves must be educated and placed in the agencies so that one day they can run their own clinics. It is very difficult to find Native Americans who have received the right education and want to return to this reservation. Now, you are faced with a management dilemma. Nurse Bennett has said that either Nurse Mikiou must go, or she will go. She has asked you to decide.

ASSIGNMENT:

List the factors bearing on this decision. What (if any) power issues are involved? Which choice will be the least damaging? Justify your decision.

LEARNING EXERCISE 13.10

Power Struggle

You are a team leader on a medical unit of a small community hospital. Your shift is 3:00 to 11:00 PM. When leaving the report room, John, the day-shift team leader, tells you that Mrs. Jackson, a patient who is terminally ill with cancer, has decided to check herself out of the hospital "against medical advice." John states that he has already contacted Mrs. Jackson's doctor, who expressed his concern that the patient would have inadequate pain control at home and undependable family support. He believes that she will die within a few days if she leaves the hospital. He did, however, leave orders for home prescriptions and a follow-up appointment.

You immediately go into Mrs. Jackson's room to assess the situation. She tells you that the doctor has told her she will probably die within 6 weeks and that she wants to spend what time she has left at home with her little dog who has been her constant companion for many years. In addition, she has many things "to put in order." She states that she is fully aware of her doctor's concerns and that she was already informed by the day-shift nurse that leaving "against medical advice" may result in the insurance company refusing to pay for her current hospitalization. She states that she will be leaving in 15 minutes when her ride home arrives.

When you go to the nurse's station to get a copy of the home prescriptions and follow-up doctor's appointment for the patient, the unit clerk states, "The hospital policy says that patients who leave against medical advice have to contact the physician directly for prescriptions and an appointment because they are not legally discharged. The hospital has no obligation to provide this service. She made the choice—now let her live with it." She refuses to give a copy of the orders to you and places the patient's chart in her lap. Short of physically removing the chart from the clerk's lap, you clearly have no immediate access to the orders.

You confront the charge nurse, who is unsure what to do and who states that the hospital policy does give that responsibility to the patient. The unit director, who has been paged, appears to be out of the hospital temporarily.

You are outraged. You believe that the patient has the "right" to her prescriptions because the doctor ordered them, assuming she would receive them before she left. You also know that if the medications are not dispensed by the hospital, there is little likelihood that Mrs. Jackson will have the resources to have the prescriptions filled. Five minutes later, Mrs. Jackson appears at the nurse's station, accompanied by her friend. She states that she is leaving and would like her discharge prescriptions.

ASSIGNMENT:

The power struggle in this scenario involves you, the unit clerk, the charge nurse, and organizational politics. Does the unit clerk in this scenario have informal or formal power? What alternatives for action do you have? What are the costs or consequences of each possible alternative? What action would you take?

LEARNING EXERCISE 13.11

Ego and the Chain of Command

You are the day-shift charge nurse for the intensive care unit. One of your nurses, Carol, has just requested a week off to attend a conference. She is willing to use her accrued vacation time for this and to pay the expenses herself. The conference is in 1 month, and you are a little irritated with her for not coming to you sooner. Carol's request conflicts with a vacation that you have given another nurse. This nurse requested her vacation 3 months ago.

You deny Carol's request, explaining that you will need her to work that week. Carol protests, stating that the educational conference will benefit the intensive care unit and repeating that she will bear the cost. You are firm but polite in your refusal. Later, Carol goes to the supervisor of the unit to request the time. Although the supervisor upholds your decision, you are upset because you believe that Carol has gone over your head inappropriately in handling this matter.

ASSIGNMENT:

Were Carol's actions appropriate? Does ego impact your response? How are you going to deal with Carol? Decide on your approach and support it with political rationale.

LEARNING EXERCISE 13.12

When You Have a Large Authority–Power Gap

You are a fairly recent registered nurse (RN) graduate. Prior to becoming an RN, you were a licensed vocational nurse (LVN)/licensed practical nurse (LPN) for 8 years and worked at the same hospital in that capacity as you do now as an RN. One of your closest friends, Jina, is an LVN/LPN under your span of control. Although Jina has told you that she is proud of you and glad that you returned to school to obtain your RN license, some of her actions have bothered you. She openly questions some of your instructions and often takes an extra 10 minutes for her breaks. She sometimes laughingly makes remarks about your new status, implying being an RN has "gone to your head."

Today, while doing your end-of-shift charting, you noticed that Jina had not recorded intake and output amounts or vital signs on some of her patients. When you question her, she says, "Oh, you gave me too much to do today and I thought I would leave those for you to do for me."

You feel hurt and betrayed by Jina because you believe that she is directly challenging your new status of team leader. You are not sure what you should do to narrow the authority–power gap because it is becoming obvious that Jina is openly defiant. For you to be successful in your role as team leader, you must take some action to solve this dilemma.

ASSIGNMENT:

How should you proceed? What are the political ramifications if this incident is not handled properly? How should you use your power and authority when dealing with this problem?

REFERENCES

American Association of Colleges of Nursing. (2022). *DNP factsheet*. Retrieved April 30, 2022, from https://www.aacnnursing.org/News-Information/Fact-Sheets/DNP-Fact-Sheet

American Nurses Association. (2022). *Nurses Serving in Congress*. Retrieved April 30, 2022, from http://www.nursingworld.org/MainMenuCategories/Policy-Advocacy/Federal/Nurses-in-Congress

Cardillo, D. (2022). *Nurses, politics, power*. DonnaCardillo.com. https://donnacardillo.com/articles/nursespoliticspower/

Huston, C. J. (2023). The nursing profession's historic struggle to increase its power base. In C. J. Huston (Ed.), *Professional issues in nursing: Challenges and opportunities* (6th ed., pp. 338–352). Wolters Kluwer.

Mind Tools Content Team. (2022). *French and Raven's five forms of power. Understanding where power comes from in the workplace*. Emerald Works Limited. http://www.mindtools.com/pages/article/newLDR_56.htm

National Academy of Medicine. (2021). *The future of nursing 2020–2030: Charting a path to achieve health Equity*. National Academies Press. https://nap.nationalacademies.org/read/25982/chapter/1

Nurses on Boards Coalition. (2022). *Welcome to the Nurses on Boards Coalition Website*. Retrieved May 1, 2022, from https://www.nursesonboardscoalition.org/

U.S. Department of Labor. (2022). *Occupational employment and wage statistics*. Occupational employment and wages, May 2021. 29–1141 Registered Nurses. Retrieved May 1, 2022, from https://www.bls.gov/oes/current/oes291141.htm

14

Organizing Patient Care

... patients now more than ever need reassurance that they are indeed the focus of the healthcare team.—**Joan Shinkus Clark**

... nurses have gone beyond the role of caregivers to become key integrators, care coordinators and efficiency experts who are redesigning the patient experience through new, innovative healthcare delivery models.—**Linda Beattle**

... take care of the patient and everything else will follow.—**Thomas Frist**

CROSSWALK

This chapter addresses:

- **AACN Essentials Domain 2:** Person-centered care
- **AACN Essentials Domain 3:** Population health
- **AACN Essentials Domain 5:** Quality and safety
- **AACN Essentials Domain 6:** Interprofessional partnerships
- **AACN Essentials Domain 7:** Systems-based practice
- **AACN Essentials Domain 9:** Professionalism
- **AACN Essentials Domain 10:** Personal, professional, and leadership development
- **AONL Nurse Executive Competency 1:** Communication and relationship building
- **AONL Nurse Executive Competency 2:** A knowledge of the health care environment
- **ANA Standard of Professional Performance 8:** Advocacy
- **ANA Standard of Professional Performance 9:** Communication
- **ANA Standard of Professional Performance 11:** Collaboration
- **ANA Standard of Professional Performance 12:** Leadership
- **ANA Standard of Professional Performance 15:** Quality of practice
- **ANA Standard of Professional Performance 16:** Professional practice evaluation
- **ANA Standard of Professional Performance 17:** Resource stewardship
- **ANA Standard of Professional Performance 18:** Environmental health
- **QSEN Competency:** Teamwork and collaboration
- **QSEN Competency:** Patient-centered care
- **QSEN Competency:** Quality improvement
- **QSEN Competency:** Safety

LEARNING OBJECTIVES

The learner will:

- differentiate among various types of patient care delivery systems, including total patient care, functional nursing, team nursing, modular nursing, primary nursing, and case management
- discuss the historical events that led to the evolution of different types of patient care delivery models

- debate the driving and restraining forces for reserving the primary nurse role for the registered nurse
- describe the challenges as well as the benefits of using interprofessional health care teams in the delivery of patient care
- reflect on how interprofessional education might better prepare multidisciplinary health care providers to collaborate in planning and implementing care
- delineate new roles that are expanding the role of nurses beyond caregivers to key integrators, care coordinators, and efficiency experts such as case managers, nurse navigators, and clinical nurse-leaders (CNLs)
- describe the role competencies expected of the CNL, as described by the American Association of Colleges of Nursing
- differentiate between case management and population-based health care management
- identify desired outcomes in disease management programs and the role the case manager plays in achieving those outcomes
- differentiate between nurse case managers and nurse navigators
- discuss how work redesign may affect social relationships on a unit
- explain what effect staff mix has on work design and patient care organization
- identify factors that must be evaluated before initiating a change in a patient care delivery system

Introduction

Top-level managers are most likely to influence the philosophy and resources needed for any effective care delivery system because without a supporting philosophy and adequate resources, the most well-intentioned delivery system will fail. It is the first- and middle-level managers, however, who generally have the greatest influence on the organizing phase of the management process at the unit or department level. It is here that leader-managers organize how work is to be done, shape the organizational climate, and determine how patient care delivery is organized.

In addition, the unit leader-manager determines how best to plan work activities so that organizational goals are met effectively and efficiently. This involves using resources wisely and coordinating activities with other departments because how activities are organized can impede or facilitate communication, flexibility, and job satisfaction.

For organizing functions to be productive and meet the organization's needs, the leader must also know the organization and its members well. Activities will be unsuccessful if their design does not meet group needs and capabilities. The roles and functions of the leader-manager in organizing groups for patient care are shown in Display 14.1.

Traditional Models of Patient Care Organization

Five traditional means of organizing nursing are total patient care, functional nursing, team and modular nursing, primary nursing, and case management (Display 14.2). Each of these models has undergone many modifications, often resulting in new terminology. For example, primary nursing was once called case method nursing and is now frequently referred to as a *professional practice model*. Team nursing is sometimes called *partners in care* or *patient service partners*, and case managers assume different titles depending on the setting in which they provide care.

Even many of the newer models of patient care delivery systems are recycled, modified, or retitled versions of these older models. It is rare to find a delivery system that has never changed or one that does not have parts of others in its design.

LEADERSHIP ROLES AND MANAGEMENT FUNCTIONS ASSOCIATED WITH ORGANIZING PATIENT CARE

DISPLAY **14.1**

Leadership Roles

1. Evaluates periodically the effectiveness of the organizational structure for the delivery of patient care
2. Determines if adequate resources and support exist before making any changes in the organization of patient care
3. Examines the human element in work redesign and supports personnel during adjustment to change
4. Inspires the work group toward a team effort
5. Inspires subordinates to achieve higher levels of education, clinical expertise, competency, and experience in differentiated practice
6. Ensures that chosen nursing care delivery models advance the practice of professional nursing
7. Encourages and supports the use of nursing care delivery models that maximize the abilities of each member on the health care team
8. Assures congruence between the organizational mission and philosophy and the patient care delivery system selected for use
9. Assures that each member of the interprofessional/multidisciplinary team participates in team planning and feels their expertise is valued
10. Assures that the patient and family are the focus of patient care delivery, regardless of which patient care delivery system is used

Management Functions

1. Makes changes in work design to facilitate meeting organizational goals
2. Selects a patient care delivery system that is most appropriate to the needs of the patients being served as well as the expertise of the staffing mix
3. Uses scientific research and current literature to analyze proposed changes in nursing care delivery models
4. Uses a patient care delivery system that maximizes human and physical resources as well as time
5. Ensures that nonprofessional staff are appropriately trained and supervised in the provision of care
6. Organizes work activities to attain organizational goals
7. Groups activities in a manner that facilitates communication and coordination within and between departments
8. Organizes work to be as time-effective and cost-effective as possible
9. Appropriately identifies cost drivers in high-cost, high-resource utilization diseases and organizes patient care to address these with efficiency across care settings
10. Establishes interprofessional/multidisciplinary health care teams to improve patient outcomes
11. Provides opportunities for different health care professionals to complete interprofessional education
12. Explores opportunities to use case managers, nurse navigators, and clinical nurse-leaders to better integrate and coordinate care

DISPLAY **14.2**   **TRADITIONAL PATIENT CARE DELIVERY METHODS**

Total patient care
Functional nursing
Team and modular nursing

Primary nursing
Case management

Although some of these care delivery systems were developed to organize care in hospitals, most can be adapted to other settings. The choice of an organization model involves staff skills, availability of resources, patient acuity, and the nature of the work to be performed.

> Some newer models of patient care delivery systems are merely recycled, modified, or retitled versions of older models.

Total Patient Care Nursing or Case Method Nursing

Total patient care is the oldest mode of organizing patient care. With total patient care, a care provider assumes total responsibility during their time on duty for meeting all the needs of assigned patients. A structural diagram of total patient care in an acute care setting is shown in Figure 14.1.

Total patient care nursing is sometimes referred to as the *case method of assignment* because patients may be assigned as cases, much like the way private duty nursing was historically carried out. Indeed, at the turn of the 19th century, total patient care was the predominant nursing care delivery model. Care was generally provided in the patient's home, and in addition to traditional nursing care, the nurse was responsible for cooking, house cleaning, and other activities specific to the patient and family. During the Great Depression of the 1930s, however, people could no longer afford private duty nurses and care shifted to hospitals instead. As hospitals grew over the next two to three decades, total care continued to be the primary means of organizing patient care.

This method of assignment is still widely used in hospitals and home health agencies today because of its advantages. For example, total patient care provides caregivers with high autonomy and responsibility. Assigning patients is simple and direct and does not require the planning that other methods of patient care delivery require. In addition, the lines of responsibility and accountability are clear, so the patient theoretically receives holistic and unfragmented care during the caregiver's time on duty.

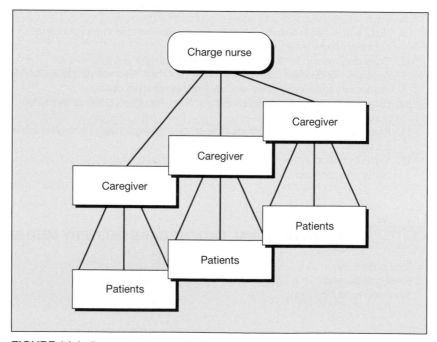

FIGURE 14.1 Case method or total patient care structure.

LEARNING EXERCISE 14.1

How Many Patients Are Too Many?

You are totally responsible for a patient's care, including bathing; bed making; vital signs; all medications; managing intravenous line; updating the patient care plan; and carrying out all ordered treatments, dressing changes, patient teaching, and discharge planning, etc. How many patients do you feel you could manage while providing good quality patient care? When you observe nurses in your clinical facility, how many patients do they care for? Write a one- to two-page essay detailing your response.

There are, however, disadvantages to this model as well. Each caregiver caring for the patient can theoretically modify the care regimen. Therefore, if there are three shifts, the patient could receive three different approaches to care, often confusing the patient. In addition, to maintain quality care, this method requires highly skilled personnel and thus may cost more than some other forms of patient care. Indeed, some tasks performed by the primary caregiver might be accomplished by someone with less training and therefore at a lower cost.

The greatest disadvantage of total patient care delivery, however, occurs when the caregiver is inadequately prepared or too inexperienced to provide total care to the patient. In the early days of nursing, only registered nurses (RNs) provided total patient care; now some hospitals assign licensed vocational nurses (LVNs)/licensed practical nurses (LPNs) as well as unlicensed health care workers to provide much of the nursing care. Because the co-assigned RN may have a heavy patient load, there may be little opportunity for supervision, which could cause unsafe care.

Functional Method

The *functional method* of delivering nursing care evolved primarily because of World War II and the rapid construction of hospitals associated with the Hill–Burton Act. Because nurses were in great demand overseas and at home, a nursing shortage developed, and ancillary personnel were needed to assist in patient care.

In functional nursing then, personnel were assigned to complete certain tasks rather than care for specific patients, and relatively unskilled workers were able to gain proficiency by task repetition. Examples of functional nursing tasks were checking blood pressures, administering medication, changing linens, and bathing patients. RNs became managers of care rather than direct care providers, and "care through others" became the phrase used to refer to this method of nursing care. Functional nursing structure is shown in Figure 14.2.

The functional form of organizing patient care was thought to be temporary, as it was assumed that when the war ended, hospitals would not need ancillary workers. However, the baby boom and resulting population growth immediately following World War II left the country short of nurses. Thus, employment of personnel with various levels of skill and education proliferated as new categories of health care workers were created. Currently, most health care organizations continue to employ health care workers of many educational backgrounds and skill levels.

Most administrators consider functional nursing to be an economical and efficient means of providing care. This is true if quality care and holistic care are not the highest priority. A major advantage of functional nursing is its efficiency; tasks are completed quickly, with little confusion regarding responsibilities. In addition, functional nursing allows care to be provided with a minimal number of RNs, and in many areas, such as the operating room, the functional structure works well and is still very much in evidence. Long-term care facilities also frequently use a functional approach to nursing care.

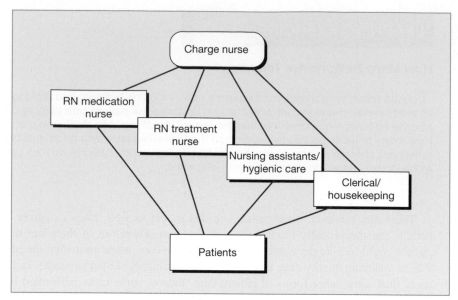

FIGURE 14.2 Functional nursing organization structure. RN, registered nurse.

During the past decade, however, the use of *unlicensed assistive personnel* (UAP), also known as *nursing assistive personnel*, in health care organizations has increased. Many nurse administrators believe that assigning low-skill tasks to UAP frees the professional nurse to perform more highly skilled duties and is therefore more economical; however, others argue that the time needed to supervise the UAP negates any time savings that may have occurred. Most modern administrators would undoubtedly deny that they are using functional nursing; yet, the trend of assigning tasks to workers, rather than assigning workers to the professional nurse, resembles, at least in part, functional nursing.

Functional nursing may, however, lead to fragmented care and the possibility of overlooking patient priority needs. In addition, because some workers feel unchallenged and understimulated in their roles, functional nursing may result in low job satisfaction. Employees may also focus only on their own efforts and be less interested in overall results. Functional nursing may also not be cost-effective due to the need for many coordinators.

Team Nursing

Despite a continued shortage of professional nursing staff in the 1950s, many believed that a patient care system had to be developed that reduced the fragmented care that accompanied functional nursing. *Team nursing* was the result. In team nursing, ancillary personnel collaborate in providing care to a group of patients under the direction of a professional nurse. As the team leader, the nurse is responsible for knowing the condition and needs of all the patients assigned to the team and for planning individual care. The team leader's duties vary depending on the patient's needs and the workload. These duties may include assisting team members, giving direct personal care to patients, teaching, and coordinating patient activities. Team nursing structure is illustrated in Figure 14.3.

One of the greatest advantages of team nursing is that through extensive team communication, comprehensive care can be provided for patients despite a relatively high proportion of ancillary staff. This communication occurs informally between the team leader and the individual team members and formally through regular team planning conferences. A team should consist of not more than five people or it will revert to more functional lines of organization.

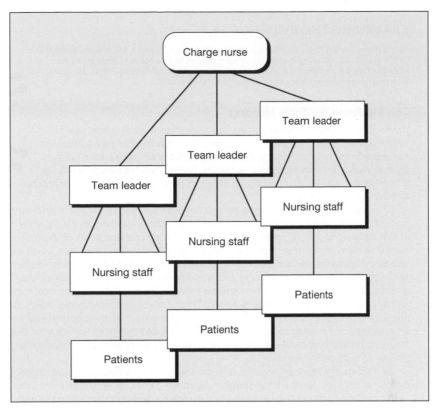

FIGURE 14.3 Team nursing organization structure.

Team nursing is also usually associated with democratic leadership. Group members are given as much autonomy as possible when performing assigned tasks, although the team shares responsibility and accountability collectively.

Team nursing also allows members to contribute their own special expertise or skills. Team leaders, then, should use their knowledge about each member's abilities when making patient assignments. Recognizing the individual worth of all employees and giving team members autonomy results in high job satisfaction.

Disadvantages to team nursing arise primarily because of improper implementation rather than the philosophy itself. For team nursing to be effective then, the team leader must be an

LEARNING EXERCISE 14.2

Transitioning to Total Patient Care

Most nursing students begin their clinical training by doing some form of functional nursing care and then advancing to total patient care for a small number of patients. Reflect on your earliest clinical experiences as a student nurse. Which tasks were easiest for you to learn? How did you gain mastery of those tasks? Was task mastery a time-consuming process for you? Was it difficult to make the transition to total patient care? If so, why? What skills were most difficult for you to learn in providing total patient care? Do you anticipate having to learn additional skills to feel comfortable in the role of total care provider as a registered nurse? What higher level skills do you think will be the hardest to learn and be confident with?

EXAMINING THE EVIDENCE 14.1

Source: From Beckett, C. D., Zadvinskis, I. M., Dean, J., Iseler, J., Powell, J. M., & Buck-Maxwell, B. (2021, August 6). An integrative review of team nursing and delegation: Implications for nurse staffing during COVID-19. *World Views on Evidence-Based Nursing, 18*(4), 251–260. https://sigmapubs.onlinelibrary.wiley.com/doi/10.1111/wvn.12523

The Evidence for Team Nursing

An integrative review of team nursing and delegation was completed using Whittemore and Knafl's (2005) methodology to review the evidence for team nursing as a model of patient care and delegation and determine how it affects patient, nurse, and organizational outcomes. Twenty-two team nursing articles, 21 delegation articles, and two papers about US nursing laws and scopes of practice for delegation were reviewed.

The researchers found that team nursing had both positive and negative outcomes for patients, nurses, and the organization. Overall, the team nursing model did not show a statistically significant difference in patient satisfaction compared with other models of care. One study reported desirable patient outcomes such as decreased pain scores and decreased seclusion and restraints compared with other nursing care models. Another study reported decreased medication errors and fewer emergency codes outside the ICU after implementing a modified team nursing model (with more licensed practical nurses [LPNs] and unlicensed assistive personnel [UAP] and fewer registered nurses [RNs]). Two studies reported decreased falls with team nursing compared with the patient allocation or modified team nursing model with fewer RNs, although another study reported that the evidence surrounding team nursing had inconsistent findings on falls and medication errors compared with other care models.

Several studies reported negative outcomes with team nursing such as increased adverse events compared with the patient allocation model, decreased mobility compared with a modified primary nursing model, and decreased quality of care compared with primary nursing. Delegation education, however, improved team nursing care.

In addition, 10 studies examined the effect of team nursing on RN job satisfaction and engagement. Findings across these studies were inconsistent. Three studies reported an improvement in job satisfaction; three studies reported a reduction; and three studies reported no difference. The systematic review by Fernandez et al. (2012) also found conflicting evidence about RN satisfaction.

Organizational outcomes were also examined. When compared with other models of care, team nursing had mixed effects on cost. Two studies reported on care quality; one reported that quality of care scores improved twice as much with a primary nursing model compared with team nursing. A systematic review contained two papers that reported quality of care. The first paper compared primary and team nursing models and found no difference between the two models regarding quality of patient care and the second compared numerous models of care and found no difference in quality of patient care between the models.

The researchers concluded that although there is a body of evidence about team nursing, the lack of consistent effects on outcomes makes it challenging to recommend it as a model of care.

excellent practitioner and have good communication, organizational, management, and leadership skills.

A recent integrative review found overall, however, that there was no statistically significant difference in patient outcomes between team nursing compared with other models of care (Beckett et al., 2021). Similarly, most of the evidence about nursing and organizational outcomes was conflicted. The researchers concluded that although there is a body of evidence about team nursing, the lack of consistent effects on outcomes makes it challenging to recommend it as a primary model of care (see Examining the Evidence 14.1).

Modular Nursing

Team nursing, as originally designed, has undergone much modification since its inception. Most team nursing was never practiced in its purest form but was instead a combination of team and functional structure. More recent attempts to refine and improve team nursing have resulted in many models including *modular nursing*.

> Most team nursing was never practiced in its purest form but was instead a combination of team and functional structure.

Modular nursing uses a *mini-team* (two or three members with at least one member being an RN), with members of the modular nursing team sometimes being called *care pairs*. In modular nursing, patient care units are typically divided into modules or districts, and assignments are based on the geographical location of patients.

Keeping the team small in modular nursing and attempting to assign personnel to the same team as often as possible should allow the professional nurse more time for planning and coordinating team members. In addition, a small team requires less communication, allowing members better use of their time for direct patient care activities.

LEARNING EXERCISE 14.3

Reorganizing to Accommodate a Change in Staffing Mix

You are the head nurse of an oncology unit. At present, the patient care delivery method on the unit is total patient care. You have a staff composed of 60% registered nurses (RNs), 35% licensed practical nurses (LPNs)/licensed vocational nurses (LVNs), and 5% clerical staff. Your bed capacity is 28, but your average daily census is 24. An example of day-shift staffing follows:

- One charge nurse who notes orders, talks with physicians, organizes care, makes assignments, and acts as a resource person and problem solver
- Three RNs who provide total patient care, including administering all treatments and medications to their assigned patients, giving intravenous (IV) medications to the LVNs/LPNs' assigned patients, and acting as a clinical resource person for the LVNs/LPNs
- Two LVNs/LPNs assigned to provide total patient care except for administering IV medications

Your supervisor has just told all head nurses that due to financial difficulties, the hospital has decided to increase the number of nursing assistants in the staffing mix. The nurses on your unit will have to assume more supervisory responsibilities and focus less on direct care. Your supervisor has asked you to reorganize the patient care management on your unit to best use the following day-shift staffing: three RNs, which will include the present charge nurse position; two LVNs/LPNs; and two nursing assistants. You may delete the past charge nurse position and divide charge responsibility among all three nurses or divide up the work any way you choose.

ASSIGNMENT:

Draw a new patient care organization diagram. Who would be most affected by the reorganization? Evaluate your rationale for both the selection of your choice and the rejection of others. Explain how you would go about implementing this planned change.

Primary Nursing

Primary nursing (also known as *relationship-based nursing*) was developed in the late 1960s, uses some of the concepts of total patient care, and brings the RN back to the bedside to provide clinical care. In inpatient primary nursing, the *primary nurse* assumes 24-hour responsibility for planning the care of one or more patients from admission or the start of treatment to discharge or the treatment's end. During work hours, the primary nurse provides total direct care for that patient. When the primary nurse is not on duty, *associate nurses*, who follow the care plan established by the primary nurse, provide care. Most experts have suggested that the role of the primary nurse should be limited to RNs. Primary nursing structure is shown in Figure 14.4.

Although originally designed for use in hospitals, primary nursing lends itself well to home health nursing, hospice nursing, and other outpatient health care delivery enterprises as well. An integral responsibility of the primary nurse is to establish clear communication among the patient, the physician, the associate nurses, and other team members. Although the primary nurse establishes the care plan, feedback is sought from others in coordinating the patient's care. The combination of clear interdisciplinary group communication and consistent, direct patient care by relatively few nursing staff allows for holistic, high-quality patient care.

Although job satisfaction is high in primary nursing, this method is difficult to implement because of the degree of responsibility and autonomy required of the primary nurse. However, for these same reasons, once nurses develop skill in primary nursing care delivery, they often feel challenged and rewarded.

Disadvantages to this method, as in team nursing, lie primarily in improper implementation. An inadequately prepared or incompetent primary nurse may be incapable of coordinating a multidisciplinary team or identifying complex patient needs and condition changes. Some nurses may be uncomfortable in this role or initially lack the experience and skills necessary. In addition, although an all-RN nursing staff has not been proved to be more costly than other modes of nursing, it sometimes has been difficult to recruit and retain enough RNs to be primary nurses, especially in times of nursing shortages.

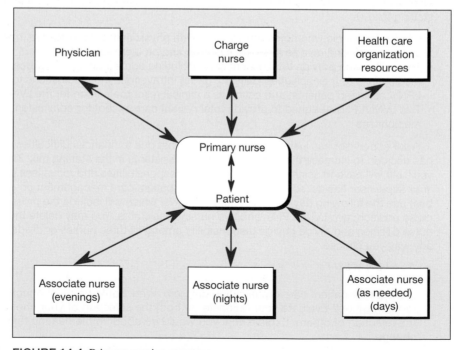

FIGURE 14.4 Primary nursing structure.

Interprofessional/Multidisciplinary Health Care Teams

A newer model of health care delivery is the *interprofessional or multidisciplinary health care team*. Interdisciplinary teamwork is a complex process involving two or more health professionals with complementary backgrounds and skills. In this process, team members share common health goals in assessing, planning, or evaluating patient care, which are accomplished through interdependent collaboration, open communication, and shared decision making (Venzin, 2022). Thus, it is about melding clinical expertise from each team member to best serve patients. One of the recommendations of the 2010 Institute of Medicine report, *The Future of Nursing: Leading Change, Advancing Health*, was to expand the opportunities for nurses to lead and diffuse collaborative improvement efforts with physicians and other members of the health care team to improve practice environments. Similarly, *The Future of Nursing 2020–2030* (National Academies of Sciences, Engineering, and Medicine & National Academy of Medicine, 2021) suggests that nurses should serve as leaders in a variety of interprofessional contexts within health care.

Primary health care teams (PHCTs) are interprofessional teams that include, but are not limited to, physicians, nurse practitioners, nurses, physical therapists, dentists, occupational therapists, and social workers who work collaboratively to deliver coordinated primary patient care. The desired outcomes for PHCTs are reduced mortality and improved quality of life for patients, a reduction in health care costs, and a more rewarding professional experience for the health care worker.

The challenges in implementing interdisciplinary health care teams mirror many of the challenges seen in more traditional primary care, including hurdles in their formation, overcoming the traditional physician-dominated hierarchy in determining who should lead the team, role confusion, and determination of structure and function of the team. In addition, because the interprofessional team brings together differing viewpoints, life experiences, and knowledge of evidence-based practices, determining what knowledge is most important in caring for the patient can be confusing.

Indeed, implementation problems are common on multidisciplinary teams, as having experts on teams is different than having expert teams. Each discipline may believe that their perspective is most important and undervalue the contributions of other team members. In addition, like traditional team nursing, multidisciplinary teams require an efficient means of communication about patient goals, progress, and problems. It is difficult to find opportunities for the entire team to meet because of work shift patterns or other work commitments. Venzin (2022) recommends strategies for health care professionals to increase the likelihood of successful interdisciplinary teams. These are shown in Display 14.3.

> A team of experts is not the same thing as an expert team. Successful interprofessional teams understand and appreciate the unique contributions each member of the team brings to patient care coordination.

DISPLAY 14.3 STRATEGIES FOR WORKING WITH AN INTERDISCIPLINARY HEALTH CARE TEAM

1. Know your role and expertise as well as that of your team members.
2. Know the end goal/the purpose of your interdisciplinary team.
3. Communicate compassionately so that all members of the interdisciplinary team feel comfortable in voicing their opinions.
4. Establish a support structure whereby all members feel like they play an important role.

Source: Extracted from Venzin, K. (2022). 4 Things to know when working with an interdisciplinary healthcare team. *Core Medical Group*. https://www.coremedicalgroup.com/blog/4-tips-interdisciplinary-healthcare-team

In addition, the challenge of interprofessional care planning could be minimized if more students participated in interprofessional education (IPE) efforts. Unfortunately, most health care professionals complete their education isolated from each other and thus may fail to appreciate the unique contributions every member of the interprofessional team brings.

Registered Nurse Primary Care Coordinators in Patient-Centered Medical Homes

Another interprofessional model for organizing patient care, enacted as part of the Patient Protection and Affordable Care Act (PPACA) was the establishment of the *patient-centered medical home* (PCMH). The PCMH delivers cost-effective primary care, utilizing care coordination, ensuring high value, and improving health outcomes. RNs are increasingly serving as the front-line primary care leaders in PCMHs alongside physicians and advanced practice nurses. Unfortunately, neither urban nor rural settings have developed a comprehensive definition of what RN primary care coordination is, nor is it being implemented in a uniform manner.

Case Management

Case management is another work design proposed to meet patient needs. Case management is defined by the Case Management Society of America (CMSA, 2021) as "a collaborative process of assessment, planning, facilitation, care coordination, evaluation and advocacy for options and services to meet an individual's and family's comprehensive health needs through communication and available resources to promote patient safety, quality of care, and cost effective outcomes" (para. 1).

In case management, nurses address each patient individually, identifying the most cost-effective providers, treatments, and care settings possible. In addition, the case manager helps patients access community resources, helps patients learn about their medication regimens and treatment plans, and ensures that they have recommended tests and procedures.

Although case management referrals often begin in the hospital inpatient setting, with length of stay and profit margin per confinement used as measures of efficiency, case management now frequently extends to outpatient settings as well. Indeed, the new medical homes created as part of the PPACA use case managers extensively.

Historically, however, the focus of case management has been episodic or component style orientation to the treatment of disease in inpatient settings and postacute care settings for insured individuals. *Acute care case management* integrates utilization management and discharge planning functions and may be unit based, assigned by patient, disease based, or primary nurse case managed. Indeed, because many admissions in most hospitals enter via the emergency department, case management often begins there in the acute care setting.

Case managers often manage care using *critical pathways* (see Chapter 10) and *multidisciplinary action plans* (MAPs) to plan patient care. The care MAP is a combination of a *critical pathway* and a *nursing care plan*. In addition, the care MAP indicates times when nursing interventions should occur. All health care providers follow the care MAP to facilitate expected outcomes. If a patient deviates from the normal plan, a *variance* is indicated. A variance is anything that occurs to alter the patient's progress through the normal critical path.

Because the role expectations and scope of knowledge required to be a case manager are extensive, some experts have argued that this role should be reserved for the advance practice nurse or RN with advanced training, although this is not usually the case in the practice setting today. In fact, board certification as a case manager is available to any individual with either a current, active, and unrestricted licensure or certification in a health or human services discipline.

> Some feel that the role of case manager should be reserved for the advance practice nurse or registered nurse (RN) with advanced training.

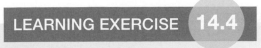

LEARNING EXERCISE 14.4

Developing a Case Management Plan

Jimmy Jansen is a 44-year-old man with type 1 diabetes mellitus. He was recently referred to your home health agency for case management follow-up at home. He is experiencing multiple complications from his diabetes, including the recent onset of blindness and peripheral neuropathy. His left leg was amputated below the knee last year because of a gangrenous infection of his foot. He is unable to wear his prosthesis at present because he has a small ulcer at the stump site. His chart states that he has been only "intermittently compliant" with blood glucose testing or insulin administration in the past despite weekly visits from a community health nurse over the past year. His renal function has become progressively worse over the past 6 months, and it is anticipated that he will need to begin hemodialysis soon.

His social history reveals that he recently separated from his wife and has no contact with an adult son who lives in another state. He has not worked for more than 10 years and has no insurance other than Medicaid, although he will qualify for Medicare if he needs regular dialysis. His house is small, and he says that he has not been able to maintain it with his wife gone. No formal safety assessment of his home has been conducted. He also acknowledges that he is not eating right because he now must do his own cooking. He cannot drive and states, "I don't know how I'm going to get to the clinic to have my blood cleaned by the kidney machine."

ASSIGNMENT:

Mr. Jansen has many problems that would likely benefit from case management intervention.
1. Make a list of five nursing diagnoses for Mr. Jansen that you would use to prioritize your interventions.
2. Then make a list of at least five goals that you would like to accomplish in planning Mr. Jansen's care. Make sure that these goals reflect realistic patient outcomes.
3. What referrals would you make? What interventions would you implement yourself? Would you involve other disciplines in his plan of care?
4. What is your plan for follow-up and evaluation?

Case management nursing is challenging to implement because case management roles and functions differ by setting, leading to confusion about what the job of a case manager entails. For example, in some settings, case managers participate in direct care or have direct communication with patients. In others, the case manager is an advocate for patients, although the patient may have no direct knowledge or interaction with that individual.

Case Management of Disease Management Programs

One role assumed by case managers is coordinating *disease management* (DM) programs. DM, also known as *population-based health care* and *continuous health improvement*, is a comprehensive, integrated approach to the care and reimbursement of high-cost, chronic illnesses.

The goal of DM is to address such illnesses or conditions with maximum efficiency across treatment settings regardless of typical reimbursement patterns. Thus, a continuum of chronic illness care is established that includes early detection and early intervention. This prevents or reduces exacerbation of the disease, acute episodes (known as *cost drivers*), and the use of expensive resources such as hospital inpatient care, making prevention and proactive case management two important areas of emphasis.

In DM programs, common high-cost, high-resource utilization diseases are identified, and population groups are targeted for implementation. This is one of the most important differences between case management and DM. In DM, the focus is on "covered lives" or

DISPLAY 14.4 COMMON FEATURES OF DISEASE MANAGEMENT PROGRAMS

1. Provide a comprehensive, integrated approach to the care and reimbursement of common, high-cost, chronic illnesses
2. Focus on prevention as well as early disease detection and intervention to avoid costly acute care episodes but provide comprehensive care and reimbursement
3. Target population groups (population based) rather than individuals
4. Employ a multidisciplinary health care team, including specialists
5. Use standardized clinical guidelines—clinical pathways reflecting best practice research to guide providers
6. Use integrated data management systems to track patient progress across care settings and allow continuous and ongoing improvement of treatment algorithms
7. Frequently employ professional nurses in the role of case manager or program coordinator

populations of patients, rather than on the individual patient. The goal in DM is to service the optimal number of covered lives required to reach operational and economic efficiency. In other words, DM is effective when cost drivers are reduced, whereas patient needs are met.

> Providing optimum, cost–effective care to individual patients is critical to the success of a disease management (DM) program; however, the focus for planning, implementation, and evaluation is population based.

Other primary features of DM programs include the use of a multidisciplinary health care team, including specialists; the selection of large population groups to reduce adverse selection; the use of standardized clinical guidelines—clinical pathways reflecting best practice research to guide provider practice—and the use of integrated data management systems to track patient progress across care settings and allow continuous and ongoing improvement of treatment algorithms. In addition, DM programs include comprehensive tracking of patient outcomes. Thus, the goals for DM are focused on integrating components and improving long-term outcomes. Common features of DM programs are shown in Display 14.4.

One thing is clear—DM continues to grow as a means of organizing patient care. This is particularly true in the government sector, which did not really begin embracing DM demonstration projects until early in the 21st century, many of which are now mainstream initiatives to deliver better outcomes at better prices. In addition, DM continues to be a promising

LEARNING EXERCISE 14.5

Researching Disease Management Programs

Search the internet for disease management programs. What chronic diseases were most commonly represented in the DM programs that you identified? What entities (private insurance companies, managed care insurers, government, pharmaceutical companies, private companies, etc.) sponsored these programs? What is the process for referral? Are the programs accredited? Are registered nurses used as case managers or program coordinators? What standardized clinical guidelines are used in the programs, and are they evidence based?

ASSIGNMENT:

Select one of the programs that you found and write a one-page summary of your findings.

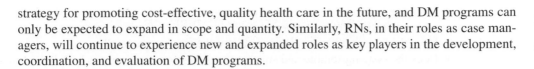

strategy for promoting cost-effective, quality health care in the future, and DM programs can only be expected to expand in scope and quantity. Similarly, RNs, in their roles as case managers, will continue to experience new and expanded roles as key players in the development, coordination, and evaluation of DM programs.

Selecting the Optimum Mode of Organizing Patient Care

Most health care organizations use one or more modes to organize patient care. Although not all care must be provided by RNs, the care delivery system chosen should be based on patient acuity and not on economics alone. In addition, the knowledge and skill required to care for specific populations should always be the true driver in determining appropriate care delivery models. Nursing departments need to organize delivery of patient care based on the best method for their needs.

> Many nursing units have a history of selecting methods of organizing patient care based on the most current popular mode rather than objectively determining the best method for a specific unit or department.

If evaluation of the present system reveals deficiencies, the manager needs to examine available resources and determine which are still needed for the change. Nursing managers often elect to change to a system that requires a high percentage of RNs, only to discover resources are inadequate, resulting in a failed planned change. One of the leadership responsibilities in organizing patient care is to determine the availability of resources and support for proposed changes. Top-level administration and the nursing staff must commit to the change for it to be successful. Because health care is multidisciplinary, the care delivery system used will have a heavy impact on many others outside the nursing unit; therefore, those affected by a system change must be involved in its planning. Change affects other departments, the medical staff, and the health care consumer. Perhaps most importantly, the philosophy of the nursing services division must support the delivery model selected.

Another mistake frequently made when changing modes of patient care delivery is to not fully understand how the new system should function or be implemented. Managers must carry out adequate research and be well versed in the system's proper implementation if the change is to be successful. It is important also to remember that not every nurse desires a challenging job with the autonomy of personal decision making. Many forces interact simultaneously in employee job design situations. Satisfaction does not occur only because of role fulfillment; it also results from social and interpersonal relationships. Therefore, the nurse leader-manager needs to be aware that redesigning work that disrupts group cohesiveness may result in increased levels of job dissatisfaction.

> Not every nurse desires a challenging job with the autonomy of personal decision making.

Such change should not be taken lightly. The leader-manager should consider the following when evaluating the current system and considering a change.

- Is the method of patient care delivery providing the level of care that is stated in the organizational philosophy? Does the method facilitate or hinder other organizational goals?
- Is the delivery of nursing care organized in a cost-effective manner?
- Does the care delivery system satisfy patients and their families? (Satisfaction and quality care differ; either may be provided without the other being present.)

- Does the organization of patient care delivery provide some degree of fulfillment and role satisfaction to nursing personnel?
- Does the system allow implementation of the nursing process?
- Does the system promote and support the profession of nursing as both independent and interdependent?
- Does the method facilitate adequate communication among all members of the health care team?
- How will a change in the patient care delivery system alter individual and group decision making? Who will be affected? Will autonomy decrease or increase?
- How will social interactions and interpersonal relationships change?
- Will employees view their unit of work differently? Will there be a change from a partial unit of work to a whole unit (e.g., total patient care would be a whole unit of work, whereas team nursing would be a partial unit)?
- Will the change require a wider or more restricted range of caregiver skills and abilities?
- Will the redesign change how employees receive feedback on their performance, either by self-evaluation or by others?
- Will communication patterns change?

The most appropriate organizational model to deliver patient care for each unit or organization depends on the skill and expertise of the staff, the availability of registered professional nurses, the economic resources of the organization, the acuity of the patients, and the complexity of the tasks to be completed.

New Roles in the Changing Health Care Arena: Nurse Navigators and Clinical Nurse-Leaders

Health care delivery models that expand the role of nurses beyond direct caregivers are continuing to emerge. Nurses form the backbone of almost all these new models. In addition, there are consistent themes regarding the focus, value, and cost in these newer care delivery models (Display 14.5). Two emerging roles are detailed in this chapter: nurse navigators and CNLs.

Nurse Navigators

The *nurse navigator* role is a relatively new role for professional nurses. Nurse navigators help patients and families navigate the complex health care system by providing information and support.

Nurse navigation commonly occurs in targeted clinical settings such as oncology, whereby a breast cancer nurse navigator might work with a patient from the time they are first diagnosed

---

DISPLAY 14.5 COMMON THEMES FOUND AMONG NEWER CARE DELIVERY MODELS

1. Elevating the role of nurses and transitioning from caregivers to "care integrators"
2. Taking a team approach to interdisciplinary care
3. Bridging the continuum of care outside of the primary care facility
4. Defining the home as a setting of care
5. Targeting high users of health care, especially older adults
6. Sharpening focus on the patient, including an active engagement of the patient and their family in care planning and delivery and a greater responsiveness to the patient's wants and needs
7. Leveraging technology
8. Improving satisfaction, quality, and cost

Source: From Beattie, L. (2017, June 15). *New health care delivery models are redefining the role of nurses.* American Mobile. https://www.americanmobile.com/mobile/NZArticle/?articleId=2205

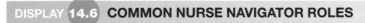

DISPLAY 14.6   COMMON NURSE NAVIGATOR ROLES

- Participates in the continuum of patient care activities including assessment, screening, diagnosis, treatment, supportive care, and end-of-life care
- Serves as a clinician, care coordinator, educator, and provider of emotional support for patients and families
- Monitors patient symptoms and progress
- Collaborates and coordinates care with other health care providers
- Provides appropriate referrals
- Offers education and information to empower patients and families in health care decision making
- Helps the patient and family identify and access acute care as well as community-based resources
- Eliminates barriers to access and treatment in the health care system
- Ensures safe transitions of care
- Is a primary contact for patients, families, and caregivers throughout an illness

and then follow them throughout the course of the illness. At Community Health Network (n.d.), the nurse navigator acts as a guide, resource, advocate, educator, and liaison for newly diagnosed cancer patients and their families. The navigator is the consistent caregiver through the cancer journey, coordinating appointments and schedules while keeping the patient and family actively involved in their plan of care. The importance of the navigator role in providing both patient care continuity and high-quality care cannot be understated. Common nurse navigator roles are shown in Display 14.6.

Nurse navigators became more visible with the Insurance Exchanges (Healthcare Marketplace) that rolled out with the PPACA. In this case, consumers were advised to consult with nurse navigators to learn about and purchase an insurance plan from the Exchanges. Critics suggest, however, that further role definition is needed to differentiate between the role case managers and nurse navigators will play in the coming decade.

The Clinical Nurse-Leader

Many of the newer patient care delivery models include the nurse as a clinical expert leading other members of a team of partners. For example, the American Association of Colleges of Nursing (AACN) identified a new nursing role in the early 1990s, that of the CNL, that is more responsive to the realities of the modern health care system. The CNL, as an advanced generalist with a master's degree in nursing, is a leader in the health care delivery system in all settings in which health care is delivered. CNL practice will vary across settings (AACN, 2022).

The CNL role, however, is not one of administration or management. Instead, the CNL "assumes accountability for patient-care outcomes through the assimilation and application of evidence-based information to design, implement, and evaluate patient-care processes and models of care delivery. The CNL is a provider and manager of care at the point of care to individuals and cohorts of patients anywhere health care is delivered" (AACN, 2022, para. 4). The CNL also plays a key role in collaborating with interdisciplinary teams.

The Veterans Health Administration became an early adopter of the CNL role, implementing the CNL initiative across all Veterans Affairs (VA) settings. At the VA, CNLs serve as the point person on patient care teams and are leaders in the health care delivery system.

Integrating Leadership Roles and Management Functions in Organizing Patient Care

Organizing care is an all-important management function. The work must be organized so that organizational goals are sustained, and activities must be grouped so that resources, people, materials, and time are used fully. The integrated leader-manager understands that the organization's and unit's nursing philosophy and the availability of resources greatly influence the type of patient care delivery system that should be chosen and the potential success of future work redesign.

The integrated leader-manager, then, is responsible for selecting and implementing a patient care delivery system that facilitates the accomplishment of unit goals. All members of the work group should be assisted with role clarification, especially when work is redesigned, or new systems of patient care delivery are implemented. This team effort in work activity increases productivity and worker satisfaction. The emphasis is on seeking solutions to poor organization of work rather than finding fault.

There is no one "best" mode for organizing patient care. Integrating leadership roles and management functions ensures that the type of patient care delivery model selected will provide quality care and staff satisfaction. It also ensures that change in the mode of delivery will not be attempted without adequate resources, appropriate justification, and attention to how it will affect group cohesiveness. Historically, nursing has frequently adopted models of patient care delivery based on societal events (e.g., a nursing shortage and a proliferation of types of health care workers) rather than on well-researched models with proven effectiveness that promote professional practice. The leadership role demands that the primary focus of patient care delivery be on promoting a professional model of practice that also reduces costs and improves patient outcomes. Increasingly, this requires the collaboration of an interprofessional team of health care experts.

Given projected health care worker shortages, many health care organizations are concerned there will be too few health care workers to deliver care with the same models used now. Health care agencies must begin now to explore how newer nursing roles such as case managers, nurse navigators, and CNLs might be used to better integrate and coordinate care—before, not after, investigating other solutions to health care shortages. In addition, there is increasing recognition that care should be planned and implemented by interdisciplinary/interprofessional teams and that IPE will likely be required to prepare health care providers for this role. As many forces come together to change the future of health care, it behooves all health care professionals to think smarter, to think outside the box, and to discover innovative ways to organize and deliver care that is patient- and family-centered to clients both inside and outside the acute care setting.

Key Concepts

- Total patient care, utilizing the case method of assignment, is the oldest form of patient care organization and is still widely used today.
- Functional nursing organization requires the completion of specific tasks by different nursing personnel.
- Team nursing typically uses a nurse-leader who coordinates team members of varying educational preparation and skill sets in the care of a group of patients.
- Modular nursing uses mini-teams, typically an RN and unlicensed health care workers, to provide care to a small group of patients, usually centralized geographically.
- Primary care nursing is organized so that one health care provider (typically the RN) has

24-hour responsibility for care planning and coordination.
- The use of interprofessional teams in planning and implementing care increases the likelihood that care will be comprehensive and holistic.
- Implementation problems may occur with interprofessional teams when one health care discipline perceives that their perspective is more important than other team members.
- Case management is a collaborative process that assesses, plans, implements, coordinates, monitors, and evaluates options and services to meet an individual's health needs through communication and the use of available resources to promote quality and cost-effective outcomes.

- Although the focus historically for case management has been the individual patient, the case manager employed in a DM program plans the care for populations or groups of patients with the same chronic illness.
- The care MAP is a combination of a critical path and a nursing care plan, except that it shows times when nursing interventions should occur as well as variances.
- Delivery systems may have elements of the various designs present in the system in use in any organization.
- Each unit's care delivery structure should facilitate meeting the goals of the organization, be cost-effective, satisfy the patient, provide role satisfaction to nurses, allow implementation of the nursing process, and provide for adequate communication among health care providers.

- When work is redesigned, it frequently has personal consequences for employees that must be considered. Social interactions, the degree of autonomy, the abilities and skills necessary, employee evaluation, and communication patterns are often affected by work redesign.
- The *nurse navigator* assists patients and families to navigate the complex health care system by providing information and support as they traverse their illnesses.
- The CNL is an experienced nurse possessing a graduate degree who provides clinical leadership in all health care settings, implements outcomes-based practice and quality improvement strategies, engages in clinical practice, and creates and manages microsystems of care that are responsive to the health care needs of individuals and families.

Additional Learning Exercises and Applications

LEARNING EXERCISE 14.6

Creating a Plan to Reduce Resistance

You work in an intensive care unit where there is an all-registered nurse (RN) staff. The staff work 12-hour shifts, and each nurse is assigned one or two patients, depending on the nursing needs of the patient. The unit has always used total patient care delivery assignments. Recently, your unit manager informed the staff that all patients in the unit would be assigned a case manager to maximize the use of resources and to reduce length of stay in the unit. Many of the unit staff resent the case manager and believe that this has reduced the RN's autonomy and control of patient care. They resist the need to document variances to the care multidisciplinary action plans and are generally uncooperative but not to the point that they are insubordinate.

Although you feel some loss of autonomy, you also think that the case manager has been effective in coordinating care to speed patient discharge. You believe that at present, the atmosphere in the unit is very stressful. The unit manager and case manager have come to you and requested that you assist them in convincing the other staff to go along with this change.

ASSIGNMENT:

Using your knowledge of planned change and case management, outline a plan for reducing resistance.

LEARNING EXERCISE 14.7

Types of Patient Care Delivery Models Used in Your Area

In a group, investigate the types of patient care delivery models used in your area. Do not limit your investigation to hospitals. If possible, conduct interviews with nurses from a variety of delivery systems. Share the report of your findings with your classmates. How many different models of patient care delivery did you find? What is the most widely used method in health care facilities in your area? Does this vary from models identified most frequently in current nursing literature?

LEARNING EXERCISE 14.8

Implementing a Managed Care System

You are the director of a home health agency that has recently become part of a managed care system. In the past, only a physician's order was required for authorization for treatment from Medicare, but now, approval must come from the managed care organization (MCO). In the past, public health certified nurses (all Bachelor of Science in Nursing graduates) have acted as case managers for their assigned caseload. Now, the MCO case manager has taken over this role, creating much conflict among the staff. In addition, there is pressure from your board to cut costs by using more nonprofessionals who are less skilled for some of the home care. You realize that unless you do so, your agency will not survive financially.

You have visited other home health agencies and researched your options carefully. You have decided that you must use some type of team approach.

ASSIGNMENT:

Develop a plan, objectives, and a time frame for implementation. In your plan, discuss who will be most affected by your changes. As a change agent, what will be your most important role?

LEARNING EXERCISE 14.9

The Clinical Nurse-Leader Application

You are the unit coordinator of a medical/surgical unit in a small acute care hospital. One of your greatest management challenges has been implementing evidence-based practice at the unit level. Your staff nurses have access to many health care resources via their computer workstations. In addition, computerized provider order entry is used in your hospital, which includes links to best practices and standardized clinical guidelines. Yet, you are aware that some of your staff continue to do things as they have always been done, despite repeated workshops on how best to integrate new evidence into their clinical practice. You hope to address this problem by hiring someone with the leadership skills needed to champion the change effort and the management skills necessary to direct staff in their new roles.

When you return to your office today, you find an application for employment from a clinical nurse-leader (CNL). She recently completed her CNL program as part of a master's entry program, so her clinical experience is limited to what she received in nursing school. You are aware, though, that her educational background will have prepared her to lead a change effort on the unit to foster evidence-based decision making and outcomes-focused practice.

You also have an employment application from a master's-prepared nurse with many years of clinical experience as a staff and charge nurse, although she is just returning from a 5-year leave of absence to care for a sick family member. She completed a master's thesis as part of her graduate nursing education 20 years ago, so you know she has at least some expertise in nursing research and its translation to practice. Given your budget constraints, you can hire only one of these individuals.

ASSIGNMENT:

Identify the driving and restraining forces for hiring the CNL or for hiring the experienced nurse with clinical and research expertise. Do you believe that the limited clinical experience of the CNL would impact her ability to serve as a leader and change agent on the floor? Would the CNL have the management skill set you also want in your new hire? Do you believe that the CNL would be better prepared as a leader in this change effort? Justify which employee you would choose to hire and suggest strategies you might use to help this individual acquire the leadership, management, and change skill sets the individual may be lacking to achieve your desired outcomes.

LEARNING EXERCISE 14.10

Permanent or Rotating Assignments

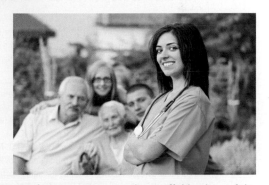

You are a registered nurse in a home health agency and have been employed at the agency for 2 years. Most of the agency's clients contract with the agency for home care services and are either paid personally by the client or by third-party payers such as the government or private insurance. Although some of the clients have short-term needs for care only, others require ongoing care for cancer or a chronic disease diagnosis. Presently, the agency rotates assignments among the staff. You have felt for some time that if the long-term clients were assigned a permanent nurse for their care, it would benefit the clients. You realize not all of the nurses would like this reorganization of care and that it might be difficult for the agency to balance workload appropriately.

ASSIGNMENT:

Develop a plan to present to the director of the agency that would show how the reorganization would work. If the agency implemented this change, what would be the driving and restraining forces and how could you strengthen the driving forces to make the plan succeed?

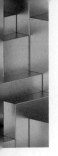

LEARNING EXERCISE 14.11

Leading an Interprofessional Team

You are a registered nurse (RN) and are a part of an interprofessional team organized to plan and deliver care to an acutely ill patient with multiple comorbidities. The team meeting today became tense when the pulmonologist and the cardiologist expressed having significantly different care priorities and treatment plans. When they could not agree, both unsuccessfully asserted themselves as the leader of the team, so that their priority would be upheld. In addition, the dietician on the team complained that her participation was not being valued and the social worker expressed frustration that while the patient was very sick and had multiple treatment needs, that the patient's family felt ignored, uninformed, and frustrated. She asked that a plan be established to address the family's needs, but team members were so frustrated and angry by this point that the meeting ended abruptly, and no action was taken.

ASSIGNMENT:

What is happening in this interprofessional team? Are issues of power, authority, trust, and respect common in interprofessional teams? Can a clearly stated, shared, and measurable purpose for the interprofessional team be identified? How can or should leadership on the team be determined? How can understanding of and appreciation for the unique contributions of each team member be increased? How should the team deal with differences in opinions when competencies are overlapping? What strategies might be used at this point to build an expert team, rather than a team of experts?

REFERENCES

American Association of Colleges of Nursing. (2022). *Competencies and curricular expectations for clinical nurse leader education and practice.* https://www.aacnnursing.org/News-Information/Position-Statements-White-Papers/CNL

Beckett, C. D., Zadvinskis, I. M., Dean, J., Iseler, J., Powell, J. M., & Buck-Maxwell, B. (2021, August 6). An integrative review of team nursing and delegation: Implications for nurse staffing during COVID-19. *Worldviews on Evidence-Based Nursing, 18*(4), 251–260. https://doi.org/10.1111/wvn.12523

Case Management Society of America. (2021). *What is a case manager?* Retrieved September 22, 2021, from https://cmsa.org/who-we-are/what-is-a-case-manager/

Community Health Network. (n.d.). *Oncology navigators.* https://www.ecommunity.com/services/cancer-care/oncology-navigators

Fernandez, R., Johnson, M., Tran, T. D., & Miranda, C. (2012, November 23). Models of care in nursing: A systematic review. *International Journal of Evidence-Based Healthcare, 10*(4), 324–337. https://onlinelibrary.wiley.com/doi/full/10.1111/j.1744-1609.2012.00287.x

National Academies of Sciences, Engineering, and Medicine & National Academy of Medicine. (2021, May 11). *The Future of Nursing 2020–2030: Charting a Path to Achieve Health Equity.* Flaubert JL, Le Menestrel S, Williams DR, et al. (Eds). National Academies Press (US). https://www.ncbi.nlm.nih.gov/books/NBK573918/

Venzin, K. (2022). 4 Things to know when working with interdisciplinary healthcare teams. *Core Medical Group.* https://www.coremedicalgroup.com/blog/4-tips-interdisciplinary-healthcare-team

Whittemore, R., & Knafl, K. (2005, November 2). The integrative review: Updated methodology. *Journal of Advanced Nursing, 52*(5). https://doi.org/10.1111/j.1365-2648.2005.03621.x

Roles and Functions in Staffing

15

Employee Recruitment, Selection, Placement, and Onboarding

*… Employee selection is so crucial that nothing else—not leadership, not team building, not training, not pay incentives, not total quality management—can overcome poor hiring decisions…—**Gerald Graham***

*… I have always surrounded myself with the best people to do their jobs, because I do not want to learn what they already know better than I do.—**Shirley Sears Chater***

*… If you pick the right people and give them the opportunity to spread their wings and put compensation as a carrier behind it, you almost don't have to manage them.—**Jack Welch***

CROSSWALK

This chapter addresses:

- **AACN Essentials Domain 5:** Quality and safety
- **AACN Essentials Domain 6:** Interprofessional partnerships
- **AACN Essentials Domain 7:** Systems-based practice
- **AACN Essentials Domain 8:** Information and health care technologies
- **AACN Essentials Domain 9:** Professionalism
- **AACN Essentials Domain 10:** Personal, professional, and leadership development
- **AONL Nurse Executive Competency 1:** Communication and relationship building
- **AONL Nurse Executive Competency 2:** A knowledge of the health care environment
- **AONL Nurse Executive Competency 5:** Business skills
- **ANA Standard of Professional Performance 8:** Advocacy
- **ANA Standard of Professional Performance 9:** Respectful and equitable practice
- **ANA Standard of Professional Performance 10:** Communication
- **ANA Standard of Professional Performance 11:** Collaboration
- **ANA Standard of Professional Performance 12:** Leadership
- **ANA Standard of Professional Performance 16:** Professional practice evaluation
- **ANA Standard of Professional Performance 17:** Resource stewardship
- **QSEN Competency:** Teamwork and collaboration
- **QSEN Competency:** Safety

LEARNING OBJECTIVES

The learner will:

- recognize the need for workforce diversity to meet the unique cultural and linguistic needs represented in the patient populations served
- determine the number and types of personnel needed to fulfill an organizational philosophy, meet fiscal planning responsibilities, and carry out a chosen patient care delivery system
- describe demand and supply factors leading to nursing shortages

- identify variables that impact an organization's ability to recruit candidates successfully for job openings
- delineate the relationship between recruitment and retention
- describe interview techniques that reduce subjectivity and increase reliability and validity during the interview process
- develop appropriate interview questions to determine whether an applicant is qualified and willing to meet the requirements of a position
- differentiate between legal and illegal interview inquiries
- analyze how personal values and biases affect employment selection decisions
- consider organizational needs and employee strengths in making placement decisions
- select appropriate activities to be included in the recruitment, selection, placement, and onboarding of employees

Introduction

After planning and organizing, staffing is the third phase of the management process. In staffing, the leader-manager recruits, selects, places, and onboards personnel to accomplish the goals of the organization. These steps, which are depicted in Display 15.1, are typically sequential, although each step has some interdependence with all staffing activities.

Staffing is an especially important phase of the management process in health care organizations because they are usually *labor intensive* (i.e., numerous employees are required for an organization to accomplish its goals). In addition, many health care organizations are open 24 hours a day, 365 days a year, and client needs are often variable.

The large workforce needed to staff health care organizations must have an appropriate balance of highly skilled, competent professionals and ancillary support workers. In addition, the workforce should reflect the diversity of the communities that the organization serves. To provide the best possible care for all patients and help minimize racial disparities, health care professionals need to acknowledge and recognize differences among varying populations. A lack of diversity in the workforce limits the capabilities of medical care, containing it within a single ethnic lens and a particular set of values. The more diverse the people who provide medical care, the better they can respectfully and knowledgeably assist their patients (The Importance of Diversity, 2021).

A lack of diversity in the health care workforce has been linked to *health disparities* in the populations served (Huston, 2023a). Brooks (2021) agrees, noting that the lack of diverse representation is about far more than appearances; it is tied to negative health outcomes. For example, Black, American Indian, and Alaska Native women are two to three times more likely to die from pregnancy-related causes than White women. In addition, racial disparities in hospitalization and death from the COVID-19 virus are well documented, with a disproportionate number of Black, Native American, and Alaska Native population deaths and infections (Brooks, 2021).

DISPLAY 15.1 SEQUENTIAL STEPS IN STAFFING

1. Determine the number and types of personnel needed to fulfill the philosophy, meet fiscal planning responsibilities, and carry out the chosen patient care delivery system selected by the organization
2. Recruit, interview, select, and assign personnel based on established job description performance standards
3. Use organizational resources for induction and orientation
4. Assure that each employee is adequately socialized to organization values and unit norms
5. Use creative and flexible scheduling based on patient care needs to increase productivity and retention

DISPLAY 15.2 LEADERSHIP ROLES AND MANAGEMENT FUNCTIONS ASSOCIATED WITH PRELIMINARY STAFFING FUNCTIONS

Leadership Roles

1. Is knowledgeable regarding historical and current staffing variables
2. Stays abreast of changes in the health care field that may impact future staffing needs and human resources
3. Identifies and recruits talented people to the organization
4. Encourages and actively seeks diversity in staffing
5. Is self-aware regarding personal biases during the preemployment process
6. Seeks to find the best possible fit between employees' unique talents and organizational staffing needs
7. Creates an interviewing process where all applicants believe that they are treated fairly
8. Reviews induction and orientation programs periodically to ascertain they are meeting unit needs
9. Ensures that each new employee understands appropriate organizational policies
10. Promotes hiring based on preferred criteria rather than minimum criteria
11. Aspires continually to create a work environment that promotes employee retention and worker satisfaction

Management Functions

1. Plans for future staffing needs proactively to ensure an adequate skilled workforce to meet the goals of the organization
2. Shares responsibility for the recruitment of staff with organization recruiters
3. Selects and uses preemployment selection tools that are reliable and valid, yielding consistent results that predict success on the job
4. Plans and structures appropriate interview activities
5. Uses techniques that increase the validity and reliability of the interview process
6. Applies knowledge of the legal requirements of interviewing and selection to ensure that the organization's hiring practices meet expected standards
7. Develops established criteria for employment selection purposes
8. Uses knowledge of organizational needs and employee strengths to make placement decisions
9. Interprets information in employee handbook and provides input for handbook revisions
10. Participates actively in employee orientation
11. Assures that adequate organizational resources are available for induction and orientation

As Schafir (n.d.) points out, the world has its eyes on systemic racism, and now, more than ever, there is widespread commitment to dismantling discrimination. But with heightened attention comes awareness of the complexity surrounding inequality. Diversity is complicated, and that's why most companies fail to meet their *Diversity, Equity, and Inclusion* goals. Many organizations report difficulty in recruiting diverse candidates, but organizations may not be looking in the right places or doing a very good job of retaining their diverse hires (Schafir, n.d.).

This chapter examines national and regional trends for professional nurse staffing. It also addresses preliminary staffing functions, namely, determining staffing needs and recruiting, interviewing, selecting, and placing personnel. It also reviews two employee onboarding processes: induction and orientation. The management functions and leadership roles inherent in these staffing responsibilities are shown in Display 15.2.

Predicting Staffing Needs

Accurately predicting staffing needs is a crucial management skill because it enables managers to avoid staffing crises. Managers should know the source of their nursing pool, the number of students enrolled in local nursing schools, the usual length of employment of newly hired staff, peak staff resignation periods, and times when the patient census is highest. In addition, they must consider the patient care delivery system in place, the education and knowledge level of needed staff, budget constraints, historical staffing needs and availability, and the diversity of the patient population to be served.

Managers also need to understand third-party insurer reimbursement because this can impact staffing in contemporary health care organizations. For example, as government and private insurer reimbursements declined in the 1990s, many health care organizations— hospitals in particular—began downsizing by replacing registered nurse (RN) positions with unlicensed assistive personnel. Even hospitals that did not downsize during this period often did little to recruit qualified RNs. This downsizing and shortsightedness regarding recruitment and retention contributed to the beginning of an acute shortage of RNs in many health care settings by the late 1990s.

The health care quality and safety movement also exacerbated this shortage in the late 1990s as research emerged to demonstrate the relationship between nurse staffing and patient outcomes and the public became aware of how important an adequately sized workforce was to patient safety.

National and local economics also play a significant role in staffing. Historically, nursing shortages occur when the economy is on the upswing and decline when the economy recedes. This is only a guideline, however, as some workforce shortages have occurred regardless of the economic climate.

> Historically, when the economy improves, nursing shortages occur. When the economy declines, nursing vacancy rates decline as well.

Is There a Nursing Shortage?

Health care managers have long been sensitive to the importance of physical (technology and space) and financial resources to the success of service delivery The shortage of human resources, however, likely poses the greatest challenge to most health care organizations today. At the close of the first decade of the 21st century, many experts suggested that the United States would be facing a profound nursing shortage by 2020.

The profound shortage, however, did not occur, at least until the COVID-19 pandemic. Economists suggest that the shortage was muted in part by the recession beginning in 2008, which caused many nurses to put off their retirements. In addition, many nurses who were working part time increased their employment to full time, and some nurses who had been out of the profession for 5 years or more returned to the workforce. Thus, the most recent economic crisis both eased the nursing shortage and obscured its depth and breadth. As the economy improved, however, fears of a shortage reemerged, although many experts felt that increases in supply due to increased nursing school enrollments would likely keep up with the projected retirement of baby boomer (those born between 1946 and 1964) nurses (Caruso, 2020).

Concerns renewed, however, with the onset of the COVID-19 pandemic in 2020, due to a wave of earlier-than-planned retirements (Arends, 2020). Fears rose that the virus could diminish the supply of new nurses at the exact time the workforce needed to grow. In addition, as hospitals began seeing an influx of patients with COVID-19, the older experienced nurses who were desperately needed to help lead their younger colleagues through the crisis were the ones at a higher risk for severe outcomes from COVID-19, increasing the likelihood they would be unable to care for patients or lead younger staff (Caruso, 2020).

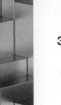

The current situation suggests shortages will continue or worsen as demand increases, an aging workforce retires, and the pandemic continues to consume nursing resources. The extent of any projected shortage, however, is hard to determine.

Supply and Demand Factors Leading to a Potential Nursing Shortage

To more accurately assess the depth or significance of any projected nursing shortage, data must be examined regarding both the demand for RNs and the supply.

Demand

As of 2020, RNs held about 3.1 million jobs (Bureau of Labor Statistics, 2022b). Even with declining vacancy rates, particularly at hospitals, there may not be enough RNs to meet either short- or long-term needs in hospitals or other health care settings. Indeed, according to the Bureau of Labor Statistics (2022a), the employment of registered nursing is projected to grow by 9% from 2020 to 2030.

Demand for RNs also is expected to continue or accelerate. This demand will be driven by technologic advances in patient care and by the increasing emphasis on preventive health care. In addition, Huston (2023b) notes that as life expectancy in the United States increases, more nurses will be needed to assist the individuals who are surviving serious illnesses and living longer with chronic diseases. The American Association of Colleges of Nursing (AACN, 2022b) concurs, predicting that larger numbers of older adults will increase the need for geriatric care, including care for individuals with chronic diseases and comorbidities.

Supply

The number of nurses available to meet demands, however, will lag. Although the RN workforce is expected to grow from 3,080,100 in 2020 to 3,356,800 in 2030, an increase of 9% (Bureau of Labor Statistics, 2022a), the AACN (2022b) notes that according to the 2018 "United States Registered Nurse Workforce Report Card and Shortage Forecast: A Revisit," a shortage of RNs will spread across the country between 2016 and 2030, with the shortage being felt most intensely in the Southern and Western United States.

The problem is not a lack of interest in nursing school enrollment. Enrollment in nursing schools has steadily increased every year for almost two decades (Huston, 2023b). Unfortunately, however, these increases do not appear to be adequate to replace those nurses who will be lost to retirement in the coming decade. Ironically, the problem is no longer a lack of nursing school applicants. The problem is that there are inadequate resources to provide nursing education to those interested in pursuing nursing as a career, including an insufficient number of clinical sites, classroom space, nursing faculty, and clinical preceptors. As a result, qualified applicants are turned away, despite the current shortage of nurses. In fact, the AACN (2022a) reported that 80,407 qualified applicants were turned away from baccalaureate and graduate nursing programs alone in 2019.

Most nursing schools responding to the survey pointed to faculty shortages as a reason for not accepting all qualified applicants into their programs (AACN, 2021a). According to a Special Survey on Vacant Faculty Positions released by AACN in October 2019, a total of 1,637 faculty vacancies were identified in a survey of 892 nursing schools with baccalaureate and/or graduate programs across the country, creating a national nurse faculty vacancy rate of 7.2% (AACN, 2022a). Inadequate numbers of doctorally prepared faculty and noncompetitive salaries compared with positions in the practice arena are fueling the problem. One must question where the faculty will come from to teach the new nurses who will be needed to address nursing shortages in the coming decade.

> The nursing faculty shortage may well be the greatest obstacle to solving the projected nursing shortage (Huston, 2023b).

In addition, Huston (2023b) notes that nursing is a "graying" population—even more so than the population at large. This means that the nursing workforce is retiring at a rate faster than it can be replaced. According to a 2018 National Sample Survey of Registered Nurses conducted by the Health Resources and Services Administration, the average age for an RN is 50 years old, which may signal a large retirement wave over the next 15 years (AACN, 2022b). In addition, in 2017, Dr. Peter Buerhaus and colleagues projected that more than 1 million RNs will leave the workforce by 2030 (AACN, 2022b).

Recruitment

Recruitment is the process of actively seeking out or attracting applicants for existing positions and should be an ongoing process. In complex organizations, work must be accomplished by groups of people; therefore, the organization's ability to meet its goals and objectives relates directly to the quality of its employees. Wise leader-managers surround themselves with people of ability, motivation, and promise. Unfortunately, some managers feel threatened by bright and talented people and surround themselves with mediocrity.

In addition, organizations must remember that nonmonetary factors are just as important, if not more so, in recruiting new employees. Before recruiting begins, organizations must identify reasons a prospective employee would choose to work for them over a competitor. Organizations considered best places to work typically are financially sustainable and focused on quality.

The Nurse-Recruiter

The manager may be greatly or minimally involved with recruiting, interviewing, and selecting personnel depending on (a) the size of the institution, (b) the existence of a separate personnel department, (c) the presence of a nurse-recruiter within the organization, and (d) the use of centralized or decentralized nursing management.

In general, the more decentralized nursing management and the less complex the personnel department is, the greater the involvement of lower-level managers in selecting personnel for individual units or departments. When deciding whether to hire a nurse-recruiter or decentralize the responsibility for recruitment, the organization needs to weigh benefits against costs. Costs include more than financial considerations. For example, an additional cost to an organization employing a nurse-recruiter might be the eventual loss of interest by managers in the recruiting process.

Therefore, when organizations use nurse-recruiters, there must be a collaborative relationship between managers and recruiters. Managers must be aware of recruitment constraints, and the recruiter must be aware of individual department needs and culture. Both parties must understand the organization's philosophy, benefit programs, salary scale, and other factors that influence employee retention.

The Relationship Between Recruitment and Retention

Recruiting adequate numbers of nurses is less difficult if the organization is in a progressive community with several schools of nursing and if the organization has a good reputation for quality patient care and fair employment practices. It is much more difficult to recruit nurses to rural areas that historically have experienced less appropriation of health care professionals per capita than urban areas. In addition, some health care organizations find it necessary to do external recruitment, partly because of their lack of attention to retention.

Because most recruitment is expensive, health care organizations often seek less costly means to achieve this goal. One of the best ways to maintain an adequate employee pool is by word of mouth—the recommendation of the organization's own satisfied and happy staff.

Recruitment, however, is not the key to adequate staffing in the long term—retention is, and it only occurs when the organization is able to create a work environment that makes staff want to stay. Such environments have been called *healthy work environments* (*HWEs*). According to the American Nurses Association (n.d.), "a *healthy work environment* is a place of 'physical, mental, and social well-being,' supporting optimal health and safety" (para. 3). The American Association of Critical-Care Nurses (n.d.) says that healthy work environments are characterized by six things: skilled communication, true collaboration, effective decision making, appropriate staffing, meaningful recognition, and authentic leadership. This leads to less moral distress, lower rates of workplace violence, and better nurse staffing and retention.

Some organizational turnover, however, is normal and, in fact, desirable. *Turnover* infuses the organization with fresh ideas. It also reduces the probability of *groupthink* in which everyone shares similar thought processes, values, and goals. However, excessive or unnecessary turnover reduces the ability of the organization to achieve its goals and is expensive. Such costs generally include human resource expenses for advertising and interviewing; recruitment fees such as sign-on bonuses; increased use of traveling nurses, overtime, and temporary replacements for the lost worker; lost productivity; and the costs of training time to bring the new employee up to desired efficiency.

Indeed, the replacement cost for an RN typically ranges from $22,000 to more than $64,000, a sum reflecting expenses associated with filling temporary vacancies and hiring and training new staff (Robert Wood Johnson Foundation [RWJF], 2001–2022). With estimated national annual turnover rates for RNs ranging from 8% to 14%, this can add up to a significant financial burden on hospitals and health care systems.

In addition, the RWJF (2001–2022) notes that the loss of veteran nurses is especially costly because nursing expertise takes years to develop. When experienced nurses leave, health care systems pay a heavy price because less-experienced nurses may not recognize symptoms as quickly, understand systems, or know the best ways to avoid certain medical errors.

The leader-manager recognizes the link between retention and recruitment. The middle-level manager often has the greatest impact in creating a positive social climate to promote retention. In addition, the closer the fit between what the nurse is seeking in employment and what the organization can offer, the greater the chance that the nurse will be retained.

LEARNING EXERCISE 15.1

Examining Recruitment Advertisements

Select one of the following:

1. In small groups, examine several nursing journals that carry job advertisements. Select three advertisements that particularly appeal to you. What do these advertisements say or what makes them stand out? Are similar key words used in all three advertisements? What bonuses or incentives are being offered to attract qualified professional nurses?
2. Select a health care agency in your area. Write an advertisement or recruitment poster that accurately depicts the agency and the community. Compare your completed advertisement or recruitment flyer with those created by others in your group.

Interviewing as a Selection Tool

An *interview* may be defined as a verbal interaction between individuals for a particular purpose. Although other tools such as testing and reference checks may be used, the interview is frequently accepted as the foundation for hiring, despite its well-known limitations in terms of reliability and validity.

The purposes or goals of the selection interview are threefold: (a) the interviewer seeks to obtain enough information to determine the applicant's suitability for the available position; (b) the applicant obtains adequate information to make an intelligent decision about accepting the job, should it be offered; and (c) the interviewer seeks to conduct the interview in such a manner that regardless of the interview's result, the applicant will continue to have respect for and goodwill toward the organization.

There are many types of interviews and formats for conducting them. For example, interviews may be unstructured, semistructured, or structured. The *unstructured interview* requires little planning because the goals for hiring may be unclear, questions are not prepared in advance, and often, the interviewer does more talking than the applicant. The lack of a standardized approach coupled with the low interrater reliability (the degree to which people agree) suggests the unstructured, unblinded interview should be replaced or augmented with a more rigorous interview strategy, yet the unstructured interview continues to be a frequently used selection tool today.

Semistructured interviews require some planning because the flow is focused and directed at major topic areas, although there is flexibility in the approach. The *structured interview* requires even greater planning time. Questions that address the specific job requirements must be developed in advance, information about the skills and qualities being sought must be offered, examples of the applicant's experience must be received, and the willingness or motivation of the applicant to do the job must be determined. The interviewer who uses a structured format would ask the same essential questions of all applicants.

> As a predictor of job performance and overall effectiveness, the structured interview is more reliable than the unstructured interview.

Limitations of Interviews

Interview bias is common. Forms of interview bias include stereotyping, forming an opinion about an applicant based on first impressions; identifying with a candidate personally rather than examining the position criteria; and asking different questions of different candidates (Lahr, 2021). In addition, in a recent survey of medical school applicants, gender, age, race, religion, and sexual orientation were all reported as sources of implicit bias in the medical school interview (Chatterjee et al., 2020). Participants also reported bias regarding education and income level, height, weight, and age. Indeed, one of every five medical school applicants reported having experienced interview bias (see Examining the Evidence 15.1).

The most significant defect of the hiring interview, however, is likely subjectivity. Indeed, research findings regarding the validity and reliability of interviews vary; however, the following findings are generally accepted:

- The same interviewer will consistently rate the interviewee the same. Therefore, the *intrarater reliability* is said to be high.
- If two different interviewers conduct unstructured interviews of the same applicant, their ratings will not be consistent. Therefore, *interrater reliability* is extremely low in unstructured interviews.
- Interrater reliability is better if the interview is *structured* and the same format is used by both interviewers.

EXAMINING THE EVIDENCE 15.1

Source: From Chatterjee, A., Greif, C., Witzburg, R., Henault, L., Goodell, K., & Paasche-Orlow, M. K. (2020). US medical school applicant experiences of bias on the interview trail. *Journal of Health Care for the Poor & Underserved, 31*(1), 185–200. https://doi-org.mantis.csuchico.edu/10.1353/hpu.2020.0017

One in Five Medical School Applicants Reports Interview Bias

A literature review suggests that the medical school interview is vulnerable to implicit bias. This study invited all 2018 to 2019 interviewees (n = 1,175) at one US medical school (Boston University School of Medicine) to complete the eight-item Everyday Discrimination Scale (EDS) to explore their experiences of bias during interview experiences. Three hundred forty-seven (30%) completed the survey.

Seventy-two (21%) responded affirmatively to one or more EDS items. Gender, age, race, religion, and sexual orientation were all sources of discrimination. Participants also reported bias due to a variety of additional factors, including education and income level, height, weight, and age.

Participants with a higher number of interviews were more likely to report an incident of bias. Most likely, this is because these participants had more opportunities to experience bias; however, it may also be that there may be a temporal aspect to expressions of bias— that later in the season, due to interviewer fatigue or other factors, expressions of bias are more likely to emerge.

Those reporting bias were also more likely to be Latinx than their counterparts. Two (14.3%) Black/African American respondents, 22 (33%) Latinx respondents, and 44 (22%) women answered yes to at least one question on the EDS. Of those responding yes to a question on the EDS, 35% reported experiencing this form of bias at more than one school. When asked what they did if they experienced bias on the interview trail, 52 (68%) reported telling friends or family members, whereas 23 (30%) reported doing nothing; only 3 (4%) indicated that they had reported the incident of bias to the medical school where it occurred.

The researchers concluded that formal but anonymous mechanisms to allow applicants to report bias are needed. In addition, developing effective bias-reduction trainings for the faculty, staff, and students participating in the admissions process will be important.

- Even if the interview has *reliability* (i.e., it measures the same thing consistently), it still may not be valid. *Validity* occurs when the interview measures what it is supposed to measure, which in this case, is the potential for productivity as an employee. Structured interviews have greater validity than unstructured interviews and thus should be better predictors of job performance and overall effectiveness than unstructured interviews.
- High interview assessments are not related to subsequent high-level job performance.
- Validity increases when there is a team approach to the interview.
- The attitudes and biases of interviewers greatly influence how candidates are rated. Although steps can be taken to reduce subjectivity, it cannot be eliminated entirely.
- The interviewer is more influenced by unfavorable information than by favorable information. Negative information is weighed more heavily than positive information about the applicant.
- Interviewers tend to make up their minds about hiring applicants very early in the job interview. Decisions are often formed in the first few minutes of the interview.
- In unstructured interviews, the interviewer tends to do most of the talking, whereas in structured interviews, the interviewer talks less. The goal should always be to have the interviewee do most of the talking.

Overcoming Interview Limitations

Interview research has helped managers develop strategies for overcoming its limitations. The following strategies will assist the manager in developing an interview process with greater reliability and validity.

Use a Team Approach

Having more than one person interview the job applicant reduces individual bias. When hiring a manager, using a staff nurse as part of the interview team is effective, especially if the staff nurse is mature enough to represent the interests and needs of the unit rather than personal interests.

Develop a Structured Interview Format for Each Job Classification

Managers should obtain a copy of the job description and know the educational and experiential requirements for each position prior to the interview. In addition, because each job has different position requirements, interviews must be structured to fit the position. The same structured interview should be used for all employees applying for the same job classification. A well-developed structured interview uses open-ended questions and provides ample opportunity for the interviewee to talk. The structured interview is advantageous because it allows the interviewer to be consistent and prevents the interview from becoming sidetracked. Display 15.3 provides sample questions that might be used for a structured interview.

Use Scenarios to Determine Decision-Making Ability

Scenarios may also be used as a tool to assess problem-solving and decision-making abilities. The same set of scenarios should be used with each category of employee. For example, a set could be developed for new graduates, critical care nurses, unit secretaries, and licensed practical nurses. Patient care situations, as shown in Display 15.4, require clinical judgment and are very useful for this purpose.

Conduct Multiple Interviews

Candidates should be interviewed more than once on separate days. This prevents applicants from being accepted or rejected merely because they were having a good or bad day. Regardless of the number of interviews held, the person should be interviewed until all the interviewers' questions have been answered and they feel confident that they have enough information to make the right decision.

Provide Training in Effective Interviewing Techniques

Interview training should focus on communication skills and advice on planning, conducting, and controlling the interview. It is unfair to expect a manager to make appropriate hiring

---

LEARNING EXERCISE 15.2

Creating Additional Interview Criteria

You are a home health nurse with a large caseload of families from low-income areas of the city. Because of your spouse's job transfer, you have just resigned from your position of 3 years to take a similar position in another public health district. Your agency supervisor has asked you to assist her with interviewing and selecting your replacement. Five applicants meet the minimum criteria. They each have at least 2 years of acute care experience, a baccalaureate nursing degree, and a state public health credential. Because you know the job requirements better than anyone, your supervisor has asked that you develop additional criteria and a set of questions to ask each applicant.

ASSIGNMENT:

1. Use a decision grid (refer to Fig. 1.3 in Chapter 1) to develop additional criteria. Weight the criteria so that the applicants will have a final score.
2. Develop an interview guide of six appropriate questions to ask the applicants.

DISPLAY 15.3 SAMPLE STRUCTURED INTERVIEW

Motivation

Why did you apply for employment with this organization?

Education

What was your grade point average in nursing school?
What were your extracurricular activities, offices held, awards conferred?
For verification purposes, are your school records listed under the name on your application?

Professional

In what states are you licensed to practice?
Do you have your license with you?
What certifications do you hold?
What professional organizations do you currently participate in that would be of value in the job for which you are applying?

Military Experience

What are your current military obligations?
Which military assignments do you think have prepared you for this position?

Present Employer

How did you secure your present position?
What is your current job title? What was your title when you began your present position?
What supervisory responsibilities do you currently have?
What are some examples of success at your present job?
How would you describe the work culture at your current place of employment?
What do you like most about your present job?
What do you like least about your present job?
May we contact your present employer?
Why do you want to change jobs?
For verification purposes only, is your name the same as it was while employed with your current employer?

Previous Position(s)

Ask similar questions about recent past employment. Depending on the time span and type of other positions held, the interviewer does not usually review employment history that took place beyond the position just before the current one.

Specific Questions for Registered Nurses

What do you like most about nursing?
What do you like least about nursing?
What is your philosophy of nursing?

Personal Characteristics

Which personal characteristics are your greatest assets?
Which personal characteristics cause you the most difficulty?
How do you handle conflict?
Can you provide an example of a successful conflict resolution intervention you were involved in?
What specific skill sets will you bring to this job that will be most helpful?

Professional Goals

What are your career goals?
Where do you see yourself 5 years from now?

Contributions to Organization

What can you offer this organization? This unit or department?

General Questions

What questions do you have about the organization?
What questions do you have about the position?
What other questions do you have?

DISPLAY 15.4 SAMPLE INTERVIEW QUESTIONS USING CASE SITUATIONS

Each recent graduate applying for a position at Country Hospital will be asked to respond to the following:

Case 1

You are working on the evening shift of a surgical unit. Mr. Jones returned from the postanesthesia care unit following a hip replacement 2 hours ago. While in the recovery room, he received 10 mg of morphine sulfate intravenously for incisional pain. Thirty minutes ago, he complained of mild incisional pain but then drifted off to sleep. He is now awake and complaining of moderate to severe incisional pain. His orders include the following pain relief order: morphine sulfate 8 to 10 mg, IV push every 3 hours for pain. It has been 2.5 hours since Mr. Jones's last pain medication. What would you do?

Case 2

One of the licensed practical nurses/licensed vocational nurses on your team seems especially tired today. She later tells you that her new baby kept her up all night. When you ask her about the noon finger-stick blood glucose level on Mrs. White (82 years old), she looks at you blankly and then says quickly that it was 150. Later, when you are in Mrs. White's room, she tells you that she does not remember anyone checking her blood glucose level at noon. What do you do?

---

decisions without adequate training in interview techniques. Unskilled interviewers often allow subjective data rather than objective data to affect their hiring evaluation. In addition, unskilled interviewers may ask questions that could be viewed as discriminatory or that are illegal.

> Many people think they are better interviewers than they really are.

Planning, Conducting, and Controlling the Interview

Planning the interview in advance is vital to its subsequent success as a selection tool. If other interviewers are to be present, they should be available at the appointed time. The plan also should include adequate time for the interview. Before the interview, all interviewers should review the application, noting questions concerning information supplied by the applicant. Although it takes considerable practice, consistently using a planned sequence in the interview format will eventually yield a relaxed and spontaneous process. The following is a suggested interview format:

1. Introduce yourself and greet the applicant.
2. Make a brief statement about the organization and the available positions.
3. Clarify the position for which the person is applying.
4. Discuss the information on the application and seek clarification or amplification as necessary.
5. Discuss employee qualifications and proceed with the structured interview format.
6. If the applicant appears qualified, discuss the organization and the position further.
7. Explain the subsequent procedures for hiring, such as employment physicals, and hiring date. If the applicant is not hired at this time, discuss how and when they will be notified of the interview results.
8. Terminate the interview.

Try to create and maintain a comfortable environment throughout the interview, but do not forget that the interviewer should control the interview. If the interview has begun well and the applicant is at ease, the interview will usually proceed smoothly. During the meeting, the manager should pause frequently to allow the applicant to ask questions. The format should always encourage and include ample time for questions from the applicant. Often, interviewers can infer much about applicants by the types of questions that they ask.

> Remember that the interviewer should have control of the interview and set the tone.

Moving the conversation along, covering questions on a structured interview guide, and keeping the interview pertinent but friendly becomes easier with experience. Methods that help reach the goals of the interview follow:

- Ask only job-related questions.
- Use open-ended questions that require more than a "yes" or "no" answer.
- Pause a few seconds after the applicant has seemingly finished before asking the next question. This gives the applicant a chance to talk further.
- Return to topics later in the interview on which the applicant offered little information initially.
- Ask only one question at a time.
- Restate part of the applicant's answer if you need elaboration.
- Ask questions clearly, but do not verbally or nonverbally indicate the correct answer. Otherwise, by watching the interviewer's eyes and observing other body language, the astute applicant may learn which answers are desired.
- Always appear interested in what the applicant has to say. The applicant should never be interrupted, nor should the interviewer's words ever imply criticism of or impatience with the applicant.
- Use language that is appropriate for the applicant. Terminology or language that makes applicants feel the interviewer is either talking down to them or talking over their heads is inappropriate.
- Keep a written record of all interviews. Note-taking ensures accuracy and serves as a written record to recall the applicant. Keep note-taking or use of a checklist, however, to a minimum so that you do not create an uncomfortable climate.

In addition, McNamara (2022) suggests that:

- Applicants should be involved in the interview as soon as possible.
- Factual data should be elicited before asking about controversial matters (such as feelings and conclusions).
- Fact-based questions should be interspersed throughout the interview to avoid having respondents disengage.
- The interviewer should ask questions about the present before questions about the past or future.
- Applicant should be allowed to close the interview with information they want to add or to comment regarding their impressions of the interview.

As the interview draws to a close, the interviewer should make sure that all questions have been answered and that all pertinent information has been obtained. Usually, applicants are not offered a job at the end of a first interview unless they are clearly qualified, and the labor market is such that another applicant would be difficult to find. In most cases, interviewers need to analyze their impressions of the applicant, compare these perceptions with members of the selection team, and incorporate those impressions with other available data about the applicant. It is important, however, to let applicants know if they are being seriously considered for the position and how soon they can expect to hear an outcome.

When the applicant is obviously not qualified, the interviewer should tactfully advise the person as soon as possible that they do not have the proper qualifications for the position. Such applicants should believe that they have been treated fairly. The interviewer should, however, maintain records of the exact reasons for rejection in case of later questions.

Regardless of the inherent defects, interviewing continues to be widely used as a selection tool. By knowing the limitations of interviews and using findings from current research evidence, interviewers should be able to conduct interviews so that they will have an increased predictive value.

Evaluation of the Interview

Interviewers should plan postinterview time to evaluate the applicant's interview performance. Interview notes should be reviewed as soon as possible, and necessary points clarified or amplified. Using a form to record the interview evaluation is a good idea. The final question on the interview report form is a recommendation for or against hiring. In answering this question, two aspects must carry the most weight:

- *The requirements for the job.* Regardless of how interesting or friendly people are, unless they have the basic skills for the job, they will not be successful at meeting the expectations of the position. Likewise, those overqualified for a position will usually be unhappy in the job.
- *Personal bias.* Because completely eliminating the personal biases inherent in the interview is impossible, it is important for the interviewer to examine any negative feelings that occurred during the interview. Often, the interviewer discovers that the negative feelings have no relation to the criteria necessary for success in the position.

Legal Aspects of Interviewing

The organization must be sure that the application form does not contain questions that violate various employment acts. Likewise, managers must avoid unlawful inquiries during the interview. Table 15.1 lists subjects that are most frequently part of the interview process or applicant form, with examples of acceptable and unacceptable inquiries.

> Interview inquiries regarding age, marital status, children, race, sexual orientation, financial or credit status, national origin, or religion are illegal because they are deemed discriminatory.

Managers who maintain interview records and receive applicants with an open and unbiased attitude have little to fear regarding charges of discrimination. Remember that each applicant should feel good about the organization when the interview concludes and be able to recall the experience as a positive one. It is a leadership responsibility to see that this goal is accomplished.

Tips for the Interviewee

Just as there are things that the interviewer should do to prepare and conduct the interview, there are things interviewees should do to increase the likelihood that the interview will be a mutually satisfying and enlightening experience. The interviewee must also prepare in advance for the interview. Obtaining copies of the philosophy and organization chart of the organization to which you are applying should give you some insight as to the organization's priorities and help you to identify questions to ask the interviewer. In addition, speaking to individuals who already work at the organization should be helpful in determining whether the organization's philosophy is implemented in practice.

TABLE 15.1 ACCEPTABLE AND UNACCEPTABLE INTERVIEW INQUIRIES

Subject	Acceptable Inquiries	Unacceptable Inquiries
Name	If applicant has worked for the organization under a different name; if school records are under another name; if applicant has another name	Inquiries about name that would indicate lineage, national origin, or marital status
Marital and family status	Whether applicant can meet specified work schedules or has commitments that may hinder attendance requirements; inquiries as to anticipated stay in the position	Any question about applicant's marital status or number or age of children; information about childcare arrangements; any questions concerning pregnancy
Address or residence	Place of residence and length resided in city or state	Former addresses, names or relationships of people with whom applicant resides, or if owns or rents home
Age	If older than 18 years or statement that hire is subject to age requirement; can ask if the applicant is between 18 and 70 years	Inquiry of specific age or date of birth
Birthplace	Can ask for proof of US citizenship	Birthplace of the applicant or spouse or any relative
Religion	No inquiries allowed	
Race or color	Can be requested for affirmative action but not as employment criteria	All questions about race are prohibited
Character	Inquiry into actual convictions that directly relate to ability to be licensed or fitness to perform job	Questions relating to arrests or conviction of a crime not directly related to ability to be licensed or fitness to perform job
Relatives	Relatives employed in organization; names and addresses of parents if the applicant is a minor	Questions about who the applicant lives with or the number of dependents
Notify in case of emergency	Name and address of a *person* to be notified	Name and address of a *relative* to be notified
Organizations	Professional organizations	Requesting a list of all memberships
References	Professional or character reference	Religious references
Physical condition	All applicants can be asked if they are able to carry out the physical demands of the job	Employers must be prepared to justify any mental or physical requirements. Specific questions regarding disabilities are forbidden
Photographs	Statement that a photograph may be required *after* employment	Requirement that a photograph be taken *before* interview or hiring
National origin	If necessary to perform job, languages applicant speaks, reads, or writes	Inquiries about birthplace, native language, ancestry, date of arrival in the United States, or native language
Education	Academic, vocational, or professional education; schools attended; ability to read, speak, and write foreign languages	Inquiries about racial or religious affiliation of a school; inquiry about dates of schooling
Sex	Inquiry or restriction of employment is only for bona fide occupational qualification, which is interpreted very narrowly by the courts	Cannot ask sex on application. Sex cannot be used as a factor for hiring decisions
Credit rating	No inquiries	Questions about car or home ownership are also prohibited
Other	Notice may be given that misstatements or omissions of facts may be cause for dismissal	

Schedule an appointment for the interview. Do not allow yourself to be drawn into an impromptu interview when you are dropping off an application or seeking information from the human resource department. You will want to be professionally dressed and will likely need time to reflect and prepare for the interview.

> Practice responses to potential interview questions. It is difficult to spontaneously answer interview questions about your personal philosophy of nursing, your individual strengths and weaknesses, and your career goals if you have not given them advance thought.

On the day of the interview, arrive about 10 minutes early to allow time for you to collect your thoughts and be mentally ready. Anticipate some nervousness (this is perfectly normal). Greet the interviewer formally (not by first name) but do not sit down before the interviewer does unless given permission to do so. Be sure to shake the interviewer's hand on entering the room and to smile. Smiling will reduce both your anxiety and the interviewer's. Remember that many interviewers make up their mind early in the interview process, so first impressions count.

During the interview, maintain eye contact, sit quietly, be attentive, and take notes only if necessary. Do not chew gum; fidget; slouch; or play with your hair, keys, or pen. Dress conservatively and make sure that you are neatly groomed. Keep jewelry to a minimum and do not wear perfume or aftershave. Ask appropriate questions about the organization or the specific job for which you are applying. Questions about wages, benefits, and advancement opportunities should likely come later in the interview. Avoid a "what can you do for me?" approach and focus instead on whether your unique talents and interests are a fit with the organization. Answer interview questions as honestly and confidently as possible. Avoid rambling and never lie. If you do not know the answer to a question, say so. Also, if you need a few moments to reflect on a complex question before answering, state that as well.

At the close of the interview, shake the interviewer's hand and thank them for taking time to talk with you. It is always appropriate to clarify at that point when hiring decisions will be made and how you will be notified about the interview's outcome. You may want to send a brief thank-you note to the interviewer as well, so be sure to note their correct title and the spelling of their name before you leave.

The Connecticut Department of Labor (2002–2022) advises candidates to assess the interview itself as soon as it is completed. This assessment should include reactions to the interview, including what went well and what went poorly. In addition, candidates should assess what they learned from the experience and what they might do differently in future interviews. Interviewing tips for applicants are summarized in Display 15.5.

Selection

After applicants have been recruited, completed their applications, and been interviewed, the next step in the preemployment staffing process is selection. *Selection* is the process of choosing the best qualified individual or individuals for a job or position. This process involves verifying the applicant's qualifications, checking their work history, and deciding if a good match exists between the applicant's qualifications and the organization's expectations. Determining whether a "fit" exists between an employee and an organization is seldom easy but hiring the wrong person often comes at significant cost to both the organization and the individual who has been hired. Structured interviews and background checks can help employers form an accurate picture of an applicant's past behavior, but preemployment screening for a potential employee is a more accurate predictor of future behavior.

DISPLAY 15.5 INTERVIEWING TIPS FOR APPLICANTS

1. Prepare in advance for the interview.
2. Review the philosophy and organization chart of the organization to which you are applying.
3. Schedule an appointment for the interview.
4. Dress professionally and conservatively. Jewelry should be modest. Do not wear perfume or aftershave.
5. Practice responses to potential interview questions in advance and out loud to increase your confidence in responding.
6. Arrive early on the day of the interview.
7. Greet the interviewer formally and do not sit down before they do unless given permission to do so.
8. Shake the interviewer's hand on entering the room and smile.
9. Maintain eye contact throughout the interview.
10. Sit quietly, be attentive, and take notes only if absolutely necessary during the interview.
11. Do not chew gum; fidget; slouch; or play with your hair, keys, or pen.
12. Ask appropriate questions about the organization or the specific job for which you are applying.
13. Avoid a "what can you do for me?" approach and focus instead on whether your unique talents and interests are a fit with the organization.
14. Answer interview questions as honestly and confidently as possible.
15. Shake the interviewer's hand at the close of the interview and thank them for their time.
16. Send a brief thank-you note to the interviewer within 24 hours of the interview.

Educational and Credential Requirements

Consideration should be given to educational requirements and credentials for each job category if a relationship exists between these requirements and success on the job. If requirements for a position are too rigid, the job may remain unfilled for some time. In addition, people who might be able to complete educational or credential requirements for a position are sometimes denied the opportunity to compete for the job. Therefore, many organizations have a list of *preferred criteria* for a position and a second list of *minimum criteria*. In addition, frequently, organizations will accept *substitution criteria* in lieu of preferred criteria. For example, a position might require a bachelor's degree, but a master's degree is preferred. However, 5 years of nursing experience might be substituted for the master's degree.

Clearly, there is a movement among health care employers to hire more nurses with at least a Bachelor of Science in Nursing degree and to urge staff to pursue higher degrees. Nurse executives value what all nurses bring to patient care, but they want to ensure staff can meet the challenges that continue to come their way and that patient care is optimized. With research supporting that educational entry level matters and that improvements in patient outcomes correlate with the number of baccalaureate or higher educated nurses (AACN, 2019), it is difficult to oppose having higher education levels as preferred criteria, if not required criteria for nursing hires. In addition, the American Nurses Credentialing Center's Magnet Recognition Program requires nurse-managers and leaders to have a degree in nursing at either the baccalaureate or graduate level.

Reference Checks and Background Screening

All applications should be examined to see if they are complete and to ascertain that the applicant is qualified for the position. It is very important to check the academic and professional credentials of all job applicants. In a competitive job market, candidates may succumb to the pressure of "embellishing" their qualifications. After determining that an applicant is qualified, references are requested, and employment history is verified. In addition, a background check is often required.

Clearly, a strong application and excellent references do not necessarily guarantee excellent job performance; however, carefully reviewing applications and checking references may help prevent a bad hiring decision. Ideally, whenever possible, these actions as well as verifying work experience and credentials should be done before the interview. Some managers prefer to interview first so that time is not wasted in processing the application if the interview results in a decision not to hire, and this is a personal choice.

> Positions should never be offered until information on the application has been verified and references have been checked.

Occasionally, reference calls will reveal unsolicited information about the applicant. Information obtained by any method may not be used to reject an applicant unless a justifiable reason for disqualification exists. For example, if the applicant volunteers information about their driving record or if this information is discovered by other means, it cannot be used to reject a potential employee unless the position requires driving.

Mandatory background checks have also become commonplace in health care settings. This has occurred because health care providers have access to vulnerable patients or protected health and financial information. Some concerns exist, however, as to who may be overseeing this screening and whether they are truly qualified to assess the risk. Complicating the issue are guidelines issued in 2012 by the U.S. Equal Employment Opportunity Commission (EEOC) that stopped short of banning criminal background checks but said that refusing to hire someone with a criminal record could constitute illegal discrimination if such decisions disproportionately affected minority groups. The EEOC (n.d.) went on to suggest that any decision not to hire must be job related and consistent with business necessity and consider factors such as the nature and gravity of the criminal offense, the amount of time since the conviction, and the relevance of the offense to the job being sought.

Preemployment Testing

The Society for Human Resource Management (SHRM, 2018) notes that employment tests typically are standardized devices designed to measure skills, intellect, personality, or other characteristics, and they yield a score, rating, description, or category. However, according to the Uniform Guidelines on Employee Selection Procedures of 1978 issued by the EEOC, any employment requirement set by an employer could be considered a "test." Thus, "preemployment tests need to be selected and monitored with care since employers run the risk of litigation if a selection decision is challenged and determined to be discriminatory or in violation of state or federal regulations. In addition, tests used in the selection process must be legal, reliable, valid, and equitable" (SHRM, 2018, para. 2).

Currently, there are many preemployment tests used to assess potential employee fit in an organization. Preemployment testing, however, is generally used only when such testing is directly related to the ability to perform a specific job, although the use of *personality tests* is becoming much more common in health care organizations. Indeed, a survey from the SHRM found that one third of human resource professionals currently use personality tests and preemployment testing to vet candidates in the hiring process (Feldman, 2022).

Personality tests are designed to reveal specific aspects of a candidate's personality and estimate the likelihood that they will excel in such a position (Feldman, 2022). For example, the questions "Do you become irritated when others criticize you?" or "How do you typically respond in a crisis?" might be used to assess emotional stability.

Although testing is not a stand-alone selection tool, when coupled with interviewing and reference checking, it can provide additional information about candidates to make a selection decision. Lawsuits, however, have resulted from allegedly improper implementation and interpretation of preemployment testing, and this makes some employers shy away from doing it.

Physical Examination as a Selection Tool

A medical examination is often a requirement for hiring. This examination determines if the applicant can meet the requirements for a specific job and provides a record of the physical condition of the applicant at the time of hiring.

Only those selected for hire can be required to have a physical examination, which is nearly always conducted at the employer's expense. If the physical examination reveals information that disqualifies the applicant, they are not hired. Most employers make job offers contingent on meeting certain health or physical requirements.

Making the Selection

When determining the most appropriate person to hire, the leader must be sure that the same standards are used to evaluate all candidates. Final selection should be based on established criteria, not on value judgments and personal preferences.

Frequently, positions are filled with internal applicants. These positions might be entry level or management. Internal candidates should be interviewed in the same manner as newcomers to the organization; however, some organizations give special consideration and preference to their own employees. Every organization should have guidelines and policies regarding how transfers and promotions are to be handled.

Finalizing the Selection

Once a final selection has been made, the manager is responsible for closure of the preemployment process as follows:

1. Follow-up with applicants as soon as possible, thanking them for applying and informing them when they will be notified about a decision.
2. Candidates not offered a position should be notified of this as soon as possible. Reasons should be provided when appropriate (e.g., insufficient education and work experience), and candidates should be told whether their application will be considered for future employment or if they should reapply.
3. Applicants offered a position should be informed in writing of the benefits, salary, and placement. This avoids misunderstandings later regarding what employees think they were promised by the nurse-recruiter or the interviewer.
4. Applicants who accept job offers should be informed of preemployment procedures such as physical examinations and supplied with the date to report to work.
5. Applicants who are offered positions should be requested to confirm in writing their intention to accept the position.

Because selection involves a process of reduction (i.e., diminishing the number of candidates for a particular position), the person making the final selection has a great deal of responsibility. These decisions have far-reaching consequences, both for the organization and for the people involved. For these reasons, the selection process should be as objective as possible. The selection process is shown in Figure 15.1.

LEARNING EXERCISE 15.3

Making a Hiring Selection and Assessing Its Impact

You are the director of an outpatient, senior community center, a position that you have held for 6 years. You are comfortable with your role and know your staff well. Recently, your lead registered nurse resigned. Two of your staff, Nancy and Sally, have applied for her position.

Nancy, an older nurse, has been with the organization for 8 years part time. Most of her work experience prior to her hire at the senior community center was in acute care nursing. She performs her job competently and has good interpersonal relationships with the other staff and with patients and physicians. Although her motivation level is adequate for her current job, she has demonstrated little creativity or initiative in helping the center establish a reputation for excellence, nor has she demonstrated specific skills in predicting or planning for the future.

Sally, a nurse in her mid-30s, has been with the organization and the unit for 2 years. She has been a positive driving force behind many of the changes that have occurred. She is an excellent clinician and is highly respected by physicians and staff. The older staff, however, appear to resent her because they feel that she attempted too much change early in her employment. Both nurses have baccalaureate degrees and meet all the qualifications for the job. Both nurses can be expected to work at least another 5 years in the new position. There is no precedent for your decision.

You must make a selection. If you do not use seniority as a primary selection criterion, many of the long-term employees may resent both Sally and you, and they may become demotivated. You are aware that Nancy is limited in her futuristic thinking and that the center may not grow and develop under her leadership as it could under that of Sally.

ASSIGNMENT:

Identify how your own values will affect your decision. Rank your selection criteria and make a decision about what you will do. Determine the personal, interpersonal, and organizational impact of your decision.

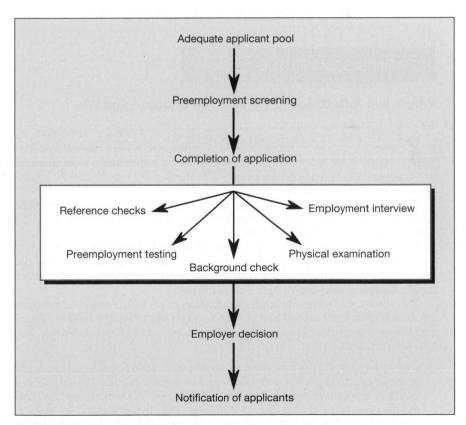

FIGURE 15.1 The selection process.

Placement

Research shows that if an employee is placed in a position that doesn't match their skillset, personal values, or if the employee cannot form an interpersonal connection with other workers, it often leads to lower work engagement, which in turn leads to lower productivity and greater turnover (Feldman, 2022). The astute leader can, however, assign a new employee to a position within their sphere of authority, where the employee will have a reasonable chance for success. This requires the leader to recognize that nursing units and departments develop subcultures with their own norms, values, and methods of accomplishing work. It is possible for one person to fit in well with an established group, whereas another equally qualified person would never become part of that group.

In addition, many positions within a unit or department require different skills. For example, in a hospital, decision-making skills might be more important on a shift where leadership is weaker; communication skills might be the most highly desired skill on a shift where there is a great deal of interaction among a variety of nursing personnel.

Frequently, newcomers suffer feelings of failure because of inappropriate placement within the organization. This can be as true for the newly hired experienced employee as for the novice nurse. Appropriate placement is as important to the organization's functioning as it is to the new employee's success. Faulty placement can result in reduced organizational efficiency, increased attrition, threats to organizational integrity, and frustration of personal and professional ambitions.

Conversely, proper placement fosters personal growth, provides a motivating climate for the employee, maximizes productivity, and increases the probability that organizational goals will be met. Leaders who can match employee strengths to job requirements facilitate unit functioning, accomplish organizational goals, and meet employee needs.

LEARNING EXERCISE 15.4

Which Two New Graduates Would You Choose—and Why?

You are the supervisor of a critical care surgical unit. For the past several years, you have been experimenting with placing four newly graduated nurses directly into the unit, two from each spring and fall graduating class. These nurses are from the local Bachelor of Science in Nursing program. You consult closely with the nursing faculty and their former employers before making a selection.

Overall, this experiment has worked well. Only two new graduates were unable to develop into critical care nurses. Both of these nurses later transferred back into the unit after 2 years in a less intensive medical-surgical area.

Because of the new graduates' motivation and enthusiasm, they have complemented your experienced critical care staff nicely. You believe that your success with this program has been due to your well-planned and structured 4-month orientation and education program, careful selection, and appropriate shift placement.

This spring, you have narrowed the selection down to four qualified candidates. You plan to place one on the 3 PM to 11 PM shift and one on the 11 PM to 7 AM shift. You sit in your office and review the culture of each shift and your notes on the four candidates. You have the following information:

3 PM to 11 PM shift: A very assertive, all-female staff; 85% registered nurses and 15% licensed practical nurses (LPNs)/licensed vocational nurses (LVNs). This is your most clinically competent group. They are highly respected by everyone, and although the physicians often have confrontations with them, the physicians also tell you frequently how good they are. The nurses are known as a group that lacks humor and does not welcome newcomers. However, once the new employee earns their trust, they are very supportive. They are intolerant of anyone not living up to their exceptionally high standards. Your two unsuccessful new graduate placements were assigned to this shift.

11 PM to 7 AM shift: A very cohesive and supportive group. Although overall these nurses are competent, this shift has some of your more clinically weak staff. However, it is also the shift that rates the highest with families and patients. They are caring and compassionate. Every new graduate that you have placed on this shift has been successful. Of the nurses on this shift, 30% are men. The group tends to be very close and has a number of outside social activities.

Your four applicants consist of the following:

- *John*: He has had a great deal of emergency department (ED) experience as a medical emergency technician. He appears somewhat aloof. His definite career goals are 2 years in critical care, 3 years in ED, and then flight crew. Instructors praise his independent judgment but believe that he was somewhat of a loner in school. Former employers have rated him as an independent thinker and very capable.
- *Sally*: She recently graduated at the top of her class clinically and academically. She has not had much work experience other than the last 2 years as a summer nursing intern at a medical center where her performance appraisal was very good. Instructors believe that she lacks some maturity and interpersonal skills but praise her clinical judgment. She does not want to work in a regular medical-surgical unit. She believes that she can adapt to critical care.
- *Joan*: She has had a great deal of health-related work experience in counseling and has had limited clinical work experience (only nursing school). Former employers praise her attention to detail and her general competence. Instructors praise her interpersonal skills, maturity, and intelligence. She is quite willing to work elsewhere if not selected. She has a long-term commitment to nursing.
- *Mary*: She was previously an LPN/LVN and returned to school to get her degree. She did not do as well academically due to working and family commitments. Former employers and instructors speak of her energy, organization, and interpersonal skills. She appears to have fewer independent decision-making skills than the others do. She previously worked in a critical care unit.

ASSIGNMENT:

Select the two new graduates and place them on the appropriate shift. Support your decisions with rationale.

Onboarding

As a management function, *onboarding* refers to the process by which "new employees are introduced to the social and performance aspects of their new job, with the goal of getting new hires adjusted quickly, increasing productivity and job satisfaction, and reducing turnover" (Valamis, 2022, para 4). Although the words "induction" and "orientation" are frequently used to describe this function, socialization is also a critical component. Because socialization is part of the staff development and team-building process, it is covered in the next chapter.

When onboarding is done well, it can establish favorable employee attitudes toward the organization, unit, and department; provide the necessary information and education for success in the position; and instill a feeling of belonging and acceptance. Effective onboarding also results in higher productivity, fewer rule violations, reduced attrition, and greater employee satisfaction (Valamis, 2022). Onboarding begins as soon as a person has been selected for a position and continues until the employee has been socialized to the norms and values of the work group. An example of employee onboarding content is shown in Display 15.6. Effective onboarding programs assist employees to have successful employment tenure. Much of this

DISPLAY 15.6 EMPLOYEE ONBOARDING CONTENT

1. Organization history, mission, and philosophy
2. Organizational structure, including department heads, with an explanation of the functions of the various departments
3. Employee responsibilities to the organization
4. Organizational responsibilities to the employee
5. Payroll information, including how increases in pay are earned and when they are given (Progressive or unionized companies publish pay scales for all employees)
6. Rules of conduct
7. Tour of the facility and of the assigned department
8. Work schedules, staffing, and scheduling policies
9. When applicable, a discussion of the collective bargaining agreement
10. Benefit plans, including life insurance, health insurance, pension, and unemployment
11. Safety and fire programs
12. Staff development programs, including in-service, and continuing education for relicensure
13. Promotion and transfer policies
14. Employee appraisal system
15. Workload assignments
16. Introduction to paperwork/forms used in the organization
17. Review of selection in policies and procedures
18. Specific legal requirements, such as maintaining a current license and reporting of accidents
19. Electronic health record training
20. Fire and safety training
21. Health Insurance Portability and Accountability Act training
22. Blood-borne pathogen training
23. Introduction to fellow employees
24. Establishment of a feeling of belonging and acceptance, showing genuine interest in the new employee

content could be provided in an online or print employee handbook, and the fire and safety regulations could be handled by a media presentation. Appropriate use of DVDs or electronic resources can be very helpful in the design of a good orientation program. All onboarding programs should be monitored to see if they are achieving their goals. Most programs need to be revised at least annually.

Induction

Induction, the first phase of onboarding, takes place after the employee has been selected but before performing the job role. The process includes all activities that educate the new employee about the organization and employment and personnel policies and procedures.

Induction activities are often performed during the placement and preemployment functions of staffing or may be included with orientation activities. However, induction and orientation are often separate entities, and new employees suffer if content from either program is omitted. The most important factor is to provide the employee with adequate information.

Employee handbooks, an important part of induction, are usually developed by the personnel department. Managers, however, should know what information the employee handbooks contain and should have input into their development. Most employee handbooks contain a form that must be signed by the employee, verifying that they have received and read it. The signed form is then placed in the employee's personnel file.

The handbook is important because employees cannot assimilate all the induction information at one time, so they need a reference for later. However, providing an employee with a personnel handbook is not sufficient for real understanding. The information must be followed with discussion by various people during the employment process, such as the personnel manager and staff development personnel during orientation. The most important link in promoting real understanding of personnel policies is the first-level manager.

Orientation

Induction provides the employee with general information about the organization, whereas *orientation* activities are more specific for the position. A sample 2-week orientation schedule is shown in Table 15.2. Organizations may use a wide variety of orientation programs. For example, a first-day orientation could be conducted by the hospital's personnel department, which could include a tour of the hospital and all of the induction items listed in Display 15.6.

TABLE **SAMPLE 2-WEEK ORIENTATION SCHEDULE FOR EXPERIENCED NURSES**

Week 1	
Day 1, Monday:	
8:00 AM–10:00 AM	Welcome by personnel department; employee handbooks distributed and discussed
10:00 AM–10:30 AM	Refreshments served; welcome by staff development department
10:30 AM–11:30 AM	General orientation by staff development
11:30 AM–12:15 PM	Blood-borne pathogen training
12:15 PM–12:45 PM	Lunch
12:45 PM–1:30 PM	Tour of the organization
1:30 PM–3:00 PM	Fire and safety training; HIPAA training
3:00 PM–4:00 PM	Afternoon refreshments and introduction to each unit supervisor
Day 2, Tuesday:	
8:00 AM–9:00 AM	Report to individual units. Time with unit supervisor; introduction to assigned preceptor
9:00 AM–10:00 AM	General orientation of policies and procedures
10:00 AM–12:00 PM	Electronic health record orientation (part I)
12:00 PM–12:30 PM	Lunch
12:30 PM–4:30 PM	Electronic health record orientation (part II)
Day 3, Wednesday:	
8:00 PM–4:30 PM	Skills certifications/competence assessments
Day 4, Thursday:	Assigned all day to unit with preceptor
Day 5, Friday:	Morning with preceptor; afternoon with supervisor and staff development for wrap-up
Week 2	
Monday to Wednesday:	Work with preceptor on shift and unit assigned, gradually assuming greater responsibilities
Thursday:	Assign 80% of normal assignment with assistance and supervision from preceptor
Friday:	Carry normal workload. Have at least a 30-minute meeting with immediate supervisor to discuss progress

HIPAA, Health Insurance Portability and Accountability Act.

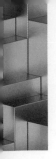

DISPLAY 15.7 COMMON RESPONSIBILITIES FOR ORIENTATION

1. Personnel or human resources department: Performs salary and payroll functions, insurance forms, physical examinations, income withholding forms, tour of the organization, employee responsibilities to the organization and vice versa, additional labor–management relationships, and benefit plan
2. Staff development department: Hands out and reviews employee handbook; discusses organizational philosophy and mission; reviews history of the organization; shows media presentation of various departments and how they function (if a media presentation is not available, introduces various department heads and shares how departments function); discusses organizational structure, fire and safety programs, blood-borne pathogen training, Health Insurance Portability and Accountability Act certification, and electronic health record training; discusses available educational and training programs; and reviews selected policies and procedures, including medication, treatment, and charting policies
3. The individual unit: Tour of the department; introductions; review of specific unit policies that differ in any way from general policies; review of unit scheduling and staffing policies and procedures, work assignments, and promotion and transfer policies; and establishment of a feeling of belonging, acceptance, and socialization

The next phase of the orientation program could take place in the staff development department, where aspects of concern to all employees such as fire safety, accident prevention, and health promotion would be presented. The third phase would be the individual orientation for each department. At this point, specific departments such as dietary, pharmacy, and nursing would each be responsible for developing their own programs. A sample distribution of responsibilities for orientation activities is shown in Display 15.7.

Because induction and orientation involve many different people from a variety of departments, they must be carefully coordinated and planned to achieve preset goals. The overall goals of induction and orientation include helping employees by providing them with information that will smooth their transition into the new work setting and health care team.

> The purpose of the orientation process is to make the employee feel like a part of the team. This will reduce burnout and help new employees become independent more quickly in their new roles.

It is important to look at productivity and retention as the orientation program is planned, structured, and evaluated. Organizations should periodically assess their induction and orientation program considering organizational goals; programs that are not meeting organizational goals should be restructured. For example, if employees consistently have questions about the benefit program, this part of the induction process should be evaluated.

Too often, various people having partial responsibility for induction and orientation "pass the buck" regarding failure of or weaknesses in the program. It is the joint responsibility of the personnel/human resources department, the staff development department, and each nursing service unit to work together to provide an onboarding program that meets the needs of employees and the organization.

For some time, managers in health care organizations, especially hospitals, did not fulfill their proper role in the orientation of new employees. Managers assumed that between the personnel/human resources and staff development, or in-service departments, the new employee would become completely oriented. This often frustrated new employees because although they received an overview of the organization, they received little orientation to the specific unit. Because each unit has many idiosyncrasies, the new employee was left feeling inadequate and incompetent. The latest trend in orientation is for the nursing unit to take a greater responsibility for individualizing orientation.

The unit leader-manager must play a key role in the orientation of the new employee. An adequate orientation program minimizes the likelihood of rule violations, grievances, and misunderstandings; fosters feelings of belonging and acceptance; and promotes enthusiasm and morale.

Integrating Leadership Roles and Management Functions in Employee Recruitment, Selection, Placement, and Onboarding

Productivity is directly related to the quality of an organization's personnel. Active recruitment allows institutions to bring in the most qualified personnel for a position. After those applicants have been recruited, managers—using specified criteria—have a critical responsibility to see that the best applicant is hired. To ensure that all applicants are evaluated by using the same standards and that personal bias is minimized, the nurse-manager must be skilled in interviewing and other selection processes.

Leadership roles in preliminary staffing functions include planning for future staffing needs and keeping abreast of changes in the health care field. Predicted nursing shortages will pose staffing challenges for some time to come. Leadership is also necessary in the preemployment interview process to ensure that all applicants are treated fairly and that the interview terminates with applicants having positive attitudes about the organization. Because leaders are fully aware of nuances, strengths, and weaknesses within their sphere of authority, they can assign newcomers to areas that offer the greatest potential for success.

The integration of leadership roles and management functions in the organization ensures positive public relations because applicants know that they will be treated fairly. In addition, there is greater likelihood that the pool of applicants will be sufficient because future needs are planned for proactively. The leader-manager uses the selection and placement process to increase productivity and retention, accomplish the goals of the organization, and meet the needs of new employees.

The integrated leader-manager also knows that a well-planned and implemented induction and orientation program is a wise investment of organizational resources. It provides the opportunity to mold a team effort and infuse employees with enthusiasm for the organization. New employees' impressions of an organization during this period will stay with them for a long time. If the impressions are positive, they will be remembered in the difficult times that will ultimately occur during any long tenure of employment.

 Key Concepts

- The first step in the staffing process is to determine the type and number of personnel needed.
- Numerous factors are contributing to significant future nursing shortages, including the aging of the nursing workforce, accelerating demand for professional nurses, inadequate enrollment in nursing programs of study, the aging of nursing faculty, and the COVID-19 pandemic.

- Successfully recruiting an adequate workforce depends on many variables, including financial resources, an adequate nursing pool, competitive salaries, the organization's reputation, the location's desirability, and the status of the national and local economy.
- A healthy work environment is one in which the nursing staff feels supported physically and emotionally as well as safe, respected, and empowered.

- Despite their limitations in terms of reliability and validity, interviews continue to be widely used as a method of selecting employees for hire.
- The limitations of interviews are reduced when a structured approach is used in asking questions of applicants.
- The interview should meet the goals of both the applicant and the manager.
- Managers must be skilled in planning, conducting, and controlling interviews.
- Because of numerous federal acts that protect the rights of job seekers, interviewers must be cognizant of the legal constraints on interview questions.
- Selection should be based on the requirements necessary for the job; these criteria should be developed before beginning the selection process.
- Leaders should seek to proactively recruit and hire staff with age, gender, cultural, ethnic, and language diversity to better mirror the rapidly increasing diversity of the communities they serve.
- New employees should be placed on units, departments, and shifts where they have the best chance of succeeding.
- Onboarding consists of induction, orientation, and socialization of employees.
- A well-prepared and executed orientation program educates the new employee about the desired behaviors and expected goals of the organization and actively involves the new employee's immediate supervisor.

Additional Learning Exercises and Applications

LEARNING EXERCISE 15.5

Assessing Personal Bias in Interviewing

You are a new evening charge nurse on a medical floor in an acute care hospital. This is your first management position. You graduated 18 months ago from the local university with a bachelor's degree in nursing. Your immediate supervisor has asked you to interview two applicants who will be graduating from nursing school in 3 months. Your supervisor believes that they both are qualified. Because the available position is on your shift, she wants you to make the final hiring decision.

Both applicants seem equally qualified in academic standing and work experience. Last evening, you interviewed Lisa and were very impressed. Tonight, you interviewed John. During the meeting, you kept thinking that you knew John from somewhere but could not recall where. The interview went well, however, and you were equally impressed with John.

After John left, you suddenly remembered that one of your classmates used to date him and that he had attended some of your class parties. You recall that on several occasions, he appeared to engage in unhealthy alcohol use. This recollection bothers you, and you are not sure what to do. You know that tomorrow your supervisor wants to inform the applicants of your decision.

ASSIGNMENT:

Decide what you are going to do. Support your decision with appropriate rationale. Explain how you would determine which applicant to hire. How great a role did your personal values play in your decision?

LEARNING EXERCISE 15.6

How Would You Strengthen This Orientation Process?

As a new unit manager, one of your goals is to reduce attrition. You plan to do this by increasing retention, thus reducing costs for orienting new employees. In addition, you believe that the increased retention will provide you with a more stable staff.

In studying your notes from exit interviews, you notice it appears that new employees seldom develop a loyalty to the unit but instead use the unit to gain experience for other positions. You believe that one difficulty with socializing new employees might be your unit's orientation program. The agency allows 2 weeks of orientation time (80 hours) when the new employee is not counted in the nursing care hours. These are referred to as *nonproductive hours* and are charged to the education department. Your unit has the following 2-week schedule for new employees:

Week 1		
Monday, Tuesday	9:00 AM to 5:00 PM	Classroom
Wednesday, Thursday, Friday	7:00 AM to 3:30 PM	Assigned to work with someone on the unit
Week 2		
Monday, Tuesday	7:00 AM to 3:30 PM	Assigned to unit with an employee
Wednesday, Thursday, Friday		Assigned to shift they will be working for orientation to shift

Following this 2-week orientation, the new employee is expected to function at 75% productivity for 2 or 3 weeks and then perform at full productivity. The exception to this is the new graduate (registered nurse) orientation. These employees spend 1 extra week on 7 AM to 3 PM and 1 extra week assigned to their particular shift before being counted as staff.

Your nursing administrator has stated that you may alter the orientation program in any way you wish as long as you do not increase the nonproductive time and you ensure that the employee receives information necessary to meet legal requirements and to function safely.

ASSIGNMENT:

Is there any way for you to strengthen the new employee orientation to your unit? Outline your plans (if any) and state the rationale for your decision.

LEARNING EXERCISE 15.7

Choosing Your Place in the Workforce

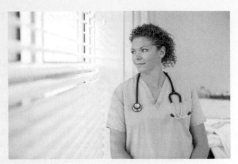

Y ou are a nursing student who will graduate in 3 months. You are aware that most of the acute care hospitals in the immediate area are not hiring new graduates, although there are a few openings in a small, rural hospital about 40 miles from where you live. There are some openings in home health, public health, community health, telehealth, and case management in the local community as well. You need to get a job as soon as possible as you are a single parent and have accrued significant debt in your educational degree quest.

Your career goal is to work in a high-paced, skill-intensive, acute care hospital environment like the emergency department, intensive care unit, or trauma, but you have not yet achieved the specialty certifications you need to do so, and there are no openings in these units for new graduates at present anyway. You enjoyed the autonomy and patient interaction that you experienced in your public health practicum as part of school, and the Monday-to-Friday work schedule of public health nurses appeals to you because you have small children. The salary, however, would be significantly lower than if you worked in an acute care setting, and you are not sure that this would be enough to make ends meet. Moreover, the orientation period at the public health facility would be fairly brief.

Finally, you also are interested in pediatric oncology, a specialty not available to you unless you relocate to a regional medical center almost 200 miles from where you currently live. There are opportunities for advancement and professional development there, but it would likely be necessary for you to take a job on the night shift on a general medical-surgical unit first, to get your foot in the door.

ASSIGNMENT:

1. Determine how you will move forward in making a decision about where you will seek employment.
2. Make a list of 10 factors that you need to consider in weighting conflicting wants, needs, and obligations.
3. What evaluation criteria can you generate to look at both the process you used to make your decision and the decision itself?

LEARNING EXERCISE 15.8

Ethical Issues in Hiring

Y ou are the head nurse of an intensive care unit and are interviewing Sam, a prospective charge nurse for your evening shift. Sam is currently the unit supervisor at Memorial Hospital, which is the other local hospital and your organization's primary competitor. He is leaving Memorial Hospital for personal reasons.

Sam, well qualified for the position, has strong management and clinical skills. Your evening shift needs a strong manager with the excellent clinical skills, which Sam also has. You feel fortunate that Sam is applying for the position.

Just before the close of the interview, however, Sam shuts the door, lowers his voice secretively, and tells you that he has vital information regarding Memorial's plans to expand and reorganize its critical care unit. He states that he will share this information with you if you hire him.

ASSIGNMENT:

How would you respond to Sam? Should you hire him? Identify the major issues in this situation. Support your hiring decision with rationale from this chapter and other readings.

LEARNING EXERCISE 15.9

Reducing Your Anxiety About Possible Hiring Interview Questions

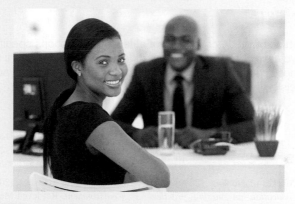

ASSIGNMENT:

Make a list of three or four interview questions you may face in your new graduate interview, which you feel most insecure about answering. Then share your questions with a small group of your peers. Work together to identify strong and weak responses to those interview questions. Make sure that every individual in the group has a chance to get feedback about the interview questions they are most anxious about.

LEARNING EXERCISE 15.10

Your Best Interview

ASSIGNMENT:

Do you remember your first interview for a job? How would you evaluate your abilities as someone being interviewed? Have you ever had the responsibility to interview someone for an employment position? What would you identify as your strengths and weaknesses in the interview process as both interviewer and interviewee? If you hired people in the past, how would you rate their performance as employees? Were they more competent or less competent than they seemed at the time you interviewed them?

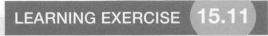

LEARNING EXERCISE 15.11

Designing an Interview Guide

You are a new evening charge nurse on a pediatric floor in an acute care hospital. This is your first management position, having just graduated 18 months ago. Your immediate supervisor has asked you to interview two applicants who will be graduating from nursing school in 3 months. Your supervisor believes that they both are qualified. Because the available position is on your shift, she wants you to make the final hiring decision.

You feel a great responsibility to be fair especially because you know both of these candidates personally. You took a chemistry course with one of them and an anatomy class with the other. Although you don't know either of them well, you do know how rigorous your academic program was and feel that they would each be well qualified.

You decide to develop an interview guide and several case scenarios to use in interviewing each applicant. You base the interview guide questions and the case scenarios on qualities that, in your experience, a new registered nurse needs to have to be successful in your unit.

ASSIGNMENT:

Write an interview guide consisting of at least 12 questions specific to your unit and develop two case scenarios for nursing decision making that will allow you to determine which of these two new graduates to recommend for hire. Did your personal values play in your decision?

REFERENCES

American Association of Colleges of Nursing. (2019). *Fact sheet: The impact of education on nursing practice.* https://www.aacnnursing.org/Portals/42/News/Factsheets/Education-Impact-Fact-Sheet.pdf

American Association of Colleges of Nursing. (2022a). *Nursing faculty shortage.* Retrieved January 3, 2022, from https://www.aacnnursing.org/News-Information/Fact-Sheets/Nursing-Faculty-Shortage

American Association of Colleges of Nursing. (2022b). *Nursing shortage.* Retrieved January 3, 2022, from https://www.aacnnursing.org/News-Information/Fact-Sheets/Nursing-Shortage

American Association of Critical-Care Nurses. (n.d.). *Healthy work environments.* https://www.aacn.org/nursing-excellence/healthy-work-environments

American Nurses Association. (n.d.). *Healthy work environment.* https://www.nursingworld.org/practice-policy/work-environment/

Arends, B. (2020, May 2). Opinion: COVID-19 crisis sparks 'early retirement' wave. *Market Watch.* https://www.marketwatch.com/story/covid-19-crisis-sparks-early-retirement-wave-2020-04-30

Brooks, A. (2021, April 5). Cultural diversity in healthcare: Why it matters, and what's next. *Rasmussen University Nursing Blog.* https://www.rasmussen.edu/degrees/nursing/blog/lack-of-cultural-diversity-in-healthcare/

Bureau of Labor Statistics. (2022a). *Registered nurses. Job outlook.* Retrieved May 28, 2022, from http://www.bls.gov/ooh/healthcare/registered-nurses.htm#tab-6

Bureau of Labor Statistics. (2022b). *Registered nurses. Work environment.* Retrieved May 28, 2022, from http://www.bls.gov/ooh/healthcare/registered-nurses.htm#tab-3

Caruso, M. (2020, April 11). Outlook for nurse supply and demand shifting amid COVID-19. *Modern Healthcare, 50*(15), 14. https://www.modernhealthcare.com/labor/outlook-nurse-supply-and-demand-shifting-amid-covid-19

Chatterjee, A., Greif, C., Witzburg, R., Henault, L., Goodell, K., & Paasche-Orlow, M. K. (2020). US medical school applicant experiences of bias on the interview trail. *Journal of Health Care for the Poor and Underserved, 31*(1), 185–200. https://doi-org.mantis.csuchico.edu/10.1353/hpu.2020.0017

Connecticut Department of Labor. (2002–2022). *Tips for job seekers. Employment interviewing.* Retrieved May 28, 2022, from https://www.ctdol.state.ct.us/progsupt/jobsrvce/intervie.htm

Feldman, J. (2022). *How to pass a pre-employment personality test.* Top Resume. https://www.topresume.com/career-advice/how-to-pass-the-pre-employment-personality-test

Huston, C. J. (2023a). Diversity in the nursing workforce (chapter 9). In C. J. Huston (Ed.), *Professional issues in nursing: Challenges and opportunities* (6th ed., pp. 121–135). Wolters Kluwer.

Huston, C. J. (2023b). Is there a nursing shortage (chapter 6)? In C. J. Huston (Ed.), *Professional issues in nursing: Challenges and opportunities* (6th ed., pp. 80–91). Wolters Kluwer.

The importance of diversity in healthcare: Medical professionals weigh in. (2021, August 19). *The SGU Pulse Medical School Blog*. https://www.sgu.edu/blog/medical/pros-discuss-the-importance-of-diversity-in-health-care/

Lahr, E. (2021, September 17). *Forms of interview bias*. Thread. https://threadhcm.com/forms-of-interview-bias/

Lewis, G. (2018). 5 New interviewing techniques that you should start using. *LinkedIn Talent Blog*. https://business.linkedin.com/talent-solutions/blog/interview-questions/2018/5-new-interviewing-techniques-that-you-need-to-know-about

McNamara, C. (2022, January 18). *General guidelines for conducting interviews*. Management Library. https://managementhelp.org/businessresearch/interviews.htm

Robert Wood Johnson Foundation. (2001–2022). *Business case/cost of nurse turnover*. Retrieved May 28, 2022, from https://www.rwjf.org/en/library/research/2009/07/business-case-cost-of-nurse-turnover.html

Schafir, H. (n.d.). *Why diversity hiring is important*. Exact Hire. https://www.exacthire.com/workforce-management/why-diversity-hiring-is-important/

Society for Human Resource Management. (2018). *Screening by means of pre-employment testing*. https://www.shrm.org/resourcesandtools/tools-and-samples/toolkits/pages/screeningbymeansofpreemploymenttesting.aspx

U.S. Equal Employment Opportunity Commission. (n.d.). *Background checks: What employers need to know*. https://www.eeoc.gov/publications/background_checks_employers.cfm

Valamis. (2022, January 17). *Employee onboarding process*. Retrieved May 28, 2022, from https://www.valamis.com/hub/employee-onboarding

16

Educating and Socializing Staff in a Learning Organization

*… environments rich in continuing education ripen staff development, morale and retention.—**Diane Postlen-Slattery and Kathryn Foley***

*… as part of the lifelong learning process, nurse leaders will increasingly use mentors and personal coaches to help them refine their tools and skills and to identify new lenses through which to view current concerns or issues.—**Karen S. Haase-Herrick***

*… An organization's ability to learn and translate that learning into action rapidly is the ultimate competitive advantage.—**Jack Welch***

CROSSWALK

This chapter addresses:

- **AACN Essentials Domain 1:** Knowledge for nursing practice
- **AACN Essentials Domain 4:** Scholarship for nursing practice
- **AACN Essentials Domain 5:** Quality and safety
- **AACN Essentials Domain 6:** Interprofessional partnerships
- **AACN Essentials Domain 7:** Systems-based practice
- **AACN Essentials Domain 9:** Professionalism
- **AACN Essentials Domain 10:** Personal, professional, and leadership development
- **AONL Nurse Executive Competency 1:** Communication and relationship building
- **AONL Nurse Executive Competency 3:** Leadership
- **AONL Nurse Executive Competency 4:** Professionalism
- **ANA Standard of Professional Performance 9:** Respectful and equitable practice
- **ANA Standard of Professional Performance 11:** Collaboration
- **ANA Standard of Professional Performance 12:** Leadership
- **ANA Standard of Professional Performance 13:** Education
- **ANA Standard of Professional Performance 14:** Scholarly Inquiry
- **ANA Standard of Professional Performance 15:** Quality of practice
- **ANA Standard of Professional Performance 17:** Resource stewardship
- **QSEN Competency:** Evidence-based practice
- **QSEN Competency:** Teamwork and collaboration

LEARNING OBJECTIVES

The learner will:

- describe characteristics of learning organizations
- differentiate between education and training
- select an appropriate sequence of events for educational planning
- identify problems that may occur when the responsibility for staff development is shared

- select appropriate educational strategies that facilitate learning in a variety of situations
- discuss criteria that should be used to evaluate staff development activities
- demonstrate knowledge of the needs of the adult learner and describe teaching strategies that best meet these needs
- explain the difference between motivation to learn and readiness to learn
- apply principles of social learning theory
- identify strategies that could be used to help staff deal successfully with role transitions
- describe strategies that could be used to assist the new graduate nurse with socialization to the nursing role
- explain why experienced nurses may have difficulty in role transition
- contrast the roles of role model, preceptor, mentor, and coach
- choose criteria for the selection of preceptors that would likely result in effective role transition for the protégé
- develop coaching techniques that enhance learning
- address the unique challenges of building a cohesive team through education and socialization, when a diverse workforce exists

Introduction

Health care organizations face major challenges in upgrading workforce skills and in maintaining a competent staff. This is especially true in times of exponential knowledge growth, significant change, and limitless new technology applications. Educating staff and assuring continuing competency then is a critical and difficult task for most 21st-century organizations and only those who are flexible, adaptive, and productive will excel.

In 2012, the Institute of Medicine (IOM), now called the National Academies of Science, Engineering, and Medicine (NASEM), released a seminal 4,000-page report, *Best Care at Lower Cost: The Path to Continuously Learning Health Care in America* (NASEM, 2013). In this report, the IOM outlined potential strategies to accelerate health care organizations' capabilities for continuous learning and improvement. One of the key recommendations was to reward providers for continuous learning and quality so that the health care delivery system learns from and evolves with every patient interaction. The task of fundamentally changing any organization's capacity to learn and adapt to shifting consumer needs and requirements is daunting, but it can be accomplished with an effective and systematic approach.

This chapter begins by introducing the concept of the *learning organization* (LO). Education and training are differentiated, as are role models, preceptors, mentors, and coaches. The needs of the adult learner are explored. The role of the organization, leader-managers, and staff development departments in creating a culture that supports and promotes evidence-based practice (EBP) is emphasized. Finally, the need to build a cohesive team through education and socialization, including the needs of a culturally diverse workforce, is explored. The leadership roles and management functions associated with educating and socializing staff are shown in Display 16.1.

The Learning Organization

A growing body of literature supports the concept that knowledge building should go beyond the boundaries of individual learning. Organizations that incorporate lifelong learning as a major part of their philosophy will be more successful. This concept was first introduced by

---

DISPLAY 16.1 LEADERSHIP ROLES AND MANAGEMENT FUNCTIONS ASSOCIATED WITH EDUCATION AND SOCIALIZING STAFF IN A LEARNING ORGANIZATION

Leadership Roles

1. Clarifies unit norms and values to all new employees
2. Infuses a team spirit among employees
3. Serves as a role model to all employees and a mentor to select employees
4. Encourages mentorship between all levels of staff
5. Observes carefully for signs of knowledge or skill deficit in new employees and intervenes appropriately
6. Assists employees in developing personal strategies to cope with role transition
7. Applies adult learning principles when helping employees learn new skills or information
8. Coaches employees spontaneously regarding knowledge and skill deficits
9. Is sensitive to the unique socialization and education needs of a culturally and ethnically diverse staff
10. Continually promotes aspects of the learning organization to employees
11. Assists nursing staff in overcoming organization barriers to effective evidence-based practice
12. Encourages and supports workers as they pursue lifelong learning individually and collectively

Management Functions

1. Is aware of and clarifies organizational and unit goals for all employees
2. Clarifies role expectations for all employees
3. Uses positive and negative sanctions appropriately to socialize new employees
4. Carefully selects preceptors and encourages positive role modeling by experienced staff
5. Provides methods of meeting the special orientation needs of new graduates, international nurses, and experienced nurses changing roles
6. Works with the education department to delineate shared and individual responsibility for staff development
7. Ensures that there are adequate resources for staff development and makes appropriate decisions regarding resource allocation during periods of fiscal restraint
8. Assumes responsibility for quality and fiscal control of staff development activities
9. Ensures that all staff are competent for roles assigned
10. Provides input in formulating staff development policies
11. Ensures that the organization provides resources to promote evidence-based nursing practice

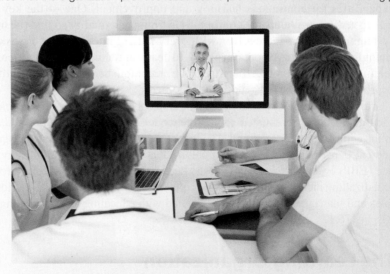

DISPLAY 16.2 SENGE'S FIVE DISCIPLINES OF A LEARNING ORGANIZATION

- *Systems thinking*. The organization encourages staff to see themselves as connected to the whole organization, and work activities are seen as having an impact beyond the individual. This creates a sense of community and builds a commitment on the part of individual workers not only to the organization but also to each other. Consequently, one of the main goals of the learning organization (LO) is to construct an organizational culture of learning.
- *Personal mastery*. Each member of the staff has a commitment to improve their personal abilities. This personal and professional learning is then integrated into the team and organization.
- *Team learning*. It is through the collaboration of team members that LOs achieve their goals. Values, such as trust and openness, commitment to one another's learning, and acknowledgment that mistakes are part of the learning process, are important characteristics of a LO.
- *Mental models*. A mental model is the set of assumptions and generalizations (or even pictures or images) that influence how we understand the world and how we take actions (The Busy Lifestyle, 2020). The goal in the LO is to foster organizational development through diverse thinking. Assumptions held by individuals then are challenged because this releases individuals from traditional thinking and promotes the full potential of individuals to learn.
- *Shared vision*. When all the employees of the LO share a common vision, they are more willing to put their personal goals and needs aside and instead focus on teamwork and collaboration.

Source: From Senge, P. (2006). *The fifth discipline: The art and practice of the learning organization.* Currency Doubleday.

Senge (2006, p. 3), who called such organizations *LOs*. Senge defined a LO as a place "where people continually expand their capacity to create the results they truly desire, where new and expansive patterns of thinking are nurtured, where collective aspiration is set free, and where people are continually learning to see the whole together." In essence, LOs are places where people are continually learning how to learn together.

The key characteristics of Senge's model of LOs (five disciplines) are shown in Display 16.2. These disciplines allow for the creation of an infrastructure that promotes continuous learning, adaptation, and growth since LOs view learning as the key to the future for individuals as well as for organizations.

Since Senge, many theorists have furthered our understanding of LOs. As Nichols (2021) explains, LOs embrace an organizational framework that relies on active and continuous learning as the foundation for an engaged and productive workforce. Thus, the overall aim of the LO is to create a more agile learning culture by building learning capabilities in teams and individuals (Liimatainen, 2021). This requires not only applying learnings continuously in daily work, but also continuously co-developing the learning process with fellow learners.

> "LOs are dependent on the systematic and duly classified archiving of successively generated knowledge, and the more intense is the sharing of this knowledge internally among its members, as well as externally within the society, then the greater is the development of the organization" (Lopes and Fernandes, 2021, p. 33).

LOs also promote recruitment and retention by allowing employees to grow and learn with and from each other. In addition, the LO fosters a shared vision and collective learning to create positive and needed organizational change. The key aspects of a LO are an open culture with a shared vision for the work, ongoing habits of feedback and assessment, an encouragement of individual mastery and expertise, adoption of accepted best practices, and a willingness to experiment and take risks (Spas, 2021). These elements allow an organization to be framed constructively, oriented toward the future, and generative of individual and collective accomplishments.

Staff Development

Because a LO recognizes that learning is never ending, the organization has at least some responsibility for developing workers through staff development programs. A LO, however, cannot just meet licensure requirements for education and training; it must also encourage individual growth and support staff development activities both financially and philosophically.

However, this fostering of growth and learning in employees is driven by more than altruistic motives. The staff's knowledge level and capabilities often determine the number of staff required to meet organizational goals. Therefore, having better trained and more competent staff can save the organization money by increasing productivity and positive outcomes.

An organization's ability to learn, and to translate that learning into action rapidly, then can create a competitive business advantage. For example, during the COVID-19 pandemic, organizations and leaders had to pause, wait, adapt, innovate, and reimagine the way to achieve their missions (Spas, 2021). These activities are what enabled successful LOs to learn and move ahead into an unknown future. Spas (2021) notes that the changes that occurred during the pandemic resulted in disruptions that were so significant that the former context is gone. Sustainability became possible only through forward motion and new learning.

> With the COVID-19 pandemic upending workplace norms the world over, even learning and development teams in LOs faced unprecedented challenges in cultivating true employee engagement and reducing remote burnout (Nichols, 2021).

Training Versus Education

Education and training are two components of staff development in LOs. Managers historically had a greater responsibility for seeing that staff were properly trained than they did for meeting educational needs. A more equal balance has been achieved in the past few decades.

Training is an organized method of ensuring that people have knowledge and skills for a specific purpose (in this case, to perform the duties of the job). To assist employees with their training needs, the manager must first determine what those needs are. This also includes future planning needs related to product line development and implementation of best practice exemplars. This is a leadership role. When such deficiencies are not corrected early or there is a lack of leadership support, a climate of nonacceptance can develop that prevents assimilation of the new employee.

Education is more formal and broader in scope than training. Whereas training has an immediate application, education is designed to develop individuals in a broader sense. Recognizing educational needs and encouraging educational pursuits are roles and responsibilities of the leader. Managers may appropriately be requested to teach classes; however, unless they have specific expertise, they would not normally be responsible for an employee's formal education.

Responsibilities of the Education Department

Staff development is a broad area of responsibility and is borne by many people in the organization. Its official functions are often housed, however, within an education department. Because most education departments have staff or advisory authority rather than line authority on the organizational chart, education personnel generally have little or no formal authority over those they teach. Likewise, the unit manager may have little authority over personnel in the education department. Because of the ambiguity of overlapping roles and difficulties inherent in line and staff positions, it is important that those responsible for educating and training be identified and given the authority to carry out the programs.

> If staff development activities are to be successful, it is necessary to delineate and communicate the authority and responsibility for all components of education and training.

In some organizations, the responsibility for staff development is decentralized. Some difficulties associated with decentralized staff development include the conflict created by *role ambiguity* whenever two people share responsibility. Role ambiguity is sometimes reduced when staff development personnel and managers delineate the difference between training and education.

Other difficulties arising from the shared responsibility for the onboarding, education, and training of personnel may include a lack of cost-effectiveness evaluation and limited accountability for the quality and outcomes of the educational activities. These suggestions can help overcome the difficulties inherent in a staff development system in which authority is shared:

- The education department must ensure that all parties involved in the onboarding, education, and training of nursing staff understand and carry out their responsibilities in that process.
- If a non-nursing administrator is responsible for the staff development department, there must be input from the nursing department in formulating staff development policies and delineating duties.
- An education advisory committee should be formed with representatives from top-, middle-, and first-level management; staff development; and the Human Resources department. Representatives from all classifications of employees receiving training or education should be part of this committee.
- Accountability for each area of the staff development program must be clearly communicated; follow-up on the process is essential.
- Some method of determining the cost and benefits of various programs should be used.

Learning Theories

All managers have a responsibility to improve employee performance through teaching. Therefore, they must be familiar with basic learning theories. Understanding teaching–learning theories allows managers to structure training and use teaching techniques to change employee behavior and improve competence, which is the goal for all staff development.

Adult Learning Theory

Many managers attempt to teach adults with pedagogical learning strategies. This type of teaching is usually ineffective for mature learners because adults have special needs. Knowles (1970) developed the concept of *andragogy*, or *adult learning*, to separate adult learner strategies from *pedagogy*, or *child learning*. Knowles suggested that the point at which an individual achieves a self-concept of essential self-direction is the point at which they psychologically become an adult. Table 16.1 shows how pedagogical and andragogical learning environments typically differ.

Adult learners are mature, self-directed people who have learned a great deal from life experiences and are focused on solving problems in their immediate environments. Therefore, adult learners need to know why they need to learn something before they are willing to learn it. Adult learning theory has strongly influenced how adults are currently taught in staff development programs. Based on the individual's needs, a combination of approaches may be required. Display 16.3 identifies the implications of Knowles's work for trainers and educators.

Although most adults enjoy and take pride in being treated as an adult in terms of learning, there are some obstacles to learning for adults that do not exist in children. Because learning tends to become problem centered as we age, adults often miss out on opportunities to enjoy

TABLE 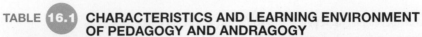 **16.1 CHARACTERISTICS AND LEARNING ENVIRONMENT OF PEDAGOGY AND ANDRAGOGY**

Pedagogy	Andragogy
Characteristics	
Learner is dependent	Learner is self-directed
Learner needs external rewards and punishment	Learner is internally motivated
Learner's experience is inconsequential or limited	Learner's experiences are valued and varied
Subject centered	Task or problem centered
Teacher directed	Self-directed
Learning Environment	
The climate is authoritative	The climate is relaxed and informal
Competition is encouraged	Collaboration is encouraged
Teacher sets goals	Teacher and class set goals
Decisions are made by teacher	Decisions are made by teacher and students
Teacher lectures	Students process activities and inquire about projects
Teacher evaluates	Teacher, self, and peers evaluate

learning for the sheer sake of learning itself. Similarly, adults often experience more external obstacles to learning, including time, energy, and institutional barriers. These and other obstacles to adult learning are shown in Display 16.4 as are the assets, or driving forces, that encourage learning in the adult.

Social Learning Theory

Social learning theory is also an important part of LOs because it suggests we learn from our interactions with others in a social context. (This is a part of the teamwork and mental model development in LOs.) Albert Bandura, a social psychologist, is often credited with developing social learning theory in the 1970s. Bandura (1977) believed that direct reinforcement could not account for all types of learning and that, instead, most people learn their behavior by direct experience and observation, known as *observational learning* or *modeling* (Cherry, 2021).

DISPLAY 16.3 IMPLICATIONS OF KNOWLES'S (1970) WORK FOR TRAINERS AND EDUCATORS

- A climate of openness and respect will assist in the identification of what the adult learner wants and needs to learn.
- Adults enjoy taking part in and planning their learning experiences.
- Adults should be involved in the evaluation of their progress.
- Experiential techniques work best with adults.
- Mistakes are opportunities for adult learning.
- If the value of the adult's experience is rejected, the adult will feel rejected.
- Adults' readiness to learn is greatest when they recognize that there is a need to know (such as in response to a problem).
- Adults need the opportunity to apply what they have learned very quickly after the learning.
- Assessment of need is imperative in adult learning.

DISPLAY 16.4 OBSTACLES AND ASSETS TO ADULT LEARNING

Obstacles to Learning

Institutional barriers
Time
Self-confidence
Situational obstacles
Family reaction
Special individual obstacles

Assets for Learning

High self-motivation
Self-direction
A proven learner
Knowledge experience reservoir
Special individual assets

Indeed, Bandura (1977) felt that four separate processes were involved in social learning. First, people learn because of the direct experience of the effects of their actions. Second, knowledge is frequently obtained through vicarious experiences, such as by observing someone else's actions. Third, people learn by judgments voiced by others, especially when vicarious experience is limited. Fourth, people evaluate the soundness of the new information by reasoning through inductive and deductive logic. If observational learning is to succeed, individuals must be motivated to imitate the behavior that has been modeled (Cherry, 2021). Figure 16.1 depicts Bandura's social learning theory process.

Other Learning Concepts

The following learning concepts may also help the leader-manager meet the learning needs of staff in LOs:

- *Readiness to learn*. This refers to the maturational and experiential factors in the learner's background that influence learning; it is not the same as motivation to learn. *Maturation* means that the learner has received the prerequisites for the next stage of learning. The

---

LEARNING EXERCISE 16.1

Changing Learning Needs

Learning needs and the maturity of those in a class often influence course content and teaching methods. Look back at how your learning needs and maturity level have changed since you were a beginning nursing student. When viewed as a whole, were you and the other beginning nursing students child or adult learners? Compare Knowles's (1970) pedagogy and andragogy characteristics to determine this.

ASSIGNMENT:

Are pedagogical teaching strategies appropriate for beginning nursing students? If so, when does the nursing student make the transition to adult learner? What teaching modes do you believe would be most conducive to learning for a beginning nursing student? Would this change as students progressed through the nursing program? Support your beliefs with rationale.

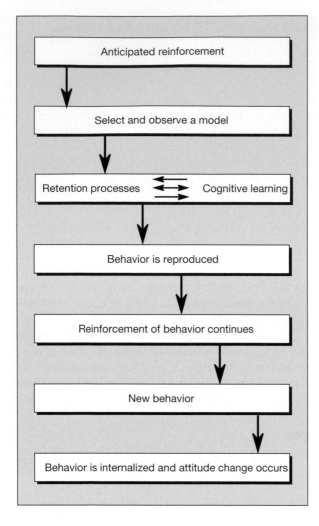

FIGURE 16.1 The social learning theory process.

prerequisites could be behaviors or prior learning. *Experiential factors* are skills previously acquired that are necessary for the next stage of learning.

- *Motivation to learn*. If learners are informed in advance about the benefits of learning specific content and adopting new behaviors, they are more likely learn. Telling employees why and how specific educational or training programs will benefit them personally (to gain buy in) is a vital management function in staff development.

- *Reinforcement*. Because a learner's first attempts are often unsuccessful, good preceptors are essential to reinforce desired behavior. Once the behavior or skill is learned, it needs continual reinforcement until it becomes internalized.

- *Task learning*. The learning of complex tasks is facilitated when tasks are broken into parts, beginning with the simplest and continuing to the most difficult. When learning motor skills, *spaced practice* (short time periods but multiple sessions) is more effective than *massed practice* (a single longer session).

- *Transfer of learning*. The goal of training is to transfer new learning to the work setting. For this to occur, there should first be as much similarity between the training context and the job as possible. Second, adequate practice is mandatory, and *overlearning* (learning repeated to the degree that it is difficult to forget) is recommended. Third, the training should include a variety of different situations so that the knowledge is generalized. Fourth, whenever possible, important features or steps in a process should be identified.

Finally, the learner must understand the basic principles underlying the tasks and how a variety of situations will modify how the task is accomplished. Learning in the classroom will not be transferred without adequate practice in a simulated or real situation and without an adequate understanding of underlying principles.

- *Span of memory*. The effectiveness of staff development activities depends to some extent on the ability of the participants to retain information. Effective strategies include the chance for repeated rehearsal, grouping items to be learned (three or four items for oral presentations and four to six visually), having the material presented in a well-organized manner, and *chunking*.
- *Chunking*. This occurs when two independent items of information are presented and then grouped together into one unit. Although the mind can remember only a limited number of chunks of data, experienced nurses can include more data in those chunks than can novice nurses. For example, experienced nurses are typically better able to recognize subtle changes in a patient's condition based on the assessments they have made or changes in lab values, whereas the novice nurse may take a bit longer to connect these pieces of information.
- *Knowledge of results*. Research has demonstrated that people learn faster when they are informed of their progress. The knowledge of results must be automatic, immediate, and meaningful to the task at hand. People need to experience a feeling of progress, and they need to know how they are doing when measured against expected outcomes.

Assessing Staff Development Needs

Although managers may not be involved in implementing all educational programs, they are responsible for identifying learning needs. If educational resources are scarce, staff desires for specific educational programs may need to be sacrificed to fulfill competency and new learning needs. Because managers and staff may identify learning needs differently, an educational needs assessment should be carried out before developing programs.

> Staff development activities are normally carried out for one of three reasons: to establish competence, to meet new learning needs, and to satisfy interests the staff may have in learning in specific areas.

Many staff development activities are generated to ensure that workers at each level are competent to perform the duties assigned to the position. *Competence* is defined as having the abilities to meet the requirements for a specific role. Health care organizations use many resources to determine competency. State board licensure, national certification, and performance review are some of the methods used to satisfy competency requirements (Huston, 2023a). In addition, self-administered competency checklists, record audits, direct observation, and peer review may be used. Many of these methods are explained in Unit VII. For staff development purposes, it is important to remember that in the case of deficient competencies, some staff development activity must be implemented to correct the deficiencies. Another learning need that frequently affects health care organizations is the need to meet new technologic and scientific challenges. Many of a manager's educational resources will be used to meet these new learning needs.

Some organizations implement training programs because they are faddish and have been advertised and marketed well. Educational programs are expensive, however, and should not be undertaken unless a demonstrated need exists. Organizational development targeted to the specific needs of the facility may be the most cost-effective approach.

In addition to developing rationale for educational programs, the use of an assessment plan will be helpful in meeting learner needs. The sequence that should be used in developing an educational program is shown in Display 16.5.

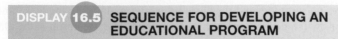

DISPLAY **16.5** **SEQUENCE FOR DEVELOPING AN EDUCATIONAL PROGRAM**

1. Identify the desired knowledge or skills that the staff should have.
2. Identify the present level of knowledge or skill.
3. Determine the deficit of desired knowledge and skills.
4. Identify the resources available to meet needs.
5. Make maximum use of available resources.
6. Evaluate and test outcomes after use of resources.

Evaluation of Staff Development Activities

Because staff development includes participation and involvement from many departments, it may be very difficult to control the evaluation of staff development activities effectively. It would be easy for the personnel department, middle-level managers, and the education department to "pass the buck" among one another for accountability regarding these activities.

In addition, the evaluation of staff development must consist of more than merely having class participants fill out an evaluation form at the end of the class session. Evaluation of staff development should include the following four criteria:

- *Learner's reaction.* How did the learner perceive the orientation, the class, the training, or the preceptor?
- *Behavior change.* What behavior change occurred because of the learning? Was the learning transferred? Testing someone at the end of a training or educational program does not confirm that the learning changed behavior. There needs to be some method of follow-up to observe if behavior change occurred.
- *Organizational impact.* Although it is often difficult to measure how staff development activities affect the organization, efforts should be made to measure this criterion. Examples of measurements are assessing quality of care, medication errors, accidents, quality of clinical judgment, turnover, and productivity.
- *Cost-effectiveness.* All staff development activities should be quantified in some manner. This is perhaps the most neglected aspect of accountability in staff development. All staff development activities should be evaluated for quality control, impact on the institution, and cost-effectiveness.

Shared Responsibility for Implementing Evidence-Based Practice

The IOM (2009) Roundtable on Evidence-Based Medicine set a goal that 90% of all clinical decisions would be supported by accurate, timely, and up-to-date information based on the best available evidence by the year 2020. Yet, the literature is replete with anecdotes suggesting that many providers do not yet implement EBP consistently or follow developed guidelines.

Chapter 11 discussed the individual's responsibility for a professional practice that was evidence based. However, the organization, as well as the individual, has a responsibility to promote best practices. Unfortunately, organizational cultures often do not support the nurse who seeks out and uses research to change long-standing practices rooted in tradition (Ford & Graves, 2023). The integrated leader-manager must create and support an organizational culture that values and uses research to improve clinical practice.

One way that health care organizations can demonstrate their commitment to becoming a LO is to promote and facilitate professional practice that is evidence based because nurses

---

DISPLAY 16.6 **STRATEGIES FOR PROMOTING EVIDENCE-BASED DECISION MAKING IN ESTABLISHING CLINICAL BEST PRACTICES**

- Develop and refine research-based policies and procedures.
- Build consensus from the interdisciplinary team through the development of protocols, decision trees, standards of care and institutional clinical practice guidelines, and other such mechanisms.
- Make research findings accessible through libraries and computer resources.
- Provide organization support such as time to do research and educational assistance in showing staff how to interpret research statistics and use findings.
- Encourage cooperation among professionals.
- When possible, hire nurse researchers or consultants to assist staff.

Source: Ford, C. D., & Graves, B. A. (2023). Evidence-based best practice (chapter 5). In C. J. Huston (Ed.), *Professional issues in nursing: Challenges and opportunities* (6th ed., pp. 67–79). Wolters Kluwer.

---

often find that barriers to EBPs exist within organizations. Such barriers include organizational culture and a lack of EBP knowledge and skills. Ford and Graves (2023) note that inadequate access to research findings and poor administrative support also contribute to the problem. They suggest strategies for organizations to encourage the use of evidence-based decision making in establishing clinical best practices (shown in Display 16.6).

> Facilitating EBP is a shared responsibility of the professional nurse, the organization, leader–managers, and the education or staff development department.

Socialization and Resocialization

In addition to training and educating staff, the leader-manager is also responsible for socializing employees to their roles and to the organization. This is not limited, however, to the leader-manager; the education department (especially during orientation), other employees, and many members of an organization are also expected to assist with employee socialization. *Socialization* then refers to a learning of the behaviors that accompany each role by instruction, observation, and trial and error.

Socialization of the New Nurse: Overcoming Reality Shock

The first socialization to the nursing role occurs during nursing school and continues after graduation. Nurse administrators and nursing faculty may hold different values as well as priorities in terms of what skills and knowledge new graduates need to know to be successful in their new role. In fact, numerous studies for decades have shown a significant gap between the perceptions of educators and clinician nurse-leaders regarding the adequacy of preparation of newly graduated nurses. Huston et al. (2018) note that academe is criticized for producing nurses insufficiently prepared to fully participate in patient care, and practice settings are criticized for having unrealistic expectations of new graduates. The perceived competence gaps among newly employed RN graduates appear to span the domains of critical thinking, communication, clinical knowledge, managing time and responsibilities, professionalism, technical or psychomotor skills, physical assessment, and teamwork (Huston et al., 2018). All these skill sets are critical to safe and effective nursing practice.

These gaps in academic and practice expectations provide fertile ground for the new graduate to feel overwhelmed, conflicted, and frustrated, a reaction often termed *reality shock* (Kramer, 1974). Indeed, 25% of new nurses leave a position within the first year of employment (National Council of State Boards of Nursing, 2022).

Several mechanisms exist, however, to ease this role transition of new graduates. *Anticipatory socialization* carried out in educational settings can help prepare new nurses for their professional role. However, managers should not assume that such anticipatory socialization has occurred. Instead, they should build opportunities for sharing and clarifying values and attitudes about the nursing role into orientation programs. Use of the group process is an excellent way to promote the sharing that provides support for new graduates and assists them in recovering from reality shock.

In addition, managers should be alert for signs and symptoms of role stress and role overload in new nurses; they should intervene by listening to these graduates and helping them to develop appropriate coping behaviors. A leadership shadowing experience may also be helpful to novice nurses so that they can explore how nurse-leaders deal with stress in their own jobs. In addition, managers must recognize the intensity of new nurses' practice experience, encourage them to have a balanced life, foster a work environment that has zero tolerance for disrespect, and strive to create work relationship models that promote interdependency of physicians and nursing staff.

Managers should also ensure that the new nurse's values are supported and encouraged so that work and academic values can blend. New professionals need to understand the universal nature of role transition and know that it is not limited to nurses. Providing a class on role transition also may assist new graduates in socialization. In addition, pairing new nurses with mentors who work outside the new nurses' place of employment can provide a safe place for these new graduates to disclose workplace issues and concerns as well as personal struggles they are experiencing in their new role (Austin & Halpin, 2021) (see Examining the Evidence 16.1).

> It is important to remember that no one is immune to a loss of idealism and commitment in response to stress in the workplace.

EXAMINING THE EVIDENCE 16.1

Source: From Austin, C., & Halpin, Y. (2021, June 10). Evaluation of a personal professional mentor scheme for newly qualified nurses. *British Journal of Nursing, 30*(11), 672–676. https://doi-org.mantis.csuchico.edu/10.12968/bjon.2021.30.11.672

The Value of Mentoring to New Graduate Nurses

New graduate nurses experience a range of feelings and fears the first year after licensure. This study examined the impact of professional mentoring from the perspective of 10 new graduate nurses working in pediatrics. A thematic analysis was used to review data from participant semistructured interviews.

Each new graduate nurse was paired with a personal professional mentor (PPM): an experienced nurse working outside the new graduate's job location, who was available and accessible to the new graduate, and with whom it was possible to talk confidentially. Participants met face to face with their mentors between zero and three times during a 12-month period in addition to e-mail exchanges.

The new graduate nurses expressed concerns to their PPMs about poor confidence, feeling overwhelmed, and feeling daunted and nervous, especially when they started their first job and in the initial few months. Through talking with their PPM these feelings were expressed in a supportive and confidential arena and the PPM was able to help the novice nurses manage and work through the feelings as opposed to continuing with them unabated, in isolation.

The researchers concluded that PPMs were able to counteract some aspects of transition isolation for the new graduate nurses. They also noted that the PPM constitutes an important addition to the portfolio of staff support roles in that their independent employment status enabled these new graduates to disclose to or confide workplace issues and concerns they might not have been able to, to colleagues/preceptors in their place of employment.

LEARNING EXERCISE 16.2

Investigating Emotional Exhaustion in New Graduates

Talk with at least four nursing graduates who have been working as nurses for at least 3 months and no more than 3 years. Make sure at least two of them are recent graduates and two of them have been working at least 18 months. Ask them about their socialization to nursing after graduation. Did any of them have trouble transitioning from academe to clinical practice? If so, how long did it last? Did they recover? If so, how? Did the COVID pandemic impact their orientation and socialization experience? Share your findings with other members of your group.

Most hospitals have developed prolonged orientation periods for new graduates that last from 6 weeks to 6 months. This extended orientation, or *internship*, contrasts sharply with the routine 2-week orientation that is normal for most other employees. During this time, graduate nurses are usually assigned to work with a preceptor and gradually take on a patient assignment equal to that of the preceptor. Even longer internships, known as *nurse residencies*, or transition-to-practice programs, were discussed in Chapter 11.

Resocialization of the Experienced Nurse

Resocialization occurs when experienced individuals must learn new values, skills, attitudes, and social rules because of changes in the type of work they do, the scope of responsibility they hold, or in the work setting itself. Assumptions may be made that such individuals already have expertise they do not, because the knowledge and skills to assume the new role may be very different. Individuals who frequently need resocialization include experienced nurses who change work settings, either within the same organization or in a new organization, and nurses who undertake new roles.

For example, the *transition from expert to novice* is very difficult. Many nurses transfer or change jobs because they no longer find their present job challenging. However, this results in the need to assume a learning role in their new environment. The employee assigned to orient the nurse in role transition should be aware of the difficulties that this nurse will experience. Transferred employees' lack of knowledge in the new area should never be belittled, and whenever possible, the special expertise they bring from their former work area should be acknowledged and utilized.

Another difficult transition is from the *familiar to the unfamiliar*. In new positions, employees must not only learn new job skills, typically they must work in an unfamiliar environment. Special orientation materials should be developed and updated frequently to reflect current practices and made available in departments to which nurses transfer most often. In addition to providing necessary staff development content, these orientation programs should focus on

LEARNING EXERCISE 16.3

Great Influences

Who or what has been the greatest influence on your socialization to the nursing role? Were positive or negative sanctions used? Write a short essay (three or four paragraphs) describing this socialization. If appropriate, share this in a group.

efforts to promote the self-esteem of these nurses as they learn the skills necessary for their new role.

> The managers of departments that receive frequent transfers should prepare a special orientation for experienced nurses transferring to the department.

Transitioning into a new job would cause less role strain if programs were designed to facilitate role modification and role expansion. For example, when a nurse transfers from a medical floor to labor and delivery, the nurse does not know the group norms, is unsure of expected values and behaviors, and may go from being an expert to a novice. All of this creates a great deal of *role strain*. This same type of *role stress* occurs when experienced nurses move from one organization to another or from an inpatient setting to a community setting. Often, nurses feel powerless during role transitions, which may culminate in anger and frustration as they seek socialization to a different role.

Programs to assist nurses with the transition to a new position should do more than just provide an orientation to the new position; they also should address specific values and behaviors necessary for the new roles. The values and attitudes expected in a hospice nursing role may be quite different from those expected of a trauma nurse. Managers should not assume that the experienced nurse is aware of the new role's expected attitudes.

In addition, employees adopting new values often experience role strain, and managers need to support employees during this value resocialization. Members of the reference group may use negative sanctions, saying things such as "Well, we don't believe in doing that here." This can make new, experienced employees feel as though the values held in other nursing roles were bad or wrong. Therefore, the manager should make efforts to see that formerly held values are not belittled. Excellent companies have leaders who take responsibility for shaping the values of new employees. By instilling and clarifying organizational values, managers promote a homogeneous staff that functions as a team.

> Values and attitudes may be a source of conflict as nurses learn new roles.

The Socialization and Orientation of New Managers

Probably no other aspect of an employee's work life has as great an influence on productivity and retention as the quality of supervision exhibited by the immediate manager. Unfortunately, the orientation and socialization of new managers is often neglected by organizations. In addition, many restructured hospital organizational designs have created different and expanded roles for existing managers without ensuring that managers are adequately prepared for these new roles.

> There is a growing recognition that good managers do not emerge from the workforce without a great deal of conscious planning on the part of the organization.

A management development program should be ongoing, and individuals should receive some management development instruction before their appointment to a management position. When an individual is filling a position where the previous manager is still available for orientation, the orientation period should be relatively short. The previous manager usually spends no longer than 1 week working directly with the new manager, especially when the new manager is familiar with the organization. A short orientation by the outgoing manager allows the newly appointed manager to gain control of the unit quickly and establish a personal management style. If the new manager has been recruited from outside the organization, the orientation period may need to be extended.

Frequently, a new manager will be appointed to a vacant or newly established position. In either case, no one will be readily available to orient the new manager. In such cases, the new manager's immediate superior should appoint someone to assist the new manager in learning the role. This could be a manager from another unit, the manager's supervisor, or someone from the unit who is familiar with the manager's duties and roles.

A new manager's orientation does not cease after the short introduction to the various tasks. Every new manager needs guidance, direction, and continued orientation and development during the first year in this new role. This direction comes from several sources in the organization:

- *The new manager's immediate superior.* This could be the unit supervisor if the new manager is a charge nurse, or it could be the chief nursing executive if the new manager is a unit supervisor. The immediate superior should have regularly scheduled sessions with the new manager to continue the ongoing orientation process.
- *A group of the new manager's peers.* There should be a management group in the organization with which the new manager can consult. The new manager should be encouraged to use the group as a resource.
- *A mentor.* If someone in the organization decides to mentor the new manager, it will undoubtedly benefit the organization. Although mentors cannot be assigned, the organization can encourage experienced managers to seek out individuals to mentor. Mentoring is discussed further later in this chapter.

Clinical nurses who have recently assumed management roles often experience role confusion when they decrease their involvement with direct patient care. When employees and physicians see a nurse-manager assuming the role of caregiver, they often make disparaging remarks such as "Oh, you're working as a real nurse today." This tends to reinforce the nurse's value conflict in the new role.

Nurses moving into positions of increased responsibility also experience role stress created by *role ambiguity* and role overload. Role ambiguity describes the stress that occurs when job expectations are unclear. *Role overload*, often a major stress for nurse-managers, occurs when the demands of the role are excessive. In addition, as nurses move into positions with increased status, their job descriptions may become more general. Therefore, clarifying job roles becomes an important tool in the resocialization process.

Socializing International Nurses

One solution to nursing shortages has been the active recruitment of nurses from other countries. Huston (2023c) argues that the ethical obligation to the foreign nurse does not end with their arrival in a new country. Instead, the sponsoring country must do whatever it can to see that the migrant nurse is assimilated into the new work environment as well as the new culture.

For example, language skills are often a significant issue for foreign nurses, and this is made even more challenging with American slang and the abbreviations that are a common part of nursing. Differing interpretations of nonverbal behavior may further cloud the picture. In addition, foreign-born nurses may find it difficult to fit into a unit's organization culture and thus fail to establish a sense of community life within the organization. Finally, many foreign nurses experience cultural, professional, and psychological dissonance that are associated with anxiety, homesickness, and isolation.

Clarifying Role Expectations Through Role Models, Preceptors, Mentors, and Coaches

One additional strategy for promoting both socialization and resocialization as well as the clarification of role expectations is the use of role models, preceptors, mentors, and coaches.

Role Models

YourDictionary (n.d.) defines a *role model* as someone who is unusually effective or inspiring in some social role, job, etc. and thus serves as a model for others. Role models in nursing are experienced, competent employees. The relationship between the new employee and the role model, however, is a passive one (i.e., employees see that role models are skilled and attempt to emulate them, but the role model does not actively seek this emulation). One of the exciting aspects of role models is their cumulative effect. The greater the number of excellent role models available for new employees to emulate, the greater the possibilities for new employees to perform well.

Unfortunately, professionals in clinical practice are often unaware that students and even other staff might see them as role models, and not all modeled behavior is positive or beneficial. In fact, sometimes, we learn as much from poor role models as we do positive ones, but ultimately, this can be damaging to the profession and to patients.

Preceptors

A *preceptor* is an experienced nurse who provides knowledge and emotional support, as well as a clarification of role expectations, on a one-to-one basis with a less experienced nurse. In most institutions, the designation of preceptor is an acknowledgment by management and peers of a high level of skill, ability, positivity, and other interpersonal attributes conducive to education (Wakefield, 2021). An effective preceptor can role model and adjust teaching to each learner as needed and appropriately apply adult learning theory.

Precepting can provide significant gratification for preceptors as they watch novice nurses gain confidence and skill in the clinical setting. It does, however, take additional time and energy. In addition, preceptorships may be assigned with little or no preparation and many preceptors feel unprepared for the role (Wakefield, 2021). Also, occasionally, the fit between a preceptor and preceptee is poor. This risk is lower if preceptors willingly seek out this responsibility and if they have attended educational courses outlining preceptor duties and responsibilities.

Organizations that use preceptors to help new employees clarify their roles and improve their skill level then should be careful not to overuse preceptors to the point that they become tired or demotivated. In addition, workload assignments for the preceptor should be decreased whenever possible so that adequate time can be devoted to helping the preceptee problem solve and learn. Incentive pay for preceptors reinforces that the organization values this role.

Finally, most organizations can avoid many of the potential hazards of preceptorship programs by (a) carefully selecting the preceptors, (b) selecting only preceptors who have a strong desire to be role models, (c) preparing preceptors for their role by giving formal classes in adult learning and other social learning concepts, (d) having either experienced staff development or supervisory personnel monitor the preceptor and preceptee closely to ensure that the relationship continues to be beneficial and growth producing for both, and (e) ensuring that good communication and mutual goal setting are an expectation of the preceptored relationship.

Mentors

Mentors take on an even greater role in using education as a means for role clarification. Mentoring is an intense reciprocal development relationship traditionally fostered between a senior, more experienced individual, and a junior, less experienced individual, although age is less relative than experience. A mentor, as no other, can instill the values and attitudes that accompany each role. This is because mentors lead by example. A mentor's strong moral and ethical fiber encourages mentees to think critically and take a stand on ethical dilemmas in the workplace. Becoming a mentor requires committing to a personal relationship. It also requires teaching skills and a genuine interest and belief in the capabilities of others.

LEARNING EXERCISE 16.4

Criteria for Preceptorship

You have been selected to represent your unit on a committee to design a preceptor program for your department. One of the committee's first goals is to develop criteria for selecting preceptors.

ASSIGNMENT:

In groups, select a minimum of five and a maximum of eight criteria that would be appropriate for selecting preceptors on your unit. Would you have minimum education or experience requirements? What personality or behavioral traits would you seek? Which of the criteria that you identified are measurable?

Although some individuals use the terms *preceptor* and *mentor* interchangeably, they are not the same. For example, preceptors are usually assigned, but mentorship involves choice. The mentor makes a conscious decision to assist the protégé in attaining expert status and in furthering their career, and the mentee chooses to work with the mentor. In addition, preceptors have a relatively short relationship with the person to whom they have been assigned, but the relationship between the mentor and mentee is longer and more encompassing.

Although mentoring relationships can vary significantly, typically, there are seven phases. The first phase includes determining whether a mentoring relationship would be helpful and if so, then finding and connecting with the right person (the second phase). Having mutual respect and an understanding is critical for a successful relationship. A successful mentoring relationship can be established only when a "chemistry" is present that fosters reciprocal trust and openness. This process is not automatic; it is intentional.

The third phase is negotiating a mentoring agreement, including boundaries, goals, and deadlines. Setting goals is important because the mentor must understand what the mentee wants to accomplish and what their expectations are of the mentor in helping this to occur. This leads to developing rapport and building trust (phase 4). Deadlines should also be established. At some point, the mentee should outgrow the need for the type of intensive coaching and support that is a big part of the mentoring relationship.

The fifth phase is implementing the agreement. The intensity of the relationship escalates to high levels during this learning, listening, and growing phase. In phase 6, goals and objectives are reviewed continuously to assess progress.

The final phase is summarizing and formally concluding the mentoring relationship. The intensity of the relationship wanes as the mentee begins to move toward independence. Mentees should be able to articulate the change and growth that has occurred as part of the mentoring relationship. The last stage finds both the mentee and the mentor achieving a different, independent relationship, hopefully based on positive, collegial characteristics. Display 16.7 depicts these phases of the mentoring relationship.

> Not every nurse will be fortunate to have a mentor to facilitate each new career role. Most nurses will be lucky if they have one or two mentors throughout their lifetimes.

Unfortunately, the literature suggests that many women have experienced reduced access to mentoring and may be disadvantaged to men when it comes to compensation, unconscious biases, and resources. In addition, traditional mentor–mentee relationships may not be as effective for

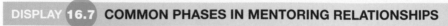

DISPLAY 16.7 COMMON PHASES IN MENTORING RELATIONSHIPS

1. Contemplate whether to begin a mentoring relationship.
2. Initiate contact to ascertain joint desire to participate.
3. Establish/negotiate goals and deadlines.
4. Develop rapport and build trust.
5. Implement mentoring to achieve growth and maintenance.
6. Periodically review progress made.
7. Summarize lessons learned and celebrate the conclusion of the mentoring relationship.

women. A recent study by Rabinowitz et al. (2021) found that women preferred a mentor of the same gender but less often had one. Women also reported having more difficulty finding a mentor than men and cited inability to identify a mentor of the same gender as a contributing factor. Anyone attempting to set up a mentoring program must keep in mind that its success will be greatly affected by the extent to which it incorporates gender and cultural factors.

So, how does someone select a mentor? This selection typically depends on the goals the mentee wishes to accomplish. The mentor may be a role model and a visionary for the mentee. Mentors may also open doors in the organization, be someone who the mentee can use to bounce ideas off of, or be a supporter or problem solver. The mentor is also often a teacher or counselor, especially in career advice.

Sometimes, a mentor is chosen because of that person's ability to assume an advocacy role. This may mean speaking on behalf of, or in some cases speaking for, the mentee. In extreme cases, mentors can even intervene on behalf of the mentee to resolve conflicts or secure projects, work assignments, or promotions.

Just as one would query a potential employer about the benefits of working for an organization, the same care must be taken when engaging with someone as a potential mentor. A strong mentor can help shape one's work style, habits, and communication practices for years to come. Consuming time and effort in finding a mentor may seem unnecessary but failing to take this step and choosing the wrong person for the wrong reason could have long-term ramifications.

A mentor, as no other, can instill the values and attitudes that accompany each role. This is because mentors lead by example. A mentor's strong moral and ethical fiber encourages mentees to think critically and take a stand on ethical dilemmas in the workplace. Becoming a mentor requires committing to a personal relationship. It also requires teaching skills and a genuine interest and belief in the capabilities of others.

Coaches

Although the terms coach and mentor are often used interchangeably, there is a difference. Coaching is generally thought to be an approach to attain short-term performance goals, whereas mentoring addresses longer-term career goals (Drake, 2021). Davis (2021) agrees, noting that coaching is often performance- and result-driven, typically lasting on a short-term or per-project basis with a specific outcome in mind.

Mentors may wait to be asked questions, allowing the mentee to take charge of what they want to know. Conversely, in coaching, the coach often asks questions to provoke the person to make decisions that require action (Drake, 2021). Coaches can also offer solutions or ideas to address problems or conflicts. The coach may suggest the best ways to approach someone, preferred communication styles, and tips to work with someone who may have a challenging personality.

Coaching is an important tool for empowering employees, changing behavior, and developing a cohesive team. It may, however, be a difficult role for a manager to master. Coaching is one person helping the other to reach an optimum level of performance. The emphasis is always on assisting the employee to recognize greater options, to clarify statements, and to grow.

Coaching may be long term or short term. Short-term coaching is effective as a teaching tool, for assisting with socialization, and for dealing with short-term problems. Long-term coaching as a tool for career management and in dealing with disciplinary problems is different and is discussed in other chapters. Short-term coaching frequently involves spontaneous teaching opportunities. Learning Exercise 16.5 illustrates how a manager can use short-term coaching to guide an employee in a new role.

LEARNING EXERCISE 16.5

Paul's Complaint

Paul is the charge nurse on a surgical floor from 3:00 PM to 11:00 PM. One day, he comes to work a few minutes early, as he occasionally does, so that he can chat with his supervisor, Mary, before taking patient reports. Usually, Mary is in her office around this time. Paul enjoys talking over some of his work-related management problems with her because he is fairly new in the charge nurse role, having been appointed 3 months ago. Today, he asks Mary if she can spare a minute to discuss a personnel problem.

Paul: Sally is becoming a real problem to me. She is taking long breaks and has not followed through on several medication order changes lately.
Mary: What do you mean by "long breaks" and not following through?
Paul: In the last 2 months, she has taken an extra 15 minutes for dinner three nights a week and has missed changes in medication orders two times.
Mary: Have you spoken to Sally?
Paul: Yes, and she said that she had been an RN on this floor for 4 years, and no one had ever criticized her before. I checked her personnel record, and there is no mention of those particular problems, but her performance appraisals have only been mediocre.
Mary: What do you recommend doing about Sally?
Paul: I could tell her that I won't tolerate her extended dinner breaks and her poor work performance.
Mary: What are you prepared to do if her performance does not improve?
Paul: I could give her a written warning notice and eventually fire her if her work remains below standard.
Mary: Well, that is one option. What are some other options available to you? Do you think that Sally really understands your expectations? Do you feel that she might resent you?
Paul: I suppose I should sit down with Sally and explain exactly what my expectations are. Since my appointment to charge nurse, I've talked with all the new nurses as they have come on shift, but I just assumed that the old-timers knew what was expected on this unit. I've been a little anxious about my new role; I never thought about her resenting my position.
Mary: I think that is a good first option. Maybe Sally interpreted you not talking to her, as you did with all the new nurses, as a rejection. After you have another talk with her, let me know how things are going.

Analysis

The supervisor has coached Paul toward a more appropriate option as a first choice in solving this problem. Although Mary's choice of questions and guidance assisted Paul, she never "took over" or directed Paul but instead let him find his own better solution. As a result of this conversation, Paul had a series of individual meetings with all his staff and shared with them his expectations. He also enlisted their assistance in his efforts to have the shift run smoothly. Although he began to see an improvement in Sally's performance, he realized that she was a marginal employee who would need a great deal of coaching. He reported back to Mary and outlined his plans for improving Sally's performance further. Mary reinforced Paul's handling of the problem by complimenting his actions.

Overcoming Motivational Deficiencies

Sometimes, difficulties in socialization or resocialization occur because an employee lacks the motivation to overcome the educational and personal challenges inherent in learning a new role. A planned program should be implemented to correct the deficiencies by using positive and negative sanctions.

Positive Sanctions

Positive sanctions can be used as an interactional or educational process of socialization. If deliberately planned, they become educational. However, sanctions given informally through the group process or reference group use the social interaction process. The reference group sets behavior norms and then applies sanctions to ensure that new members adopt these norms before acceptance into the group. These informal sanctions offer an extremely powerful tool for socialization and resocialization in the workplace. Managers should become aware of what role behavior they reward and what new employee behavior the senior staff is rewarding.

Negative Sanctions

Negative sanctions, like rewards, provide cues that enable people to evaluate their performance consciously and to modify behavior when needed. For positive or negative sanctions to be effective, they must result in the role learner internalizing the values of the organization.

Negative sanctions are often applied in very subtle and covert ways. Making fun of a new graduate's awkwardness with certain skills or belittling a new employee's desire to use nursing care plans are examples of inappropriate, negative sanctions that may be used by group members to mold individual behavior to group norms. These actions constitute bullying and should never be condoned. This is not to say, however, that negative sanctions should never be used. New employees should be told when their behavior is not an acceptable part of their role. However, the sanctions used should be constructive and not destructive.

> The manager should know what the group norms are, be observant of sanctions used by the group to make newcomers conform and intervene if group norms are not appropriate.

Meeting the Educational Needs of a Diverse Staff

In the 21st century, nurse-leaders should expect to work with a more diverse workforce. According to Huston (2023b), there are many types of diversity in the workforce although most organizations consciously focus on ethnicity, gender, and generational differences. However, increased attention must also be given to diversity in sexual orientation and identity. Current literature on diversity often fails to address the 4% of the population self-identifying as lesbian, gay, bisexual, transgender, and/or queer (LGBTQ) (Cole, 2020). In addition, LGBTQ and intersex (LGBTQI+) people experience high rates of discrimination in health care settings worldwide, which have been linked to poor health outcomes and delays in seeking care (Sherman et al., 2021).

Creating an organization that celebrates a diverse workforce rather than merely accepting it is a leadership role and requires well-planned learning activities. There should also be opportunities for small groups so that personnel can begin recognizing their own biases and prejudices.

Heterogeneity of staff in a teaching–learning setting may add strength or create difficulty. Factors such as gender, age, English language proficiency, and culture may affect success and cooperative learning of groups. Although meeting the educational needs of a heterogeneous staff may be more time-consuming and beset with communication challenges, the educational needs must be met. The ability of all nurses to work well with a culturally diverse staff is essential. Managers should respect cultural diversity and recognize the desirability of having nurses from various cultures on their staff.

Educational staff should be open to exploring diversity and be aware that learners with diverse learning styles and cultural backgrounds may perceive both the classroom and instruction differently from learners who have only experienced mainstream US culture. Managers should also consider the learning styles of their more mature nurses and preceptor needs. These nurses often learn best in a different manner than do new graduates and respond well

LEARNING EXERCISE 16.6

Cultural Considerations in Teaching

You are the evening charge nurse for a large surgical unit. Recently, your longtime and extremely capable unit clerk retired, and the manager of the unit replaced the clerk with 23-year-old Nan, who does not have a health care background and is a recent immigrant from Southeast Asia. She speaks English with an accent but can be easily understood. She is intelligent, but shy, and seems to have trouble asserting herself.

Nan received a 2-week unit clerk orientation that consisted of actual classroom time and working directly with the retiring clerk. She has been functioning on her own for 2 weeks, and you realize that her orientation was insufficient. Last evening, after her 10th mistake, you became rather sharp with her, and she broke down in tears.

You are frustrated by this situation. Your unit is very busy in the evening with returning surgeries and surgeons making rounds and leaving a multitude of orders. On the other hand, you believe that Nan has great potential. You realize that, for a person without a health care background, learning the terminology, physicians' names, and unit routine is difficult. You spend the morning devising a training plan for Nan.

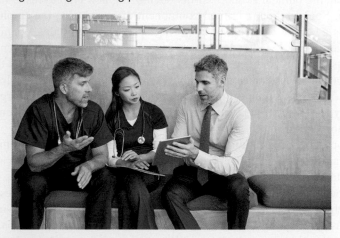

ASSIGNMENT:

Using your knowledge of learning theories, explain your teaching plan and support your plan with appropriate rationale. How might Nan's lack of an American education and socialization influence her learning?

to sharing anecdotal case histories. In addition, whether teaching in a classroom or at the bedside, there are several things that staff development personnel can do to facilitate the learning process, such as giving the learner plenty of time to respond to questions and restating information that is not understood.

Integrating Leadership and Management in Team Building Through Socializing and Educating Staff in a Learning Organization

There is momentum in organizations to provide a continual supportive learning environment. Health care science and technology change so rapidly that without adequate teaching–learning skills and educational services, organizations will be left behind. Likewise, it has become obvious in the new millennium that teams, rather than individuals, function more efficiently. Learning together and for the organization makes the sum of the team more important than the individual, and the workplace becomes more productive when there is team compatibility.

The integrated leader-manager knows that a well-planned and well-implemented staff development program is an important part of being a LO. The leader-manager accepts the ultimate responsibility for staff development and uses appropriate teaching theories to assist with teaching and training staff. In addition, they share the responsibility for assessing educational needs, educational quality, and fiscal accountability of all staff development activities.

The integrated leader-manager is also one who encourages continuous learning from all individuals in the organization and is a role model of the lifelong learner. This is especially important in promoting evidence-based nursing practice. The nurse-leader should use EBP and make research resources available to the staff. They understand that by building and supporting a knowledgeable team, the collective knowledge generated will be greater than any single individual's contribution.

There is perhaps no other part of management, however, that has as great an influence on reducing burnout as successfully socializing new employees to the values of the organization. Socialization, a critical component of introducing the employee into the organization, is a complex process of acquiring appropriate attitudes, cognition, emotions, values, motivations, skills, knowledge, and social patterns necessary to cope with the social and professional environment. It differs from and has a greater impact than either induction or orientation on subsequent productivity and retention. It can also help build loyalty and team spirit. This is the time to instill the employee with pride in the organization and the unit. This type of affective learning becomes the foundation for subsequent increased satisfaction and motivation.

As part of socialization, the integrated leader-manager supports employees during difficult role transitions. Mentoring, precepting, coaching, and role modeling are encouraged, and role expectations are clarified. The manager recognizes that employees who are not supported and socialized to the organization will not develop the loyalty necessary in the competitive marketplace. Leaders understand that creating a positive work environment where there is interdisciplinary respect will assist employees in their role transitions.

Finally, the manager ensures that resources for staff development are used wisely. A focus of staff development should be keeping staff updated with new knowledge and ascertaining that all personnel remain competent to perform their roles. By integrating the leadership role with the management functions of staff development, the manager can collaborate with education personnel and others so that the learning needs of unit employees are met.

Key Concepts

- The philosophy of LOs is the concept that collective learning goes beyond the boundaries of individual learning and releases gains for both the individual and the organization.
- The leader is a role model of the lifelong learner and seeks to encourage lifelong learning in others.
- Training, education, and onboarding are important parts of staff development and should be evaluated for purpose, quality control, and fiscal accountability.
- The promotion and use of evidence-based nursing practice is an organization-wide responsibility.
- Managers and education department staff have a shared responsibility for the education, training, and onboarding of staff. The roles that each play must be clearly delineated and communicated for staff development activities to be successful.
- Theories of learning and principles of teaching must be considered if staff development activities are to be successful.

- Social learning theory suggests that people learn most behavior by direct experience and observation.
- The socialization of people into roles occurs with all professions and is a normal sociologic process.
- Socialization and resocialization are often neglected areas of the onboarding process.
- New graduates, international nurses, new managers, and experienced nurses in new roles have unique socialization needs.
- Difficulties with resocialization usually center on unclear role expectations (role ambiguity), an inability to meet job demands, or deficiencies in motivation. Role strain and role overload contribute to the problem.
- The terms *role model, preceptor, mentor,* and *coach* are not synonymous, and all play an important role in assisting with the socialization of employees.
- Successful mentoring relationships can result in increased productivity, career advancement, and career satisfaction.
- People from different cultures and age groups may have different socialization and learning needs.

Additional Learning Exercises and Applications

LEARNING EXERCISE 16.7

Accepting Additional Responsibility

You are an experienced staff nurse on an inpatient specialty unit. Today, a local nursing school instructor approaches you and asks if you would be willing to become a preceptor for a nursing student as part of his 10-week leadership–management clinical rotation. The instructor relays that there will be no instructor on site and that the student has had only minimal exposure to acute care clinical skills. The student will have to work very closely with you on a one-to-one basis. The school of nursing can offer no pay for this role, but the instructor states that she would be happy to write a thank you letter for your personnel file and that she would be available at any time to address questions that might arise.

The unit does not reduce workload for preceptors, although credit for service is given on the annual performance review. The unit supervisor states that the choice is yours but warns that you may also be called on to assist with the orientation of a nurse who will transfer to the unit in 6 weeks' time. You have mixed feelings about whether to accept this role. Although you enjoy having students on the unit and being in the teaching role, you are unsure if you can do both your normal, heavy workload and give this student and the new

(continues on page 418)

LEARNING EXERCISE 16.7

Accepting Additional Responsibility (continued)

employee the time that they will undoubtedly need to learn. You do feel a "need to give back to your profession" and personally believe that nurses need to be more supportive of each other, but you are significantly concerned about role overload.

ASSIGNMENT:

Decide if you will accept this role. Would you place any constraints on the instructor, the student, the new employee, or your supervisor as a condition of accepting the role? What were the strongest driving forces for your decision? What were the greatest restraining forces? What evaluation criteria would you develop to assess whether your final decision was a good one?

LEARNING EXERCISE 16.8

Addressing Resocialization Issues

You are one of the care coordinators for a home health agency. One of your duties is to orient new employees to the agency. Recently, the chief nursing executive hired Brian, an experienced acute care nurse, to be one of your team members. Brian seemed eager and enthusiastic. He confided in you that he was tired of acute care and wanted to be more involved with long-term patient and family caseloads.

During Brian's orientation, you became aware that his clinical skills were excellent, but his therapeutic communication skills were inferior to those of the rest of your staff. You discussed this with Brian and explained how important communication is in gaining the trust of agency patients and that trust is necessary if the needs of the patients and the goals of the agency are to be met. You referred Brian to some literature that you believed might be helpful to him.

After a 3-week orientation program, Brian began working unsupervised. It is now 4 weeks later. Recently, you received a complaint from one of the other nurses and one from a patient regarding Brian's poor communication skills. Brian seems frustrated and has not gained acceptance from the other nurses in your work group. You suspect that some of the nurses resent Brian's superior clinical skills, whereas others believe that he does not understand his new role, and they are becoming impatient with him. You are genuinely concerned that Brian does not seem to be fitting in.

ASSIGNMENT:

Could this problem have been prevented? Decide what you should do now. Outline a plan to resocialize Brian into his new role and make him feel like a valued part of the staff.

LEARNING EXERCISE	16.9

Effective Interpersonal Problem Solving When Incivility Occurs

You are a new graduate nurse and have been working at Memorial Hospital for 9 months and have begun to feel somewhat confident in your new role. However, one of the older nurses working on your shift constantly belittles your nursing education. Whenever you request assistance in problem solving or in learning a new skill, she says, "Didn't they teach you anything in nursing school?" Your charge nurse has given you satisfactory 3- and 6-month evaluations, but you are becoming increasingly defensive regarding the comments of the other nurse.

ASSIGNMENT:

Explain how you plan to evaluate the accuracy of the older nurse's comments. Might you be contributing to the problem? How will you cope with this situation? Would you involve others? What efforts can you make to improve your relationship with this coworker?

REFERENCES

Austin, C., & Halpin, Y. (2021, June 10). Evaluation of a personal professional mentor scheme for newly qualified nurses. *British Journal of Nursing, 30*(11), 672–676. https://doi-org.mantis.csuchico.edu/10.12968/bjon.2021.30.11.672

Bandura, A. (1977). *Social learning theory.* Prentice-Hall.

The Busy Lifestyle. (2020, May 5). *A learning organization has these 5 key elements.* https://thebusylifestyle.com/learning-organization-peter-senge/

Cherry, K. (2021, July 28). *How social learning theory works.* Verywell Mind. https://www.verywell.com/social-learning-theory-2795074

Cole, K. A. (2020). Health disparities and diversity in the nursing workforce: A call to action. *Kansas Nurse, 95*(1), 18–20,

Davis, N. E. (2021). How mentorship and coaching can unlock one's full potential. *Journal of Legal Nurse Consulting, 32*(1), 8–12.

Drake, K. (2021, August). Coaching vs. mentoring. *Nursing Management, 52*(8), 56.

Ford, C. D., & Graves, B. A. (2023). Evidence-based best practice (chapter 5). In C. J. Huston (Ed.), *Professional issues in nursing: Challenges and opportunities* (6th ed., pp. 67–79). Wolters Kluwer.

Huston, C. J. (2023a). Assuring provider competence through licensure, continuing education, and certification (chapter 20). In C. J. Huston (Ed.), *Professional issues in nursing: Challenges and opportunities* (6th ed., pp. 288–301). Wolters Kluwer.

Huston, C. J. (2023b). Diversity in the nursing workforce (chapter 9). In C. J. Huston (Ed.), *Professional issues in nursing: Challenges and opportunities* (6th ed., pp. 121–135). Wolters Kluwer.

Huston, C. J. (2023c). Foreign nurse migration (chapter 7). In C. J. Huston (Ed.), *Professional issues in nursing: Challenges and opportunities* (6th ed., pp. 92–108). Wolters Kluwer.

Huston, C. L., Phillips, B., Jeffries, P., Todero, C., Rich, J., Knecht, P., & Lewis, M. P. (2018). The academic-practice gap: Strategies for an enduring problem. *Nursing Forum, 53*(1), 27–34.

Institute of Medicine. (2009). *Roundtable on evidence-based medicine. Leadership commitments to improve value in healthcare: Finding common ground: Workshop summary.* National Academies Press (US). https://www.ncbi.nlm.nih.gov/books/NBK52847/

Knowles, M. (1970). *The modern practice of adult education: Andragogy versus pedagogy.* Association Press.

Kramer, M. (1974). *Reality shock: Why nurses leave nursing.* Mosby.

Liimatainen, H. (2021, August 24). 3 Great examples of organizational learning in 2021. *Howspace.* https://www.howspace.com/resources/3-great-examples-organizational-learning-in-2021

Lopes, M. C., & Fernandes, G. L. (2021, July). Knowledge management and its role in universities as learning organizations: The case of ISEG. *IUP Journal of Knowledge Management, 19*(3), 32–48.

National Academies of Science, Engineering, and Medicine. (2013). *Best care at lower cost: The path to continuously learning health care in America.* Retrieved November 26, 2021, from http://www.nationalacademies.org/hmd/Reports/2012/Best-Care-at-Lower-Cost-The-Path-to-Continuously-Learning-Health-Care-in-America.aspx

National Council of State Boards of Nursing. (2022). *Transition to practice. Why transition to practice (TTP)?* Retrieved May 28, 2022, from https://www.ncsbn.org/transition-to-practice.htm

Nichols, R. (2021). Why 2021 is the year of the 'learning organization.' *360Learning.* https://360learning.com/blog/learning-organization-model-2021/

Rabinowitz, L. G., Grinspan, L. T., Zylberberg, H., Dixon, R., David, Y, Aroniadis, O, Chiang, A., Christie, J., Fayad, N. F.,

Ha, C., Harris, L. A., Ko, C. W., Kolb, J., Kwah, J., Lee, L., Lieberman, D., Raffals, L. E., Rex, D. K., Shah, S. C., … Greenwald, D. A. (2021, September). Survey finds gender disparities impact both women mentors and mentees in gastroenterology. *The American Journal of Gastroenterology, 116*(9), 1876–1884. https://doi.org/10.14309/ajg.0000000000001341. https://journals.lww.com/ajg/Abstract/2021/09000/Survey_Finds_Gender_Disparities_Impact_Both_Women.18.aspx

Senge, P. (2006). *The fifth discipline: The art and practice of the learning organization.* Currency Doubleday.

Sherman, A. D. F., Cimino, A. N., Clark, K. D., Smith, K., Klepper, M., & Bower, K. M. (2021, February). LGBTQ+ health education for nurses: An innovative approach to improving nursing curricula. *Nursing Education Today.* https://pubmed.ncbi.nlm.nih.gov/33341526/

Spas, M. (2021, October 12). Learning organizations and sustainability. *IUPUI Lilly Family School of Philanthropy.* https://philanthropy.iupui.edu/news-events/insights-newsletter/2021-issues/oct-2021-issue-1.html

Wakefield, E. (2021, October–December). Preceptoring the preceptors: Empowering and sustaining our profession. *Australian Nursing & Midwifery Journal, 27*(5), 40–41.

YourDictionary. (n.d.). Role model. In *YourDictionary.* Retrieved May 28, 2022, from http://www.yourdictionary.com/role-model

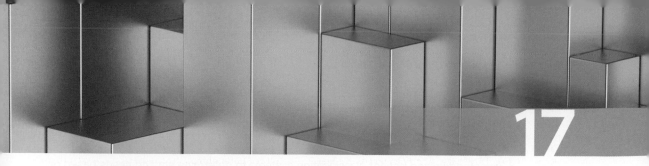

Staffing Needs and Scheduling Policies

*… Nursing leaders must understand data-driven nurse staffing plans to communicate clearly and budget appropriately for nursing resources.—**Bob Dent***

*… Acuity systems that capture actual patient data automatically, as part of the documentation process, resolve objectively the level-of-care issues that contribute to accidents, mortality and readmissions, reducing preventable adverse events and the high costs associated with them.—**Harris Healthcare***

*… Think of people as individuals. What do they need on a day to day basis? Who is everyone beyond their title?—**Andrew Graff***

This chapter addresses:

- **AACN Essentials Domain 1:** Knowledge for nursing practice
- **AACN Essentials Domain 2:** Person-centered care
- **AACN Essentials Domain 3:** Population health
- **AACN Essentials Domain 4:** Scholarship for nursing practice
- **AACN Essentials Domain 5:** Quality and safety
- **AACN Essentials Domain 7:** Systems-based practice
- **AACN Essentials Domain 8:** Information and health care technologies
- **AONL Nurse Executive Competency 2:** A knowledge of the health care environment
- **AONL Nurse Executive Competency 3:** Leadership
- **AONL Nurse Executive Competency 5:** Business skills
- **ANA Standard of Professional Performance 8:** Advocacy
- **ANA Standard of Professional Performance 9:** Respectful and equitable practice
- **ANA Standard of Professional Performance 10:** Communication
- **ANA Standard of Professional Performance 15:** Quality of practice
- **ANA Standard of Professional Performance 17:** Resource stewardship
- **ANA Standard of Professional Performance 18:** Environmental health
- **QSEN Competency:** Patient-centered care
- **QSEN Competency:** Teamwork and collaboration
- **QSEN Competency:** Quality improvement
- **QSEN Competency:** Safety
- **QSEN Competency:** Informatics

LEARNING OBJECTIVES

The learner will:

- use an evidence-based approach in determining staffing needs
- differentiate between centralized and decentralized staffing, citing the advantages and disadvantages of each

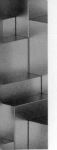

- identify organizational variables that impact the numbers of staff needed to carry out the goals of the organization
- identify common staffing and scheduling options currently used in health care organizations
- use standardized patient classification systems to determine staffing needs based on patient acuity
- calculate nursing care hours per patient-day if given total hours of care in a 24-hour period as well as the patient census
- use staffing formulas accurately to avoid over- and understaffing
- explain the relationship of flex time and self-scheduling to increased job satisfaction
- identify the driving and restraining forces for the implementation of mandatory minimum staffing ratios in acute care hospitals
- provide examples of how generational (the veteran generation, baby boomers, generation X, generation Y, and generation Z) value differences may impact staffing and scheduling needs and wants
- select appropriate staffing policies for a given situation
- discuss the minimum written staffing and scheduling policies a health care organization should have

Introduction

In addition to selecting, developing, and socializing staff, managers must be certain that adequate numbers and an appropriate mix of personnel are available to meet unit needs and organizational goals. These staffing determinations should be based on existing research evidence that correlates staffing mix, numbers of staff needed, and patient outcomes.

In addition, because staffing patterns and scheduling policies directly affect the daily lives of all personnel, they must be administered fairly as well as economically. This chapter examines different methods for determining staffing needs, communicating staffing plans, and developing and communicating scheduling policies. In addition, unit fiscal responsibility for staffing is discussed, with sample formulas and instructions for calculating daily staffing needs.

The manager's responsibility for adequate and well-communicated staffing and scheduling policies is stressed, as is the need for periodic reevaluation of the staffing philosophy. There is a focus on the leadership responsibility for developing trust through fair staffing and scheduling procedures. Existing and proposed legislation regarding mandatory staffing requirements are also discussed, including the manager's role for ensuring that the organization can facilitate the changes required by law. The leadership roles and management functions inherent in staffing and scheduling are shown in Display 17.1.

Management's Responsibilities in Meeting Staffing Needs

Harris Healthcare (2017) notes that the "Accountable Care Act triggered a host of changes in healthcare, from risk-based reimbursement and accountable care organizations to value-based, patient-centric care models. This gave rise to an increased focus on quality and transparency, especially as it relates to acute care. Achieving the optimum balance between nurse staffing and patient acuity is also key to a healthcare organization's financial viability" (para. 1). Five driving forces for developing effective nurse staffing are shown in Display 17.2.

In addition, the requirement for night, evening, weekend, and holiday work that is frequently necessary in health care organizations can be stressful and frustrating. Management should do what they can for employees to feel they have some control over scheduling, shift

DISPLAY 17.1 LEADERSHIP ROLES AND MANAGEMENT FUNCTIONS ASSOCIATED WITH STAFFING AND SCHEDULING

Leadership Roles

1. Identifies creative and flexible staffing methods to meet the needs of patients, staff, and the organization
2. Is knowledgeable regarding contemporary methods and tools used in staffing and scheduling
3. Assumes a responsibility toward staffing that builds trust and encourages a team approach
4. Role models the use of evidence in making appropriate staffing and scheduling decisions
5. Is alert to extraneous factors that have an impact on unit and organizational staffing
6. Is ethically accountable to patients and employees for adequate and safe staffing
7. Encourages diversity of thought, gender, age, and culture in nursing staffing
8. Proactively plans for staffing shortages so that patient care goals will be met
9. Communicates work schedules as well as scheduling policies clearly and effectively to staff
10. Assesses if and how workforce intergenerational values impact staffing needs and responds accordingly

Management Functions

1. Provides adequate staffing to meet patient care needs according to the philosophy of the organization and evidence-based needs
2. Uses organizational goals and patient classification tools to minimize understaffing and overstaffing as patient census and acuity fluctuate
3. Schedules staff in a fiscally responsible manner
4. Periodically examines the unit standard of productivity to determine if changes are needed
5. Ascertains that scheduling policies are not in violation of state and national labor laws, organizational policies, or union contracts
6. Assumes accountability for quality and fiscal control of staffing
7. Evaluates scheduling and staffing procedures and policies on a regular basis
8. Develops and implements fair and uniform scheduling policies and communicates these clearly to all staff
9. Selects acuity-based staffing tools that reduce subjectivity and promote objectivity in patient acuity determinations

options, and staffing policies. Creating safe staffing practices continues, however, to be a challenge for nurse-leaders.

In addition, each organization has different expectations regarding the unit manager's responsibility in long-range human resource planning and in short-range planning for daily staffing. Although many organizations now use staffing clerks and computers to assist with

DISPLAY 17.2 DRIVING FORCES FOR THE DEVELOPMENT OF EFFECTIVE NURSE STAFFING

1. *Staffing can make—or break—the relationship between finance and nursing.* Acuity systems have improved accountability, but patient acuity is still a subjective measure.
2. *Staffing can blow a budget.* Nursing accounts for most of an acute care facility's total payroll.
3. *Staffing affects the cost of care.* Patient mortality, readmission, and unsafe care increase both human and monetary costs. Adequate staffing helps mitigate these problems, thereby reducing cost.
4. *Staffing affects the quality of care.* Research shows that higher nurse staffing levels lead to better clinical outcomes.
5. *Staffing matters to nursing.* Staffing impacts all aspects of nurses' personal and professional lives. It influences the quality of their patients' care; their job satisfaction, perception of the workplace, and desire to remain in the profession; and their physical, emotional, and mental health.

Source: Adapted from Harris Healthcare. (2017). *Five reasons why CFOs should care about staffing and acuity.* https://www.harrishealthcare.com/wp-content/uploads/2017/11/Five-Reasons_whitepaper_FINAL-1.pdf

staffing, the overall responsibility for scheduling continues to be an important function of first- and middle-level managers.

Centralized and Decentralized Staffing

Some organizations decentralize staffing by having unit managers make scheduling decisions. Other organizations use *centralized staffing* where staffing decisions are made by a central office or staffing center. Such centers may or may not be staffed by registered nurses (RNs), although someone in authority should be a nurse even when a staffing clerk carries out the day-to-day activity.

In organizations with *decentralized staffing*, the unit manager is often responsible for covering all scheduled staff absences, reducing staff during periods of decreased patient census or acuity, adding staff during periods of high patient census or acuity, preparing monthly unit schedules, and preparing holiday and vacation schedules. Advantages of decentralized staffing are that the unit manager understands the needs of the unit and staff intimately, which leads to the increased likelihood that sound staffing decisions will be made. In addition, the staff feels more in control of their work environment because they can take personal scheduling requests directly to their immediate supervisor. Decentralized scheduling and staffing also lead to increased autonomy and flexibility, thus decreasing nurse attrition.

Decentralized staffing, however, carries the risk that employees will be treated unequally or inconsistently. For example, some employees may have more staffing requests granted than others or be given preferential schedules. In addition, the unit manager may be viewed as granting rewards or punishments through the staffing schedule. Decentralized staffing also is time-consuming for the manager and often promotes more "special pleading" than centralized staffing. However, undoubtedly, the greatest difficulty with decentralized staffing is ensuring high-quality staffing decisions throughout the organization.

In centralized staffing, the manager's role is limited to making minor adjustments and providing input. For example, the manager would communicate special staffing needs and assist with obtaining staff coverage for illness and sudden changes in patient census. Therefore, the manager in centralized staffing continues to have ultimate responsibility for seeing that adequate personnel are available to meet the needs of the organization.

Centralized staffing is generally fairer to all employees because policies tend to be applied more consistently and impartially. In addition, centralized staffing frees the middle-level manager to complete other management functions. Centralized staffing also allows for the most efficient (cost-effective) use of resources because the more units that can be considered together, the easier it is to deal with variations in patient census and staffing needs. Centralized staffing, however, does not provide as much flexibility for the worker. Nor can it account as well for a worker's desires or special needs. In addition, managers may be less responsive to personnel budget control if they have limited responsibility in scheduling and staffing matters. The strengths and limitations of decentralized and centralized staffing are summarized in Table 17.1.

It is important, though, to remember that centralized and decentralized staffing are not synonymous with centralized and decentralized decision making. For example, a manager can work in an organization that has centralized staffing but decentralized organizational decision making. Regardless of whether the organization has centralized or decentralized staffing, all unit managers should understand scheduling options and procedures and accept fiscal responsibility for staffing.

> Decentralized scheduling and staffing lead to increased autonomy and flexibility, but centralized staffing is fairer to all employees because policies tend to be employed more consistently and impartially.

TABLE STRENGTHS AND LIMITATIONS OF DECENTRALIZED AND CENTRALIZED STAFFING

	Strengths	Limitations
Decentralized staffing	• Manager retains greater control over unit staffing • Staff can take requests directly to their manager • Provides greater autonomy and flexibility for the individual staff member	• Can result in more special pleading and arbitrary treatment of employees • May not be cost-effective for organization because staffing needs are not viewed holistically • More time-consuming for the unit manager
Centralized staffing	• Provides organization-wide view of staffing needs, which encourages optimal utilization of staffing resources • Staffing policies tend to be employed more consistently and impartially • More cost-effective than decentralized staffing • Frees the middle-level manager to complete other management functions	• Provides less flexibility for the worker and may not account for a specific worker's desires or special needs • Managers may be less responsive to personnel budget control in scheduling and staffing matters

Staffing and Scheduling Options

Because it is beyond the scope of this book to discuss all the creative staffing and scheduling options available, only a few are discussed here. Some of the more frequently used creative staffing and scheduling options are shown in Display 17.3. There are advantages and disadvantages to each type.

Ten- or Twelve-Hour Shifts

Ten- or 12-hour shifts have become commonplace in acute care hospitals even though there continues to be debate about whether extending the length of shifts causes increased judgment errors related to fatigue and more care left undone. Many studies suggest that when nurses work more than 8 hours a day, patients are at risk. This is because more medication errors and sentinel events occur when nurses are fatigued, and the numbers rise exponentially when nurses work past 12 hours (Bucceri Androus, 2022). Indeed, Bae (2021) found a conclusive relationship between excessive nurse work hours (more than 40 hours per week or 12 hours per day) and adverse

DISPLAY 17.3 COMMON STAFFING AND SCHEDULING OPTIONS IN HEALTH CARE ORGANIZATIONS

- 10- and 12-hour shifts
- Premium pay for weekend work
- Part-time staffing pool for weekend shifts and holidays
- Cyclical staffing, which allows long-term knowledge of future work schedules because a set staffing pattern is repeated every few weeks (Fig. 17.1 shows a master staffing pattern of 8 hour shifts that repeats every 4 weeks)
- Staggered shift scheduling
- Job sharing
- Allowing nurses to exchange hours of work among themselves
- Flextime
- Use of supplemental staffing from outside registries, agencies, and float pools
- Travel nurses
- Staff self-scheduling
- Shift bidding, which allows nurses to bid for shifts rather than requiring mandatory overtime

Position	Name	Week I								Week II								Week III								Week IV							
		S	M	T	W	T	F	S	S	M	T	W	T	F	S	S	M	T	W	T	F	S	S	M	T	W	T	F	S
Full-time	RN 1				X			X	X					X					X			X	X					X	
Full-time	RN 2	X				X						X			X	X				X						X			X
Full-time	RN 3			X			X		X			X						X			X	X				X			
Full-time	RN 4	X				X					X			X		X				X					X				X
Full-time	RN 5			X			X		X					X					X			X	X					X	
Full-time	RN 6	X				X				X				X		X				X					X				X
Full-time	RN 7		X				X		X			X					X				X		X			X			
Full-time	RN 8	X				X					X			X		X			X						X				X
Part-time	8 hr/wk RN 9	On													On	On													On
Part-time	8 hr/wk RN 10							On	On													On	On						
Part-time	8 hr/wk RN 11	On													On	On													On
Part-time	8 hr/wk RN 12							On	On													On	On						
Total RNs on duty each day		6	7	7	6	6	6	6	6	7	7	6	6	6	6	6	7	7	6	6	6	6	6	7	6	7	6	6	6

Elements: Every other weekend off   Number of split days off each period: 2   X: Scheduled day off
            Maximum days worked: 4   Operates in multiples of 4, 8, 12 . . .
            Minimum days worked: 2   Schedule repeats itself every 4 weeks

FIGURE 17.1 Four-week cycle master time sheet.

patient outcomes, such as medication errors, nosocomial infections, falls with injuries, and errors or near misses, and suggested that nursing shifts longer than 12 hours should be prohibited.

In addition, most nurses who work 12-hour shifts do not get enough sleep, tallying around 5.5 hours per night and even less for night-shift workers. Lack of sleep and fatigue are known to cause poor judgment and significantly high rates of errors (Bucceri Androus, 2022). Working abnormally extended periods in a health care environment may also cause nurses to exceed the safe limits for exposure to a variety of hazards, including ergonomic stressors and chemical agents, increasing the risk for both mental and physical health conditions (Stasik, 2022).

In addition, drowsy driving following 12-hour night shifts is persistent among nurses, resulting in elevated rates of vehicle crashes and crash-related injuries and deaths (Smith et al., 2020). Indeed, Olson (2021) notes that nursing is among occupations with the highest workplace fatalities (105 incidents per 10,000 fulltime workers), which may be a consequence of long, cumulative work schedules. Fatigue may accumulate across multiple shifts and lead to performance impairments, which in turn may be linked to injury risks.

LEARNING EXERCISE 17.1

Choosing 8- or 12-Hour Shifts

You are the manager of an intensive care unit. Many of the nurses have approached you requesting 12-hour shifts. Other nurses have approached you stating that they will transfer out of the unit if 12-hour shifts are implemented. You are exploring the feasibility and cost-effectiveness of using both 8- and 12-hour shifts so that staff could select which type of scheduling they wanted.

ASSIGNMENT:

Would this create a scheduling nightmare? Will you limit the number of 12-hour shifts that staff could work in a week? Would you pay overtime for the last 4 hours of the 12-hour shift? Would you allow staff to choose freely between 8- and 12-hour shifts? What other problems may result from mixing 8- and 12-hour shifts?

EXAMINING THE EVIDENCE 17.1

Source: From How 12-hour nursing shifts impact burnout and job satisfaction. (2020). *DailyNurse*. Retrieved November 26, 2021, from https://dailynurse.com/how-12-hour-nursing-shifts-impact-burnout-and-job-satisfaction/#:~:text=One%20of%20the%20major%20results%20was%20that%20nurses,nurses%20working%20shifts%20of%20eight%20hours%20or%20less

Twelve-Hour Work Shifts Linked With Burnout and Job Dissatisfaction by Nurses

In a large European study involving more than 31,000 nurses in 488 hospitals across 12 countries, hospital nurses who worked 12-hour shifts experienced more adverse outcomes like burnout and job dissatisfaction. Most notably, nursing shifts of at least 12 hours increased the odds of high emotional exhaustion by 26% compared with nurses working shifts of 8 hours or less. Nurses who worked longer shifts were also more likely to experience high depersonalization (a dreamlike or detached state of mind) and low personal accomplishment.

Another important finding was the connection with job dissatisfaction. Nurses who worked shifts of 12 hours or more were 40% more likely to report being dissatisfied with their job—and 31% were more likely to plan to leave their job—compared with nurses working shifts of 8 hours or less.

The researchers also noted a paradox; nurses prefer longer shifts because of the perception that they improve job satisfaction, but longer shifts may have the opposite effect. Nurses may be choosing to sacrifice work satisfaction for benefits in other spheres of life; however, this type of choice is likely to compromise nurses' recovery sleep, physical and psychological well-being: the stress of those long workdays and the recovery time needed may counterbalance any perceived benefit.

Yet, many nurses report a higher level of satisfaction with 12-hour shifts because they work less days each week and have more consecutive time for leisure and personal obligations, all leading to potentially improved work–life balance. However, researchers in a large European study involving more than 31,000 nurses in 488 hospitals across 12 countries noted a paradox: The choice to work 12-hour shifts is likely to compromise nurses' recovery sleep as well as physical and psychological well-being, so the stress of those long workdays and the recovery time needed may counterbalance any perceived benefit (see Examining the Evidence 17.1).

For employers, longer shifts mean fewer benefitted employees and overtime scheduling (only two shifts to cover). Extended work shifts also provide a solution for difficulties with childcare because they reduce the number of working days. In addition, some agencies pay overtime for any shift over 8 hours, whereas others do not. Furthermore, fewer shift changes mean more time spent with patients and better communication because of fewer handoffs.

How long can nurses work safely? Given the variability in each situation, there is no one answer to this question. There is little doubt, however, that after a certain point of protracted work time, fatigue becomes a factor and the likelihood of errors, near errors, mistakes, and lapses in judgment increases.

Agency and Travel Nurses

Another increasingly common staffing and scheduling alternative is the use of supplemental nursing staff such as *agency nurses* and *travel nurses*. These nurses are usually directly employed by an external broker and work for premium pay (often two to three times that of a regularly employed staff nurse), without benefits. Although such staff provide scheduling relief, especially in response to unanticipated increases in census or patient acuity, their continuous use is expensive and can result in poor continuity of nursing care.

Travel nurses were in high demand across the United States as hospitals worked to treat surges of coronavirus (COVID-19) patients early this decade (The Risks to Travel, 2021). Data from different staffing platforms show that throughout the pandemic, travel nurses were in highest demand in areas most impacted by the coronavirus, like New York and Washington State, and certain nursing specialties like ICU/Critical Care, ER/Trauma, and Medical/Surgical care.

Travel nurses need to ensure that their licenses will allow them to practice in whatever state/ jurisdiction they are seeking employment in. Multi-state licenses are available for nurses who meet the requirements and temporary licenses are also generally reserved for travel nurses who have accepted a job in another state and are awaiting their permanent license (The Risks to Travel, 2021).

Per Diem Employment and Float Pools

In addition, some hospitals have created their own internal supplemental staff by hiring per diem employees and creating float pools. *Per diem* staff generally have the flexibility to choose when they want to work. In exchange for this flexibility, they receive a higher rate of pay but usually no benefits. As of July 2022, the average hourly pay for a per diem nurse in the United States was $40.89 an hour (Zip Recruiter, 2022). Like agency or travel nurses, however, high use of per diem workers may increase risks to patient safety because they are less likely to be familiar with organizational policies and procedures.

Float pools are generally composed of employees who agree to cross-train on multiple units so that they can work additional hours during periods of high census or worker shortages. These pools are adequate for filling intermittent staffing holes, but like agency or registry staff, they are not an answer to the ongoing need to alter staffing according to census because they result in a lack of staff continuity. In addition, many staff feel uncomfortable with floating if they have not been adequately oriented to the new unit.

> Float staff must be able to perform the core competencies of the unit they are floating to meet their legal and moral obligations as caregivers.

Flextime Scheduling

Other organizations have tried to combat staffing shortages by using flextime. *Flextime* is a system that allows employees to select the time schedules that best meet their personal needs while still meeting work responsibilities. In the past, most flextime has been possible only for nurses in roles that did not require continuous coverage. However, staff nurses recently have been able to take part in a flextime system through prescheduled shift start times. Variable start times may be used to schedule shifts longer or shorter than the normal 8-hour workday. When a hospital uses flextime, units have employees coming and leaving the unit at many different times. Although flextime staffing creates greater employee choices, it may be difficult for the manager to coordinate and could easily result in overstaffing or understaffing.

Self-Scheduling

Self-scheduling allows nurses in a unit to work together to construct their own schedules rather than have schedules created by management. With self-scheduling, employees typically are given 4- to 6-week schedule worksheets to fill out several weeks in advance of when the schedule is to begin. The nurse-manager then reviews the worksheet to make sure that all guidelines or requirements have been met. Although self-scheduling offers nurses greater control over their work environment, it is not easy to implement. Success depends on the leadership skills of the manager to support the staff and demonstrate patience and perseverance throughout the implementation.

Shift Bidding

Another newer method of reducing staff shortages and mandatory overtime, as well as allowing nurses some control over scheduling extra shifts, is *shift bidding*. In most organizations that use shift bidding, the organization sets the opening price for a shift. For example, this may be at a higher rate of pay than the hourly wage of some nurses, and nurses may bid down the price to be assigned the overtime shift. In general, organizations will choose the nurse with the lowest bid to work the shift, but some organizations may deny bids to nurses who work too much overtime.

Evaluating Changes to Staffing and Scheduling Policies

Obviously, all scheduling and staffing patterns, from traditional to creative, have shortcomings. Therefore, any changes in current policies should be evaluated carefully as they are implemented. Because all scheduling and staffing patterns have a heavy impact on employees' personal lives, productivity, and budgets, it is wise to have a 6-month trial of new staffing and scheduling changes, with an evaluation at the end of that time to determine the impact on financial costs, retention, productivity, risk management, and employee and patient satisfaction.

LEARNING EXERCISE 17.2

Self-Scheduling Holiday Dilemma

You graduated last year from your nursing program and were excited to obtain the job that you wanted most. The unit where you work has a very progressive supervisor who believes in empowering the nursing staff. Approximately 6 months ago, after considerable instruction, the unit began self-scheduling. You have enjoyed the freedom and control that this has given you over your work hours. There have been some minor difficulties among staff, and occasionally, the unit was slightly overstaffed or understaffed. However, overall, the self-scheduling has seemed to work well.

Today (September 15), you come to work on the 3:00 PM to 11:00 PM shift after 2 days off and see that the schedule for the upcoming Thanksgiving and Christmas holiday period has been posted, and many of the staff have already scheduled their days on and their days off. When you take a close look, it appears that no one has signed up to work Christmas Eve, Thanksgiving Day, or Christmas Day. You are very concerned because self-scheduling includes responsibility for adequate coverage. There are still a few nurses, including yourself, who have not added their days to the schedule, but even if all of the remaining nurses work all three holidays, it will provide only scant coverage.

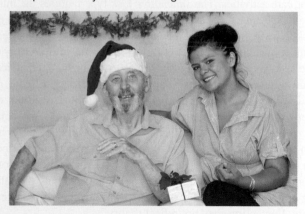

ASSIGNMENT:

What leadership role (if any) should you take in solving this dilemma? Should you ignore the problem and schedule yourself for only one holiday and let your supervisor deal with the issue? Remember, you are a new nurse, both in experience and on this unit. List the options for decision making available to you and, using rationale to support your decision, plan a course of action.

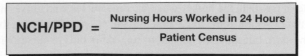

$$NCH/PPD = \frac{\text{Nursing Hours Worked in 24 Hours}}{\text{Patient Census}}$$

FIGURE 17.2 Standard formula for calculating nursing care hours per patient-day (NCH/PPD).

Workload Measurement Tools

Requirements for staffing are based on whatever standard unit of measurement for productivity is used in each unit. A formula for calculating *nursing care hours per patient-day* (NCH/PPD) is reviewed in Figure 17.2. This is a simple formula that continues to be used widely. In this formula, all nursing and ancillary staff are treated equally for determining hours of nursing care, and no differentiation is made for differing acuity levels of patients. These two factors alone may result in an incomplete or even inaccurate picture of nursing care needs, and the use of NCH/PPD as a workload measurement tool may be too restrictive because it may not represent the reality of today's inpatient care setting, where staffing fluctuates not only among shifts but within shifts as well.

As a result, *patient classification systems* (PCSs), also known as *workload management*, or *patient acuity tools*, were developed in the 1960s. A PCS groups patients according to specific characteristics that measure acuity of illness to determine both the number and mix of the staff needed to adequately care for those patients. A sample classification system is illustrated in Table 17.2.

Because other variables within the system have an impact on NCH, it is usually not possible to transfer a PCS from one facility to another. Instead, each basic classification system must be modified to fit a specific institution.

> PCSs are institution specific and must be modified to reflect the unique staff and patient population of each health care organization.

There are several types of PCS measurement tools. The *critical indicator* PCS uses broad indicators such as bathing, diet, intravenous fluids and medications, and positioning to categorize patient care activities. The *summative task* type requires the nurse to note the frequency of occurrence of specific activities, treatments, and procedures for each patient. For example, a summative task–type PCS might ask the nurse whether a patient required nursing time for teaching, elimination, or hygiene. Both types of PCSs are generally filled out prior to each shift, although the summative task type typically has more items to fill out than the critical indicator type.

Once an appropriate PCS is adopted, hours of nursing care must be assigned for each patient classification. Although an appropriate number of hours of care for each classification is generally suggested by companies marketing PCSs, each institution is unique and must determine to what degree that classification system must be adapted for that institution. With objective data, organizations can staff according to documented need rather than perceived convenience, decreasing distrust, fostering collaboration, and moving finance and patient management toward a common goal. It is important, though, to remember that staffing according to a PCS does not always mean that staffing is adequate or that it will be perceived as adequate. Perception may not reflect reality.

> It is not uncommon to have staffing perceived as adequate one day and considered inadequate the next day, even if there are the same number of patients and staff.

As long as managers realize that all staffing systems have weaknesses and they periodically evaluate the tools used, needed change can be initiated. It is crucial, however, for managers to

TABLE 17.2 **PATIENT CARE CLASSIFICATION USING FOUR LEVELS OF NURSING CARE INTENSITY**

Area of Care	Category 1	Category 2	Category 3	Category 4
Eating	Feeds self or needs little food	Needs some help in preparing food tray; may need encouragement	Cannot feed self but is able to chew and swallow	Cannot feed self and may have difficulty swallowing
Grooming	Almost entirely self-sufficient	Needs some help in bathing, oral hygiene, hair combing, and so forth	Unable to do much for self	Completely dependent
Excretion	Up and to bathroom alone or almost alone	Needs some help in getting up to bathroom or using urinal	In bed, needs bedpan or urinal placed; may be able to partially turn or lift self	Completely dependent
Comfort	Self-sufficient	Needs some help with adjusting position or bed (e.g., tubes and IVs)	Cannot turn without help, get drink, adjust position of extremities, and so forth	Completely dependent
General health	Good—for diagnostic procedure, simple treatment, or surgical procedure (D&C, biopsy, and minor fracture)	Mild symptoms—more than one mild illness, mild debility, mild emotional reaction, and mild incontinence (not more than once per shift)	Acute symptoms—severe emotional reaction to illness or surgery, more than one acute illness, medical or surgical problem, severe or frequent incontinence	Critically ill—may have severe emotional reaction
Treatments	Simple—supervised ambulation, dangle, simple dressing, test procedure preparation not requiring medication, reinforcement of surgical dressing, x-pad, vital signs once per shift	Any Category 1 treatment more than once per shift, Foley catheter care, I&O, bladder irrigations, sitz bath, compresses, test procedures requiring medications or follow-ups, simple enema for evacuation, vital signs every 4 hours	Any treatment more than twice per shift, IV medications, complicated dressings, sterile procedures, care of tracheostomy, Harris flush, suctioning, tube feeding, vital signs more than every 4 hours	Any complex procedure requiring two nurses, vital signs more often than every 2 hours
Medications	Simple, routine, not needing preevaluation or postevaluation; medications no more than once per shift	Diabetic, cardiac, hypotensive, hypertensive, diuretic, anticoagulant medications, PRN medications more than once per shift; medications needing preevaluation or postevaluation	High amount of Category 2 medications; control of refractory diabetes (need to be monitored more than every 4 hours)	Extensive Category 3 medications; IVs with frequent, close observation and regulation

continues on page 432

TABLE 17.2 **(CONTINUED)**

Area of Care	Category 1	Category 2	Category 3	Category 4
Teaching and emotional support	Routine follow-up teaching; patients with no unusual or adverse emotional reactions	Initial teaching of care of ostomies; patients newly diagnosed with diabetes; tubes that will be in place for periods of time; conditions requiring major change in eating, living, or excretory practices; patients with mild adverse reactions to their illness (e.g., depression and being overly demanding)	More intensive Category 2 items; teaching of patients who are apprehensive or mildly resistive; care of patients who are moderately upset or apprehensive; patients who are confused and disoriented	Teaching of patients who are resistive; care and support of patients with severe emotional reaction

IV, intravenous; D&C, dilation and curettage; I&O, input and output; PRN, as needed.

make every effort to base unit staffing on their organization's workload management system. This will allow for more consistent staffing and an improved ability to identify overstaffing and understaffing on a timelier basis. In addition, this is a fairer method of allocating staff.

The greater the degree of objectivity and accuracy in any system, however, the longer the time required to make staffing computations. Perhaps the greatest danger in staffing by acuity is that many organizations are unable to supply the extra staff when the system shows unit understaffing. However, the same organization may use the acuity-based staffing system to justify reducing staff on an overstaffed unit. Therefore, a staffing classification system can be demotivating if used inconsistently or incorrectly.

Clearly, PCSs will not solve all staffing problems, as all systems have special features and faults as well. Although such systems improve definition of problems, it is up to people in the organization to make judgments and use the information obtained by the system appropriately to solve staffing problems. Managers must not just focus on numbers of personnel; they must also examine nursing duties, job descriptions, patient care organization, staffing mix, and staff competency levels.

Saville and Griffiths (2021) agree, noting that using a PCS staffing tool without applying professional judgment or triangulating against other methods can lead to inaccurate estimates of staffing requirements and unsafe staffing levels. Staffing then must be flexible and consider patient acuity as well as the expertise/experience of the workers available. Thus, although staffing precision is always the goal, the responsibility for determining safe staffing ultimately requires nursing judgment.

In addition, the middle-level manager must be alert to internal or external forces affecting unit needs that may not be reflected in the organization's patient care classification system. Examples could be a sudden increase in nursing or medical students using the unit, a lower skill level of new graduates, or cultural and language differences of recently hired foreign nurses. The organization's classification system may prove to be inaccurate, or the hours allotted for each category or classification of patient may be inaccurate (too high or too low).

Some futurists have suggested that eventually, *workload measurement systems* may replace acuity-based staffing systems or that the two will be used as a hybrid tool for determining staffing needs. Workload measurement is a technique that evaluates work performance as well as necessary resource levels. Therefore, it goes beyond patient diagnosis or acuity level and examines the specific number of care hours needed to meet a given population's care needs. Thus, workload measurement systems typically capture census data, care hours, patient acuity, and patient activities. Although complicated, workload measurement systems do hold promise for more accurately predicting the nursing resources needed to staff hospitals effectively.

LEARNING EXERCISE 17.3

Calculating Staffing Needs

You use a patient classification system to assist you with your daily staffing needs. The following are the hours of nursing care needed for each acuity level patient per shift:

	Category I Acuity Level	Category II Acuity Level	Category III Acuity Level	Category IV Acuity Level
Nursing care hours per patient-day (NCH/PPD) needed for day shift (7 AM–3 PM)	2.3	2.9	3.4	4.6
Nursing care hours per patient-day (NCH/PPD) needed for PM shift (3 PM–11 PM)	2.0	2.3	2.8	3.4
Nursing care hours per patient-day (NCH/PPD) needed for night shift (11 PM–7 AM)	0.5	1.0	2.0	2.8

When you came on duty this morning, you had the following patients:

- One patient in category I acuity level
- Two patients in category II acuity level
- Three patients in category III acuity level
- One patient in category IV acuity level

Note that you must be overstaffed or understaffed by more than half of the hours a person is working to reduce or add staff. For example, for nurses working 8-hour shifts, the staffing must be over or under more than 4 hours to delete or add staff.

ASSIGNMENT:

Calculate your staffing needs for the day shift. You have on duty one registered nurse and one licensed vocational nurse/licensed practical nurse working 8-hour shifts and a ward clerk for 4 hours. Are you understaffed or overstaffed?

If you had the same number of patients but the acuity levels were the following, would your staffing needs be the same?

- Two patients in category I acuity level
- Three patients in category II acuity level
- Two patients in category III acuity level
- Zero patients in category IV acuity level

Regardless of the workload measurement tool used (NCH/PPD, PCS, workload measurement system, etc.), the units of workload measurement need to be reviewed periodically and adjusted as necessary. This is both a leadership role and a management responsibility.

The Relationship Between Nursing Care Hours, Staffing Mix, and Quality of Care

The literature is replete with studies examining the relationship between NCH, staffing mix, quality of care, and patient outcomes over the past three decades. Although early research lacked standardization in terms of tools used and measures examined, a plethora of better funded and more rigorous scientific study followed. Methods for studying the relationship between these three variables have become dramatically more sophisticated. Still, there are issues related to how outcomes are defined, what operational definitions should be used, and who should be counted in nurse staffing. A current review of the current literature, however, generally suggests that as RN hours decrease in NCH/PPD, adverse patient outcomes generally increase, including increased errors and patient falls as well as decreased patient satisfaction (Huston, 2023b).

Should Minimum Registered Nurse to Patient Staffing Ratios Be Mandated?

As the current health care system is evaluated, nurse-managers must be cognizant of new recommendations and legislation affecting staffing. Some US states, with the backing of professional nursing organizations, have moved toward imposing mandatory licensed staffing requirements.

Still, as of March 2022, only 16 states had passed some form of safe staffing laws (American Nurses Association [ANA], n.d.; King University Online, 2019). Some states, however, continue to pursue such legislation. For example, New York passed "safe staffing" legislation for nursing homes in May 2021, though staffing standards are yet to be established by the Commissioner of Health, as are the civil penalties for nursing homes that fail to adhere to the new minimum standards (Reyes, 2021). In addition, Pennsylvania nurses went to the state capitol in 2021 to argue for the need for a state policy requiring minimum nurse-to-patient staffing ratios, a need made even more urgent by the COVID-19 pandemic (Sholtis, 2021).

Also in 2021, the Connecticut General Assembly undertook a human resource and cost analysis to consider the adoption of minimum nurse staffing ratios for state nursing homes. The analysis suggested that Connecticut nursing homes by themselves would be highly unlikely to be able to cover the costs associated with minimum staffing ratios but noted that finding individuals to fill the positions would likely be the most challenging aspect of implementing a minimum staffing threshold. This is because nursing homes must compete with hospitals and others for a workforce that was already low in numbers before the pandemic and has been further dwindling since (Hawk & Sreenivas, 2021).

In addition, as of mid-2019, seven states (Connecticut, Illinois, Nevada, New York, Ohio, Oregon, Texas) and Washington, DC now require hospitals to have staffing committees responsible for plans and staffing policy, and five states require some form of disclosure and/or public reporting—Illinois, New Jersey, New York, Rhode Island, and Vermont (ANA, n.d.).

Legislation to impose government-mandated staffing ratios in Massachusetts was defeated in the November 2018 election. The Massachusetts Nurses Association supported the ballot question, whereas hospitals and doctors' groups opposed it.

California is the only state that has enacted legislation requiring mandatory staffing ratios that affect hospitals and long-term care facilities. Under Assembly Bill 394 ("Safe Staffing Law"), passed in 1999 and crafted by the California Nurses Association (CNA), all hospitals in California had to comply with the minimum staffing ratios shown in Table 17.3 by January 1, 2004, with subsequent modifications following in the next few years. These ratios, developed by the California Department of Health Care Services with assistance from the University of California, Davis, represented the maximum number of patients an RN could be assigned to care for, under any circumstance. The National Nurses United (NNU, 2010–2021) advocated for even lower ratios as of 2021 (see Table 17.3).

Proponents of legislated minimum staffing ratios say that ratios are needed because many hospitals' current staffing levels are so low that both RNs and their patients are negatively affected (Huston, 2023b). In addition, numerous articles have appeared in the media attesting to grossly inadequate staffing in hospitals and nursing homes, and professional nursing organizations have expressed concern about the effect poor staffing has on nurses' health and safety and

TABLE **MINIMUM REGISTERED NURSE STAFFING RATIOS FOR HOSPITALS IN CALIFORNIA IN 2004, 2008 REVISIONS, AND NATIONAL NURSES UNITED (NNU) RECOMMENDATIONS FOR 2021**

Unit	Minimum Registered Nurse–Patient Ratio Required in California in 2004 as a Result of AB 394 and 2008 Revisions	Minimum Registered Nurse–Patient Ratio Recommended by NNU in 2021
Critical care/ICU	1:2	1:2
Neonatal ICU	1:2	1:2
Operating room	1:1	1:1 (plus at least one additional scrub assistant)
Postanesthesia		1:2
Labor and delivery	1:2	1:2
Antepartum	1:4	1:3
Postpartum couplets	1:4	1:3
Combined labor and delivery and postpartum		1:3
Postpartum women only	1:6	1:3
Intermediate care nursery		1:4
Pediatrics	1:4	1:3
ER	1:4	1:3
Trauma patient in ER		1:1
ICU patient in ER		1:2
Step-down	1:4 initially; 1:3 as of 2008	1:3
Telemetry		1:3
Medical/surgical	1:6 initially; 1:5 as of 2005	1:4
Oncology	1:5 initially; 1:4 as of 2008	
Coronary care		1:2
Acute respiratory care		1:2
Burn unit		1:2
Other specialty care units		1:4
Psychiatry	1:6	1:4
Rehabilitation		1:5
Skilled nursing facility		1:5

AB, Assembly Bill; ICU, intensive care unit; ER, emergency room.

Source: Data from National Nurses United. (2010–2021). *National campaign for safe RN-to-patient staffing ratios.* Retrieved November 28, 2021, from http://www.nationalnursesunited.org/issues/entry/ratios

on patient outcomes. Adequate staffing, then, is needed to ensure that care provided is at least safe and hopefully high-quality. Proponents also suggest that such ratios protect the most basic elements of the public health we take for granted and argue that the government must take on this responsibility to ensure that safe health care is provided to all Americans (Huston, 2023b).

However, there are arguments against staffing ratios. Huston (2023b) explains that nursing shortages make it difficult to fill the slots when ratios exist, and ratios may merely serve as a

Comparing Staffing Ratios

Many states are currently considering the adoption of minimum staffing legislation and as such are closely monitoring the outcomes in states that have already taken such action.

ASSIGNMENT:

Compare the current staffing ratios used at the facility in which you work or do clinical practicums with those shown in Table 17.3. How do they compare? Is there an effort to legislate minimum staffing ratios in the state in which you live? Who or what would you anticipate is the greatest barrier to implementation of staffing ratios in your state?

Band-Aid to the greater problems of quality of care. In addition, numbers alone do not ensure improved patient care, as not all RNs have equivalent clinical experience and skill levels. Some also argue that staffing could decline with ratios because they might be used as the ceiling or as ironclad criteria if institutions are not willing to adjust for patient acuity or RN skill level.

In addition, some critics suggest that mandatory staffing ratios create significant opportunity costs that may restrict employers and payers from responding to market forces; subsequently, they may be unable to take advantage of improved technologic support or respond to changes in patient acuity. Mandatory staffing ratios also may cause conflicts between nurses and hospitals that might otherwise not exist.

Even nurses are split on whether government-mandated staffing ratios are needed and what those ratios should be. In the Massachusetts November 2018 ballot question on whether ratios were needed, a poll of 500 RNs before the election showed that 48% planned to vote for the ballot question and 45% said they would vote against the measure. Seven percent were undecided (Bebinger, 2018). Forty-one percent of respondents said all or most of the six nurse-to-patient ratios spelled out in the ballot question were appropriate, from one-to-one in intensive care to six patients per nurse after a birth with no complications, but 38% didn't agree with many or any of the proposed ratios, and 20% didn't know or declined to say. In addition, 56% of the nurses felt the state did not have enough nurses to make the law work (Bebinger, 2018).

It is still unclear whether mandated ratios have improved care or created new cost burdens for California. The CNA says the ratios improved nurse retention, raised the numbers of qualified nurses willing to work, reduced burnout, and improved morale (Huston, 2023b). Other studies have shown mixed results.

Efforts are under way, however, in both California and the rest of the nation, to explore alternatives to improving nurse staffing that do not require legislated minimum staffing ratios. In fact, many leading health care and professional nursing organizations do not support the need for legislated minimum staffing ratios (Huston, 2023b). For example, The Joint Commission, one of the most powerful accrediting bodies for hospitals in the United States, has been reluctant to endorse nationally mandated minimum staffing ratios, suggesting that they would not be flexible enough to allow for staffing that reflects the patient diversity in hospitals across the United States.

In addition, the ANA does not support fixed nurse–patient ratios, arguing that evidence does not exist to support legislated ratios (Arthur L. Davis Publishing Agency, 2022). Instead, it advocates an evidence-based workload system that considers the many variables that exist to ensure safe staffing. Indeed, the ANA (n.d.) has recommended three general approaches to assure adequate nurse staffing at the state level, arguing that this type of approach better accommodates changes in patients' needs, available technology, and the preparation and experience of staff (Display 17.4). In addition, the ANA argues that what may be established

1. The formation of nurse-driven staffing committees to create staffing plans that reflect the needs of the patient population and match the skills and experience of the staff.
2. Legislators mandate specific nurse-to-patient ratios in legislation or regulation.
3. Facilities are required to disclose staffing levels to the public and/or a regulatory body.

through legislation today as an appropriate minimum nurse-to-patient ratio may be obsolete by the next shift or 2 years from now and that disclosure of staffing plans without evaluation and recourse for inadequate levels is futile.

Recent research by Han et al. (2021) further clouds the issue. Their research compared the effects of three types of staffing laws (mandatory ratios, staffing committees, and public reporting legislation) on different levels of nurse staffing in hospitals. The researchers found that California's mandate had a significant positive effect on RNs and nursing assistive personnel (NAP). Neither the staffing committee nor the public reporting approach alone were effective in increasing hospital RN staffing, although the public reporting approach appeared to have a positive effect on LPN staffing. When California was excluded from the model, public reporting also had a positive effect on RN staffing (see Examining the Evidence 17.2).

EXAMINING THE EVIDENCE 17.2

Source: From Han, X., Pittman, P., & Barnow, B. (2021, October). Alternative approaches to ensuring adequate nurse staffing: The effect of state legislation on hospital nurse staffing. *Medical Care, 59,* S463–S470. https://doi-org.mantis.csuchico.edu/10.1097/MLR.0000000000001614

Do State Legislative Interventions Improve Nurse Staffing in Hospitals?

The objective of this quasi experimental study was to address whether legislative approaches are effective in encouraging hospitals to increase nurse staffing. Using 16 years of nationally representative hospital-level data from the American Hospital Association (AHA) annual survey, the researchers employed a difference-in-difference design to compare changes in productive hours per patient day for registered nurses (RNs), licensed practical/vocational nurses (LPNs), and nursing assistive personnel (NAP) in California with mandated staffing ratios, in states that legislated staffing committees, in states that legislated public reporting, and in states that did not implement nurse staffing legislation.

Compared with states with no legislation, the state, California, with legislated minimum staffing ratios had a 0.996 (P < 0.01) increase in RN hours per patient day and 0.224 (P < 0.01) increase in NAP hours after legislation was implemented. No statistically significant changes in RN or NAP hours were found in states that legislated a staffing committee or public reporting.

The staffing committee approach, however, had a negative effect on LPN hours (difference-in-difference = −0.076, P < 0.01), whereas the public reporting approach had a positive effect on LPN hours (difference-in-difference = 0.115, P < 0.01). There was no statistically significant effect of staffing mandate on LPN hours.

The researchers suggested that staffing committee laws may not result in higher RN staffing due to variations in nurses' power within hospitals. This type of legislation does not give staffing committees control over the hospital budget, and if resources are limited, committees may be forced to plan cuts, rather than increases. Findings suggested that cutting LPNs, rather than RNs, may indeed be an area where committees found the most palatability.

The researchers concluded that neither the staffing committee nor the public reporting approach alone were effective in increasing hospital RN staffing, although the public reporting approach appeared to have a positive effect on LPN staffing. When California was excluded from the model, public reporting also had a positive effect on RN staffing.

The implementation and subsequent evaluation of mandatory staffing ratios in California should provide greater insight into the ongoing debate about the need for mandatory staffing ratios.

> Minimum staffing ratios would not have been proposed in the first place had staffing abuses and the resultant declines in the quality of patient care not occurred.

Establishing and Maintaining Effective Staffing Policies

Unit managers must understand the effect that major restructuring and redesign have on their staffing and scheduling policies as well. As new practice models are introduced, there must be a simultaneous examination of the existing staff mix and patient care assessments to ensure that appropriate changes are made in staffing and scheduling policies.

For example, decreasing licensed staff, increasing numbers of unlicensed assistive personnel (UAP), and developing new practice models have a tremendous impact on patient care assignment methods. Past practices of relying on part-time staff, responding to staff preferences for work, and providing a variety of shift lengths and shift rotations may no longer be enough. Administrative practices also have saved money in the past by sending staff members home when there was low census; they have also floated staff to other areas to cover other unit needs, not scheduled staff for consecutive shifts because of staff preferences, and had scheduling policies that were unreasonably accommodating. Finally, patient assignments in the past were often made without attention to patient continuity and were assigned by numbers rather than workload. Some of these past practices benefited staff, and some benefited the organization, but few of them benefited the patient. Indeed, assigning a different nurse to care for a patient each day of an already reduced length of stay may contribute to negative patient outcomes.

Therefore, an honest appraisal of current staffing, scheduling, and assignment policies is needed while organizations are restructured and new practice models are engineered. Changing these policies often has far-reaching consequences, but this must be done for new models of care to be successfully implemented. For example, if primary nursing is to be effective, then nurses must work several successive days with a client to ensure that there is time to formulate and evaluate a plan of care. In this example, floating policies and requests for days off may need to be changed or modified to fit the philosophy of primary nursing care delivery.

Determining an appropriate skill mix depends on the patient care setting, acuity of patients, and other factors. There is no national standard to determine whether staffing decisions are suitable for a given setting. In addition, many of the tools and methods used to determine staffing have been unreliable and invalid, either in their development or their application. However, some formulas allow for adjustment for variations in the skill mix of staff. These formulas are still relatively new but may be better tools to use when making staffing decisions. Having an adequate number of knowledgeable, trained nurses, however, will be imperative to attaining desired patient outcomes.

The Impact of Nursing Staff Shortages on Staffing

As discussed in Chapter 15, nursing shortages have occurred periodically, whether nationally, regionally, or locally. It has been difficult for the profession to accurately predict exactly when and where there will be a short supply of professional nurses, but all nurse-managers will at some time face a short supply of staff—both RNs and others.

Health care organizations have used many solutions to combat this problem. Advanced planning and recruitment have already been discussed. Another long-term solution is *cross-training*. Cross-training involves giving personnel with varying educational backgrounds and expertise the skills necessary to take on tasks normally outside their scope of work and to move between units and function knowledgeably.

However, staffing shortages frequently occur on a day-to-day basis due to an increase in patient census, an unexpected increase in client needs, or an increase in staff absenteeism or illness. Health care organizations often address the problem through closed-unit staffing, drawing from a central pool of nurses for additional staff, requesting volunteers to work extra duty, and mandatory overtime. *Closed-unit staffing* occurs when the staff members on a unit make a commitment to cover all absences and needed extra help themselves in return for not being pulled from the unit in times of low census. In *mandatory overtime*, employees are forced to work additional shifts, often under threat of being charged with patient abandonment should they refuse to do so. Some hospitals routinely use mandatory overtime to keep fewer people on the payroll.

A health care worker who is in an exhausted state represents a risk to public health and patient safety. Although mandatory overtime is neither efficient nor effective in the long term, it has an even more devastating short-term impact on staff perceptions of a lack of control and subsequently, an impact on mood, motivation, and productivity. Nurses who are forced to work overtime do so under the stress of competing duties—to their job, their family, their own health, and their patients' safety (Huston, 2023c). Regardless of how the manager chooses to deal with an inadequate number of staff, the criteria outlined in Display 17.5 must be met.

> Mandatory overtime should be a last resort, not standard operating procedure because an institution does not have enough staff.

Employees have the right to expect a reasonable workload. Managers must ensure that adequate staffing exists to meet the needs of staff and patients. Managers who constantly expect employees to work extra shifts, stay overtime, and carry unreasonable patient assignments are not being ethically accountable.

Uncomplaining nursing staff have often put forth superhuman efforts during periods of short staffing simply because they believed in their supervisor and in the organization. However, just as often, the opposite has occurred: Nurses on units that were only moderately understaffed spent an inordinate amount of time and wasted energy complaining about their plight. The difference between the two examples has much to do with trust that such conditions are the exception, not the norm; that real solutions and not Band-Aid approaches to problem solving will be used to plan for the future; that management will work just as hard as the staff in meeting patient needs; and that the organization's overriding philosophy is based on patient interest and not financial gain.

DISPLAY 17.5 MINIMUM CRITERIA FOR SAFE STAFFING

- Decisions made must meet state and federal labor laws and organizational policies.
- Staff must not be demoralized or excessively fatigued by frequent or extended overtime requests.
- Long-term as well as short-term solutions must be sought.
- Patient care must not be jeopardized.

Fiscal and Ethical Accountability for Staffing

Leader-managers are fiscally accountable to the organization for appropriate staffing. Accountability for a prenegotiated budget is a management function. Growing federal and state budget deficits have caused increased pressure for all health care organizations to reduce costs. Because personnel budgets are large in health care organizations, a small percentage cut in personnel may result in large savings. Thus, managers must increase staffing when patient acuity rises as well as decrease staffing when acuity is low; to do otherwise is demoralizing to the unit staff. It is important for managers to use staff to provide safe and effective care economically.

> Fiscal accountability to the organization for staffing is not incompatible with ethical accountability to patients and staff. The manager's goal is to stay within a staffing budget and meet the needs of patients and staff.

Generational Considerations for Staffing

Managers must be alert to how generational diversity may impact staffing needs. Four generations of nurses are now working together. In previous years, earlier retirement from nursing and shorter life spans kept the workforce typically to three generations.

Some researchers suggest that the different generations represented in nursing today have different value systems that may impact staffing (Table 17.4). For example, most experts now identify five generational groups in today's workforce: the veteran generation (also called the silent generation or the traditionalist), the baby boomers, generation X, generation Y (also called the millennials), and generation Z.

The veteran generation is typically recognized as those nurses from the generation born between 1925 and 1942. Having lived through several international military conflicts (World War II, Korean War, and Vietnam War) and the Great Depression, they tend to be more risk averse, highly respectful of authority, supportive of hierarchy, and disciplined. They are also called the silent generation because they tend to support the status quo rather than protest or push for rapid change. As a result, these nurses are less likely to question organizational practices and more likely to seek employment in structured settings. Their work values are traditional, and they are often recognized for their loyalty to their employers.

The baby boomer generation (born 1943 to early 1960s), representing just under half of the current workforce, also displays traditional work values; however, they tend to be more materialistic and thus are willing to work long hours at their jobs to get ahead. Indeed, this generation, which includes many of today's nursing leaders, is more apt than any other to

TABLE 17.4 GENERATIONAL WORK GROUPS

Generation	Year of Birth
Silent generation or veteran generation	1925–1942
Baby boomer or boom	1943 to early 1960s
Generation X	Early 1960s to early 1980s
Generation Y	Early 1980s to mid-1990s
Generation Z	1996–2015

be called "workaholics." Yet, many baby boomers are caring for family members from both sides. In addition, many boomers volunteer their time to advance environmental, cultural, or educational causes.

In contrast, "Generation Xers" (born between early 1960s and early 1980s), a smaller cohort than the baby boomers who preceded them, or the Generation Yers who follow them, may lack the interest in lifetime employment at one place that prior generations have valued, instead valuing greater work hour flexibility and opportunities for time off. This likely reflects the fact that because many individuals born in this generation had both parents working outside their home as they were growing up, they want to put more emphasis on family and leisure time in their own family units. Thus, this generation may be less economically driven than prior generations and may define success differently than the veteran generation or the baby boomers.

Generation Y, also known as the millennials (born early 1980s to mid-1990s), represents the first cohort of truly global citizens. They are known for their optimism, self-confidence, relationship orientation, volunteer mindedness, and social consciousness. They are also highly sophisticated in their use of technology. Therefore, some people call this generation "digital natives." Generation Y is known to work together well in teams, exhibit a high degree of altruism, have a higher eco-awareness, and far greater multicultural ease than their older coworkers.

Finally, Generation Z, also known as the Homeland Generation, iGeneration, Gen Tech, or The Founders, includes those born between 1996 and 2015. The older members of this generation are just now entering the workforce. Sociologists suggest this generation will resemble the silent generation. Having grown up with social unrest and economic insecurity, they will be more likely to value security, comfort, and familiar activities and environments.

Given these attitudinal and value differences, it is not surprising that some workplace conflict results between different generations of workers (Huston, 2023a). Each generation exhibits differing levels of formality. Generation X workers also report higher levels of burnout as compared with baby boomers, related to incivility from colleagues and cynicism. In addition, there may also be conflicts related to competencies and strategies for knowledge acquisition.

Although this type of generational diversity poses management challenges, it also provides a variety of perspectives and outlooks that can enhance productivity and result in the creation of new ideas. Generational diversity also allows patients to receive care from both the most experienced nurses as well as those with the most recent education and likely greater technologic expertise.

Developing Staffing and Scheduling Policies

Nurses will be more satisfied in the workplace if staffing and scheduling policies and procedures are thoughtfully developed, fairly applied, and clearly communicated to all employees. Personnel policies represent the standard of action that is communicated in advance so that employees are not caught unaware regarding personnel matters. Written policies generally provide a means for greater consistency and fairness. In addition to being standardized, personnel policies should be written in a manner that allows some flexibility. A leadership challenge for the manager is to develop policies that focus on outcomes rather than constraints or rules that limit responsiveness to individual employee needs.

Scheduling and staffing policies should be reviewed and updated periodically. When formulating policies, management must examine its own philosophy and consider prevailing community practices. Unit-level managers will seldom have complete responsibility for formulating organizational personnel policies but should have some input as policies are reviewed. There are, however, nursing department and unit personnel policies that supervisors develop and implement.

DISPLAY 17.6 UNIT CHECKLIST OF EMPLOYEE STAFFING POLICIES

1. Name of the person responsible for the staffing schedule and the authority of that individual if it is other than the employee's immediate supervisor
2. Type and length of staffing cycle used
3. Rotation policies, if shift rotation is used
4. Fixed shift transfer policies, if fixed shifts are used
5. Time and location of schedule posting
6. When shift begins and ends
7. Day of week schedule begins
8. Weekend off policy
9. Tardiness policy
10. Low census procedures
11. Policy for trading days off
12. Procedures for days off requests
13. Absenteeism policies
14. Policy regarding rotating to other units
15. Procedures for vacation time requests
16. Procedures for holiday time requests
17. Procedures for resolving conflicts regarding requests for days off, holidays, or requested time off
18. Emergency request policies
19. Policies and procedures regarding requesting transfer to other units
20. Mandatory overtime policy

The policies in Display 17.6 should be formalized by the manager and communicated to all personnel. To ensure that unit-level staffing policies do not conflict with higher-level policies, there should be adequate input from the staff, and they should be developed in collaboration with personnel and nursing departments. For example, some states have labor laws that prohibit 12-hour shifts. Other states allow workers to sign away their rights to overtime pay for shifts greater than 8 or 12 hours. In addition, in organizations with union contracts, many staffing and scheduling policies are incorporated into the union contract. In such cases, staffing changes might need to be negotiated at the time of contract renewal.

LEARNING EXERCISE 17.5

Implementing a New Nursing Care Delivery Model

You are serving on an ad hoc committee to examine ways to improve the continuity of patient assignments because your unit is thinking about switching from total patient care to a primary nursing care delivery model. The committee is having a difficult time formulating policy because you currently have a great number of nurses who work part-time, 2 days on and 2 days off. In addition, your unit has a census that goes up and down unexpectedly, resulting in nurses being floated out of the unit often. The committee is committed to providing continuity of care in the new patient care delivery system.

ASSIGNMENT:

Develop several scheduling and staffing policies that have the probability of increasing continuity of assignment and will not result in a financial liability to the unit. How will these polices be fairly executed, and do they have the potential to cause staff to leave the unit?

Integrating Leadership Roles and Management Functions in Staffing and Scheduling

The manager is responsible for providing adequate staffing to meet patient care needs. The leader assumes an ethical accountability to patients and employees for adequate and appropriate staffing. The leader-manager then must pay attention to fluctuations in patient census and workload units to ensure that understaffing or overstaffing is minimized and to ensure fiscal accountability to the organization.

Using evidence and evidence-based tools in making these staffing decisions is critical for contemporary nurse leader-managers. The prudent leader-manager is also cognizant of the need to have comprehensive scheduling and staffing policies that are not only fair but also in compliance with organizational policies, union contracts, and labor laws. When possible, employees should be involved in developing these staffing and scheduling policies. This helps establish the trust needed to build team spirit when dealing with temporary staff shortages.

Unit staffing and scheduling policies should be reviewed and revised on a timely basis to reflect changes in community and national trends as well as contemporary methods of staffing and scheduling. In addition, the leader should be alert for factors that affect the standard of productivity and negotiate changes in the standard when appropriate.

The leader also looks for innovative methods to overcome staffing difficulties. Knowing that staff needs are in part related to work design, the prudent leader-manager looks for ways to redesign work to reduce staffing needs. When leadership roles are integrated with management functions, creative staffing and scheduling options can occur.

Key Concepts

- The manager has both a fiscal and an ethical duty to plan for adequate staffing to meet patient care needs.
- In *centralized staffing*, staffing decisions are made by personnel in a central office or staffing center. In *decentralized staffing*, each department is responsible for its own staffing.
- Innovative and creative methods of staffing and scheduling should be explored to avoid understaffing and overstaffing as patient census and acuity fluctuate.
- Ten- and 12-hour shifts have become commonplace in acute care hospitals even though there continues to be debate about whether extending the length of shifts results in increased judgment errors related to fatigue, increased sick time, and job dissatisfaction.
- Agency nurses and travel nurses, who are typically employed by an external broker, can provide scheduling relief in response to unanticipated increases in census or patient acuity, but their continuous use is expensive and can result in poor continuity of nursing care.

- Per diem staff, who receive a higher rate of pay, but no benefits, have the flexibility to choose when they want to work.
- Flextime is a system that allows employees to select the time schedules that best meet their personal needs while still meeting work responsibilities.
- Self-scheduling allows nurses in a specific unit or department to work together to construct their own schedules rather than have schedules created by management.
- Workload measurement systems, which typically capture census data, care hours, patient acuity, and patient activities, can evaluate work performance as well as required resource levels.
- Workload measurement tools include NCH/PPD, PCS, and workload measurement systems.
- All workload measurement tools should be periodically reviewed to determine if they are valid and reliable tools for measuring staffing needs in each organization.
- Mandatory overtime should be a last resort, not standard operating procedure because an institution does not have enough staff.

- Research suggests that as professional nursing representation in the skill mix increases, patient outcomes generally improve, and adverse incidents decline.
- California is the only state in the United States that has enacted legislation requiring mandatory staffing ratios in hospitals and long-term care facilities. It is still unclear whether mandated ratios have improved care or created new cost burdens for California.
- Those with staffing responsibility must remain cognizant of mandatory staffing ratios and comply with such mandates.
- Managers should attempt to have a diverse staff who will meet the cultural and language needs of the patient population.

- Staffing and scheduling policies must not violate labor laws, state or national laws, or union contracts.
- Fair and uniform staffing and scheduling policies and procedures must be written and communicated to all staff.
- Existing staffing policies must be examined periodically to determine if they still meet the needs of the staff and the organization.
- Generational diversity in the workforce allows patients to receive care from both the most experienced nurses as well as those with the most recent education and likely greater technologic expertise; however, the different generations represented in nursing today have different value systems that may impact staffing.

Additional Learning Exercises and Applications

LEARNING EXERCISE 17.6

Making Sound Staffing Decisions

You are the staffing coordinator for a small community hospital. It is now 12:30 PM, and your staffing plan for the 3:00 PM to 11:00 PM shift must be completed no later than 1:00 PM. (The union contract stipulates that any "call offs" required for low census must be done at least 2 hours before the shift begins; otherwise, employees will receive a minimum of 4 hours of pay.) You do, however, have the prerogative to call off staff for only half a shift (4 hours). If they are needed for the last half of the shift (7:00 PM to 11:00 PM), you must notify them by 5:00 PM tonight. A local outside registry is available for supplemental staff; however, their cost is two and a half times that of your regular staff, so you must use this resource sparingly. Mandatory overtime is also used but only as a last resort.

The current hospital census is 52 patients, although the emergency department (ED) is very busy and has four possible patient admissions. There are also two patients with confirmed discharge orders and three additional potential discharges on the 3:00 PM to 11:00 PM shift. All units have just submitted their patient classification system (PCS) calculations for that shift.

You have five units to staff: the intensive care unit (ICU), pediatrics, obstetrics (includes labor, delivery, and postpartum), medical, and surgical departments. The ICU must be staffed with a minimum of a 1:2 nurse–patient ratio. The pediatric unit is generally staffed at a 1:4 nurse–patient ratio and the medical and surgical departments at a 1:6 ratio. In obstetrics, a 1:2 ratio is used for labor and delivery, and a 1:6 ratio is used in postpartum. On reviewing the staffing, you note the following:

Intensive Care Unit

Census = 6. Unit capacity = 8. The PCS shows a current patient acuity level requiring 3.2 staff. One of the potential admissions in the ED is a patient who will need cardiac monitoring. One patient, however, will likely be transferred to the medical unit on 3:00 PM to 11:00 PM shift. Four registered nurses (RNs) are assigned for that shift.

Pediatrics

Census = 8. Unit capacity = 10. The PCS shows a current acuity level requiring 2.4 staff. There are two RNs and one certified nursing assistant assigned for the 3:00 PM to 11:00 PM shift. There are no anticipated discharges or transfers.

Obstetrics

Census = 6. Unit capacity = 8. Three patients are in active labor, and three patients are in the postpartum unit with their babies. Two RNs are assigned to the obstetrics department for the 3:00 PM to 11:00 PM shift. There are no in-house staff on that shift who have been cross-trained for this unit.

Medical Floor

Census = 19. Unit capacity = 24. The PCS shows a current acuity level requiring 4.4 staff. There are two RNs, one licensed vocational nurse, and two certified nursing assistants assigned for the 3:00 PM to 11:00 PM shift. Three of the potential ED admissions will come to this floor. Two of the potential patient discharges are on this unit.

Surgical Floor

Census = 13. Unit capacity = 18. The PCS shows a current acuity level requiring 3.6 staff. Because of sick calls, you have only one RN and two certified nursing assistants assigned for the 3:00 PM to 11:00 PM shift. Both confirmed patient discharges as well as one of the potential discharges are from this unit.

ASSIGNMENT:

Answer the following questions:
1. Which units are overstaffed, and which are understaffed?
2. Of those units that are overstaffed, what will you do with the unneeded staff?
3. How will you staff units that are understaffed? Will outside registry or mandatory overtime methods be used?
4. How did staffing mix and PCS acuity levels factor into your decisions, if at all?
5. What safeguards can you build into the staffing plan for unanticipated admissions or changes in patient acuity during the shift?

LEARNING EXERCISE 17.7

Reviewing Pros and Cons of Staffing Solutions

You are serving on a committee to help resolve a chronic problem with short staffing on your pediatric unit. Volunteer overtime, cross-training with the intensive care pediatric unit, and closed-unit staffing have been suggested as possible solutions.

ASSIGNMENT:

Make a list of the pros and cons of each of these suggestions to bring back to the committee for review. Share your list with group members.

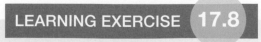

LEARNING EXERCISE 17.8

Choosing a Delivery Care Model and Staffing Pattern

You have been hired as the unit supervisor of the new rehabilitation unit at Memorial Hospital. The hospital decentralizes the responsibility for staffing, but you must adhere to the following constraints:

1. All staff must be licensed.
2. The ratio of licensed vocational nurses (LVNs)/licensed practical nurses (LPNs) to registered nurses (RNs) is 1:1.
3. An RN must always be on duty.
4. Your budgeted nursing care hours per patient-day (NCH/PPD) is 8.2.
5. You are not counted into the NCH/PPD, but ward clerks are counted.
6. Your unit capacity is seven patients, and you anticipate a daily average census of six patients.
7. You may use any mode of patient care organization.

Your patients will be chronic, not acute, but will be admitted for an active 2- to 12-week rehabilitation program. The emphasis will be in returning the patient home with adequate ability to perform activities of daily living. Many other disciplines, including occupational and physical therapy, will be part of the rehabilitation team. A waiting list for the beds is anticipated because this service is needed in your community. You anticipate that most of your patients will have had cerebrovascular accidents, spinal cord injuries, other problems with neurologic deficits, and amputations.

You have hired four full-time RNs and two part-time RNs. The part-time RNs would like to have at least 2 days of work in a 2-week pay period; in return for this work guarantee, they have agreed to cover for most sick days and vacations and some holidays for your regular RN full-time staff.

You also have hired three full-time LVNs/LPNs and two part-time LVNs/LPNs. However, the part-time LVNs/LPNs would like to work at least 3 days per week. You have decided not to hire a ward clerk but to use the pediatric ward clerk for 4 hours each day to assist with various duties. Therefore, you need to calculate the ward clerk's 4 hours into the total hours worked.

You have researched various types of patient care delivery models (Chapter 14) and staffing patterns. Your newly hired staff is willing to experiment with any type of patient care delivery model and staffing pattern that you select.

ASSIGNMENT:

Determine which patient care delivery model and staffing pattern you will use. Explain why and how you made your choice. Next, show a 24-hour and 7-day staffing pattern. Were you able to create a schedule that adhered to the given constraints? Was this a time-consuming process?

LEARNING EXERCISE 17.9

Floating Again

You are a new registered nurse, having graduated just 4 months ago from nursing school. When you arrive for work tonight, you are told that because your unit is experiencing a low census, you must once again float to another unit. This is the third night in a row that you have been required to float, and the last two nights were to two different units. When you question why it is your turn to float again, you are told that this is the last night you will work before having 3 days off and that it makes more sense to have you go than to have someone else who will be working the next few nights and could provide continuity of care. Another nurse says that this is the last night for him in a 7-day work stretch and that it would not be fair for him to have to float at this point. In addition, one of the nurses says she has not been cross-trained for the unit needing staff, and another one says that she is there only because she swapped nights with another nurse as a personal favor and therefore should not have to float. The charge nurse recognizes your frustration but says that because the current floating policy is not clear, she had to make a decision and selected you to float. She invites you, though, to help her create a written floating policy that is fairer to all.

ASSIGNMENT:

You feel that the lack of a clearly written policy about floating resulted in arbitrary and unfair treatment, and you decide to use your upcoming days off to begin work on a new policy which comprehensively covers all aspects of floating. Create such a policy. Make sure it addresses the qualifications necessary to float as well as how floating will be determined when employee needs and arguments are conflicting. Then have your peers review your floating policy. Do they feel your policy is comprehensive? Clear? Safe? Fair?

LEARNING EXERCISE 17.10

Combining a Patient Classification System and Staffing Formula

You are assigned to provide total patient care this shift for five patients. The handoff report you just received provided the following information about your patients:

1. **SB:** 54-year-old female, with a BMI of 42, admitted for cholecystectomy last night. Intravenous (IV) normal saline (NS) infusing at 150 mL/hour. Patient nauseated, unable to keep fluids down. Currently nothing by mouth. Needs order for antiemetic from medical doctor. Receives IV pain medication every 3 to 4 hours. Requires maximal assist (two persons) for turning and getting up to the chair. Requests to use the bedpan although bedside commode is ordered. Requires blood sugar checks four times a day for type 2 diabetes. Vital signs stable.

2. **LM:** 79-year-old male admitted for open reduction and internal fixation (ORIF) left hip following fall at home 2 days ago. Post-op course uneventful until earlier today when patient developed sudden onset of acute shortness of breath, which has resolved to some extent. Pleural scan ordered this shift to rule out pulmonary embolus. Currently on 4-L oxygen (O_2) with O_2 saturation of 94%. IV D5/.45 NS infusing at 75 mL/hour. Patient was assisted to chair for first time this morning with moderate assist. Indwelling Foley catheter present. History of early-onset dementia and is oriented only to person. Requires maximal assist in dressing, oral care, and grooming.

3. **CK:** 54-year-old female admitted following a fall from a ladder yesterday. Required ORIF of right wrist comminuted fracture yesterday afternoon. Also fractured right malleolus, which is in a boot cast. Circulation, sensation, and motion checks required every 2 hours on both extremities. Started on soft diet today, which she is tolerating well, although she needs maximal assist with feeding and toileting. IV lactated Ringer's infusing at 50 mL/hour. Receiving IV pain medications every 4 to 6 hours. Physical therapist will begin to work with patient this afternoon to show her how to use platform walker.

4. **SA:** 66-year-old male admitted last night to the telemetry unit with chest pain. Initial cardiac enzymes and electrocardiogram negative so was transferred to your unit this afternoon. Exhibits behavior suggesting high levels of anxiety. Frequently rings call light to make sure it is working. Has reported to staff that his father and two of his three siblings died in their 50s of heart disease. Has saline lock. On regular diet. Vital signs stable other than blood pressure 150/94. Has orders for by mouth (PO) medications every 6 hours.

(continues on page 448)

LEARNING EXERCISE 17.10

Combining a Patient Classification System and Staffing Formula (continued)

5. **PR:** 92-year-old male with multiple system failure. Admitted 3 days ago. Intermittently confused and calling out. Long history chronic obstructive pulmonary disease with recent O_2 saturation of 90% and PCO_2 level of 52. On O_2 at 2 L. Cough productive of thick yellow sputum. Receiving IV antibiotics every 6 hours as well as numerous other PO and IV medications. Also has right-sided heart failure with resultant 4+ pitting edema in ankles bilaterally. Indwelling Foley catheter placed last night with immediate return of 500 mL clear yellow urine and hourly input last night of 40 to 45 mL/hour. Urine output this last shift reduced to only 25 mL/hour—doctor yet to be notified of change in urine output. Do-not-resuscitate order is in chart. Family members gathering because physician told them this morning that patient was dying.

ASSIGNMENT:

1. Using the patient classification system (PCS) in Table 17.3, determine what acuity level you believe most closely represents your patient's need for care. Justify your choice, especially when the PCS is not a perfect fit for your patient.
2. Then, using the hours of nursing care formula shown below, for each acuity level you have identified, determine if your workload for this shift is reasonable.

	Category I Acuity Level	Category II Acuity Level	Category III Acuity Level	Category IV Acuity Level
Nursing care hours per patient-day (NCH/PPD) needed for day shift	2.2	2.6	3.2	3.6
NCH/PPD needed for pm shift	1.8	2.2	2.6	3.0
NCH/PPD needed for night shift	1.2	1.6	2.2	2.6

REFERENCES

American Nurses Association. (n.d.). *Advocating for safe staffing*. Retrieved June 5, 2022, from https://www.nursingworld.org/practice-policy/nurse-staffing/nurse-staffing-advocacy/

Arthur L. Davis Publishing Agency. (2022, June). *ANA's case for evidence-based nursing staffing. Essential for cost-effective, high-quality hospital-based care and patient safety.* Retrieved June 5, 2022, from https://www.nursingald.com/articles/20360-ana-s-case-for-evidence-based-nursing-staffing

Bae, S. (2021, August). Relationships between comprehensive characteristics of nurse work schedules and adverse patient outcomes: A systematic literature review. *Journal of Clinical Nursing, 30*(15/16), 2202–2221. https://doi.org/10.1111/jocn.15728

Bebinger, M. (2018). Nurses are split on staffing ratio ballot question, WBUR poll finds. *WBUR.* http://www.wbur.org/commonhealth/2018/10/15/wbur-poll-nurse-staffing-question-one

Bucceri Androus, A. (2022, February 1). *Are breaks and the 12-hour shift being dealt a bad hand?* RegisteredNursing.org. https://www.registerednursing.org/are-breaks-12-hour-shift-being-dealt-bad-hand/

Han, X., Pittman, P., & Barnow, B. (2021, October). Alternative approaches to ensuring adequate nurse staffing: The effect of state legislation on hospital nurse staffing. *Medical Care, 59*, S463–S470. https://doi-org.mantis.csuchico.edu/10.1097/MLR.0000000000001614

Harris Healthcare. (2017). *Five reasons why CFOs should care about staffing and acuity.* https://www.harrishealthcare.com/wp-content/uploads/2017/11/Five-Reasons_whitepaper_FINAL-1.pdf

Hawk, T., & Sreenivas, K. (2021, February 12). *Estimating the cost of minimum staffing ratios in Connecticut nursing homes.* The Center for Health Policy Evaluation in Long-Term Care. https://www.cga.ct.gov/2021/appdata/tmy/2021HB-06439-R000303-Barrett,%20

Matthew-CT%20Assoc.%20of%20Health%20Care%20 Facilities-Attachment%20-%20DSS-TMY.PDF

Huston, C. (2023a). Diversity in the nursing workforce (chapter 9). In C. Huston (Ed.), *Professional issues in nursing: Challenges and opportunities* (6th ed., pp. 121–135). Wolters Kluwer.

Huston, C. (2023b). Mandatory minimum staffing ratios (chapter 11). In C. Huston (Ed.), *Professional issues in nursing: Challenges and opportunities* (6th ed., pp. 154– 168). Wolters Kluwer.

Huston, C. (2023c). Mandatory overtime in nursing: How much? How often (chapter 12)? In C. Huston (Ed.), *Professional issues in nursing: Challenges and opportunities* (6th ed., pp. 169–180). Wolters Kluwer.

King University Online. (2019, March 12). *Nurse-to-patient ratio: How many is too many?* https://online.king.edu/ news/nurse-to-patient-ratio/

National Nurses United. (2010–2021). *National campaign for safe RN-to-patient staffing ratios.* Retrieved June 5, 2022, from http://www.nationalnursesunited.org/issues/entry/ratios

Olson, N. (2021, May 19). *Your guide to workplace injury statistics for 2021.* Safesite. https://safesitehq.com/2021- workplace-injury-statistics/

Reyes, A. (2021, May 4). NYS Assembly and Senate pass 'safe staffing' legislation for nursing homes, hospitals. *WKBW.* https://www.wkbw.com/news/state-news/ nys-assembly-and-senate-pass-safe-staffing-legislation- for-nursing-homes-hospitals

The risks to travel nurses during the pandemic. (2021). *Arizona Nurse, 74*(1), 14.

Saville, C., & Griffiths, P. (2021, October). Ward staffing guided by a patient classification system: A multi-criteria analysis of "fit" in three acute hospitals. *Journal of Nursing Management (John Wiley & Sons, Inc.), 29*(7), 2260–2269. https://doi-org.mantis.csuchico.edu/10.1111/jonm.13341

Sholtis, B. (2021, May 10). Facing burnout, worker shortages, nurses say COVID-19 shows need for staffing ratios. *WLVR.* https://wlvr.org/2021/05/facing-burnout-worker- shortages-nurses-say-covid-19-shows-need-for-staffing- ratios/#.YaK4NrqIaUk

Smith, A., McDonald, A. D., & Sasangohar, F. (2020, December). Night-shift nurses and drowsy driving: A qualitative study. *International Journal of Nursing Studies, 112.* https://doi.org/10.1016/j.ijnurstu.2020.103600

Stasik, S. (2022, January 6). The dangers of mandated overtime for nurses. *Onward Healthcare.* Retrieved June 5, 2022, from https://www.onwardhealthcare.com/nursing- resources/the-dangers-of-mandated-overtime-for-nurses/

Zip Recruiter. (2022). *Per diem nurse salary.* Retrieved July 18, 2022 from https://www.ziprecruiter.com/Salaries/ Per-Diem-Nurse-Salary

Roles and Functions in Directing

18

Creating a Motivating Climate

… how we feel about and enjoy our work is crucial to how we perceive the quality of our lives.—**Jo Manion**

… whether you think you can or whether you think you can't, you're right.—**Henry Ford**

… It's only after you've stepped outside your comfort zone that you begin to change, grow, and transform.—**Roy T. Bennett**

LEARNING OBJECTIVES

The learner will:

- describe the relationship between motivation and behavior
- differentiate between intrinsic and extrinsic motivation
- recognize the need to create a work environment in which both organizational and individual needs can be met
- delineate how the work of individual motivation theorists has contributed to the understanding of what motivates individuals inside and outside the work setting
- describe the links between risk taking, innovation, creativity, and employee empowerment
- recognize the complexity of using incentives and rewards so that they motivate rather than demotivate
- recognize the need to individualize reward systems for each subordinate
- differentiate between employee engagement and employee satisfaction
- develop strategies for creating a motivating work environment
- identify positive reinforcement techniques that may be used by a manager in an organization

- describe the constraints managers face in creating a climate that will motivate employees
- develop increased self-awareness about personal motivation and the need for "self-care" to remain motivated in a leadership or management role

Introduction

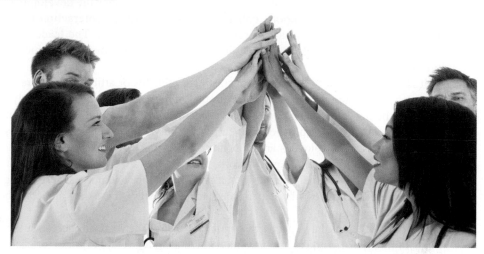

This unit reviews the fourth phase of the management process: *directing*. This phase also may be referred to as *coordinating* or *activating*. Regardless of the nomenclature, this is the "doing" phase of management, requiring the leadership skills and management functions necessary to accomplish the goals of the organization. Managers direct the work of their subordinates during this phase, and leaders support them, so they can achieve desired outcomes. Components of the directing phase discussed in this unit include creating a motivating climate, fostering organizational communication, managing conflict, facilitating collaboration, negotiating, and responding to collective bargaining practices and employment laws.

In planning and organizing, leader-managers attempt to establish an environment that is conducive to getting work done. In directing, the leader-manager sets those plans into action. This chapter focuses on creating a motivating climate as a critical element in meeting employee and organizational goals.

The amount and quality of work accomplished by managers directly reflects their motivation and that of their subordinates. Why are some managers or employees more motivated than others? How do demotivated managers affect their subordinates? What can the manager do to help the employee who is demotivated? The motivational problems encountered by the manager are complex. To respond to demotivated staff, managers need an understanding of the relationship between motivation and behavior.

> "Motivated employees bring extensive benefits to the wider organization, such as increased performance, improved retention, and improved customer service performance. However, poorly motivated employees can deliver significant repercussions, including, reduced productivity, increased employee turnover, and apathy towards work" (10x Psychology, 2021, para 3).

This chapter examines motivational theories that have guided organizational efforts and resource distribution for the last 100 years. Leadership and management strategies for promoting worker engagement and encouraging a motivating work environment are emphasized.

Motivation

Motivation is the force within the individual that influences or directs behavior. Because motivation comes from within the person, managers cannot directly motivate subordinates. The leader can, however, create an environment that maximizes the development of human potential. Management support, collegial influence, and the interaction of personalities in the work group can have a synergistic effect on motivation. The leader-manager must identify those components and strengthen them in hopes of maximizing motivation at the unit level.

It is also important to examine organizational climates or attitudes that directly influence workers' morale and motivation. For example, organizations frequently overtly or covertly reinforce the image that employees are expendable and that individual recognition is in some way detrimental to the employee and their productivity within the organization. Just the opposite is true because employees are an organization's most valuable asset. When an organization gives purpose to its employees' work, it helps them see how valuable they are (Espinal, 2021). This helps them feel like they're making a difference and not just performing tasks with no real value. Employees who experience satisfaction stay where they are, contributing to an organization's retention.

All human beings have needs that motivate them. The leader focuses on the needs and wants of individual workers and uses motivational strategies appropriate for each person and situation. In addition, leaders apply techniques, skills, and knowledge of motivational theory to help workers achieve what they want out of work. At the same time, these individual goals should complement the goals of the organization.

The manager bears primary responsibility for meeting organizational goals, such as reaching acceptable levels of productivity and quality. The leader-manager, then, must create a work environment in which both organizational and individual needs can be met. Adequate tension must be created to maintain productivity while encouraging workers' job satisfaction as well as engagement in the organization. This is not an easy task. The leadership roles and management functions inherent in creating such an environment are included in Display 18.1.

Intrinsic Versus Extrinsic Motivation

Motivation involves the action people take to satisfy unmet needs. It is the willingness to put effort into achieving a goal or reward to decrease the tension caused by the need. *Intrinsic motivation* comes from within the person, driving them to be productive (Table 18.1). In a study of certified nurse aide (CNA) motivation, 92% attributed their motivation at work to intrinsic factors, such as an innate desire to help, a natural sense of duty, empathy, and work ethic (see Examining the Evidence 18.1; Lyman et al., 2021).

This does not mean, however, that others cannot influence an individual's intrinsic motivation. Parents and peers, for example, often play major roles in shaping a person's values about what they want to do and be. Parents who set high but attainable expectations for their children, and who constantly encourage them in a nonauthoritative environment, tend to impart strong achievement drives. Cultural background also has an impact on intrinsic motivation because some cultures value career mobility, job success, and recognition more than others.

Extrinsic motivation occurs when individuals are motivated to perform a behavior or engage in an activity to earn a reward or avoid punishment (Cherry, 2022b). Although all people are

DISPLAY 18.1 LEADERSHIP ROLES AND MANAGEMENT FUNCTIONS ASSOCIATED WITH CREATING A MOTIVATING WORK CLIMATE

Leadership Roles

1. Recognizes each worker as a unique individual who is motivated by different things
2. Identifies the individual and collective value system of the unit and implements a reward system that is consistent with those values
3. Fosters employee engagement and thus emotional commitment to the goals of the organization
4. Listens attentively to individual and collective work values and attitudes to identify unmet needs that can cause dissatisfaction
5. Encourages workers to "stretch" themselves in an effort to promote self-growth and self-actualization
6. Promotes a positive and enthusiastic image of self-empowerment to subordinates
7. Encourages mentoring, sponsorship, and coaching with subordinates
8. Devotes time and energy to create an environment that is supportive and encouraging to the discouraged individual
9. Is authentic rather than automatic in giving praise and positive reinforcement
10. Develops a unit philosophy that recognizes the unique worth of each employee and promotes reward systems that make each employee feel successful
11. Demonstrates through actions and words a belief in subordinates that they desire to meet organizational goals
12. Is self-aware regarding own enthusiasm for work and takes steps to remotivate self as necessary

Management Functions

1. Uses legitimate authority to provide formal reward systems
2. Uses positive feedback to reward the individual employee
3. Develops unit goals that integrate organizational and subordinate needs
4. Maintains a unit environment that eliminates or reduces job dissatisfiers
5. Promotes a unit environment that focuses on employee motivators
6. Creates the tension necessary to maintain productivity while encouraging subordinate job satisfaction
7. Communicates expectations to subordinates clearly
8. Demonstrates and communicates sincere respect, concern, trust, and a sense of belonging to subordinates
9. Assigns work duties commensurate with employee abilities and past performance to foster a sense of accomplishment in subordinates
10. Identifies achievement, affiliation, or power needs of subordinates and develops appropriate motivational strategies to meet those needs

intrinsically motivated to some degree, it is unrealistic for the organization to assume that all workers have adequate levels of intrinsic motivation to meet organizational goals. Thus, the organization must provide a climate that stimulates both extrinsic and intrinsic drives.

> The intrinsic motivation to achieve is directly related to a person's level of aspiration; however, it can be and often is influenced by others. Extrinsic motivation is motivation enhanced by the job environment or external rewards.

TABLE 18.1 INTRINSIC AND EXTRINSIC MOTIVATION

Intrinsic	Extrinsic
Comes from within the individual	Comes from outside the individual
Often influenced by family unit and cultural values	Rewards and reinforcements are given to encourage certain behaviors and/or levels of achievement

EXAMINING THE EVIDENCE 18.1

Source: From Lyman, B., Biddulph, M. E., & George, K. C. (2021). Organizational learning and motivation in certified nurse aides: A qualitative study. *Research in Gerontological Nursing, 14*(5), 255–263. https://doi–org.mantis.csuchico.edu/10.3928/19404921–20210708–02

What Motivates Certified Nurse Aides?

The unique position and expertise of certified nurse aides (CNAs) are crucial for excellent resident care in long-term care facilities; however, limited research exists as to their sources of motivation. This qualitative descriptive study, using semistructured interviews, explored sources and implications of CNA motivation, particularly as it relates to engaging in organizational learning.

Twenty-four CNAs working in a state veteran's home were interviewed. CNAs described their sources of motivation as:

- *"I'm a natural caregiver": 92% of CNAs felt their motivation was intrinsic and reported natural caregiving tendencies. They also overwhelmingly reported "loving their jobs" as well as high levels of empathy and work ethics.*
- *Support from administration: 38% of CNAs reported support from the facility's administration and reported that collaborative, relational experiences with administrators motivated them to provide excellent care to residents.*
- *Working as a team: 42% felt motivated when health care staff worked well together and problem solved as a team. When CNAs noticed their coworkers were motivated, they "naturally . . . want[ed] to step up" and improve the quality of care they provided as well.*
- *Love for residents: 92% expressed that their "love for the residents" was a significant motivator that drove them to provide high-quality care. CNAs felt motivated by their personal relationships with residents and the residents' gratitude toward them.*
- *Self-care: 17% of CNAs described a positive relationship between their efforts to engage in self-care and their feelings of motivation.*

Motivation helped CNAs feel more committed to the organization and its residents. When motivated, CNAs had more positive attitudes about their work, a higher level of engagement with residents, a stronger drive to accomplish extra tasks, and less desire to quit.

Because people have constant needs and wants, they are always motivated to some extent. In addition, because all human beings are unique and have different needs, they are motivated differently. The difference in motivation can be explained in part by our large- and small-group cultures. For example, because American culture tends to value material goods and possessions more highly than many other cultures, rewards in this country are frequently tied to those values.

> Because motivation is so complex, the leader faces tremendous challenges in accurately identifying individual and collective motivators.

LEARNING EXERCISE 18.1

Thinking About Motivation

Think back to when you were a child. What rewards did your parents use to promote good behavior? Was your behavior more intrinsically or extrinsically motivated? Were strong achievement drives encouraged and supported by your family? If you have children, what rewards do you use to influence their behavior? Are they the same rewards that your parents used? Why or why not?

Organizations also have cultures and values. Motivators vary among organizations as well as among units in organizations. Even in similar or nearly identical work environments, large variations in individual and group motivation often exist. Much research has been undertaken by behavioral, psychological, and social scientists to develop theories and concepts of motivation. Economists and engineers have focused on extrinsic fiscal rewards to improve performance and productivity, whereas human relations scientists have stressed intrinsic needs for recognition, self-esteem, and self-actualization. To better understand the current view that both extrinsic and intrinsic rewards are necessary for high productivity and worker satisfaction, one needs to look at how motivational theory has evolved over time.

Motivational Theory

Chapter 2 introduced traditional management philosophy, which emphasizes paternalism, worker subordination, and bureaucracy to promote predictable but moderate productivity. With this philosophy, high productivity means greater monetary incentives for the worker, and workers are viewed as being motivated primarily by economic factors. This traditional management philosophy is still in use today. Many factory and assembly line production jobs as well as jobs that use production incentive pay are based on these principles. The shift to a greater focus on the human element and worker satisfaction as factors in productivity began during the human relations era (1930 to 1970).

Maslow

Focus on human motivation did not continue until Abraham Maslow's work in the 1950s. Indeed, Abraham Maslow is the leading figure in the tradition of humanistic psychology, and the modern *positive psychology movement* owes a huge debt to his theories (Sze, 2017).

Many nurses are familiar with Maslow's *Hierarchy of Needs* and theory of human motivation. Maslow (1970) believed that people are motivated to satisfy certain needs, ranging from basic survival to complex psychological needs, and that people seek a higher need only when the lower needs have been predominantly met. (Maslow's Hierarchy of Needs is depicted in Fig. 18.1.)

A central belief of Maslow's theory was that people are born with the desire to self-actualize. Self-actualization, the pinnacle of the hierarchy, occurs when an individual maximizes their potential, doing the best that they can do (Sze, 2017). Maslow's portrait of the self-actualized person, however, is detailed and complex.

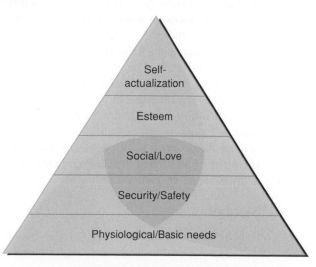

FIGURE 18.1 Maslow's hierarchy of needs.

DISPLAY 18.2 CHARACTERISTICS OF THE SELF-ACTUALIZED INDIVIDUAL

Self-Actualized People

1. Embrace the unknown and the ambiguous
2. Accept themselves, together with all their flaws
3. Prioritize and enjoy the journey, not just the destination
4. While inherently unconventional, do not seek to shock or disturb
5. Are motivated by growth, not by the satisfaction of needs
6. Have purpose
7. Are not troubled by the small things
8. Are grateful
9. Share deep relationships with a few but also feel identification and affection toward the entire human race
10. Are humble
11. Resist enculturation
12. Are not perfect

Extracted from Sze, D. (2017, December 6). Maslow: The 12 characteristics of a self-actualized person. *The Huffington Post*. http://www.huffingtonpost.com/david-sze/maslow-the-12-characteris_b_7836836.html

For example, self-actualized persons embrace the unknown, are focused on personal growth, and have an accurate perception of self. They also focus on the big picture, do not take blessings for granted, and have a mission in life or some problem outside themselves that enlists much of their energies (Sze, 2017). In addition, self-actualized individuals do not allow themselves to be passively molded by culture—they are deliberate and make their own decisions, selecting what they see as good and rejecting what they see as bad. Sze (2017) also notes that "they are the most ethical of people even though their ethics are not necessarily the same as those of the people around them [because] the ordinary ethical behavior of the average person is largely conventional behavior rather than truly ethical behavior" (para. 21). These characteristics and others of the self-actualized individual are shown in Display 18.2.

> Because of Maslow's work, managers began to realize that people are complex beings, and rather than just being motivated by economics, they have many needs motivating them at any one time.

In the workplace, Maslow's work contributed to the recognition that people are motivated by many needs other than economic security. It also became clear that motivation is internalized and that if productivity is to increase, management must help employees meet lower-level needs. The shifting focus on what motivates employees has tremendously affected how organizations value workers today.

Some contemporary theorists, however, have questioned the validity of Maslow's hierarchy, suggesting that limited empirical research has been done to support the rankings in the hierarchy or that these needs even occur in a hierarchical order (Cherry, 2022a). Many examples exist where individuals appear to be self-actualized, when indeed, many of their basic needs have not been fulfilled. In addition, self-actualization is difficult to test empirically, and much of Maslow's work on self-actualization actually came from a very small sampling of biographies of notable individuals (Cherry, 2022a). Although further testing of Maslow's work is needed, his Hierarchy of Needs theory continues to influence how many individuals and organizations view motivation and the path to fulfillment.

Skinner

B. F. Skinner was another theorist in this era who contributed to the understanding of motivation, dissatisfaction, and productivity. Skinner's (1953) research on *operant conditioning* and *behavior modification* demonstrated that people could be conditioned to behave in a certain way based on a consistent reward or punishment system. Behavior that is rewarded will be repeated, and behavior that is punished or goes unrewarded will be extinguished. Skinner's work continues to be reflected today in the way many managers view and use discipline and rewards in the work setting.

Herzberg

Frederick Herzberg (1987) believed that employees could be motivated by the work itself and that there is an internal or personal need to meet organizational goals. He believed that separating personal motivators from job dissatisfiers was possible. This distinction between *hygiene* or *maintenance factors* and *motivator factors* was called the motivation–hygiene theory or two-factor theory. Table 18.2 lists motivator and hygiene factors identified by Herzberg.

Herzberg (1987) maintained that motivators or job satisfiers are present in work itself; they give people the desire to work and to do that work well. Hygiene or maintenance factors keep employees from being dissatisfied or demotivated but do not act as real motivators. It is important to remember that the opposite of dissatisfaction may not be satisfaction. When hygiene factors are met, there is a lack of dissatisfaction, not an existence of satisfaction. Likewise, the absence of motivators does not necessarily cause dissatisfaction.

For example, salary is a hygiene factor. Although it does not directly motivate, when used with other motivators such as recognition and advancement, it can influence motivation. If, however, salary is deficient, employee dissatisfaction can result. Some theorists continue to argue, however, that money can truly be a motivator, as evidenced by people who work excessive hours at jobs they truly do not enjoy. Some theorists would argue that money in this case might be taking the place of some other unconscious need. For example, money can be correlated with power and status.

Some people in Herzberg's (1987) studies, however, did report job satisfaction solely from hygiene or maintenance factors. Herzberg asserts that these people are only temporarily satisfied when hygiene factors are improved; show little interest in the kind and quality of their work; experience little satisfaction from accomplishments; and tend to show chronic dissatisfaction with other hygiene factors such as salary, status, and job security.

Herzberg's (1987) work suggests that although the organization must build on hygiene or maintenance factors, the motivating climate must actively include the employee. The worker must be given greater responsibilities, challenges, and recognition for work well done. The reward system must meet both motivation and hygiene needs, and the emphasis given by the

TABLE 18.2   HERZBERG'S MOTIVATORS AND HYGIENE FACTORS

Motivators	Hygiene Factors
Achievement	Salary
Recognition	Supervision
Work	Job security
Responsibility	Positive working conditions
Advancement	Personal life
Possibility for growth	Interpersonal relationships and peers
	Company policy
	Status

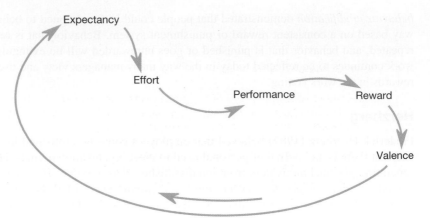

FIGURE 18.2 Vroom's expectancy model.

manager should vary with the situation and the employee involved. Although hygiene factors in themselves do not motivate, they are needed to create an environment that encourages the worker to move on to higher-level needs. Hygiene factors also combat employee dissatisfaction and are useful in recruiting an adequate personnel pool.

Vroom

Victor Vroom (1964), another motivational theorist in the human relations era, developed an *Expectancy Model*, which looks at motivation in terms of the person's valence or preferences based on social values. In contrast to *operant conditioning*, which focuses on observable behaviors, the Expectancy Model says that a person's expectations about their environment or a certain event will influence behavior. In other words, people look at all actions as having a cause and effect; the effect may be immediate or delayed, but a reward inherent in the behavior exists to motivate risk taking.

In Vroom's Expectancy Model (Fig. 18.2), people make conscious decisions in anticipation of reward; in operant conditioning, people react in a stimulus–response mode. Managers using the Expectancy Model must become personally involved with their employees to understand better the employees' values, reward systems, strengths, and willingness to take risks.

McClelland

David McClelland (1971) examined what motives guide a person to action, stating that people are motivated by three basic needs: achievement, affiliation, and power. *Achievement-oriented* people actively focus on improving what is; they transform ideas into action, judiciously and wisely, taking risks when necessary. In contrast, *affiliation-oriented* people focus their energies on families and friends; their overt productivity is less because they view their contribution to society in a different light from those who are achievement-oriented. *Power-oriented* people are motivated by the power that can be gained as a result of a specific action. They want to command attention, get recognition, and control others. McClelland theorizes that managers can identify achievement, affiliation, or power needs of their employees and develop appropriate motivational strategies to meet those needs.

Gellerman

Saul Gellerman (1968), another humanistic motivational theorist, identified several methods to motivate people positively. One such method, *stretching*, involves assigning tasks that are more difficult than what the person is used to doing. This includes personal and professional

LEARNING EXERCISE 18.2

Identifying Goals and Motivation

Identify the greatest motivator in your life currently. Has it always been the strongest motivator? Could you list the strongest motivator for the significant others in your life? If so, have you ever used this awareness to motivate those people to do something specific?

List six goals that you hope to accomplish in the next 5 years. Identify which goals are most related to achievement needs, affiliation needs, and power needs. Remember that most people are motivated in part by all three needs, and no one motivational need is better than the others. However, each person must recognize and understand which basic needs provide their motivation.

development in areas of vocational knowledge, skills, and expertise. Giving people responsibility, encouraging creativity, and empowering them to complete a task often causes them to rise to the challenge. Stretching should not, however, be a routine or daily activity. All employees need to have time to rest and regroup after being stretched.

> The challenge of "stretching" is to energize people to enjoy the beauty of pushing themselves beyond what they think they can do.

Another method, *participation*, entails actively drawing employees into decisions affecting their work. Gellerman (1968) strongly believed that motivation problems usually stem from the way the organization manages and not from the staff's unwillingness to work hard. According to Gellerman, most managers "overmanage"—they make the employee's job too narrow and fail to give the employee any decision-making power.

LEARNING EXERCISE 18.3

The Anticipated Reward

You are a new nurse who has been working on a medical-surgical unit for the 6 months since you graduated from nursing school. Your dream job is to work in the emergency department (ED), but you were told that these jobs are rarely given to new graduate nurses. Instead, you were advised by the ED manager to work on the medical unit to gain needed skills, experience as well as confidence and to work on achieving specialty certifications and training that would make you a stronger candidate for ED job openings in the future. As a result, you have been working to complete courses in pediatric and adult advanced life support training and are currently enrolled in a course that will prepare you to work as a mobile base station responder in the ED.

Today, when you return to work after 4 days off, you learn that a job was posted in the ED several days ago and that a new graduate nurse was hired for the position. You are frustrated and angry because you thought you would at least be given the opportunity to apply for any open positions and do not understand why the position was given to a new graduate, when it was denied to you initially.

ASSIGNMENT:

Using Vroom's Expectancy Model, describe the problem that has occurred here. What are the sources of your anger and frustration and whom are they directed at? How will this action influence your work motivation? Develop a plan for what you will do next.

TABLE **18.3** **McGREGOR'S THEORY X AND THEORY Y ASSUMPTIONS**

Theory X Employees	Theory Y Employees
Avoid work if possible	Like and enjoy work
Dislike work	Are self-directed
Must be directed	Seek responsibility
Have little ambition	Are imaginative and creative
Avoid responsibility	Have underutilized intellectual capacity
Need threats to be motivated	Need only general supervision
Need close supervision	Are encouraged to participate in problem solving
Are motivated by rewards and punishment	

McGregor

Douglas McGregor (1960) examined the importance of a manager's assumptions about workers on the intrinsic motivation of the workers. These assumptions, which McGregor labeled *Theory X* and *Theory Y* (depicted in Table 18.3), led to the realization in management science that how the manager views, and thus treats, the worker will have an impact on how well the organization functions.

McGregor (1960) did not consider Theory X and Theory Y as opposite points on the spectrum but rather as two points on a continuum extending through all perspectives of people. McGregor believed that people should not be artificially classified as always having Theory X or Theory Y assumptions about others; instead, most people's beliefs fall somewhere on a continuum. Likewise, McGregor did not promote either Theory X or Theory Y as being the one superior management style, although many managers have interpreted Theory Y as being the ultimate management model. No one style is effective in all situations and with all people. McGregor, without making value judgments, simply stated that in any situation, the manager's assumptions about people, whether grounded in fact or not, affect motivation and productivity.

> Theory Y is not a "better" management style than Theory X; the style which is "best" depends on the variables inherent in a given situation.

The work of all these theorists has added greatly to the understanding of what motivates people in and out of the work setting. Research reveals that motivation is extremely complex and that there is tremendous variation in what motivates different people. Therefore, managers must understand what can be done at the unit level to create a climate that allows the worker to grow, increases motivation and productivity, and eliminates dissatisfiers that drain energy and promote frustration.

Strategies for Creating a Motivating Climate

The leader-manager can do many things to help create an environment that is motivating. We often forget that the only way to achieve our goals is through the people who work with us. Therefore, although managers cannot directly motivate employees, they can create a climate that demonstrates positive regard for their employees, encourages open communication as well as growth and productivity, and recognizes achievement.

Sometimes, fostering a subordinate's motivation is as simple as establishing a supportive and encouraging environment. The cost of this strategy is only the manager's time and energy. Most managers, however, will tell you that recognition, incentives, support for making progress, and clear goals are also essential to creating motivating work environments. In addition, engaging and empowering workers are critical leadership tasks.

Worker Engagement

The term used to describe an employee's emotional commitment to the organization and its goals is *employee engagement. Engagement* occurs when workers are involved in, enthusiastic about, and committed to their work and workplace.

Bigham (2022) notes, however, that since the concept was introduced in 1990, how we view engagement in the workplace has shifted dramatically. The emphasis is no longer on the employee being happy. Instead, the focus is on the employer ensuring each employee feels fulfilled in their role, supported by their manager and leaders, and connected to the company's purpose. It is also important to note that employee engagement is not the same thing as employee satisfaction. An employee can be satisfied with their job but not be engaged.

Why is engagement important? Research from Gallup notes that low engagement goes hand in hand with poor performance and higher turnover. Engaged workers also report better health outcomes, are more productive, and are more likely to be retained (Barnhart, 2021).

Unfortunately, after wild fluctuations in 2020 (likely pandemic induced), only 36% of US workers were engaged as of 2021, although this figure is the highest level reported since Gallup began reporting the national figure in 2000 (Harter, 2021). Strategies to engage workers often include investing in work–life balance and boosting onboarding and hiring practices. In addition, employee engagement happens when the goals of the business and the ambitions of the employee are fully aligned.

> Organizations and teams with higher employee engagement and lower active disengagement perform at higher levels and have better employee retention.

Worker Empowerment

Another proven strategy for creating a motivating climate is the empowerment of workers. Leonard (2020) defines *employee empowerment* as giving employees the ability to make decisions and encouraging them to challenge the status quo, which is critical for organizations to avoid obsolescence in fast-changing, technology-driven environments. Similarly, Huston (2020, p. 87) suggests that empowerment occurs when workers are involved in planning and implementing change—and when workers believe they have some control over their future work environments.

Leader-managers then must encourage workers to think creatively within the organization and avoid the micromanaging that often stifles creativity. The reality is that creativity requires risk taking, and innovation may at least initially result in failure. Even failure, though, can lead to worker empowerment. "When employees feel that managers trust them to make choices based on sound reasoning, and a focus on business needs, they feel more confident in their ability to try, and even fail—learning in the process. This empowers them to try harder" (Richards, 2022, para. 3).

To empower workers, the leader-manager must create an environment where employees understand what is expected of them, know how their work contributes to the organization's success, and feel free to make choices and decisions about their work without having to ask for management permission (Richards, 2022). In addition, managers must be role models of empowerment and lead by example; managers who do not feel empowered will set a stage for employees to not feel empowered.

Positive Reinforcement

One of the most powerful, yet frequently overlooked or underused, strategies the manager can use to create a motivating climate is *positive reinforcement*, which validates workers' efforts.

Negative feedback makes workers feel as if they are being punished for trying, and if negative feedback is consistently provided, the person will give up trying. If not corrected, this feeling can undermine their commitment, engagement, and performance.

It is important, however, when showing appreciation, to be specific. Instead of just saying, "We really are grateful for the good job you do around here," the approach might be, "I really appreciate how you dealt with the difficult patient last night. Your effort really made a difference." It is also important that the appreciation be genuine and that it recognizes extra or exceptional effort. When praise becomes automatic and expected, it loses its meaning.

Leaders then need a variety of ways to recognize performance and show appreciation. This ability to individualize reward systems is a cardinal element in a successful motivation–reward system for an organization.

Jensen (2022) suggests strategies for creating a motivating climate in the workplace, which include hiring top performers (working with lower performers may decrease the productivity of other workers), creating and displaying goals the employee or organization could reasonably attain, showing that you trust your employees to make the right decisions for the overall well-being of the organization, and making every employee feel that their job makes a difference.

When employees feel valued and empowered, they become more engaged in the organization, and this often results in a greater willingness to invest time and energy in meeting organization's goals. Those who do not feel appreciated often move on to other places of employment where they feel their efforts will be more valued (Huston, 2020).

Incentives and Rewards

Many organizations also use incentives or rewards to foster a motivating climate. The use of incentives and rewards for this purpose, however, can be very challenging. Cherry (2022b) notes that although offering rewards can increase motivation in some cases, researchers have also found that this is not always the case. In fact, offering excessive rewards can lead to a *decrease* in intrinsic motivation. The tendency of extrinsic motivation to interfere with intrinsic motivation is known as the *overjustification effect*. This involves a decrease in intrinsically motivated behaviors after the behavior is extrinsically rewarded and the reinforcement is subsequently discontinued (Cherry, 2022b).

In addition, some individuals erroneously believe that if a small reward results in desired behavior, then a larger reward will result in even more of the desired behavior. This simply is not true. There appears to be a perceived threshold beyond which increasing the incentive results in no additional meaning or weight.

Using incentives and rewards to motivate workers can also be complicated by a view of rewards as competition. When rewards lack consistency, there is greater risk that the reward itself will become a source of competition and thereby lower morale. When employees perceive that a limited number of awards are available, and others receiving awards limits their chances of obtaining their own awards, it becomes more difficult to support their peers.

Likewise, rewarding one person's behavior and not the behavior of another who has accomplished a similar task at a similar level promotes jealousy and can demotivate. All employees should be recognized for meeting milestones.

In contrast, Stark (2021) suggests that managers consider making incentives competitive to add a little fun among the routine. An incentive challenge for teams can instill a sense of excitement and energy, further promoting the results of these efforts. Managers are often surprised by the competitiveness of their staff, a trait common to teams participating in high-demand, challenging positions. Leader-managers, however, must be careful when rewards result in competition (whether intentional or not), since the practice can result in a loss of motivation for employees and a reduction in team cohesion.

DISPLAY 18.3 STRATEGIES FOR THE EFFECTIVE USE OF INCENTIVES AND REWARDS

1. Workers need to know that management is aware of and appreciative of their unique contributions.
2. Expressed appreciation should be genuine and somewhat specific in nature.
3. One of the most powerful, yet frequently underused strategies to show appreciation is simply saying thank you for a job well done, particularly if it is done in public.
4. In formal incentive programs, the incentives should be visible.
5. Incentives offered must be meaningful to the person who is receiving them since what motivates one individual may not motivate another.
6. The value of an incentive can change over time and in different situations.
7. There appears to be a perceived threshold beyond which increasing an incentive results in no additional meaning or weight.
8. Incentivized goals should be challenging, but achievable.
9. Competition should be considered as part of an incentive program.
10. Excessive use of rewards can lead to a reduction in intrinsic motivation.

In addition, rewards and praise should be spontaneous and not relegated to predictable events, such as routine annual performance reviews and recognition dinners. Rewards and praise should be given whenever possible and whenever they are deserved. Indeed, employees want to know that their manager is aware of their unique contributions when they make extra effort. These moments of connection, of conversing with those you lead, help engender a sense of meaning with the employee (Huston, 2020).

If positive reinforcement and rewards are to be used as motivational strategies, however, rewards must represent a genuine accomplishment on the part of the person and should be somewhat individual in nature. For example, many managers erroneously consider annual merit pay increases as rewards that motivate employees. Most employees, however, recognize annual merit pay increases as a universal "given"; thus, this reward has little meaning and little power to motivate.

> Organizations must be cognizant of the need to offer incentives at a level where employees value them. This requires that the organization and its managers understand employees' collective values and devise a reward system that is consistent with that value system.

Strategies for the effective use of incentives and rewards are shown in Display 18.3.

The Relationship Between the Employee and Their Supervisor

In addition, the interpersonal relationship between an employee and their supervisor is critical to employees' motivation levels. Indeed, Custom Insight (2022) suggests that an employee's engagement with their manager is a key predictor of their engagement within the organization. Feeling valued, being treated fairly, receiving feedback and direction, and generally having a strong working relationship between an employee and their manager that is based on mutual respect is predictive of strong employee engagement with the manager.

In addition, the relationship an employee has with their boss is a key predictor of turnover. Huston (2020) notes that the deciding factor for why people stay at a job or look elsewhere often has to do with the relationship they have with their manager. Many people have left jobs where they loved the work, but simply could not work with their manager. It turns out that the opposite is true, too. An inspiring manager creates more team engagement.

Additional strategies that can be used to create a motivating climate are outlined in Display 18.4.

DISPLAY 18.4 STRATEGIES TO CREATE A MOTIVATING CLIMATE

1. Have clear expectations for workers and communicate these expectations effectively.
2. Be fair and consistent when dealing with all employees.
3. Be a firm decision maker using an appropriate decision-making style.
4. Develop the concept of teamwork. Develop group goals and projects that will build a team spirit.
5. Integrate the staff's needs and wants with the organization's interests and purpose.
6. Know the uniqueness of each employee. Let each know that you understand their uniqueness.
7. Remove traditional blocks between the employee and the work to be done.
8. Provide experiences that challenge or "stretch" the employee and allow opportunities for growth.
9. When appropriate, request participation and input from all subordinates in decision making.
10. Whenever possible, give subordinates recognition and credit.
11. Be certain that employees understand the reason behind decisions and actions.
12. Reward desirable behavior; be consistent in how you handle undesirable behavior.
13. Let employees exercise individual judgment as much as possible.
14. Create a trustful and helping relationship with employees.
15. Empower employees to have as much control as possible over their work environment and the decisions that impact it.
16. Be a positive and enthusiastic role model for employees.

LEARNING EXERCISE 18.4

Write a Detailed Plan to Motivate—Quickly!

You are the manager of a medical unit in a community hospital. The hospital has faced extreme budget cuts during the last 5 years as a result of decreased reimbursement. Your unit used to be a place where nurses wanted to work, and you rarely had openings for long, even though it was necessary for the hospital to contain costs and shorten nursing care hours per patient-day. A recent hiring freeze has accelerated worker dissatisfaction in your staff.

In the last week, five of the unit nurses, all excellent long-time employees, have stopped by your office either in tears, anger, or frustration. Their various comments have included "Working here is no longer fun," "I used to love my job," "I am tired of working with incompetent people," and "I am sick to death of calling for supplies that should be stocked on the floor." You know that funding will not increase soon, but you think that perhaps there are things you could do to make the situation better for your staff.

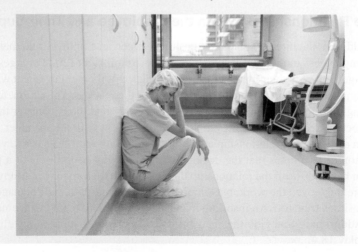

ASSIGNMENT:

• • • • • • • •

In examining the strategies for creating a motivating climate and an atmosphere that supports finding joy in work, decide what you as an individual unit manager can do to provide a more positive work environment. Avoid taking items from the list in Displays 18.3 and 18.4, but write a detailed plan that is feasible, that could be implemented fairly quickly, and that would have the potential to turn this situation around.

Self-Care

Managers can also create a motivating climate by being positive and enthusiastic role models in the clinical setting. Managers, however, must be internally motivated before they can motivate others and virtually every leader (as well as employee) has struggled with demotivation at some point in their life.

Managers who frequently project unhappiness to subordinates, however, contribute to low unit morale. A burned-out, tired manager will develop a lethargic and demotivated staff. In contrast, a positive attitude is infectious, and it can help managers and their employees start to view problems as opportunities to get creative rather than as difficulties that need to be overcome (Espinal, 2021). Therefore, managers must constantly monitor their own motivational level and do whatever is necessary to restore their motivation to be role models to staff.

> The attitude and energy level of managers directly affect the attitude and productivity of their employees.

It is imperative then that discouraged managers acknowledge their own feelings and seek assistance accordingly. Taking time off to rest and recuperate often helps managers to return refreshed and ready for action. Setting realistic expectations is also critical to avoiding feelings of failure and inadequacy. The same strategies apply to employees.

Managers are responsible to themselves and to subordinates to remain motivated to do the best job possible. Nursing is a stressful profession, and managers must practice health-seeking behaviors and find social supports when confronted with stress or else risk burnout as a result. Burnout and other forms of work-related stress are related to negative organizational outcomes such as illness, absenteeism, turnover, performance deterioration, decreased productivity, and job dissatisfaction. These outcomes cost the organization and impede quality of care.

Perhaps the most important strategy for avoiding burnout and maintaining a high motivation level is *self-care*. For self-care, the manager should seek time off on a regular basis to meet personal needs, seek recreation, form relationships outside the work setting, and have fun.

Often, friends and colleagues are essential for emotional support, guidance, and renewal. A proper diet and exercise are important to maintain physical health as well as emotional health. Finally, the manager must be able to separate their work life and personal life; the manager should remember that there is life outside of work and that time should be relished and protected. Ultimately, the decision to practice self-care rests with each nurse.

Integrating Leadership Roles and Management Functions in Creating a Motivating Climate at Work

Most human behavior is motivated by a goal that the person wants to achieve. Identifying employee goals and fostering their attainment allow the leader to create an environment that encourages employees to reach personal and organizational goals. The motivational strategy that the leader uses should vary with the situation and the employee involved; it may be formal or informal. It may also be extrinsic, although because of a limited formal power base, the leader generally focuses on other aspects of motivation. The leader must listen, support, and encourage the discouraged employee. However, perhaps the most important role that the leader has in working with the demotivated employee is that of role model. Leaders who maintain a positive attitude and high energy levels directly and profoundly affect the attitude and productivity of their followers.

When creating a motivating climate, the manager uses formal authority to reduce dissatisfiers at the unit level and to implement a reward system that reflects individual and collective value systems. This reward system may be formalized, or it may be as informal as praise. In addition, managers, by virtue of their position, can motivate subordinates by "stretching" them intermittently with increasing responsibility and assignments that they are capable of achieving. The manager's role, then, is to create the tension necessary to maintain productivity while encouraging subordinates' job satisfaction. Therefore, the success of the motivational strategy is measured by increased productivity and benefit to the organization and by growth in the person, which motivates them to accomplish again.

Key Concepts

- Because human beings have constant needs and wants, they are always motivated to some extent. However, what motivates each human being varies significantly.
- Managers cannot intrinsically motivate people because motivation comes from within the person. The humanistic manager can, however, create an environment in which the development of human potential can be maximized.
- *Engagement*, a key to retention, is the term used to describe workers who are involved in, enthusiastic about, and committed to their work and workplace.
- Maslow stated that people are motivated to satisfy certain needs, ranging from basic survival to complex psychological needs, and that people seek a higher need only when the lower needs have been predominantly met.
- Skinner's research on operant conditioning and behavior modification demonstrates that people can be conditioned to behave in a certain way based on a consistent reward or punishment system.
- Herzberg maintained that motivators, or job satisfiers, are present in the work itself and encourage people to want to work and to do that work well. Hygiene or maintenance factors keep the worker from being dissatisfied or demotivated but do not act as true motivators for the worker.
- Vroom's expectancy model says that people's expectations about their environment or a certain event will influence their behavior.

- McClelland's studies state that all people are motivated by three basic needs: achievement, affiliation, and power.
- Gellerman states that most managers in organizations overmanage by making the responsibilities too narrow, failing to give employees any decision-making power, or not "stretching" them often enough.
- McGregor points out the importance of a manager's assumptions about workers on the intrinsic motivation of the worker.
- The term used to describe an employee's emotional commitment to the organization and its goals is *employee engagement*.
- There appears to be a perceived threshold beyond which increasing reward incentives results in no additional meaning or weight in terms of productivity.
- Positive reinforcement is one of the most powerful motivators the manager can use and is frequently overlooked or underused.
- The supervisor or manager's personal motivation is an important factor affecting staff's commitment to duties and morale.
- The success of a motivational strategy is measured by the increased productivity and benefit to the organization and by the growth in the person, which motivates them to accomplish again.
- Managers must show their own positive attitude to demonstrate to employees that there is joy in work.

Additional Learning Exercises and Applications

LEARNING EXERCISE **18.5**

Why Won't Beth Apply for the Position?

You have been the evening charge nurse of a large surgical unit for the last 4 years. Each year, you schedule a career development coaching session with all your licensed staff. These sessions are held separately from the performance appraisal interviews. You have been extremely pleased with the results of these sessions. Two of your licensed vocational nurses/licensed practical nurses are now enrolled in a registered nurse (RN) program. Several of the RNs from your unit have obtained advanced clinical positions, and many have returned to school. As a result of your encouragement and support, several of the nurses have taken charge positions on other units. You are proud of your ability to recognize talent and to perform successful career counseling.

This is the last time that you will be performing career counseling because you have resigned from your position to return to graduate school. You have encouraged several of the staff to apply for your position but think that one nurse—Beth, a 34-year-old woman—would be exceptional. She is extremely capable clinically, very mature, well respected by everyone, and has excellent interpersonal skills. Beth only works 4 days a week but has been invaluable to you in the 4 years since you have been a charge nurse. However, Beth is one of the few nurses who have never acted on any of your suggestions at previous career-coaching sessions.

Last week, you had another coaching session with Beth and told her of your plans. You urged her to apply for your position and told her that you would recommend her to your supervisor, although you would not be making the final selection. Beth told you that she would think about it, and today, she told you that she does not wish to apply for the position. You are very disappointed and believe that perhaps you have failed in some way.

ASSIGNMENT:

Examine this scenario carefully. Make a list of the possible reasons that Beth declined the promotion. Be creative. Is the value of your coaching diminished by Beth's choice to decline the position? Compare your findings with others in the group. After comparison, determine what influence, if any, personal values had on the development of the lists.

LEARNING EXERCISE **18.6**

Create a Plan to Remotivate a New Employee

You are a county public health coordinator. You have grown concerned about the behavior of one of the new registered nurses assigned to work in the agency. This new nurse, Sally Brown, is a recent graduate of a local Bachelor of Science in Nursing program. She came to work for the agency immediately after her graduation 6 months ago and for the first few months appeared to be extremely hard working, knowledgeable, well liked, and highly motivated. Recently, though, several small incidents involved Sally. The agency's medical director became very angry with her over a medication error that she had made. Sally

(continues on page 470)

LEARNING EXERCISE 18.6

Create a Plan to Remotivate a New Employee (continued)

was already feeling bad about the careless error. Soon after, a patient's husband began disliking Sally for no discernible reason and refused Sally entrance to his home to care for his wife. Then, 2 weeks ago, a patient with diabetes died fairly suddenly from renal failure, and although no one was to blame, Sally thought that if she had been more observant and skilled in assessment, she would have detected subtle changes in the patient's condition sooner.

Although you have been supportive of Sally, you recognize that she is in danger of becoming demotivated. Her once flawless personal appearance now borders on being unkempt, she is frequently absent from work, and her once pleasant personality has been exchanged for withdrawal from her coworkers.

ASSIGNMENT:

Using your knowledge of new role identification, socialization, and motivational theory, develop a plan to assist this young nurse. What can you do to provide a climate that will remotivate her and decrease her job dissatisfaction? Explain what you think is happening to this nurse and the rationale behind your plan, which should be realistic in terms of the time and energy that you have to spend on one employee. Be sure to identify the responsibilities of the employee as well.

LEARNING EXERCISE 18.7

A Chief Nursing Officer's Dilemma

You are the chief nursing officer of County Hospital. Dr. Martin Jones, a cardiologist, has approached you about having an intensive care unit/critical care unit (ICU/CCU) nurse make rounds with him each morning on all of the patients in the hospital with a cardiac-related diagnosis. He believes that this will probably represent a 90-minute commitment of nursing time daily. He is vague about the nurse's exact role or purpose, but you believe that there is great potential for better and more consistent patient education and care planning.

Audrey, one of your finest ICU/CCU nurses, agrees to assist Dr. Jones. She has always wanted to have an expanded teaching role. However, for various reasons, she has been unable to relocate to a larger city where there are more opportunities for teaching. You warn Audrey that it might be some time before this role develops into an autonomous position, but she is eager to assist Dr. Jones. The other ICU/CCU staff agree to cover Audrey's patients while she is gone, although it is obviously an extension of an already full patient load.

After 3 weeks of making rounds with Dr. Jones, Audrey comes to your office. She reports that rounds frequently take 2 to 3 hours and that making rounds with Dr. Jones amounts to little more than "picking up his pages and being a personal handmaiden." She has assertively stated her feelings to him and has attempted to demonstrate to Dr. Jones how their allegiance could result in improved patient care. She states that she has not been allowed any input into patient decisions and is frequently reminded of "her position" and his ability to have her removed from her job if she does not like being told what to do. She is demoralized and demotivated. In addition, she believes that her peers resent having to cover her workload because it is obvious that her role is superficial at best.

You ask Audrey if she wants you to assign another nurse to work with Dr. Jones, and she says that she would really like to make it work but does not know what action to take that would improve the situation.

You call Dr. Jones, and he agrees to meet with you at your office when he completes rounds the following morning. At this visit, Dr. Jones confirms Audrey's description of her role but justifies his desire for the role to continue by saying, "I bring millions of dollars in business to this hospital every year in cardiology procedures. The least you can do is provide the nursing assistance I am asking for. If you are unable to meet this small request, I will be forced to consider taking my practice to a competitive hospital." However, after further discussion, he does agree that eventually, he would consider a slightly more expanded role for the nurse after he learns to trust her.

ASSIGNMENT:

Do you meet Dr. Jones's request? Does it make any difference whether Audrey is the nurse, or can it be someone else? Is the amount of revenue that Dr. Jones generates relevant in your decision making? Should you try to talk Audrey into continuing the position for a while longer? While trying to reach a goal, people must sometimes endure a difficult path, but at what point does the means not justify the end? Be realistic about what you would do in this situation. What do you perceive to be the greatest obstacles in implementing your decision?

LEARNING EXERCISE 18.8

To Work or Not to Work?

You are a nurse in a long-term care facility. The facility barely meets minimum licensing standards for professional nursing staffing. Although agency recruiters have been actively seeking to hire more licensed staff, pay at the facility for professional staff is less than at local acute care hospitals and the patient–nurse ratio is significantly higher. There appears to be little chance of improving the registered nurse staffing mix in your agency any time soon. The nursing administrator is extremely supportive of the staff's efforts but can do little to ease the current workload for licensed staff other than to turn away patients or close the agency. As a result, all of the nurses on the unit have been working at least 48 hours per week during the last 6 months; many have been working several double shifts and putting in many overtime hours each pay period.

Morale is deteriorating, and the staff has begun to complain. Most of the licensed staff are feeling burned out and demotivated. Many have started refusing to work overtime or to take on extra shifts. You feel a responsibility to the patients, community, and organization and have continued to work the extra hours, but you are exhausted as well.

Today is your first evening off in 6 days. At 2:00 PM, the phone rings, and you suspect that it is the agency calling you to come in to work. You delay answering while you decide what to do. The answering machine turns on, and you hear your administrator's voice. She says that they are desperate. Two new patients were admitted during the day, and the facility is full. She says that she appreciates all the hours you have been working but needs you once again, although she is unable to give you tomorrow off in compensation. You feel conflicting loyalties to the unit, patients, supervisor, and yourself.

ASSIGNMENT:

Decide what you will do. Will you agree to work? Will you return the administrator's telephone call or pretend that you are not at home? When do your loyalties to your patients and the organization end and your loyalties to yourself begin? Is the administrator taking advantage of you? Are the other staff being irresponsible? What values have played a part in your decision making?

LEARNING EXERCISE 18.9

Remotivating Oneself

You are a school nurse and have worked in the same school for 2 years. Before that time, you were a staff nurse at a local hospital working in pediatrics and later for a physician. You have been a registered nurse for 6 years.

When you began your job at the school, it was exciting. You believed that you were really making a difference in children's lives. You started several good health promotion programs and worked hard upgrading your health aides' education and training.

Several months ago, funding for the school was drastically cut, and several of your favorite programs were eliminated. You have been depressed about this and lately have been short tempered at work. Today, one of your best health aides gave you her 2-week notice and said, "This isn't a good place to work anymore." You realize that many of the aides and several of the schoolteachers have picked up your negative attitude.

There is much that you still love about your job, and you are not sure if the budget problems are temporary or long term. You go home early today and contemplate what to do.

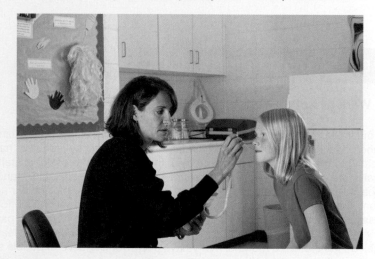

ASSIGNMENT:

Should you stay in this job or leave? If you stay, how can you get remotivated? Can you remotivate yourself if the budget cuts are long term? Make a plan about what to do.

LEARNING EXERCISE 18.10

Downsizing Panic and Anxiety

As a result of rising costs and shrinking reimbursement, some hospitals choose to downsize staff in an effort to shrink costs. Because the hospital where you are the chief nursing administrator is faced with mandatory staffing ratios, it is impossible to cut further staff nurse positions and meet requirements for state licensing.

Therefore, the chief executive officer (CEO) of the hospital has mandated that management positions be reduced by 20% (flattening the organization) throughout the hospital. The CEO has decided that department heads can reduce management positions by any method they choose as long as it is done in 6 months. Job duties are to be reassigned among the remaining managers.

This affects you significantly, as nursing has more managers than any other department. It does not appear that attrition or turnover rates in the next months will be adequate to eliminate the need for some reassignments, demotions, or termination of your group of 12 managers. This includes both house supervisors and unit managers.

The news travels rapidly through the hospital grapevine. Panic prevails, with many managers consulting you regarding whether their position is in jeopardy and what they can do to increase the likelihood of their retention. Morale is rapidly plummeting, and relationships are becoming increasingly competitive rather than cooperative.

ASSIGNMENT:

Determine how you will handle this situation. What strategies might you implement to reduce the immediate anxiety level? What advice can you give to staff who may face either a layoff or a demotion? Is it possible to preserve the morale of your managers in an uncertain situation such as this?

LEARNING EXERCISE 18.11

Just Getting By

You are a senior student in a nursing program. You are also a single mother of three grade school–aged children, currently living at home with your parents who are retired. Your recent divorce left you emotionally shattered as well as financially destitute. You work part-time as a waitress at a local coffee shop at night to help buy groceries and pay your educational expenses, but there is never enough money and you are just trying to do what you can to get by. Your barely passing grades at school reflect the recent disorganization in your life. In addition, you feel physically exhausted and increasingly depressed.

Today, one of your nursing instructors calls you into her office, noting the drop in your grades, and expresses concern that "you're not living up to your academic potential." She encourages you to try harder because she knows that you had hoped at some point to attend graduate school, and your current grades would not likely qualify you to do so.

You leave her office, feeling more discouraged than ever. There is already no time in your life for self-care, and doing better in school would require you to either work less or spend less time with your family, neither of which seems like a plausible alternative to you.

ASSIGNMENT:

Decide what you will do. Make sure the expectations you set for yourself are reasonable. Are the expectations intrinsically or extrinsically determined? Also identify whether your plan of action is more driven by achievement, affiliation, or power needs.

LEARNING EXERCISE 18.12

Men in Nursing

You are a new graduate male nurse. Lately, you have found yourself questioning your decision to become a nurse. There are many things you enjoy about nursing, including the opportunity to help others and the ability to make a good living to support your family. However, you are increasingly frustrated by the stereotypes many male nurses face regarding their sexual orientation and a perception that male nurses must not have been qualified for medicine, if "they settled for becoming a nurse." In addition, at times, you are reluctant to use therapeutic touch or to fully embrace the caring art of nursing for fear that your actions will be misinterpreted as sexual in nature. You also resent being called on to lift every heavy patient or to perform any manual labor needed on the unit just because you are often the only male nurse on the floor. Sometimes, you just feel out of place in a female-dominated profession and wonder if your career choice was a mistake.

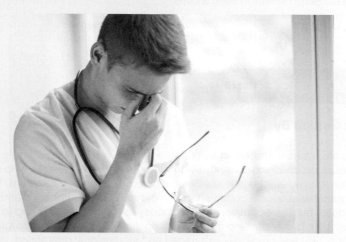

ASSIGNMENT:

Reflect on the intrinsic and extrinsic motivators and demotivators that exist in this situation. What strategies might you use to increase your intrinsic motivation? What factors might your employer use to increase your extrinsic motivation? What is the likelihood that the hygiene factors influencing your motivation may become more significant than the motivators?

REFERENCES

Barnhart, B. (2021, May 20). Employee engagement: How to keep workers engaged in a meaningful way. *Sprout Blog.* https://sproutsocial.com/insights/employee-engagement-guide/

Barnhart, B. (2022). 5 Employee engagement trends in the era of Coronavirus. *15five Blog.* https://www.15five.com/blog/7-employee-engagement-trends-2019/

Bigham, B. (2022). 5 employee engagement trends in the era of Coronavirus. *15five.* https://www.15five.com/blog/employee-engagement-trends-in-the-era-of-coronavirus/

Cherry, K. (2022a). *Maslow's hierarchy of needs.* Verywell Mind. Retrieved June 14, 2022, from https://www.verywell.com/hierarchy-of-needs-2795947

Cherry, K. (2022b). *What is extrinsic motivation?* Verywell Mind. Retrieved June 14, 2022, from https://www.verywell.com/what-is-extrinsic-motivation-2795164

Custom Insight. (2022). *What is employee engagement?* Retrieved June 14, 2022, from http://www.custominsight.com/employee-engagement-survey/what-is-employee-engagement.asp

Espinal, A. (2021). The top 14 ways to motivate employees in 2021. *Bond Collective.* Retrieved June 14, 2021, from https://www.bondcollective.com/blog/how-to-motivate-employees/

Gellerman, S. W. (1968). *Management by motivation.* American Management Association.

Harter, J. (2021, July 29). *U.S. employee engagement holds steady in first half of 2021*. Gallup. Retrieved June 14, 2022, from https://www.gallup.com/workplace/352949/employee-engagement-holds-steady-first-half-2021.aspx#:~:text=In%202021%2C%20the%20engagement%20of%20U.S.%20employees%20has,73%25%20of%20engaged%20workers%20on%20the%20same%20metric

Herzberg, F. (1987). One more time: How do you motivate employees? *Harvard Business Review, 81*, 87–96.

Huston, C. J. (2020). *The road to positive work cultures*. Sigma Theta Tau International Honor Society of Nursing.

Jensen, A. (2022, June 7). *5 Ways to create a motivating work environment*. Retrieved June 14, 2022, from http://www.andrewjensen.net/5-ways-to-create-a-motivating-work-environment/

Leonard, K. (2020, July 2). What are the benefits of employee empowerment? *Chron*. https://smallbusiness.chron.com/benefits-employee-empowerment-1177.html

Lyman, B., Biddulph, M. E., & George, K. C. (2021). Organizational learning and motivation in certified nurse aides: A qualitative study. *Research in Gerontological Nursing, 14*(5), 255–263. https://doi-org.mantis.csuchico.edu/10.3928/19404921-20210708-02

Maslow, A. (1970). *Motivation and personality* (2nd ed.). Harper & Row.

McClelland, D. C. (1971). *Assessing human motivation*. General Learning Press.

McGregor, D. (1960). *The human side of enterprise*. McGraw-Hill.

Richards, L. (2022). Employee empowerment questions for management students. *Chron*. Retrieved June 14, 2022, from http://smallbusiness.chron.com/employee-empowerment-questions-management-students-1846.html

Skinner, B. F. (1953). *Science and human behavior*. Free Press.

Stark, J. (2021, August). Organizational effectiveness, performance, and the benefit of incentives. *Case Management Monthly, 18*(8), 5–7.

Sze, D. (2017, December 6). Maslow: The 12 characteristics of a self-actualized person. *The Huffington Post*. http://www.huffingtonpost.com/david-sze/maslow-the-12-characteris_b_7836836.html

10x Psychology. (2021, November 16). Employee motivation in 2022. *Unleash*. Retrieved June 14, 2022, from https://www.unleash.ai/employee-motivation-in-2022/

Vroom, V. H. (1964). *Work and motivation*. Wiley.

19

Organizational, Interpersonal, and Group Communication in Team Building

*… effective communication is the lifeblood of a successful organization. It reinforces the organization's vision, connects employees to the business, fosters process improvement, facilitates change and drives business results by changing employee behavior.—**Watson Wyatt Worldwide***

*… the difference between the right word and the almost right word is the difference between lightning and a lightning bug.—**Mark Twain***

*… It is simply impossible to become a great leader without being a great communicator. I hope you noticed the previous sentence didn't refer to being a great talker—big difference.—**Mike Myatt***

CROSSWALK

This chapter addresses:

- **AACN Essentials Domain 2:** Person-centered care
- **AACN Essentials Domain 5:** Quality and safety
- **AACN Essentials Domain 6:** Interprofessional partnerships
- **AACN Essentials Domain 7:** Systems-based practice
- **AACN Essentials Domain 8:** Information and health care technologies
- **AACN Essentials Domain 9:** Professionalism
- **AACN Essentials Domain 10:** Personal, professional, and leadership development
- **AONL Nurse Executive Competency 1:** Communication and relationship building
- **AONL Nurse Executive Competency 2:** A knowledge of the health care environment
- **AONL Nurse Executive Competency 3:** Leadership
- **AONL Nurse Executive Competency 4:** Professionalism
- **AONL Nurse Executive Competency 5:** Business skills
- **ANA Standard of Professional Performance 10:** Communication
- **ANA Standard of Professional Performance 11:** Collaboration
- **ANA Standard of Professional Performance 12:** Leadership
- **ANA Standard of Professional Performance 15:** Quality of practice
- **ANA Standard of Professional Performance 16:** Resource utilization
- **ANA Standard of Professional Performance 17:** Resource stewardship
- **QSEN Competency:** Patient-centered care
- **QSEN Competency:** Teamwork and collaboration
- **QSEN Competency:** Quality improvement
- **QSEN Competency:** Safety
- **QSEN Competency:** Informatics

LEARNING OBJECTIVES

The learner will:

- describe the relationship between communication and team building
- identify the relationship between the sender, message, and receiver in communication
- differentiate between the internal and external climate in which communication occurs
- identify barriers to effective organizational communication
- describe strategies managers can use to increase the likelihood of clear and complete organizational communication
- diagram upward, downward, horizontal, and diagonal communication
- choose appropriate communication modes for specific situations and messages
- recognize culture and gender as significant variables impacting communication
- differentiate among assertive, passive, aggressive, and passive–aggressive communication
- recognize ISBAR, SBAR, ANTICipate, and I-PASS as structured, orderly approaches in providing accurate, relevant information, in emergent patient situations as well as routine handoffs
- demonstrate listening skills consistent with those outlined in the GRRRR (Greeting, Respectful Listening, Review, Recommend or Request More Information, and Reward) listening model
- write in a clear and concise manner using appropriate language for the receiver of the message
- describe the opportunities as well as the challenges new technologies pose for communication in contemporary organizations
- recognize the potential benefits of social media as a communication tool as well as the potential risks and identify principles for social networking use that minimize those risks
- describe the challenges encountered by health care providers in understanding and capturing relevant data in the electronic health record (EHR)
- recognize the need for confidentiality in sensitive interpersonal, group, or organizational communication
- assess accurately the stages of group formation (forming, storming, norming, and performing)
- identify specific group-building and maintenance roles that must be established for groups to accomplish work

Introduction

Although some functions of management such as planning, organizing, and controlling can be reasonably isolated, communication impacts all management activities and cuts across all phases of the management process. Indeed, the Mind Tools Content Team (2022) notes that poor communication lies at the root of many problems at work because it can lead to mistakes, quality problems, conflict, missed deadlines, and lost opportunities. That's why developing good communication skills is so important.

The nurse-leader communicates with clients, colleagues, bosses, and subordinates. In addition, because nursing practice tends to be group oriented, interpersonal communication among team members is necessary for continuity and productivity. One must have excellent interpersonal communication skills, then, to be an effective leader-manager. In fact, communication is perhaps the most critical leadership skill.

Organizational communication is even more complex than interpersonal or group communication, as there are more communication channels, more individuals to communicate with, more information to transmit, and new technologies, which both complicate and ease care delivery. Thus, organizational communication is a high-level management function; it must be systematic, have continuity, and be appropriately integrated into the organizational structure, encouraging an exchange of views and ideas. Organizational communication is complex, however, and communication failure often results in a failure to meet organizational goals. In addition, there are confidentiality risks that must be addressed.

The leader is responsible for developing a cohesive team to meet organizational goals. To do this, the leader must articulate issues and concerns so that workers will not become confused about priorities. The ability to communicate effectively often determines success as a leader-manager and developing expertise in all aspects of communication is critical. Leadership skills and management functions inherent in organizational, interpersonal, and group communication in team building are listed in Display 19.1.

This chapter examines multiple forms of communication. Barriers to communication in large organizations and managerial strategies to minimize those difficulties are presented. Channels and modes of communication are compared, and guidelines are given for managerial selection of the optimum channel or mode. In addition, assertiveness, nonverbal behavior,

---

DISPLAY 19.1 LEADERSHIP ROLES AND MANAGEMENT FUNCTIONS ASSOCIATED WITH ORGANIZATIONAL, INTERPERSONAL, AND GROUP COMMUNICATION IN TEAM BUILDING

Leadership Roles

1. Understands and appropriately uses both the formal and informal communication network in the organization
2. Communicates clearly and precisely in language that others will understand
3. Is sensitive to the internal and external climate of the sender or receiver and uses that awareness in sending and interpreting messages
4. Observes and interprets appropriately the verbal and nonverbal communication of followers
5. Role models assertive communication and active listening
6. Demonstrates congruency in verbal and nonverbal communication
7. Recognizes status, power, and authority as barriers to manager–subordinate communication and uses communication strategies to overcome those barriers
8. Role models the use of social networking principles that promote collaboration, shared decision making, and evidence-based practice, while protecting patient's rights and confidentiality
9. Seeks a balance between technologic communication options and the need for human touch; caring; and one-on-one, face-to-face interaction
10. Maximizes team functioning by keeping group members on course, encouraging the shy, controlling the garrulous, and protecting the weak

Management Functions

1. Understands and appropriately uses the organization's formal communication network
2. Determines the appropriate communication mode or combination of modes for optimal distribution of information in the organizational hierarchy
3. Prepares written communications that are clear and uses language that is appropriate for the message and the receiver
4. Consults with other departments or disciplines in coordinating overlapping roles and group efforts
5. Differentiates between "information" and "communication" and appropriately assesses the need for subordinates to have both
6. Prioritizes and protects client's and subordinate's confidentiality
7. Ensures that staff and self are trained to appropriately and fully utilize technologic communication tools
8. Establishes a technology-enabled communication infrastructure that leverages the benefits of social media while minimizing the risks
9. Uses knowledge of group dynamics for building teams, attaining shared goals, and maximizing organizational communication

and active listening as interpersonal communication factors are discussed. This chapter also includes a discussion of how standardized handoff tools, such as ISBAR, SBAR, ANTICipate, and I-PASS, can be used to provide a more structured, orderly approach in communicating client data. The impact of technology on communication in health care settings and the ever-increasing challenge of maintaining confidentiality in a system where so many people have access to so much information are discussed. Finally, communication as a vehicle to team building is threaded throughout the chapter.

The Communication Process

Answers.com (2022) defines *communication* as "to make common" or "to make known" through the exchange of thoughts, ideas, or the like. Communication can also occur on at least two levels: *verbal* and *nonverbal*. Thus, whenever two or more people are aware of each other, communication begins.

> Communication begins the moment that two or more people become aware of each other's presence.

What happens, however, when the thoughts, ideas, and information exchanged do not have the same meaning for both the sender and the receiver of the message? What if the verbal and nonverbal messages are incongruent? Does communication occur if an idea is transmitted but interpreted differently than its intent?

Because communication is so complex, many models exist to explain how organizations and individuals communicate. Basic elements common to most models are shown in Figure 19.1. In all communication, there is at least one sender, one receiver, and one message. There is also a mode or medium through which the message is sent—for example, spoken, written, or nonverbal.

An internal and an external climate also exist in communication. The *internal climate* includes the values, feelings, temperament, and stress levels of the sender and the receiver. Weather conditions, temperature, timing, and the organizational climate itself are parts of the external climate. The *external climate* also includes status, power, and authority as barriers to manager–subordinate communication (Table 19.1).

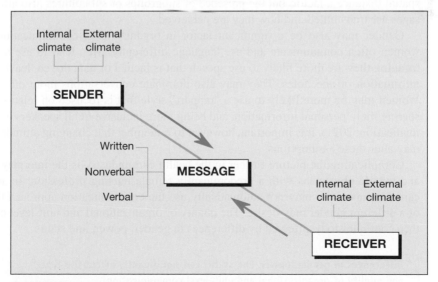

FIGURE 19.1 The communication process.

TABLE 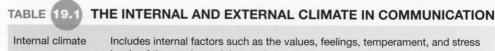 **THE INTERNAL AND EXTERNAL CLIMATE IN COMMUNICATION**

Internal climate	Includes internal factors such as the values, feelings, temperament, and stress levels of the sender and the receiver
External climate	Includes external factors such as the weather, temperature, timing, status, power, authority, and the organizational climate itself

Both the sender and the receiver must be sensitive to the internal and external climate because the perception of the message is altered greatly depending on the climate that existed at the time the message was sent or received. For example, an insecure manager who is called to meet with superiors during a period of stringent layoffs will probably view the message with more trepidation than a manager who is secure in their role.

Because each person is different and makes decisions and perceives differently, assessing external climate is usually easier than assessing internal climate. In assessing internal climate, remember that the human mind tends to perceive only what it expects to perceive. The unexpected is generally ignored or misunderstood. In other words, receivers cannot communicate if the message is incompatible with their expectations. If senders want communication to be effective, they need to be attentive to what they believe the receiver will see or hear.

> Effective communication requires the sender to validate what receivers see and hear.

Variables Affecting Organizational Communication

Formal organizational structure has an impact on communication. People at lower levels of the organizational hierarchy are at risk for inadequate communication from higher levels. As the number of employees increases (particularly more than 1,000 employees), the quantity of communication generally increases; however, employees may perceive it as increasingly closed. In large organizations, it is impossible for individual managers to communicate personally with each person or group involved in organizational decision making. Not only is spatial distance a factor, but the presence of subgroups or subcultures also affects what messages are transmitted and how they are perceived.

Gender may also be a significant factor in organizational communication, as men and women often communicate and use language differently. Men tend to use a "report" style, meaning they are more likely to use speech that is factual or data driven, leaving out personal information or anecdotes. They may also dominate conversations more often than women. Women may be more likely to use a "rapport" style that is focused on relationship-building, sharing more personal information, and being more inclusive of all speakers (Gendered Communication, 2021). It is important, however, to remember that changing attitudes about gender may alter these assumptions.

Complicating the picture further in the health care industry is the interplay between male and female physicians with a predominantly female nursing profession. In addition, health care administrators may not automatically use the communication approach that employees of a different gender may desire. The quality of organizational and unit-level communication then continues to be affected by differences in gender, power, and status.

> Differences in gender, power, and status can significantly affect the types and quality of organizational and unit-level communication.

LEARNING EXERCISE 19.1

Large Organization Communication

Have you ever been employed in a large organization? Was the communication within that organization clear and timely? What or who was your primary source of information? Were you a part of a subgroup or subculture? If so, how did that affect communication?

Power and status also impact organizational communication. When workers feel unimportant or ignored, job satisfaction and teamwork decline, and it becomes difficult for organization leaders to address the problems that are affecting the organization's ability to function and change. The importance of the manager in setting up a culture of open communication cannot be underestimated.

Organizational Communication Strategies

Although organizational communication is complex, the following strategies increase the likelihood of clear and complete communication:

- *Leader-managers must assess organizational communication*: Who communicates with whom in the organization? Is the communication timely? Does communication within the formal organization concur with formal lines of authority? Are there conflicts or disagreements about communication? What modes of communication are used?
- *Leader-managers must understand the organization's structure and recognize who will be affected by decisions*: Both formal and informal communication networks need to be considered. *Formal communication networks* follow the formal line of authority in the organization's hierarchy. *Informal communication networks* occur among people at the same or different levels of the organizational hierarchy but do not represent formal lines of authority or responsibility. For example, an informal communication network might occur between a hospital's chief executive officer (CEO) and her daughter, who is a unit clerk on a medical wing. Although there may be a significant exchange of information about unit or organizational functioning, this communication network would not be apparent on the organization chart. It is imperative, then, that managers be very careful about what they say and to whom until they have a good understanding of the formal and informal communication networks.
- *Communication is not a one-way channel*: If other departments or disciplines will be affected by a message, the leader-manager must consult with those areas for feedback before the communication occurs.
- *Communication must be clear, simple, and precise*: This requires the sender to adjust the language as necessary to the target audience.
- *Senders should seek feedback regarding whether their communication was accurately received*: One way to do this is to ask the receiver to repeat the communication or instructions. In addition, the sender should continue follow-up communication in an effort to determine if the communication is being acted on. The sender is responsible for ensuring that the message is understood.
- *Multiple communication modes should be used, when possible, if a message is important*: Using a variety of communication modes in combination increases the likelihood that everyone in the organization who needs to hear the message actually will hear it.
- *Managers should not overwhelm subordinates with unnecessary information*: *Information* is formal; impersonal; and unaffected by emotions, values, expectations, and perceptions. *Communication*, on the other hand, involves perception and feeling. It does not

depend on information and may represent shared experiences. In contrast to information sharing, superiors must continually communicate with their subordinates. For example, most staff need little information about ordering procedures or organizational supply vendors if supplies are adequate and appropriate to meet unit needs. If, however, a vendor is temporarily unable to meet unit supply needs, the use of supplies by staff becomes an issue requiring close communication between managers and subordinates. The manager must communicate with the staff about which supplies will be inadequately stocked and for how long. The manager also may choose to discuss this inadequacy of resources with the staff to identify alternative solutions.

> Although information and communication are different, they are interdependent.

Channels of Communication

Because large organizations are so complex, communication channels used by the manager may be upward, downward, horizontal, diagonal, or through the "grapevine." In *upward communication*, the manager is a subordinate to higher management. Needs and wants are communicated upward to the next level in the hierarchy. Those at this higher level make decisions for a greater segment of the organization than do the lower-level managers.

In *downward communication*, the manager relays information to subordinates. This is a traditional form of communication in organizations and helps to coordinate activities in various levels of the hierarchy.

In *horizontal communication*, managers interact with others on the same hierarchical level as themselves who are managing different segments of the organization. The need for horizontal communication increases as departmental interdependence increases.

In *diagonal communication*, the manager interacts with personnel and managers of other departments and groups such as physicians, who are not on the same level of the organizational hierarchy. Although these people have no formal authority over the manager, this communication is vital to the organization's functioning. Diagonal communication tends to be less formal than other types of communication.

The most informal communication network is often called the *grapevine*. *Grapevine communication* flows quickly and haphazardly among people at all hierarchical levels and usually involves three or four people at a time. Senders have little accountability for the message, and often, the message becomes distorted as it speeds along. Given the frequency of grapevine communication in all organizations, all managers must attempt to better understand how the grapevine works in their own organization as well as who is contributing to it. The channels of communication are summarized in Table 19.2.

> Grapevine communication is subject to error and distortion because of the speed at which it passes and because the sender has little formal accountability for the message.

TABLE 19.2 **CHANNELS OF COMMUNICATION**

Upward	From subordinate to superior
Downward	From superior to subordinate
Horizontal	From peer to peer
Diagonal	Between individuals at differing hierarchy levels and job classifications
Grapevine	Informal, haphazard, and random, usually involving small groups

LEARNING EXERCISE 19.2

When and How Will You Tell?

Assume that you are the project director of a small family planning clinic. You have just received word that your federal and state funds have been slashed and that the clinic will probably close in 3 months. Although an additional funding source may be found, it is improbable that it will occur within that time period. The board of directors informed you that this knowledge is not to be made public at this time.

You have five full-time employees at the clinic. Because two of these employees are your close friends, you feel some conflict about withholding this information from them. You are aware that another clinic in town currently has job openings and that the positions are generally filled quickly.

ASSIGNMENT:

It is important that you staff the clinic for the next 3 months. When will you notify the staff of the clinic's intent to close? Will you communicate the closing to all staff at the same time? Will you use downward communication? Should the grapevine be used to leak news to employees? When might the grapevine be appropriate to pass on information?

Communication Modes

A message's clarity is greatly affected by the mode of communication used. In general, the more direct the communication, the greater the probability that it will be clear. The more people involved in filtering the communication, the greater the chance of distortion. The manager must evaluate each circumstance individually to determine which mode or combination of modes is optimal for each situation.

Doyle (2021) agrees, suggesting that an important communication skill is simply knowing what form of communication to use. "For example, some serious conversations (layoffs, changes in salary, etc.) are almost always best done in person. You should also think about the person with whom you wish to speak—if they are very busy people (such as your boss, perhaps), you might want to convey your message through e-mail. People will appreciate your thoughtful means of communication and will be more likely to respond positively to you" (paras. 25/26).

Managers typically use the following modes of communication most frequently:

- *Written communication*: Written messages (including memos, reports, e-mail, and texting, which are discussed later in this chapter) allow for documentation. Most managers are required to do a considerable amount of this type of communication and therefore need to be able to write clearly.
- *Face-to-face communication*: Oral, in-person communication is rapid but may result in fewer people receiving the information than necessary.
- *Telephone communication*: A telephone call is rapid and allows the receiver to clarify the message at the time it is given. It does not, however, allow the receipt of nonverbal messages for either the sender or receiver of the message. Accents may be difficult to understand as well in a multicultural workforce.
- *Nonverbal communication*: Nonverbal communication includes facial expression, body movements, and gestures and is commonly referred to as *body language*. Nonverbal communication is considered more reliable than verbal communication because it conveys the emotional part of the message. There is significant danger, however, in misinterpreting nonverbal messages if they are not assessed in context with the verbal message.

In addition, gender appears to influence nonverbal communication. Research suggests that men may use fewer of the thousands of available facial expressions than women do, including smiling less. Men may also stand closer to women than to men and may prefer speaking face-to-face. Women are more likely to use touch to reassure or to build a connection, whereas men may use touch as a show of dominance, including pats, back slaps, and shoulder touches. In addition, women are more likely to use eye contact to connect with a speaker, suggesting that they are engaged and listening whereas men may listen with their eyes closed or avoid eye contact altogether as the other person speaks (Gendered Communication, 2021). All nurses must be sensitive to nonverbal clues and their importance in communication.

Effective leaders make sure that both verbal and nonverbal communications are congruent. Likewise, leaders are sensitive to nonverbal and verbal messages from followers and look for inconsistencies that may indicate unresolved problems or needs. Often, organizational difficulties can be prevented because leaders recognize the nonverbal communication of subordinates and take appropriate and timely action.

> Effective leaders are congruent in their verbal and nonverbal communication so that followers are clear about the messages they receive.

Elements of Nonverbal Communication

Nonverbal communication is the language of your body. Body language consists of 55% body movements, face, and arms, 38% voice and tone, and only 7% words (Internal Auditors Training, 2021). Nonverbal communication then must be examined in the context of the verbal content. In general, if verbal and nonverbal messages are incongruent, the receiver will believe the nonverbal message. Because nonverbal behavior can be and frequently is misinterpreted, receivers must validate perceptions with senders. The incongruence between verbal and nonverbal messages leads to many communication problems.

> Because nonverbal communication indicates the emotional component of the message, it is generally considered more reliable than verbal communication.

Silence

Silence can also be used as a means of nonverbal communication. This supports the adage that *even silence can be deafening*. The following section identifies other nonverbal clues that can occur with or without verbal communication.

Space (Proxemics)

The study of how space and territory affect communication is called *proxemics*. All of us have an invisible zone of psychological comfort that acts as a buffer against unwanted touching and attacks. The degree of space we require depends on who we are talking to as well as the situation we are in. For example, an intimate distance of less than 1.5 feet is generally reserved for romantic partners, close friends, and family whereas 1.5 to 4 feet is the personal space or "bubble" that is generally reserved for significant others and friends (Nicholson, 2021). A social distance is generally 4 to 12 feet, and a public distance is over 12 feet.

Proxemics also vary according to cultural norms. Some cultures require greater space between the sender and the receiver than others. Also, older individuals tend to prefer larger personal and intimate distances (Nicholson, 2021).

LEARNING EXERCISE 19.3

Silence Can Also Be Deafening

You are a nursing student and share an apartment with a friend who dropped out of school several months ago. Your roommate works as a bartender at a local restaurant four evenings per week and often doesn't get home until the wee hours of the morning. When she was in school, her general routine would be to come in quietly and go to bed so that she could be up early for classes the next day. Since she dropped out of school, however, she often brings home her coworkers who party all night and then sleep on the sofa or floor in your apartment. This has made it very difficult for you to get the sleep you need to be clearheaded for your early morning clinical courses, and you resent the loss of privacy in your apartment.

When the situation first began, you attempted to talk to your roommate about the problem. She became very angry and accused you of being jealous that she "gets to have fun and you don't." She refused to discuss the situation further. Since then, she has been cold and aloof, and the situation in the apartment has become worse, not better. When you come out at night and ask her to turn the music down, it is often turned up even louder as soon as you go back to your room. You can hear her and her friends mocking you. Today, you discovered toothpaste squirted inside your shoes and your stethoscope was hung on the toilet.

When you attempt to confront your roommate about the latest incidents, she states she does not have time to talk and that "this is your problem, not mine." Your lease does not end for 6 months, and you do not have the financial resources to simply walk away and find a new place to live.

ASSIGNMENT:

Develop a plan for how you will deal with the passive–aggressive and aggressive behavior of your roommate. How do you communicate with someone who doesn't want to or won't communicate with you?

Proxemics, then, may contribute to the message being sent. Distance may imply a lack of trust or warmth, whereas inadequate space, as defined by cultural norms, may make people feel threatened or intimidated. Likewise, the manager who sits beside employees during performance appraisals sends a different message than the manager who speaks to the employee from the opposite side of a large and formal desk. In this case, distance increases power and status on the part of the manager; however, the receptivity to distance and the message that it implies varies with the culture of the receiver.

Environment

There are many potential environmental barriers in communication including time, physical distance, space, climate, and place (Reference, 2020). If the temperature is too high or too cold, people can become agitated, frustrated, and uncomfortable, reducing the likelihood of good communication.

The place where communication takes place is also important. Communication that takes place in a superior's office is generally considered to be more serious than that which occurs in the cafeteria or a hallway. In addition, when there is not enough space for conversation or too many people are nearby, communication can be altered (Reference, 2020). Other problems, such as poor lighting and uncomfortable furniture may contribute to the problem.

In addition, noise levels in the environment may pose communication difficulties. For example, research by Grant et al. (2021) explored how noise affected communication between health professionals in the operating room (OR). Health professionals struggled to

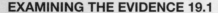

EXAMINING THE EVIDENCE 19.1

Source: From Grant, L., Nicholson, P., Davidson, B., & Manias, E. (2021). "Can you hear me?" Barriers to and facilitators of communication in the presence of noise in the operating room. *Journal of Perioperative Nursing, 34*(3), e-26–e-33. https://doi-org.mantis.csuchico.edu/10.26550/2209-1092.1132

Barriers to the Effective Use of I-PASS as a Handoff Tool

The aim of this exploratory qualitative study at a tertiary university-affiliated hospital in Northern Australia was to examine health professionals' perceptions of the impact of noise on communication in the operating room (OR). Semistructured interviews were used, transcribed, and analyzed using thematic analysis. Twenty-six health professionals participated, including anesthetists, surgeons, nurses, and theatre technicians.

Two themes were found: barriers to communication and facilitators of communication in the OR. Barriers to communication focused on difficulties health professionals experienced when attempting to communicate in the presence of noise—difficulty hearing in noisy ORs, positioning of health professionals, and inability to filter out sounds.

Participants expressed that their attitudes to noise changed as they grew older, becoming less tolerant to noise as a distractor. How the space in the OR was used when positioning the equipment influenced where health professionals were able to stand and move around during surgery, and this had an impact on their ability to communicate. In addition, the ability to clearly comprehend conversations required health professionals to filter out some of the sounds in the OR, allowing them to focus on conversations that were necessary at the time. However, when the OR was noisy, they were unable to filter out these sounds.

Facilitators of communication consisted of health professionals' adaption to the presence of noise during communication—nonverbal communication, such as gestures, and the ability to filter out unwanted sounds. Nonverbal communication was described as an effective form of communication when the OR was noisy. In addition, participants reported that filtering out sounds such as concurrent conversations and equipment, including suction or electrosurgical units, enabled them to focus their attention on the tasks at hand and essential conversations.

The researchers concluded that inexperienced health professionals may struggle with communicating effectively in noisy ORs and need to be supported until they acclimatize to the competing sounds and learn methods of effective communication. Consideration also needs to be given to the use of space and positioning of noise-emitting equipment to optimize communication in the OR. Furthermore, communication can be facilitated by the judicious use of nonverbal communication.

communicate effectively when the OR was noisy, because of how health professionals were positioned. Surgical procedures need to be undertaken in an OR that leaves adequate space for health professionals to maneuver around the equipment to better hear and communicate with each other. In addition, the ability to clearly comprehend conversations required health professionals to filter out some of the sounds in the OR, allowing them to focus on conversations that were necessary at the time. However, when the OR was noisy, they were unable to filter out these sounds (see Examining the Evidence 19.1).

Appearance

Much is communicated by our clothing, hairstyle, use of cosmetics, and grooming. Care should be exercised, however, to be sure that organizational policies regarding desired appearance are both culturally and gender sensitive.

Eye Contact

Eye contact invites interaction and emotional connection, if it is not too prolonged. Likewise, breaking eye contact suggests that the interaction is about to cease. It suggests to listeners that you may not be interested in them and are not engaged in the conversation. It may also suggest that you may be trying to conceal your real feelings. Unfortunately, eye contact is also declining because individuals focus on their smart devices when they are supposedly communicating with other people.

In addition, one must remember that like space, eye contact is often strongly influenced by cultural standards or religious practices. For example, in some cultures, prolonged eye contact may imply rudeness and, in some religions, eye contact with the opposite sex may be frowned upon (Nonverbal Communication Portal, n.d.).

Posture

Posture and the way that you control the other parts of your body are also extremely important parts of nonverbal communication. For example, sitting up straight suggests you are paying attention. Sitting with the body hunched forward, on the other hand, can imply that you are bored or indifferent. Crossing arms across one's chest may suggest defensiveness or aggressiveness. Moreover, the weight of a message is increased if the sender faces the receiver; stands or sits appropriately close; and, with head erect, leans toward the receiver.

Gestures

A message accented with appropriate gestures takes on added emphasis. Too much gesturing can, however, be distracting. For example, hand movement can emphasize or detract from the message. Gestures also have a cultural meaning. Some cultures are more tactile than others. Indeed, the use of touch is one gesture that often sends messages that are misinterpreted by receivers from different cultures.

Facial Expression and Timing

Effective communication requires a facial expression that agrees with your message. Staff perceive managers who present a pleasant and open expression as approachable. Likewise, a nurse's facial expression can greatly affect how and what clients are willing to relate. On the other hand, hesitation may diminish the effect of your statement or imply untruthfulness.

Vocal Expression

Vocal clues such as tone, volume, and inflection add to the message being transmitted. A tentative tone can make statements sound more like questions, leading listeners to think that you are unsure of yourself, and speaking quickly may be interpreted as being nervous. The goal, then, should always be to convey confidence and clarity.

Assertive, Passive, Aggressive, and Passive–Aggressive Verbal Communication Skills

Highly developed verbal communication skills are critical for the leader-manager. *Assertive communication* reduces stress, improves productivity, and contributes to a healthy workforce. With assertive communication, individuals express themselves in direct, honest, and appropriate ways that do not infringe on another person's rights. Positions are expressed clearly and firmly using "I" statements as well as direct eye contact and a calm voice. In addition, assertive communication requires that verbal and nonverbal messages be congruent.

There are many misconceptions about assertive communication. The first is that all communication is either assertive or passive. Actually, at least four possibilities for communication exist: passive, aggressive, indirectly aggressive or passive–aggressive, or assertive. *Passive communication* occurs when a person suffers in silence, although they may feel strongly about the issue. Thus, passive communicators avoid conflict, often at the risk of bottling up feelings that may lead to an eventual explosion.

Aggressive communication is generally direct, threatening, and condescending. It infringes on another person's rights and intrudes into that person's personal space. This behavior is also oriented toward "winning at all costs" or demonstrating self-importance.

Passive–aggressive communication is an aggressive message presented in a passive way. It generally involves limited verbal exchange (often with incongruent nonverbal behavior) by a person who feels strongly about a situation. This person feigns withdrawal to manipulate the situation. For example, the passive–aggressive communicator may say yes when they want to say no or be sarcastic or complain about others behind their backs. Over time, this type of behavior damages relationships and undercuts mutual respect (Mayo Clinic Staff, 1998–2022).

The second misconception is that those who communicate or behave assertively get everything they want. This is untrue. Being assertive involves both rights and responsibilities. The assertive person has the right to their own opinions and to express their thoughts in an honest and open manner, but a responsibility not to infringe on the rights of others in doing the same.

The third misconception about assertiveness is that it is unfeminine. Although the role of women in society in general has undergone tremendous change in the last 100 years, some individuals continue to find great difficulty in accepting that nurses of all genders play assertive, active, decision-making roles. Assertive communication involves conveying a message that insists on being heard. The nursing profession must be more assertive in its need to be heard. Eventually, a form of peer pressure can emerge that reshapes others and results in an assertive nursing voice.

> Assertive communication is not rude or insensitive behavior; rather, it is having an informed voice that insists on being heard.

A fourth misconception is that the terms *assertive* and *aggressive* are synonymous. To be assertive is to not be aggressive, although some cultures find the distinction blurred. Even when faced with someone else's aggression, the assertive communicator does not become aggressive. When under attack by an aggressive person, an assertive person can do several things:

- *Reflect:* Reflect the speaker's message back to them. Focus on the affective components of the aggressor's message. This helps the aggressor evaluate whether the intensity of their feelings is appropriate to the specific situation or event. For example, assume that an employee enters a manager's office and begins complaining about a newly posted staff schedule. The employee is obviously angry and defensive. The manager might use reflection by stating, "I understand that you are very upset about your schedule. This is an important issue, and we need to talk about it."
- *Repeat the assertive message*: Repeated assertions focus on the message's objective content. They are especially effective when the aggressor overgeneralizes or seems fixated on a repetitive line of thinking. For example, if a manager asks an angry employee to step into their office to discuss a problem, and the employee continues their tirade in the hallway, the manager might say, "I am willing to discuss this issue with you in my office. The hallway is not the appropriate place for this discussion."
- *Point out the implicit assumptions*: This involves listening closely and letting the aggressor know that you have heard them. In these situations, managers might repeat major points or identify key assumptions to show that they are following the employee's line of reasoning.

- *Restate the message by using assertive language*: Rephrasing the aggressor's language will defuse the emotion. Paraphrasing helps the aggressor to focus more on the cognitive part of the message. The manager might use restating by changing a "you" message to an "I" message.
- *Question*: When the aggressor uses nonverbal clues to be aggressive, the assertive person can put this behavior in the form of a question as an effective means of helping the other person become aware of an unwarranted reaction. For example, the desperate, angry employee may imply threats about quitting or transferring to another unit. The manager could appropriately confront the employee about their implied threat to see if it is real or simply a reflection of the employee's frustration.

> As in nonverbal communication, the verbal communication skills of the leader–manager in a multicultural workplace require cultural sensitivity.

SBAR, ISBAR, ANTICipate, and I-PASS as Verbal Communication Tools

Improving and standardizing professional communication are critical to quality patient care and the reduction of errors. *SBAR, ISBAR* (adds *identification* or *introduction* as the first step), ANTICipate, and I-PASS are several strategies that have been developed to address this problem.

SBAR (Situation, Background, Assessment, and Recommendation), first used in the U.S. Navy to standardize important and urgent communication in nuclear submarines and further developed by Kaiser Permanente, is an easy-to-remember tool that provides a structured, orderly approach in providing accurate, relevant information in emergent patient situations as well as routine handoffs (Table 19.3). *Handoffs* (verbal exchange of information, which occurs between two or more health care providers about a patient's condition, treatment plan, care needs, etc.) typically occur both at change of shift and when patients are transferred to different units.

Unfortunately, these transitions do not always go smoothly. Ineffective care transition processes lead to adverse events and higher hospital readmission rates and costs. It has been estimated that 80% of serious medical errors involve miscommunication during the handoff between medical providers (Healthcare Inspirations, 2022).

Using SBAR helps health care providers avoid long narrative descriptions and ensures that facts, which are essential for the proper assessment of the patient's needs, are passed on. The SBAR technique has become The Joint Commission's stated industry best practice for standardized communication in health care because of its potential for reducing communication errors, thus increasing patient safety. In addition, The Joint Commission has added standardized communication to its *Patient Safety Goals*.

Some health care organizations have chosen to add an *identification or introduction step (ISBAR)* to SBAR because they feel it is important that the clinicians start off with an introduction

TABLE 19.3 SBAR AS A COMMUNICATION TOOL

S	Situation	Introduce yourself and the patient and briefly state the issue that you want to discuss (generally the patient's condition).
B	Background	Describe the background or context (patient's diagnosis, admission date, medical diagnosis, and treatment to date).
A	Assessment	Summarize the patient's condition and state what you think the problem is.
R	Recommendation	Identify any new treatments or changes ordered and provide opinions or recommendations for further action.

if they do not actively know the person they are speaking with during a patient handoff or over the phone. This step includes an introduction of the person doing the handoff, their role in the patient's care, and the unit they are calling from if the handoff occurs over the phone.

Other organizations have moved to an *ANTICipate* (Administrative data, New clinical information, Tasks, Illness severity, Contingency plans) model for clinicians to follow as part of a standardized handoff protocol. And still, others are now using *I-PASS* (Illness severity, Patient summary, Action list, Situational awareness and contingency planning, and Synthesis by receiver [or read-back]).

Regardless of the model used, standardization of the information passed from provider to provider during handoff can improve communication and reduce errors. There are, however, barriers to implementation. Research by Miller (2021) found that despite 94% of nurses knowing where to find the I-PASS tool in the medical record and 98% feeling there was time to ask questions, interruptions during shift change were prominent barriers to the use of I-PASS. Admissions, phone calls, and families asking for assistance represented other common distractions.

LEARNING EXERCISE 19.4

Handoff With ISBAR

Today, you were assigned to provide total patient care for Mr. Dixon. He is a 73-year-old male who was admitted for a total knee replacement 2 days ago. Today, the bloody output from Mr. Dixon's Jackson–Pratt drains increased dramatically, and the incision site appears to be reddened, swollen, and hot. He has required intravenous (IV) pain medication every 3 to 4 hours, which reduces his pain from a level 6 to 8 out of 10 to a level of 2 to 3. He is refusing to use his continuous passive motion machine because he says it is too painful. He is also nauseated and refused his lunch today. His bowel sounds are diminished. Mr. Dixon's wife is at the bedside and shares with you that the patient does not normally complain, so she is worried that something might be wrong. Mr. Dixon's surgeon is not expected to see this patient until later this evening, after the close of his private practice.

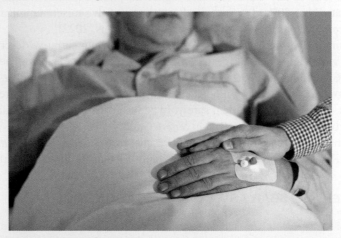

ASSIGNMENT:

Use ISBAR to prepare your handoff report for the next shift and then share what you have prepared with a peer. Ask them to critique whether you communicated all vital patient information and whether your assessment and recommendations were appropriate for the situation.

Listening Skills

Research shows that most people hear or retain only a small amount of the information given to them. In fact, communication failure is a common root cause of medical error. It is important that the leader-manager approaches listening as an opportunity to learn.

To become better listeners, leaders must first become aware of how their own experiences, values, attitudes, and biases affect how they receive and perceive messages. Second, they must overcome the information and communication overload inherent in the middle-management role. It is easy for overwhelmed managers to stop listening actively to the many subordinates who need and demand their time simultaneously.

Finally, the leader must continually work to improve listening skills by giving time and attention to the message sender. The leader's primary purpose is to receive the message being sent rather than forming a response before the transmission of the message is complete. Good listeners are better able to ask great questions—not a multitude of questions, just the ones that matter because they have been paying attention.

> The leader who actively listens gives genuine time and attention to the sender, focusing on verbal and nonverbal communication.

Boynton (2009) suggests that using a listening model such as *GRRRR* is especially helpful in organizations where disruptive behavior, toxic environments, and power struggles interfere with listening (Table 19.4). In the *Greeting* stage, a simple respectful greeting is offered to establish a professional dialogue. Next, participants demonstrate *Respectful Listening* by giving each other time to think and transmit critical information without interrupting. *Review* occurs when the speaker summarizes the information they have conveyed to make sure that the message was understood correctly. Once the speaker is finished conveying this summary and the other party has validated or clarified it, the listener has enough information to *Recommend or Request More Information*. The communication exchange ends when both parties *Reward* each other by recognizing and thanking each other for a collaborative exchange. GRRRR can be used regardless of the relative rank and status of the participants because maintaining structured communication is even more vital when power differences exist (Boynton, 2009).

Written Communication Within the Organization

Although communication may take many forms, written communication is used most often in large organizations. The written communication issued by the manager reflects greatly on both the manager and the organization. Thus, the manager must be able to write clearly and professionally and to use understandable language. Many types of written communication are used in organizations. Organizational policy, procedures, job descriptions, performance appraisals, and letters of reference are sample forms of written communication.

TABLE 19.4 GRRRR (BOYNTON, 2009) AS A LISTENING TOOL

G	Greeting	Offer greetings and establish positive environment.
R	Respectful listening	Listen without interrupting and pause to allow others to think.
R	Review	Summarize message to make sure it was heard accurately.
R	Recommend or request more information	Seek additional information as necessary.
R	Reward	Recognize that a collaborative exchange has occurred by offering thanks.

LEARNING EXERCISE 19.5

Practice Your Listening Skills

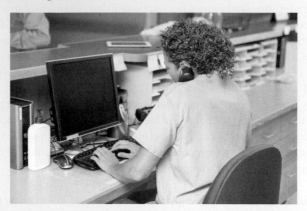

Transcript of Caller

Hi, my name is Joe Merlisch and I was a patient at the med center last week on 3 East . . . room 211 or 213, I'm not sure. Dr. Trenweth took care of me—did surgery on my left knee. My hearing aids disappeared when I was there, and Lori told me that the hospital would take care of getting them replaced, but no one has ever called me. My son Seth says that Medicare won't replace them without me paying another $850 deductible, and my private insurance says that they won't cover it at all. I think it's a problem with that "donut hole" in Medicare—isn't that what they call it? They were the Medihearing brand, and they cost me $1,700 when I bought them. I need to get them replaced because I have 60% hearing loss in my right and 70% in my left. You guys don't know what it's like when you can't hear anything anyone is saying to you. My wife, Nora, is mad at me all the time because she thinks I'm just ignoring her, and I just don't hear her. Now you guys want me to drive the 70 miles back to the hospital to look in your lost and found and see if my hearing aids are there. Well, . . . I'm not going to, and I need someone to fix this. Why don't you drive out here and show me what you've got in that lost and found? I've talked to at least 10 people today and everyone just keeps sending me from person to person. Isn't there anyone there who can fix this for me? What kind of hospital are you anyway?

ASSIGNMENT:

Form small groups. Assign a group leader and have that person quickly read the following brief telephone transcript to group members. Group members should be told to take whatever notes they would need to report the conversation to their unit manager. Group members should not be allowed to read this exercise, only listen. The group leader should read the transcript only once and then ask group members the questions at the end of the call transcript.

The group leader should then ask group members to test their listening skills by writing down answers to the following questions:

- What is the patient's name?
- What is the patient's wife's name?
- What is the doctor's name?
- What was lost?
- When was this item lost?
- What room was the patient in at the hospital?
- How much did the lost hearing aids cost?
- What brand were the hearing aids?
- How far is it from the patient's home to the hospital?
- How many people has this person spoken to today already?

Often, though, the written communication used most by managers in their daily work life is the *memo*. Purdue Online Writing Lab (2021a) suggests that business memos have a twofold purpose: They bring attention to problems, and they solve problems. Thus, it is important to choose the audience of a memo wisely and to ensure that everyone on the distribution list of the memo actually needs to read it. Typically, memos should be sent to only a small to moderate number of people. In addition, memos should not be used for highly sensitive messages, which are better communicated face-to-face or by telephone (Purdue Online Writing Lab, 2021a).

The Purdue Online Writing Lab (2021b) suggests that business memos should be composed of the following components:

- *Header* (includes the to, from, date, and subject lines): One eighth of the memo
- *Opening, context, and task* (includes the purpose of the memo, the context and problem, and the specific assignment or task): One fourth of the memo
- *Summary and discussion segment* (the details that support your ideas or plan): One half of the memo
- *Closing segment and necessary attachments* (the action that you want your reader to take and a notation about what attachments are included): One eighth of the memo

In addition, because writing is a learned skill that improves with practice, Writing Help Central (n.d.) suggests the following in writing professional correspondence:

- Keep your message short and concise. Less than one page is always preferred. Use bullets to highlight key points.
- Use the first paragraph to express the context or purpose of the memo and to introduce the problem. In the next paragraphs, address what has been done or needs to be done to address the problem at hand.
- Add a conclusion to summarize the memo, to clarify what the reader is expected to do, and to address any attachments that are a part of the memo.
- Focus on the recipient's needs. Make sure that your communication addresses the recipient's expectations and what they need to know.
- Use simple language so that the message is clear. Keep paragraphs to less than three or four sentences.
- Review the message and revise as needed. Most important communication requires several drafts. Always reread the written communication before sending it. Look for areas that might be misunderstood. Pay attention to tone. Have all the key points been made?
- Use spelling and grammar checks to be sure that the communication looks professional. Remember that your document is a direct reflection of you, and even the most important message will likely be ignored if the communication is perceived as unprofessional.

Technology as a Tool in Contemporary Organizational Communication

Technology has dramatically changed how nurses communicate and perform their work. Younger generations of nurses, who grew up using computers, cell phones, and instant messaging, recognize that technology has given us the potential for instant information access and exchange. These nurses approach and accept technology as an adjunct to their nursing cognizance and do not question its presence or use.

The Internet

Nurses are increasingly using the *internet* as both a communication tool and an information source. As an information source, the internet allows nurses to access the latest research and

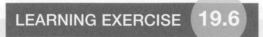

LEARNING EXERCISE 19.6

Revising a Formal Business Letter

Read the following formal business letter and assess the quality of the writing. Rewrite the letter so that it is clearly written and professional in nature. Be prepared to read your letter to the class.

Mrs. Joan Watkins
October 19, 2024
Brownie Troop 407
Anywhere, USA 00000

Dear Mrs. Watkins:

I am the official Public Relations Coordinator for County Hospital and serve as correspondence officer for requests from public service groups. We have more than 100 requests such as yours every year, so I have a very busy job! You are welcome to come and visit our hospital anytime. My assistant told me you called yesterday and wondered whether we provide tours. There is no charge for our tours. My assistant also told me that the average age of your Brownies is 8 years, so it might be most appropriate to have them visit our NICU, PICU, and ED. Please tell the girls about the units in advance so they'll be better prepared for what they will see. The philosophy at our hospital promotes community involvement, so this is one way we attempt to meet this goal. I'll be sure to arrange to have a nursing manager escort the group on your tour. Please call when you have a date and time in mind. I was a Brownie myself when I was 7 years old, so I think this is a terrific idea on your part.

Sincerely,

Ima Verbose, MSN
Public Relations Coordinator
County Hospital

best practice information so that their care can be evidence based. Indeed, the internet, which is growing faster than any other medium in the world, has enormous potential to improve Americans' health by enhancing communications and improving access to information for care providers, patients, health plan administrators, public health officials, biomedical researchers, and other health professionals (Huston, 2023).

Hospital Information Systems and Intranets

The use of *hospital information system* configurations, such as stand-alone systems, online interactive systems, networked systems, and integrative systems, has also increased. Some organizations have created internal electronic data repositories as a way of cataloging internal reference materials, such as policy and procedure manuals. This increases the likelihood that staff will be able to find such resources when they need them and that they are as up to date as possible. In such a system, references are typically converted to the portable document format (PDF) and launched electronically via an *intranet* (internal networks, not normally accessible from the internet) that allows workers and departments to share files, use websites, and collaborate (Huston, 2023).

Wireless Local Area Networking

The use of *wireless local area networking* (WLAN) is also growing. WLAN uses spread-spectrum radiofrequency modulation technology to link two or more computers or devices without using wires (Huston, 2023). This allows caregivers to access, update, and transmit critical patient and treatment information despite moving between or being located at multiple

DISPLAY 19.2 AMERICAN NURSES ASSOCIATION/NATIONAL COUNCIL OF STATE BOARDS OF NURSING PRINCIPLES FOR SOCIAL NETWORKING

1. Nurses must not transmit or place online individually identifiable patient information.
2. Nurses must observe ethically prescribed professional patient–nurse boundaries.
3. Nurses should understand that patients, colleagues, institutions, and employers may view postings.
4. Nurses should take advantage of privacy settings and seek to separate personal and professional information online.
5. Nurses should bring content that could harm a patient's privacy, rights, or welfare to the attention of appropriate authorities.
6. Nurses should participate in developing institutional policies governing online conduct.

Sources: American Nurses Association. (2011). *Principles for social networking and the nurse.* Author; National Council of State Boards of Nursing. (2011). *White paper: A nurses' guide to the use of social media.* https://www.ncsbn.org/Social_Media.pdf

sites of care. The area of outreach in the network is called the *basic service set*. Similarly, *Bluetooth* technology creates a small wireless network (called a *piconet*) between two pieces of hardware through short-range radio signals. This allows devices such as keyboards to link with personal computers and headsets to link with cell phones (Huston, 2023).

Social Media and Organizational Communication

Technologies such as social networking, texting, e-mail, and the intranet are increasing the potential for effective and efficient communication throughout the organization, and carefully utilized web-based platforms can potentially enhance practice, education, and research.

The reality, however, is that social media can be misused. It can also violate patients' rights and has been implicated in boundary violations of patients by nurses and nursing students, including blogging about specific patients and posting actual pictures of patients or body parts on Facebook. In addition, Gee and Litchman (2023) note that social media can literally expose nurses and/or their patients to billions of individuals on the internet. And although this open access may offer endless opportunities, it can also create serious breaches in privacy and exposure to internet predators and criminals. These risks have led the American Nurses Association (2011) and the National Council of State Boards of Nursing (2011) to establish the *Principles for Social Networking* shown in Display 19.2.

Gee and Litchman (2023) note, however, that if properly harnessed, social media can be a powerful tool for professional nursing practice and patient support. Nurses need to add an understanding of these new web-based platforms to their knowledge base, and nursing education is duty-bound to deliberately add social media to all levels of curriculum. Gee and Litchman conclude that social media comes with pitfalls and opportunities for both nurses and patients but suggests that now is the opportunity for nursing to embrace this new and exciting platform and use the social media tools to improve our profession and the health of our communities.

Electronic Health Records

Even health records have changed as a result of technology. The *electronic health record* (EHR) is a digital record of a patient's health history that may be made up of records from many locations and/or sources, such as hospitals, providers, clinics, and public health agencies. For example, an EHR might include immunization status, allergies, patient demographics, laboratory test and radiology results, advanced directives, current medications taken, and current health care appointments. The EHR is theoretically available 24 hours a day, 7 days a week, and has built-in safeguards to assure patient health information confidentiality and security.

In January 2004, former President George Bush set a goal that most Americans would have an EHR by 2014. This goal was endorsed by former President Barack Obama as part

LEARNING EXERCISE 19.7

Communicating on Social Networking Sites

You are part of a new graduate nurse cohort completing its residency program at a local acute care hospital. The new graduates often connect via a social networking site in the evening to share what they learned or experienced that day. Several of the group participants have discussed specific patient scenarios with the group, and although they do not share the patient's name, there is enough identifying information that you are concerned that patient confidentiality could be threatened. One nurse today shared a photo of a stage IV sacral decubitus that she took on her cell phone to demonstrate the scope and severity of such a pressure ulcer. No identifying patient information was included with the photo, but you know the photo should never have been taken in the first place, much less shared on the social networking site.

ASSIGNMENT:

Discuss what you will do. What parameters should be in place to protect patient confidentiality in groups such as these? What safeguards does the Health Insurance Portability and Accountability Act (HIPAA) provide to guide this electronic communication about patients that nurses care for?

of the American Recovery and Reinvestment Act (ARRA). At the same time, Obama offered financial incentives through Medicare and Medicaid to encourage providers and physicians to adopt certified EHRs. Providers who did not adopt an EHR by 2015 would see their Medicare reimbursements increasingly reduced over the next few years. As a result, this optional improvement really became a mandatory initiative.

LEARNING EXERCISE 19.8

When Personal and Professional Obligations Conflict

You are a registered nurse (RN) employed by an insurance company that provides workers' compensation coverage for large companies. Your job requires that you do routine health screening on new employees to identify personal and job-related behaviors that may place these clients at risk for injury or illness and then to counsel them appropriately regarding risk reduction.

One of the areas that you assess during your patient history is high-risk sexual behavior. One of the clients you saw today expressed concern that he might be positive for HIV because a former girlfriend, with whom he had unprotected sex, recently tested positive for HIV. He tells you that he is afraid to be tested "because I don't want to know if I have it." He seems firm on his refusal to be tested. You go ahead and provide him information about HIV testing and what he can do in the future to prevent transmission of the virus to himself and others.

Later that evening, you are having dinner with your 26-year-old sister, and she reveals that she has a "new love" in her life. When she tells you his name and where he works, you immediately recognize him as the client you counseled in the office today.

ASSIGNMENT:

What will you do with the information you have about this client's possible HIV exposure? Will you share it with your sister? What are the legal and ethical ramifications inherent in violating this patient's confidentiality? What are the conflicting personal and professional obligations? Would your action be the same if a casual acquaintance revealed to you that this client was her new boyfriend? Be as honest as possible in your analysis.

It has not been easy, however, to make such system-wide changes. Cost, debates about ownership of data, and communication across computer systems have posed relentless challenges.

In addition, heavy investments are required upfront, with returns that occur only over time, if at all. The 38-hospital Kaiser Permanente invested an estimated $4 billion for its system nearly 15 years ago (Pearl, 2017). Many challenges also exist in understanding and capturing relevant data electronically as part of clinical workflows, and not having the appropriate technology. Training issues also pose significant challenges.

Physicians have been especially slow to adopt EHRs. In a 2015 study, 83% of physicians expressed frustration using EHRs to support clinical communications because of poor interoperability, limited EHR messaging capabilities, and poor usability that made it difficult to find relevant clinical data (HIT Consultant, 2022).

Furthermore, the EHR may interfere with the patient–provider encounter, preventing quality information from being attained. Patients may feel less satisfied if providers focus on their computers instead of them as the face-to-face encounter may feel less personal.

Regardless of the implementation challenges, EHRs are here to stay. Most health care organizations now have EHRs, and the value of the data collected is beginning to emerge. The promise continues to be that EHRs will transform health care into a safer, more effective, and more efficient system.

Ransomware and Cyber Attacks

Ransomware is a form of malicious software that can lock and encrypt a computer or device data, and then demand a ransom to restore access (Ransomware Attacks, 2021). Anyone can unknowingly download ransomware onto a computer by opening an e-mail attachment, clicking an ad, following a link, or even visiting a website that's embedded with malware.

Between 2019 and 2020, the rate of attack on hospitals and health care facilities jumped 470%. Indeed, in 2020, more than one in three health care organizations reported ransomware threats and in the first 6 months of 2021, nearly half of all US hospitals had to disconnect their networks due to escalating ransomware attacks. Hospitals that admitted to shutting down networks due to ransomware "were a mix of those who did so proactively to avoid a damaging breach and those forced to do so because of severe malware infection" (Bilyeau, 2021, para 10).

As a result, more than 25 million patients have experienced personal health care record compromise or have otherwise seen an impact from these attacks. In addition, ransomware attacks threaten patient care and data privacy (Ransomware Attacks, 2021).

Health care organizations must proactively utilize effective security tools including antimalware software and intrusion detection/prevention solutions to help prevent, detect, and contain these attacks. Operating systems, software, and applications should be kept current and up to date and backups should be secured.

The best way for employees to avoid being exposed to ransomware—or any type of malware—is to be cautious and conscientious computer users and to avoid downloading and clicking on unknown sources (Federal Bureau of Investigation, n.d.). The protection of patient confidentiality and the assurance of safe patient care in an electronic communication environment is an essential leadership responsibility.

Communication, Confidentiality, and Health Insurance Portability and Accountability Act

Nurses have a duty to maintain confidential information revealed to them by their patients. This *confidentiality* can be breached legally only when one provider must share information about a patient so that another provider can assume care. In other words, there must be a legitimate professional need to know. The same level of confidentiality that is required to protect patient's rights is expected regarding sensitive personal communications between managers and subordinates.

> Confidentiality can be breached legally only when one provider must share information about a patient so that another provider can assume care.

The *Health Insurance Portability and Accountability Act of 1996 (HIPAA)* calls for strict protection and privacy of medical information. Enactment of HIPAA requires putting in place mechanisms and accountabilities to protect patients' privacy. Violations of HIPAA can result in significant fines for a facility. There is an ethical duty to maintain confidentiality as well.

Protecting confidentiality and privacy of personal or patient information becomes even more difficult with increased electronic communication because the information available by electronic communication is typically easier to access than traditional information-retrieval methods and because computerized databases are unable to distinguish whether the user has a legitimate right to such information. For example, the federal government has mandated computerized patient records, and many health care organizations have implemented this mandate. Unfortunately, the discussion and determination of who in the organization should have access to what information are often inadequate before such hardware is put in place, and great potential exists for violations of confidentiality. Clearly, any nurse-manager working with clinical information systems has a responsibility to see that confidentiality is maintained and that any breaches in confidentiality are dealt with swiftly and appropriately.

Group Communication

Managers must communicate with large and small groups as well as with individual employees. Because a group communicates differently than individuals do, it is essential that the manager understands group dynamics, including the sequence that each group must go through before work can be accomplished. Psychologist Bruce Tuckman, building on the work of earlier management theorists, labeled these stages—*forming*, *storming*, *norming*, and *performing*—in his classic 1965 work (Tuckman Forming, Storming, n.d.).

When people are introduced into work groups, they must go through a process of meeting each other: the *forming* stage. Here, interpersonal relationships are formed, expectations are defined, and directions are given. They then progress through a stage where there is much competition and attempts at the establishment of individual identities: the *storming* stage. Individuals in the storming stage begin to feel comfortable enough with each other to disagree, and, if managed appropriately, this discourse can lead to increased trust, positive competition, and effective bargaining. Next, the group begins to establish rules and design its work: the *norming* stage. Sometimes, norming never occurs because no one takes the time to agree on and enforce ground rules and processes. Finally, during the *performing* stage, the work gets done. Table 19.5 summarizes each stage.

Some experts suggest, however, that there another phase: *termination or closure*. In this phase, the leader guides members to summarize, express feelings, and come to closure. A celebration at the end of committee work is a good way to conclude group effort and motivates group members to participate in committees again in the future.

Tuckman's model explains that as the team develops maturity and ability, relationships establish, and the leader changes leadership style. Initially, the leader is more directive. Then they begin to move the group through coaching and delegation until the group is almost ready to detach. At this point, the team may produce a successor leader and the previous leader can move on to develop a new team (Tuckman Forming, Storming, n.d., para. 3).

TABLE **STAGES OF GROUP PROCESS**

Group Development Stage	Group Process	Task Process
Forming	Testing occurs to identify boundaries of interpersonal behaviors, establish dependency relationships with leaders and other members, and determine what is acceptable behavior.	Testing occurs to identify the tasks, appropriate rules, and methods suited to the task's performance.
Storming	Resistance to group influence is evident as members polarize into subgroups; conflict ensues and members rebel against demands imposed by the leader.	Resistance to task requirements and the differences surface regarding demands imposed by the task.
Norming	Consensus evolves as group cohesion develops; conflict and resistance are overcome.	Cooperation develops as differences are expressed and resolved.
Performing	Interpersonal structure focuses on task and its completion; roles become flexible and functional; energies are directed to task performance.	Problems are solved as the task performance improves; constructive efforts are undertaken to complete task; more of group energies are available for the task.

However, because a group's work develops over time, the addition of new members to a committee typically results in a return to the forming stage, often slowing productivity. In addition, some developmental stages will be performed again or delayed if new members join a group. Therefore, it is important when assigning members to a committee to select those who can remain until the work is finished or until their appointment time is over.

Group Dynamics

In addition to forming, storming, and norming, two other functions of groups are necessary for work to be performed. One has to do with the task or the purpose of the group, and the other has to do with the maintenance of the group or support functions. Managers should understand how groups carry out their specific tasks and roles.

Group Task Roles

There are 11 tasks that each group performs. A member may perform several tasks, but for the work of the group to be accomplished, all the necessary tasks will be carried out either by members or by the leader. These task-based roles follow:

1. *Initiator:* Contributor who proposes or suggests group goals or redefines the problem; may be more than one initiator during the group's lifetime
2. *Information seeker:* Searches for a factual basis for the group's work
3. *Information giver:* Offers an opinion of what the group's view of pertinent values should be
4. *Opinion seeker:* Seeks opinions that clarify or reflect the value of other members' suggestions
5. *Elaborator:* Gives examples or extends meanings of suggestions given and how they could work
6. *Coordinator:* Clarifies and coordinates ideas, suggestions, and activities of the group
7. *Orienter:* Summarizes decisions and actions; identifies and questions departures from predetermined goals

8. *Evaluator:* Questions group's accomplishments and compares them with a standard
9. *Energizer:* Stimulates and prods the group to act and raises the level of its actions
10. *Procedural technician:* Facilitates group action by arranging the environment
11. *Recorder:* Records the group's activities and accomplishments

Group-Building and Maintenance Roles

Group task roles contribute to the work to be done; group-building roles provide for the care and maintenance of the group. Examples of group-building roles include the following:

- *Encourager:* Accepts and praises all contributions, viewpoints, and ideas with warmth and solidarity
- *Harmonizer:* Mediates, harmonizes, and resolves conflict
- *Compromiser:* Yields their position in a conflict situation
- *Gatekeeper:* Promotes open communication and facilitates participation by all members
- *Standard setter:* Expresses or evaluates standards to evaluate group process
- *Group commentator:* Records group's process and provides feedback to the group
- *Follower:* Accepts the group's ideas and listens to discussion and decisions

Organizations need to have a mix of members—enough people to carry out the work and also people who are good at team building. One group may perform more than one function and group-building role.

Individual Roles of Group Members

Group members also carry out roles that serve their own needs. Group leaders must be able to manage members' roles so that individuals do not disrupt group productivity. The goal, however, should be management and not suppression. Not every group member has a need that results in the use of one of these roles. Eight potentially disruptive individual roles follow:

1. *Aggressor:* Expresses disapproval of others' values or feelings through jokes, verbal attacks, or envy
2. *Blocker:* Persists in expressing negative points of view and resurrects dead issues
3. *Recognition seeker:* Works to focus positive attention on themselves
4. *Self-confessor:* Uses the group setting as a forum for personal expression
5. *Playboy:* Remains uninvolved and demonstrates cynicism, nonchalance, or horseplay
6. *Dominator:* Attempts to control and manipulate the group
7. *Help seeker:* Uses expressions of personal insecurity, confusion, or self-deprecation to manipulate sympathy from members
8. *Special interest pleader:* Cloaks personal prejudices or biases by ostensibly speaking for others

LEARNING EXERCISE 19.9

Identifying Group Stages and Roles

Compile a list of the various groups with which you are currently involved. Describe the stage of each one. Did it take longer for some of your groups to get to the performing stage than others? If membership in the group changed, describe what happened to the productivity level. Can you identify which individuals in the group are fulfilling group task roles? Group maintenance and building roles? Individual roles?

> Managers must be well grounded in group dynamics and group roles because of the need to facilitate group communication and productivity within the organization.

Whereas managers must understand group dynamics and roles to facilitate communication and productivity in teams, leaders tend to make an even greater impact on group effectiveness. Dynamic leaders inspire followers toward participative management by how they work and communicate in teams. Leaders keep group members on course, draw out the shy, politely cut off the garrulous, and protect the weak.

Communication and Team Building

Melnyk et al. (2023) suggest that communication has always been an important skill for all clinicians and teams. Fagnani (2021) agrees, noting that communication and team building are intertwined because team-building activities encourage trust, cooperation, and communication within a group and improving communication enhances how workers interact with one another. It is a responsibility of the leader-manager to use communication in such a way that it builds team relationships for mutual goal attainment.

Melnyk et al. (2023) agree, noting that communication, whether effective or ineffective, is jointly owned by all members of a team, and each member is equally capable of engaging in good or bad communication tactics. Each member of the team enters the communication with different worldviews, values, fears, confidence levels, and assumed place within the hierarchy. Effective communication then requires conscious effort, shared commitment, and hard work.

Melnyk et al. (2023) note that leaders can significantly impact the success of teams and communication efforts in their organizations in a variety of ways. First, leaders must be effective communicators themselves and role model excellent communication skills in all settings. In addition, leaders are responsible to establish and uphold administrative structures to require and support effective teamwork and communication in their organizations. Finally, leaders must have the skills to effectively confront/manage conflicts that arise out of poor communication.

In addition, leader-managers must communicate what is expected of each team member. Effective leader-managers listen to what team members have to say about each other and to them in a nonjudgmental manner. If team members share a concern, steps should be taken to resolve the issue as quickly as possible and keep the team informed regarding the resolution.

When possible, leader-managers should regularly schedule team meetings to make sure everyone shares common priorities. These meetings are also a good time to recognize the progress the team has made and to build trust and cooperation. In addition, leaders should pay attention to the ways in which team members work together and take steps to improve communication, cooperation, trust, and respect in those relationships. How team members feel about their coworkers can affect how effectively a team works together (Huston, 2020).

Integrating Leadership and Management in Organizational, Interpersonal, and Group Communication in Team Building

Communication is critical to successful leadership and management. A manager has the formal authority and responsibility to communicate with many people in the organization.

Cultural diversity and rapidly flourishing communication technologies also add to the complexity of this organizational communication. Because of this complexity, the manager must understand each unique situation well enough to be able to select the most appropriate internal communication network or channel.

After selecting a communication channel, the manager faces an even greater challenge in communicating the message clearly, either verbally or in writing, in a language appropriate for the message and the receiver. To select the most appropriate communication mode for a specific message, the manager must determine what should be told, to whom, and when. Because communication is a learned skill, managers can improve their written and verbal communication with repetition.

The interpersonal communication skills are more reflective of the leadership role. Sensitivity to verbal and nonverbal communication; recognition of status, power, and authority as barriers to manager–subordinate communication; and consistent use of assertiveness techniques are all leadership skills. Nurse-leaders who are perceptive and sensitive to the environment and people around them have a keen understanding of how the unit is functioning at any time and can intervene appropriately when problems arise. Through consistent verbal and nonverbal communication, the nurse-leader can be a role model for subordinates.

The integrated leader-manager also uses groups to facilitate team communication. Group work is a tool for increasing productivity. All members of work groups should be assisted with role clarification and productive group dynamics.

Organizational communication requires both management functions and leadership skills. Management functions in communication ensure productivity and continuity through appropriate sharing of information. Leadership skills ensure appraisal and intervention in meeting expressed and tacit human resource needs. Leadership skills in communication also allow the leader-manager to clarify organizational goals and to work with teams to reach those goals. Communication within the organization would fail if both leadership skills and management functions were not present.

Key Concepts

- Communication forms the core of management activities and cuts across all phases of the management process. It is also the core of the nurse–patient, nurse–nurse, and nurse–physician relationship.
- Depending on the manager's position in the hierarchy, the majority of managerial time is often directed at some type of organizational communication; thus, organizational communication is a high-level management function.
- Because most managerial communication time is spent speaking and listening, managers must have excellent interpersonal communication skills.
- Communication in large organizations is particularly difficult due to their complexity and size.

- Managers must understand the structure of the organization and recognize whom their decisions will affect. Both formal and informal communication networks need to be considered.
- The clarity of the message is significantly affected by the mode of communication used. In general, the more direct the communication, the greater the probability of clear communication. The more people involved in filtering the communication, the greater the chance of distortion.
- Written communication is used most often in large organizations.
- A manager's written communication reflects greatly on both the manager and the organization. Thus, managers must be able to write clearly and professionally and use understandable language.

- The incongruence between verbal and non-verbal messages is a significant barrier to effective interpersonal communication.
- Effective leaders are congruent in their verbal and nonverbal communication so that followers are clear about the messages they receive. Likewise, leaders are sensitive to nonverbal and verbal messages from followers and look for inconsistencies that may indicate unresolved problems or needs.
- To be successful in the directing phase of management, the leader must have well-developed skills in assertive communication.
- SBAR, ISBAR ANTICipate, and I-PASS provide structured, orderly approaches to provide accurate, relevant information in emergent patient situations as well as routine handoffs.
- Most people hear or retain only a small amount of the information given to them.
- Active listening is an interpersonal communication skill that improves with practice.

- Using a listening model such as *GRRRR* is especially helpful in organizations where disruptive behavior, toxic environments, and power struggles interfere with listening.
- Rapidly flourishing communication technologies have great potential to increase the efficiency and effectiveness of organizational communication. They also, however, pose increasing challenges to patient confidentiality.
- Adding new members to an established group disrupts productivity and group development.
- Group members perform certain important tasks that facilitate work.
- Group members also perform roles that assist with group-building activities.
- Some group members will perform roles to meet their individual needs.
- Communication and team building are intertwined because team-building activities encourage trust, cooperation, and communication within a group and improving communication enhances how workers interact with one another.

Additional Learning Exercises and Applications

LEARNING EXERCISE 19.10

Writing a Memo

You are a school nurse. In the last 2 weeks, nine cases of head lice have been reported in four different classrooms. The potential for spread is high, and both the teachers and parents are growing anxious.

ASSIGNMENT:

Compose a memo for distribution to the teachers. Your goals are to inform, reassure, and direct future inquiries.

LEARNING EXERCISE 19.11

Identifying and Rephrasing Nonassertive Responses

Decide if the following responses are an example of assertive, aggressive, passive–aggressive, or passive behavior. Change those that you identify as aggressive, passive–aggressive, or passive into assertive responses.

Situation	Response
1. A coworker withdraws instead of saying what is on his mind. You say:	"I guess you are uncomfortable talking about what's bothering you. It would be better if you talked to me."
2. This is the third time in 2 weeks that your coworker has asked for a ride home because her car is not working. You say:	"You're taking advantage of me, and I won't stand for it. It's your responsibility to get your car fixed."
3. You note that a nursing colleague is charting her medications in the electronic medical record (EMR) before she gives them. You say:	"Your practice does not follow current best practices or hospital policy. This is placing the hospital and your patients at risk."
4. You would like to have a turn at being in charge on your shift. You say to your head nurse:	"Do you think that, ah, you could see your way clear to letting me be in charge once in a while?"
5. A committee meeting is being established. The proposed time is convenient for other people but not for you. The time makes it impossible for you to attend meetings regularly. When you are asked about the time, you say:	"Well, I guess it's OK. I'm not going to be able to attend very much, but it fits into everyone else's schedule."
6. In a conversation, a male colleague suddenly asks, "What do you women libbers want anyway?" You respond:	"Fairness and equality."
7. An employee makes a lot of mistakes in his work. You say:	"You're a lazy and sloppy worker!"
8. You are the only woman in a meeting with seven men. At the beginning of the meeting, the Chair asks you to be the secretary. You respond:	"No. I'm sick and tired of being the secretary just because I'm the only woman in the group."
9. A coworker asks to borrow your stethoscope. You say:	"Well, I guess so. A coworker walked off with mine last week, and this new one cost me $95. Be sure you return it, OK?"
10. You are interpreting the intake and output (I&O) sheet for a coworker, and he interrupts you. You say:	"You could understand this if you'd stop interrupting me and listen."

LEARNING EXERCISE 19.12

Memo to Chief Executive Officer Leads to Miscommunication

Carol White, the coordinator for the multidisciplinary mental health outpatient services of a 150-bed psychiatric hospital, feels frustrated because the hospital is very centralized. She believes that this keeps the hospital's therapists and nurse-managers from being as effective as they could be if they had more authority. Therefore, she has worked out a plan to decentralize her department, giving the therapists and nurse-managers more control and new titles. She sent her new plan to Chief Executive Officer Joe Short and has just received this memo in return.

Dear Ms. White:

The Board of Directors and I met to review your plan and think it is a good one. In fact, we have been thinking along the same lines for quite some time now. I'm sure you must have heard of our plans. Because we recently contracted with a physician's group to cover our crisis center, we believe that this would be a good time to decentralize in other ways. We suggest that your new substance abuse coordinator report directly to the new Chief of Mental Health. In addition, we believe that your new director of the suicide prevention center should report directly to the Chief of Mental Health. He then will report to me.

I am pleased that we are both moving in the same direction and have the same goals. We will be setting up meetings in the future to iron out the small details.

Sincerely,

Joe Short, CEO

ASSIGNMENT:

How and why did Carol's plan go astray? How did her mode of communication affect the outcome? Could the outcome have been prevented? What communication mode would have been most appropriate for Carol to use in sharing her plan with Joe? What should be her plan now? Explain your rationale.

LEARNING EXERCISE 19.13

Writing a Letter of Reference

Unit managers are frequently asked to write letters of reference for employees who have left their employment. The information used in writing these letters comes from performance evaluations, personal interviews with staff and patients, evidence of continuing education, and personal observations. Assume that you are a unit manager and that you have collected the following information on Mary Doe, a registered nurse (RN) who worked at your facility for 3 months before abruptly resigning with 48 hours' notice.

Performance Evaluation

Three-month evaluation scant.

- The following criteria were marked "competent": amount of work accomplished, relationships with patients and coworkers, work habits, and basic skills.
- The following criteria were identified as "needing improvement": quality of work, communication skills, and leadership skills.
- No criteria were marked unsatisfactory or outstanding.
- Narrative comments were limited to the following: "has a bit of a chip on her shoulder," "works independently a lot," and "assessment skills improving."

Interviews With Staff

- Coworker RN Judy: "She was OK. She was a little strange—she belonged to some kind of traveling religious cult. In fact, I think that's why she left her job."
- Coworker licensed vocational nurse (LVN)/licensed practical nurse (LPN) Lisa: "Mary was great. She got all her work done. I never had to help her with her meds or AM care. She took her turn at floating, which is more than I can say for some of the other RNs."
- Coworker RN John: "When I was the charge nurse, I found that I needed to seek Mary out to find out what was going on with her patients. It made me really uncomfortable."
- Coworker LVN/LPN Joe: "Mary hated it here—she never felt like she belonged. The charge nurse was always hassling her about little things, and it really seemed unfair."

(continues on page 506)

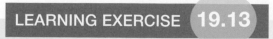

LEARNING EXERCISE 19.13

Writing a Letter of Reference (continued)

Patient Comments

- "She helped me with my bath and got all my pills on time. She was a good nurse."
- "I don't remember her."
- "She was so busy—I appreciated how efficient she was at how she did her job."
- "I remember Mary. She told me she really liked older people. I wish she had had more time to sit down and talk to me."

Notes from Personnel File

Twenty-four years old; graduated from 3-year diploma school, 2 years ago; has worked in three jobs since that time

Continuing Education

Current cardiopulmonary resuscitation (CPR) card; no other continuing education completed at this facility

ASSIGNMENT:

Mary Doe's prospective employer, with written permission from Mary to share information, has requested a letter of reference to accompany Mary's application to become a hospice nurse/counselor. No form has been provided, so you must determine an appropriate format. Decide which information you should include in your letter, and which should be omitted. Will you weigh some information more heavily than other information? Would you make any recommendations about Mary Doe's suitability for the hospice job? Be prepared to read your letter aloud to the class and justify your rationale for the content that you included.

LEARNING EXERCISE 19.14

Team Building

You are the evening charge nurse of a medical unit. The staff on your unit has voiced displeasure in how requests for days off are handled. Your manager has given you the task of forming a committee and reviewing the present policy regarding requests for days off on the unit. On your committee are four licensed practical nurses (LPNs)/licensed vocational nurses (LVNs), three certified nursing assistants, and five registered nurses (RNs). All shifts are represented. There are three men among the group members, and there is a broad range of ethnic and cultural groups.

Tomorrow will be your fourth meeting, and you are becoming a bit frustrated because the meetings do not seem to be accomplishing much to reach the objective that the group was charged with: developing a fair method of handling special requested days off that are not part of the normal rotation.

On your first meeting, you spent time getting to know group members and identified the objective. Various committee members contacted other hospitals, and others did a literature search to determine how other institutions handled this matter. During the second meeting, this material was reviewed by all members. At the last meeting, the group was very contentious. In fact, several raised their voices. Others sat quietly, and some seemed to pout. Only the three men could agree on anything. One LPN/LVN thought that the RNs were overly represented. One RN thought that the policy for day-off requests should be separated into three different policies—one for each classification. You are not sure how to bring this team together or what, if any, action you should take.

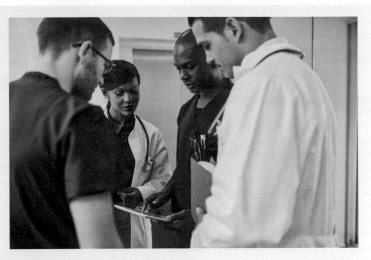

ASSIGNMENT:

• • • • • • • •

Review the section in this chapter about how groups work. Write a one-page essay on what is happening in the group and answer the following questions: Should you add members to the committee? Does your group have too many task members and not enough team-building members? What should be your role in getting the group to perform its task? What could be some strategies you could use that would perhaps bring the team together?

REFERENCES

American Nurses Association. (2011). *Principles for social networking and the nurse.* Author.

Answers.com. (2022). *What is communication?* Retrieved June 15, 2022, from http://www.answers.com/Q/What_is_communication

Bilyeau, N. (2021, August 18). Newest target of cyber attacks: America's hospitals. *The Crime Report.* https://thecrimereport.org/2021/08/18/hospitals-cyberattacks/

Boynton, B. (2009). How to improve your listening skills. *American Nurse Today, 4*(9), 50–51.

Doyle, A. (2021, March 13). Communication skills for workplace success. *The Balance Careers.* https://www.thebalancecareers.com/communication-skills-list-2063779

Fagnani, S. (2021). Team building activities on listening. *Chron.* https://smallbusiness.chron.com/team-building-activities-listening-20014.html

Federal Bureau of Investigation. (n.d.). *Scams and safety: Ransomware.* Retrieved June 15, 2022, from https://www.fbi.gov/scams-and-safety/common-scams-and-crimes/ransomware

Gee, P., & Litchman, M. L. (2023). The use of social media in nursing: Pitfalls and opportunities (chapter 14). In C. J. Huston (Ed.), *Professional issues in nursing: Challenges and opportunities* (6th ed., pp. 198–211). Wolters Kluwer.

Gendered communication: Differences in communication styles (2021, May 27). Point Park University. https://online.pointpark.edu/public-relations-and-advertising/gender-differences-communication-styles/

Healthcare Inspirations. (2022). *Hand-off communications.* Retrieved June 15, 2022, from http://www.healthcareinspirations.com/hci_hand-off_communications.html

HIT Consultant. (2022). *83% of physicians are resistant to use EHRs for clinical communications.* Study results of January 19, 2015. Retrieved June 15, 2022, from https://hitconsultant.net/2015/01/19/physicians-resistantehrs-clinical-communications/

Huston, C. J. (2020). *The road to positive work cultures.* Sigma Theta Tau International Honor Society of Nursing.

Huston, C. J. (2023). Technology in the health care workplace: Benefits, limitations, and challenges (chapter 21). In C. J. Huston (Ed.), *Professional issues in nursing: Challenges and opportunities* (6th ed., pp. 302–318). Wolters Kluwer.

Internal auditors training focuses on 'impact of non-verbal communication' (2021, November 20). Gulf Times. https://www.gulf-times.com/story/704828/Internal-auditors-training-focuses-on-impact-of-no#:~:text=Shivram%20was%20the%20semi-finalist%20of%20the%20World%20Champion,Hence%2C%20what%20you%20don%E2%80%99t%20say%20counts%20a%20lot

Mayo Clinic Staff. (1998–2022). *Being assertive: Reduce stress, communicate better.* Retrieved June 15, 2022, from http://www.mayoclinic.com/health/assertive/SR00042

Melnyk, B. M., Malloch, K., & Gallagher-Ford, L. (2023). Developing effective leaders to meet 21st-century health care challenges (chapter 3). In C. J. Huston (Ed.), *Professional issues in nursing: Challenges and opportunities* (6th ed., pp. 32–51). Wolters Kluwer.

Miller, D. (2021). I-PASS as a nursing communication tool. *Pediatric Nursing, 47*(1), 30–37.

Mind Tools Content Team. (2022). *Team building exercises— Communication. Six ways to improve communication skills.* Retrieved June 15, 2022, from https://www.mindtools.com/pages/article/team-building-communication.htm

National Council of State Boards of Nursing. (2011). *White paper: A nurses' guide to the use of social media.* https://www.ncsbn.org/Social_Media.pdf

Nicholson, J. (2021, March 2). Proxemics: How interpersonal distance communicates intimacy. *Psychology Today.* https://www.psychologytoday.com/us/blog/the-attraction-doctor/202103/proxemics-how-interpersonal-distance-communicates-intimacy#:~:text=Posted%20Mar%2002%2C%202021%20The%20study%20of%20what,of%20nonverbal%20communication%20for%20successful%20dating%20and%20relating

Nonverbal Communication Portal. (n.d.). *Eye contact.* Retrieved June 15, 2022, from https://sites.google.com/site/nonverbalcommunicationportal/forms-of-nonverbal-communication/eye-contact

Pearl, R. (2017, June 15). What health systems, hospitals, and physicians need to know about implementing electronic health records. *Harvard Business Review.* https://hbr.org/2017/06/what-health-systems-hospitals-and-physicians-need-to-know-about-implementing-electronic-health-records#:~:text=Summary.%20A%20decade%20ago%2C%20Kaiser%20Permanente%20installed%20the,time%20was%20estimated%20to%20be%20around%20%24%244%20billion

Purdue Online Writing Lab. (2021a). *Audience and purpose.* Retrieved June 15, 2022 from https://owl.purdue.edu/owl/subject_specific_writing/professional_technical_writing/memos/audience_and_purpose.html

Purdue Online Writing Lab. (2021b). *Format.* Retrieved June 15, 2022, from https://owl.purdue.edu/owl/subject_specific_writing/professional_technical_writing/memos/format.html

Ransomware attacks on hospitals 2022. (2021, August 10). Cyber Talk. https://www.cybertalk.org/2021/08/10/best-practices-to-avoid-ransomware-attacks-on-hospitals-in-2021/

Reference (Staff Writer). (2020, April 7). *What are environmental barriers in communication?* https://www.reference.com/business-finance/environmental-barriers-communication-dbffee910dd7b6e3

Tuckman: Forming, storming, norming, performing model. (n.d.). Retrieved July 26, 2022, from https://www.businessballs.com/team-management/tuckman-forming-storming-norming-performing-model/

Writing Help Central. (n.d.). *Letter writing resources.* Retrieved November 30, 2021, from http://www.writing-help-central.com/letter-writing.html

Delegation

*... I not only use all the brains I have, but all that I can borrow.—**Woodrow Wilson***

*... The best executive is one who has sense enough to pick good people to do what he wants done, and self-restraint enough to keep from meddling with them while they do it.—**Theodore Roosevelt***

*... Deciding what not to do is as important as deciding what to do.—**Jessica Jackley***

LEARNING OBJECTIVES

The learner will:

- identify specific strategies that increase the likelihood of effective delegation
- recognize delegation as a learned skill imperative to professional nursing practice
- delegate tasks using appropriate priority setting and personnel in specific situations
- differentiate between tasks that should and should not be delegated to licensed and unlicensed personnel based on skill and education level as well as individual state scope of practice guidelines

- identify common causes of underdelegation, overdelegation, and improper delegation as well as strategies to overcome these delegation errors
- describe why providing adequate information and authority to others is necessary for them to successfully complete delegated tasks
- identify factors that must be considered when determining what tasks can be safely delegated to subordinates
- discuss how the role of the registered nurse as delegator has changed with the increased use of nursing assistive personnel
- identify leadership strategies that can be used to reduce subordinate resistance to delegation
- describe cultural phenomena that must be considered when delegating to a multicultural staff or when encouraging multicultural staff to delegate
- describe actions the manager can take to reduce the liability of supervision, particularly when delegating tasks

Introduction

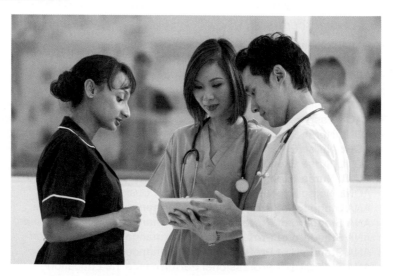

Delegation has long been a function of registered nursing. Indeed, the professional nurse (registered nurse [RN]) role has changed in many settings from one of direct care provider to one requiring the delegation of direct patient care to others (Huston, 2023).

Delegation can be defined simply as getting work done through others or as directing the performance of one or more people to accomplish organizational goals. It is not the same as *assignment*, which involves distributing work to a qualified person or persons for implementation of a specific activity or set of activities within their job description (American Nurses Association [ANA] & National Council of State Boards of Nursing [NCSBN], n.d.). In delegation, the individual transfers the authority to perform a specific activity from their own practice to an individual qualified to perform that task but retains accountability for the delegated task.

Even more complex definitions of delegation, supervision, and assignment have been created by the ANA and the NCSBN in response to the complexity of delegation in today's health care arena, where significant numbers of unlicensed workers provide direct patient care. Historically, the ANA and the NCSBN defined delegation differently, with the ANA defining delegation as the transfer of responsibility for the performance of a task from one person to another and the NCSBN defining delegation as transferring to a competent individual the authority to perform a selected nursing task in a selected situation (Huston, 2023). Both groups have come together, however, to issue a *Joint Statement on Delegation*, intended to support nurses in using delegation safely and effectively (ANA & NCSBN, n.d.). In addition, both suggest that delegation is a skill that must be taught and practiced for proficiency.

Experts also agree that delegation is an essential element of the directing phase of the management process because much of the work accomplished by managers occurs not only through their own efforts but also through those of their subordinates. Frequently, there is too much work to be accomplished by one person. In these situations, delegation becomes synonymous with productivity and is not an option—but a necessity.

There are many good reasons for delegating. Sometimes, managers must delegate routine tasks so they are free to handle problems that are more complex or require a higher level of expertise. Managers may also delegate work if someone else is better prepared or has greater expertise or knowledge about how to solve a problem. Delegation can also be used to provide learning or "stretching" opportunities for subordinates. Subordinates who are not delegated enough responsibility often become bored, nonproductive, and ineffective. Thus, in delegating, the leader-manager contributes to employees' personal and professional development.

As managers gain the maturity and self-confidence needed to delegate wisely, they increase their impact and power both within and outside the organization. Subordinates gain self-esteem and increased job satisfaction from the responsibility and authority given to them, and the organization moves a step closer toward achieving its goals. The leadership roles and management functions inherent in delegation are shown in Display 20.1.

> The mark of a great leader is when they can recognize the excellent performance of someone else and allow others to shine for their accomplishments.

DISPLAY 20.1 LEADERSHIP ROLES AND MANAGEMENT FUNCTIONS ASSOCIATED WITH DELEGATION

Leadership Roles

1. Assures that organizational guidelines regarding delegation are current, reflecting best practices
2. Functions as a role model, supporter, and resource person in delegating tasks to subordinates
3. Encourages followers to use delegation as a time management strategy and team-building tool
4. Assists followers in identifying situations appropriate for delegation
5. Communicates clearly when delegating tasks
6. Maintains patient safety as a minimum criterion in determining the most appropriate person to carry out a delegated task
7. Plans ahead and delegates proactively, rather than waiting until time urgency is present and crisis responses are required
8. Conveys a feeling of confidence and encouragement to the individual who has taken on a delegated task
9. Is an informed and active participant in the development of local, state, and national guidelines for nursing assistive personnel (NAP) scope of practice
10. Is sensitive to how cultural phenomena affect transcultural delegation
11. Uses delegation as a means for stretching and empowering workers to learn new skills and be successful
12. Works to establish a culture of mutual trust, teamwork, and open communication so that delegation becomes a strategy that health care workers feel comfortable using to achieve organizational, patient, and personal goals

continues on page 512

Management Functions

1. Creates job descriptions and scope of practice statements for all personnel, including NAP, that conform to national, state, and professional recommendations for ensuring safe patient care
2. Is knowledgeable regarding legal liabilities of subordinate supervision
3. Assesses accurately subordinates' capabilities and motivation when delegating
4. Delegates a level of authority necessary to complete delegated tasks
5. Shares accountability for delegated tasks
6. Attempts consciously to see the subordinate's perspective to reduce the likelihood of resistance in delegation
7. Develops and implements a periodic review process for all delegated tasks
8. Avoids overburdening subordinates by giving them permission to refuse delegated tasks
9. Counsels and/or disciplines employees appropriately when they fail to carry out appropriately delegated tasks
10. Provides recognition or reward as appropriate for the completion of delegated tasks
11. Provides formal education and training opportunities on delegation principles for staff

Delegating Effectively

Most delegation errors could be avoided if the five rights of delegation, identified by the ANA and NCSBN (n.d.), were followed. These are shown in Table 20.1.

Yet, delegation is not easy. It requires you to trust somebody else to perform a task that you believe to be important. It also takes effort: You must explain how you do a task, train somebody else to do it, and then oversee the delegated task. However, it is also critical to managerial productivity and efficiency. Strategies that increase the likelihood of successful and effective delegation are shown in Display 20.2. Each of these strategies is detailed in the following sections.

Identify Necessary Skill and Education Levels

Identify the skill or educational level necessary to complete the job. Often, legal and licensing statutes such as the Nurse Practice Act (NPA) determine the scope of practice for the RN in each state. The challenge is that the RN must also understand the scope of practice of others on the nursing team who are providing patient care.

For example, each state regulates what licensed practical nurses (LPNs) or licensed vocational nurses (LVNs) can do. Greenwood (2021) notes that intravenous (IV) therapy is within the scope of practice for both RNs and LPNs/LVNs in most states, but some states require LPNs/LVNs to complete a course in IV therapy to administer IV solutions. Other states allow

TABLE 20.1 THE FIVE RIGHTS OF DELEGATION

Right task	One that is delegable for a specific patient
Right circumstances	Appropriate patient setting, available resources, and other relevant factors considered
Right person	Right person is delegating the right task to the right person to be performed on the right person
Right direction/communication	Clear, concise description of the task, including its objective, limits, and expectations
Right level of supervision	Appropriate monitoring, evaluation, intervention, as needed, and feedback

Source: American Nurses Association & National Council of State Boards of Nursing. (n.d.). *Joint statement on delegation*. https://www.ncsbn.org/Delegation_joint_statement_NCSBN-ANA.pdf

DISPLAY 20.2 STRATEGIES FOR SUCCESSFUL DELEGATION

Identify necessary skill and education levels to complete the delegated task.
Plan ahead; delegate before you become overwhelmed.
Select and empower capable personnel.
Communicate the goals of the delegation clearly.
Set deadlines and monitor progress.
Monitor the delegated task and provide guidance.
Evaluate performance.
Reward the completion of successfully delegated tasks.

the LPN/LVN to add vitamins to an IV solution but not to give IV antibiotics. In some states, dialysis therapy can be delegated to LPNs/LVNs, whereas in others, it is prohibited.

In the state of California, the duties of the LVN include, but are not limited to, the provision of basic hygienic nursing care; measurement of temperature, pulse, respirations, and blood pressure; administration and documentation of basic prescribed medications; and performance of skin testing and patient education (Shasta College, 2021). In New York, however, an LPN cannot perform patient assessments independently, develop a nursing care plan, administer IV chemotherapy, or give any medications by direct IV push (Greenwood, 2021). In Nebraska, an LPN cannot perform triage, coordinate, and manage care, or perform activities that require independent nursing judgment. Nor can they insert a catheter for IV therapy or give IV fluids to pediatric patients (Greenwood, 2021).

Different rules also apply in each state for the delegation to unlicensed personnel. The California Board of Registered Nursing (2010) notes that unlicensed personnel should never be assigned tasks that require a substantial amount of scientific knowledge or technical skill. Examples of tasks that should not be delegated to unlicensed assistive personnel (UAP) include preprocedure assessment and postprocedure evaluation of the patient; handling of invasive lines, sterile technique, or procedure on a patient; parenteral medications or lines; nursing process including patient assessment, monitoring, or evaluating; triaging of patients; and patient education. Instead, UAPs should be assigned basic activities of daily living such as bathing, feeding, ambulating, vital signs, weight, assistance with elimination, and maintaining a safe environment.

Nurses then must be aware of their state NPA essential elements regarding delegation, including the following:

- The state's NPA definition of delegation
- Items that cannot be delegated
- Items that cannot be routinely delegated
- Guidelines for RNs about tasks that can be delegated
- A description of professional nursing practice
- A description of RN, LPN/LVN, and UAP scope of practice
- The degree of supervision required to complete a task
- The guidelines for lowering delegation risks
- Warnings about inappropriate delegation
- If there is a restricted use of the word *nurse* to licensed staff

In addition, the manager should know the official job description expectations for each worker classification in the organization, as they may be more restrictive than the state NPA.

Plan Ahead; Delegate Before You Become Overwhelmed

Plan ahead when identifying tasks to be accomplished. Always try to delegate before you become overwhelmed. In addition, always be sure to carefully assess the situation before delegating and to clearly delineate the desired outcomes.

Select and Empower Capable Personnel

Identify which individuals can complete the job in terms of capability and time to do so. It is a leadership role to stretch new and capable employees who want opportunities to learn and grow. Managing employee workload is critical, however, when delegating because overburdened employees may find it impossible to compete assigned tasks and will be less likely to learn the desired skills. In addition, it is important to have reasonable expectations of what the selected individual can do with the time and resources available.

Also, look for employees who are innovative and willing to take risks. The person to whom the task is being delegated should consider the task to be important. This does not suggest, however, that skill and expertise are not needed. Leader-managers should always ask the individuals to whom they are delegating if they can complete the delegated task and validate this perception by direct observation.

Delegate the authority and the responsibility necessary to complete the task. Nothing is more frustrating to a creative and productive employee than not having the resources or authority to carry out a well-developed plan.

Communicate the Goals of the Delegation Clearly

The goals for delegation and the expected deliverables should always be clearly communicated. This includes identifying any limitations or qualifications that are being imposed on the delegated task. In addition, communication should include what is being delegated, the purpose and goal of the task, any limitations for task completion including a timeline, and the expectations for reporting. The leader-manager, however, should always leave the employee room for some independent thought and creativity.

Set Deadlines and Monitor Progress

Set timelines and monitor how the task is being accomplished through informal but regularly scheduled meetings. This shows an interest on the part of the leader-manager, provides for a periodic review of progress, and encourages ongoing communication to clarify any questions or misconceptions. In doing so, staff receive appropriate feedback to be successful. In addition, this keeps the delegated task before the subordinate and the leader-manager so that both share accountability for its completion. Although the final responsibility belongs to the delegator, the subordinate doing the task accepts responsibility for completing it appropriately and is accountable to the person who delegated the task.

> While you remain responsible for delivering the results of the tasks you delegate, excessive supervision can demoralize the employee.

Monitor the Delegated Task and Provide Guidance

The leader-manager should convey a feeling of confidence and encouragement to the individual who has taken on a delegated task. If the worker is having difficulty carrying out the delegated task, the leader-manager should be available as a role model and resource in identifying alternative solutions. Leaders should encourage employees, however, to attempt to solve problems themselves first, although they should always be willing to answer questions about the task or to clarify desired outcomes as necessary.

Finding a balance between providing guidance and allowing others to best determine how to accomplish a delegated task, however, is sometimes difficult. Although the desired outcome should be specified, it is important to give the subordinate feedback and an appropriate degree of autonomy in deciding exactly how the work can be accomplished. The leader-manager should monitor the delegation but not hamper that independence unless absolutely necessary.

Reassuming the delegated task should be a manager's last resort because this action fosters a sense of failure in the employee and demotivates rather than motivates. Delegation is useless if the manager is unwilling to allow divergence in problem solving and thus redoes all work that has been delegated. However, the manager may need to delegate work previously assigned to an employee so that the employee has time to do the newly assigned task.

Evaluate Performance

Evaluate the delegation experience after the task has been completed. Include positive and negative aspects of how the person completed the task. Were the outcomes achieved? Ask the individual you delegated to what you could have done differently to facilitate their completion of the delegated tasks. This shared reflection encourages the development of a mutually trusting and productive relationship between delegators and subordinates.

Reward the Completion of Successfully Delegated Tasks

Be sure to appropriately reward a successfully completed task. Leaders are often measured by the successes of those on their teams. Therefore, the more recognition team members receive, the more recognition will be given to their leader.

> The right to delegate and the ability to provide formal rewards for successful completion of delegated tasks reflect the legitimate authority inherent in the management role.

Common Delegation Errors

Delegation is not intuitive for most people; instead, it is a critical leadership skill that must be learned. Salemme (2021) states that the major challenge in delegating is knowing what to delegate and what not to delegate. When delegation is inappropriate, significant time and energy can be spent doing the wrong tasks.

Unfortunately, only 30% of managers believe they know how to delegate tasks with efficiency, and within those, only one in three of their subordinates judge their superiors to be good delegators (Salemme, 2021). Many managers then need to improve their expertise in this specific area.

In addition, nurses in clinical roles must have highly developed delegation skills. Delegation errors can lead to patients not receiving the care that they need, increasing the risk of patient harm. It is not realistic for nurses to expect to accomplish every task that comes their way. Only so much can be accomplished in a day and trying to take on too much too often can quickly lead to fatigue and burnout. That's why learning how to successfully delegate tasks early on in one's nursing career is so important.

Frequent mistakes made in delegating include underdelegating, overdelegating, and improper delegating (Display 20.3).

DISPLAY 20.3 COMMON DELEGATION ERRORS

1. Underdelegating
2. Overdelegating
3. Improper delegating

Underdelegating

Underdelegating frequently stems from the individual's false assumption that delegation may be interpreted as a lack of ability on their part to do the job correctly or completely. Delegation does not need to limit the individual's control, prestige, and power; rather, delegation can extend their influence and capability by increasing what can be accomplished. In fact, delegation can be empowering, both to the person delegating and to the person being delegated to. That's because delegation suggests trust and belief in the person being delegated to. When people feel trusted, they are more willing to take risks and generally work harder to be successful.

Another cause of underdelegating is the individual's desire to complete the whole job personally due to a lack of trust in the subordinates; some people believe that they need the experience or that they can do it better and faster than anyone else, and indeed, sometimes, this is the case. This is especially true for individuals who are new to delegation because delegation requires them to give up some control.

Similarly, some individuals underdelegate because they have an emotional attachment to the task that must be completed. Thompson (2021) notes that some people are simply too emotionally invested in the work to assign it to someone else. For example, they may have a vision in their mind of the desired end product, and do not want someone else taking it in a different direction.

> It will likely be unnerving (at least initially) to allow a team member to complete a task for which you are ultimately responsible.

Other individuals underdelegate because there is not enough time to delegate. It takes time to delegate because the delegator must adequately explain the task or teach their team member the skills necessary to complete the delegated task. Yet, in the end, it can save time.

Individuals may also underdelegate because they lack experience in the job or in delegation itself. Others refuse to delegate because they have an excessive need to control or be perfect. The leader-manager who accepts nothing less than perfection limits the opportunities available for subordinate growth and often wastes time redoing delegated tasks.

In addition, some individuals underdelegate because they fail to anticipate how much help they will need. In an ideal situation, the best time to delegate is *before* you become overwhelmed. Although crises happen that require you to reorganize your priorities, often, you can foresee hectic or challenging times. For example, waiting until the end of your shift to delegate the tasks you didn't have time to finish is unfair to the person you're delegating to, and that individual is likely to resent your request.

Finally, some novice managers emerging from the clinical nurse role underdelegate because they find it difficult to assume the manager role. This occurs, in part, because these nurses have been rewarded in the past for their clinical expertise and not their management skills. As managers come to understand and accept the need for the hierarchical responsibilities of delegation, they become more productive and develop more positive staff relationships.

> "One of the most difficult transitions leaders have to get their head around is the shift from doing to leading" (Meyer-Cuno, 2021, para 1).

Overdelegating

In contrast to underdelegating, which overburdens the manager, some managers *overdelegate*, burdening their subordinates. Some managers overdelegate because they are poor managers of time, spending most of it just trying to get organized. Others overdelegate because they feel insecure in their ability to perform a task and some overdelegate simply because they do not want to do the work.

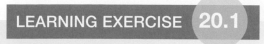

LEARNING EXERCISE   20.1

Difficulty in Delegation

Is it difficult for you to delegate to others? If so, do you know why? Are you more apt to underdelegate, overdelegate, or delegate improperly? What safeguards can you build in to decrease this delegation error? Think back to the last thing you delegated. Was this delegation successful?

It is critical that the manager is sensitive to the workload constraints of their staff. Staff should always have the right to refuse a delegated task. The servant leader always asks the person they want to delegate to if they have time to help, instead of just assuming that their needs are greater than those of the staff member. Managers also must be careful not to overdelegate to exceptionally competent employees because they may become overworked and tired, which can decrease their productivity.

When employees perceive delegation is the result of "hands-off leadership" rather than a sincere need to accomplish a task, they tend to resist their manager's directives in a passive-aggressive manner by making a half-hearted effort or pretending they forgot or don't understand the delegation request (Biddle, 2021). To successfully delegate then, leader-managers should consider the nature of the task, communicate openly, and ensure their subordinates understand the intentions, expectations, and needs for the delegation.

Improper Delegating

Improper delegation includes such things as delegating at the wrong time, to the wrong person, or for the wrong reason. It also may include delegating tasks and responsibilities that are beyond the capability of the person to whom they are being delegated or that should be done by someone with greater expertise, training, or authority.

Delegating decision making without providing adequate information is another example of improper delegation. If the manager requires a higher quality than *satisficing*, this must be made clear at the time of the delegation. Not everything that is delegated needs to be handled in a maximizing mode.

Delegation as a Function of Professional Nursing

RNs at all levels are increasingly being expected to make assignments for and supervise the work of different levels of employees. To increase the likelihood that the increased delegation does not result in an unsafe work environment, organizations should have (a) a clearly defined structure where RNs are recognized as leaders of the health care team, (b) job descriptions that clearly define the roles and responsibilities of all workers, (c) education programs that help personnel learn the roles and responsibilities of coworkers, and (d) training programs that foster the development of leadership and delegation skills (Huston, 2023).

RNs asked to assume the role of supervisor and delegator need preparation to assume these leadership tasks, including instruction in personnel supervision and delegation principles. Repeated education programs on delegation principles and role clarity are necessary for one to demonstrate consistency in delegating appropriate role activities and to begin to feel confident in delegating.

> The RN, although well trained in the role of direct care provider, may not be adequately prepared for the role of delegator.

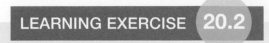

LEARNING EXERCISE   20.2

Assessing Nurses' Comfort with Delegation

Informally survey nurses in the agency in which you work or do clinical practicums. How many of them have received formal education on delegation principles? How comfortable do these nurses feel in determining what should be delegated to whom? How comfortable do you feel in delegating work to other members of the health care team?

In addition, nursing schools and health care organizations need to do a better job of preparing professional RNs for the delegator role. This includes educating them about the NPA governing the scope of practice in their state; basic principles of delegating to the right person, at the right time, and for the right reason; and actions that must be undertaken when work is delegated in an inappropriate or unsafe manner.

Finally, health care organizations need to assure that new nurses are supported in their early efforts to delegate and that these skills are not learned by trial and error. Instead, leaders must create workplace cultures where teamwork, mutual respect, and open communication are valued and where delegation is perceived as an appropriate and expected role to be assumed by nurses.

> Nurses must believe they can delegate without fearing they will be perceived as lazy or incompetent.

Delegating to Unlicensed Assistive Personnel

To contain spiraling health care costs, some health care providers have replaced RN or LVN/LPN positions with UAP *or nursing assistive personnel* (NAP). In 2007, the ANA stopped using the term *UAP* and replaced it with *NAP*, suggesting that many NAP are now certified or formally recognized in some manner. The term *UAP* is used in this chapter only when it is specified as such by the source being cited. NAP include, but are not limited to, nurse extenders, care partners, nurse's aides, orderlies, assistants, attendants, health care assistants, and technicians (Huston, 2023).

Almost all RNs in acute care institutions and long-term care facilities are currently involved in some capacity with the assignment, delegation, and supervision of the NAP in the delivery of nursing care. The primary argument for utilizing NAP is cost (although nursing shortages are a contributing factor). NAP can free professional nurses from tasks and assignments (specifically, nonnursing functions) that can be completed by less extensively trained personnel at a lower cost.

Nonnursing tasks and functions are those routine or standardized activities that can be done by an individual with minimal training and do not require a great deal of individual client assessment, independent thought, or decision making. Examples of nonnursing activities include making a bed, doing vital signs, feeding clients, measuring intakes and outputs, and obtaining a weight or height. This is significant because much of a typical nurse's time can be spent on nonnursing tasks and functions.

Assuming the role of delegator and supervisor to NAP, however, increases the scope of liability for the RN. Although there is limited case law involving nursing delegation and supervision, it is generally accepted that the RN is responsible for adequate supervision of the person to whom an assignment has been delegated. Although nurses are not automatically held liable for all acts of negligence on the part of those they supervise, they may be held liable if they were negligent in the supervision of those employees at the time that those employees committed the negligent acts. Liability is based on a supervisor's failure to determine which patient needs could safely be assigned to a subordinate or for failing to closely monitor a subordinate who requires such supervision.

Experienced nurses have traditionally been expected to work with minimal supervision. The RN who delegates care to another competent RN does not have the same legal obligation to closely supervise that person's work as when the care is delegated to NAP (Huston, 2023). In assigning tasks to NAP, however, the RN must be aware of the job description, knowledge base, and demonstrated skills of each person.

The bottom line is that RNs are always accountable for the care given and must be responsible for instructing NAP as to who needs care, what type of care is needed, and when that care should be provided. NAP should be accountable for knowing how to properly perform their segment of assigned care and for knowing when other workers should be called in for tasks beyond the limits of their knowledge and training. Indeed, NAP must refuse to carry out a delegated task if they feel they do not have the skills, knowledge, and experience to carry it out safely; if the task is something they haven't done before or isn't a part of their normal duties; or if the supervision provided is inadequate (Royal College of Nursing, 2021). As such, the NAP does bear some personal accountability for their actions. This does not, however, negate accountability for the RN who delegated the task(s). The RN continues to be accountable for both the care they deliver and for that which they delegate.

> In delegation, the responsibility for a task can be transferred from the licensed person to the NAP, but accountability is shared by both.

In addition, RNs should recognize that although the Omnibus Budget Reconciliation Act of 1987 established regulations for the education and certification of nurse's aides (minimum of 75 hours of theory and practice and successful completion of an examination in both areas), no federal or community standards have been established for training the more broadly defined NAP (Huston, 2023). Some standards and guidelines are now required for the preparation and use of NAP in certified home health agencies and skilled nursing facilities, but there are no required education standards or guidelines for the use of NAP in acute care hospitals that cross state lines and jurisdictions.

> The NAP has no license to lose for "exceeding scope of practice," and nationally established standards for scope of practice do not exist for NAP.

This does not imply that all NAP are uneducated and unprepared for the roles they have been asked to fill. Indeed, NAP educational levels vary from less than a high school graduate to those holding advanced degrees. It merely suggests that the RN, in delegating to NAP, must carefully assess what skills and knowledge that each NAP has, or risk increased personal liability for the failure to do so (Huston, 2023).

Nursing Assistive Personnel Scope of Practice

Common tasks generally considered appropriate for delegation to NAP are shown in Display 20.4. Unfortunately, many institutions do not have distinct job descriptions for NAP that clearly define their scope of practice. Although some institutions limit the scope of practice for NAP to nonnursing functions, other organizations allow NAP to perform many skills traditionally reserved for the licensed nurse. This is because some agencies interpret regulations broadly, allowing NAP a broader scope of practice than that advocated by professional nursing associations or State Boards of Nursing.

State regulations regarding NAP practice vary as well with only a few states using the ANA or NCSBN definitions for delegation, supervision, or assignment. As a result, although all states allow NAP to complete nine tasks designated by federal codes, some states allow others to do "expanded" care tasks, even though the impact on patient safety is unknown.

DISPLAY 20.4 **COMMON TASKS GENERALLY CONSIDERED APPROPRIATE FOR DELEGATION TO NURSING ASSISTIVE PERSONNEL**

- Personal hygiene care including bathing, dressing, and grooming
- Monitor vital signs including respiration rate, temperature, and blood pressure
- Weight and height measurements
- Measure and record intake and output
- Empty urinary catheter bags
- Feed clients
- Assist with ambulation and positioning
- Transfer patients to commodes, wheelchairs, or other surfaces
- Assist with toileting and other activities of daily living (ADLs)
- Noninvasive and nonsterile treatments
- Comfort care
- Change bed linens
- Transport patients

Some State Boards of Nursing, to more clearly define the scope of practice for NAP, have issued task lists. Training of the NAP is not based on the notion that such individuals will be performing activities independently. Task lists, however, suggest no need for delegation, as NAP already have a list of nursing activities that they may perform without waiting for the delegation process. But what happens when the condition of a client changes? Are NAPs with fewer than 75 hours of training astute enough to recognize that there has been a change in the client's condition and alert the RN?

In addition, in the late 1990s, the NCSBN established a *decision tree for delegation*, which includes a step-by-step analysis nurses can use to decide whether a task should be delegated. Many State Boards of Nursing have also adopted decision trees that are posted on their websites. See Figure 20.1 for an example of the decision tree created by the Kentucky Board of Nursing (2018) to guide nurses in delegating to unlicensed workers. In addition, Display 20.5 suggests criteria developed by the North Carolina Board of Nursing (2014) that may be helpful in determining what tasks can safely be delegated to NAP.

> Decision trees created by the NCSBN and State Boards of Nursing can guide RNs in determining what can safely be delegated to unlicensed workers.

One expansion of NAP scope of practice that is generating concern, however, is administering medications. NAP who administer medications are also known as *unlicensed medication*

DISPLAY 20.5 **CRITERIA FOR DELEGATION TO AN UNLICENSED ASSISTIVE PERSONNEL**

The North Carolina Board of Nursing (2014) suggests that tasks may be delegated to nursing assistive personnel only if they meet *all* of the following criteria:

1. Frequently recur in the daily care of a client or group of clients
2. Are performed according to an established (standardized) sequence of steps
3. Involve little or no modification from one client-care situation to another
4. May be performed with a predictable outcome
5. Do not inherently involve ongoing assessment, interpretation, or decision making which cannot be logically separated from the procedure(s) itself
6. Do not endanger the health or well-being of clients
7. Are allowed by agency policy/procedures

Source: North Carolina Board of Nursing. (2014, January). *Delegation—Non-nursing functions. Position statement for RN and LPN practice (Revised)*. https://www.ncbon.com/vdownloads/position-statements-decision-trees/delegation-non-nursing-functions.pdf

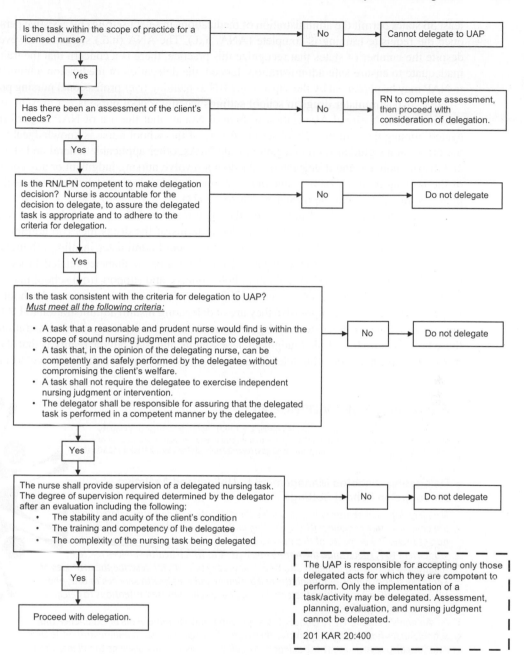

FIGURE 20.1 Kentucky Board of Nursing decision tree for delegation to unlicensed assistive personnel (UAP). LPN, licensed practical nurse; RN, registered nurse. (*Source:* Kentucky Board of Nursing. [Revised June 2018]. *Decision tree for delegation to unlicensed assistive personnel [UAP].* https://kbn.ky.gov/General/Documents/decision-tree-for-delegation-to-uap.pdf)

administration personnel, medication aides, or *medication assistant technicians.* For years, medication administration was considered a professional nursing function, requiring assessment and clinical judgment, but during the past decade, many states granted unlicensed personnel the right to pass medications, particularly in schools, assisted living facilities, and correctional institutions (Huston, 2023).

In addition, *certified medicine aides* have worked in licensed nursing home settings, residential care settings, and adult day services in this country for almost four decades. Currently, at least 36 states permit the administration of medications in select settings by assistive personnel, once the requisite training is complete (ANA, n.d.). The ANA (n.d.) suggests, however, that despite the number of states that recognize this practice, there is a concern that the training is inadequate to ensure safe administration. Indeed, the delegation of medication administration to NAP may be perceived by the supervising RN as handing over professional nursing practice.

NAP also administer drugs in school settings when a school nurse is not present. It is the position of the National Association of School Nurses that the use of NAP to perform delegated nursing tasks in the school setting is safe, if the school nurse is knowledgeable about the profession's guidance on delegation, state NPAs, other applicable federal and state laws, and district policies and if delegated tasks do not involve nursing judgment or any component of the nursing process, such as nursing assessment or developing individualized health care plans (National Association of School Nurses, 2021).

As a result, many school nurses and the organizations that represent them are waging a battle to stop the expansion of NAP practice in terms of the drugs they can administer. For example, historically, only licensed school nurses could administer insulin, although recent legislative changes in Kentucky expanded the delegation of diabetes-related tasks to unlicensed school personnel (UAP), eliciting both concern and support from school nurses there (Lineberry et al., 2021). Lineberry et al. (2021) note that the more experienced school nurses in Kentucky are, the less supportive they are of delegating insulin administration to UAP. They are more willing to delegate blood glucose monitoring and glucagon administration since these tasks require less skilled judgment, assessment, and risk, but the reality is that shortfalls in staffing have made broader delegation necessary (see Examining the Evidence 20.1).

EXAMINING THE EVIDENCE 20.1

Source: From Lineberry, M., Noland, M., & Wilson, J. F. (2021, April). Intentions of Kentucky school nurses to delegate diabetes-related tasks to unlicensed assistive personnel. *Journal of School Nursing, 37*(2), 99–108. https://eric.ed.gov/?q=%22Noland+Melody%22&id=EJ1290696

Delegating Diabetes Management to Unlicensed Assistive Personnel in School Settings

New legislation in Kentucky has expanded the delegation of diabetes-related tasks to unlicensed school personnel (UAP), eliciting both concern and support from school nurses there. The purposes of this nonexperimental, descriptive, correlational study were to (1) determine the nature and extent to which health services related to diabetes were being delegated to UAP in Kentucky schools, (2) describe the attitudes of Kentucky school nurses regarding the delegation of diabetes health services to UAP, and (3) examine the relationship of selected variables to school nurses' intentions to delegate diabetes health services.

An analysis of the 111 respondent surveys found that the more years of experience that school nurses had, the less supportive they were of delegating insulin administration to UAP. Analyses also revealed that the delegation of diabetes-related tasks seems to fall into three tiers, with most nurses having delegated blood glucose monitoring (73%) and glucagon administration (79.3%), a moderate amount having delegated carbohydrate counting (42.3%) and insulin dose verification (40.5%), and few (29.7%) having delegated insulin administration. These three tiers seem to align with the amount of skilled judgment and assessment involved with those tasks, as well as with the severity of their associated risks.

In addition, analyses suggested that nurses' intentions to delegate were higher than their support for delegation. The reason these school nurses intend to delegate some diabetes-related tasks despite their lack of support for UAP administering those services was likely insufficient resources.

The researchers concluded that anecdotal comments suggested that school nurses were passionate about their jobs and the students they serve and that they should never feel forced to compromise student safety or put their licensure in jeopardy due to policies that are unsupported by funding.

The concern in having NAP administer medications is that medication administration is much more than dispensing a pill, handing a student an inhaler, or giving a subcutaneous injection. It requires high-level assessment skills; an understanding of drug actions, interactions, and side effects; and the highly developed critical thinking skills needed to intervene when problems occur. In addition, the practice of nursing clearly requires a license under the NPA. School nurses argue that it is nonnursing tasks such as documentation that should be shifted to the NAP so that they can retain the responsibility for the administration of medications like insulin to children with complex medical issues.

Subordinate Resistance to Delegation

Resistance is a common response by subordinates to delegation. One of the most common causes of subordinate resistance to, or refusal of, delegated tasks is the failure of the delegator to see the subordinate's perspective. Workloads assigned to NAP are generally highly challenging, both physically and mentally. In addition, NAP frequently must adapt rapidly to changing priorities, often imposed on them by more than one delegator. If the subordinate is truly overwhelmed, additional delegation of tasks is inappropriate, and the RN should reexamine the necessity of completing the delegated task personally or finding someone else who is able to complete the task.

> The leader–manager should always attempt to see the delegated task from the perspective of the individual being delegated to.

Some subordinates resist delegation simply because they believe that they are incapable of completing the delegated task. If the employee is capable but lacks self-confidence, the astute leader may be able to use performance coaching to empower the subordinate and build self-confidence levels. If, however, the employee is truly at high risk for failure, the appropriateness of the delegation must be questioned and a task more appropriate to that employee's ability level should be delegated.

Another cause of subordinate resistance to delegation is an inherent resistance to authority. Some subordinates simply need to "test the water" and determine what the consequences are of not completing delegated tasks. In this case, the delegator must be calm but assertive about their expectations and provide explicit work guidelines, if necessary, to maintain an appropriate authority power gap. It is an ongoing leadership challenge to instill a team spirit between delegators and their subordinates.

Finally, resistance to delegation may be occurring because tasks are overdelegated in terms of specificity. All subordinates need to believe that there is some room for creativity and independent thinking in delegated tasks. Failure to allow for this human need results in disinterested subordinates who fail to internalize responsibility and accountability for the delegated task. When delegating to NAP, the RN should try to mix routine and boring tasks with more challenging and rewarding assignments. An additional strategy is to provide NAP with consistent, constructive feedback, both positive and negative, to foster growth and self-esteem.

When subordinates resist delegation, the delegator may be tempted to avoid confrontation and simply do the delegated task independently. This is seldom appropriate. Instead, the delegator must ascertain why the delegated task was not accomplished and take appropriate action to eliminate these restraining forces.

Delegating to a Multicultural Work Team

The increasing diversity of both the workforce and the client populations being served has ramifications for delegation. Challenges in delegation are seen for both the culturally diverse

LEARNING EXERCISE 20.3

Dealing with Resistance to Delegation

You are the registered nurse supervisor in a skilled nursing facility. Most of the direct patient care is provided by licensed vocational nurses (LVNs)/licensed practical nurses (LPNs) and nurse's aides. It is an extremely busy day, and there is a great deal of work to be done. Several times today, you have found one of the LVNs/LPNs taking long breaks in the lounge or chatting socially at the front desk despite the unmet needs of many patients. On those occasions, you have clearly delegated work tasks and timelines to her. Several hours later, you follow up on the delegated tasks and find that they were not completed. When you seek out the LVN/LPN, you find that she went to lunch without telling you or the aide. You are furious at her apparent disregard for your authority.

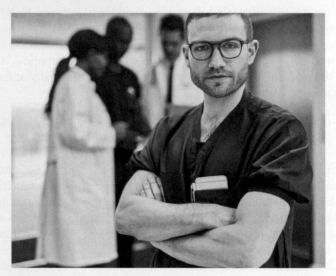

ASSIGNMENT:

What are possible causes of the LVN/LPN's failure to follow up on delegated tasks? How will you deal with this LVN/LPN? What goal serves as the basis for your actions? Justify your choice with rationale.

delegatee and the delegator. Such cultural considerations may include generational and gender differences as well as ethnic differences. For example, nurses from some cultures may require more time to develop delegation skills because assertiveness and asking for help from others may violate values that are culturally bound.

According to Giger (2017), there are six cultural phenomena that must be considered when working with staff from a culturally diverse background: communication, space, social organization, time, environmental control, and biologic variations.

Communication, the first of the cultural phenomena, is greatly affected by cultural diversity in the workforce because dialect, volume, use of touch, context of speech, and kinesics such as gestures, stance, and eye movement all influence how messages are sent and received. For example, delegation delivered in a softer tone may be perceived as less important than delegation delivered in a loud tone, even if the delegated tasks have equal importance. Similarly, a manager may make an inappropriate assumption about a person's inability to carry out an important delegated task if that person is a member of a culture that values softer speech and more passive behavior.

DISPLAY 20.6 CULTURAL PHENOMENA TO CONSIDER WHEN DELEGATING TO A TRANSCULTURAL TEAM

1. **Communication:** especially dialect, volume, use of touch, and eye contact
2. **Space:** interpersonal space differs between cultures
3. **Social organization:** family unit of primary importance in some cultures
4. **Time:** cultures tend to be past, present, or future oriented
5. **Environmental control:** cultures often have either internal or external locus of control
6. **Biologic variations:** susceptibility to diseases (e.g., Tay–Sachs) and physiologic differences (e.g., height and skin color)

Source: Giger, J. N. (2017). *Transcultural nursing: Assessment and intervention* (7th ed.). Mosby.

Space is the second cultural phenomenon influencing delegation. Space refers to the distance and intimacy techniques that are used when relating verbally or nonverbally to others. It is important that the delegator recognizes the personal space needs of each staff member and acts accordingly. If these space needs are not recognized and respected, the likelihood that a delegated task will be heard and followed through on appropriately will be reduced.

The third cultural phenomenon, *social organization*, refers to the importance of a group or unit in providing social support in a person's life. For many cultures, the family unit is the most important social organization. In some cultures, the duty to family always takes precedence over the needs of the organization. In other cultures, this values ranking is less clear, and the employee may experience great intrapersonal conflict in prioritizing delegated work tasks and obligations to the family unit. It is important, then, that the delegator is aware that employees' values differ and is sensitive in delegating critical tasks to employees who are experiencing stress in the family unit.

Time is the fourth cultural phenomenon affecting delegation. Cultural groups can be past, present, or future oriented. *Past-oriented cultures* are interested in preserving the past and maintaining tradition. *Present-oriented cultures* focus on maintaining the status quo and on daily operations. *Future-oriented cultures* focus on goals to be achieved and are more visionary in their approach to problems. For example, strategic planning might best be delegated to a person from a future-oriented culture, although the leader-manager should always be alert for opportunities to create new insight and stretching opportunities for subordinates.

Environmental control, the fifth cultural phenomenon, refers to the person's perception of control over their environment (internal *locus of control*). Some cultures believe more strongly in fate, luck, or chance than other cultures, and this may affect how a person approaches and carries out a delegated task. The person who believes that they have an internal locus of control is more likely to be creative and autonomous in decision making.

The final phenomenon, *biologic variations*, refers to the biopsychosocial differences between racial and ethnic groups, such as susceptibility to disease and physiologic differences. Display 20.6 provides a summary of considerations when delegating to a transcultural work team.

LEARNING EXERCISE 20.4

Cultural Considerations in Delegation

You are a new charge nurse working on a surgical unit and have a recently hired Filipino travel registered nurse working on your unit. This is the end of her second week of orientation on the unit. She also received a month of classroom orientation and enculturation when she was first hired. Today, you assign her as one of your team leaders, responsible for a team of licensed vocational nurses (LVNs)/licensed practical nurses (LPNs) and certified

(continues on page 526)

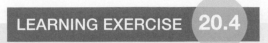

LEARNING EXERCISE 20.4

Cultural Considerations in Delegation (continued)

nursing assistants. She has been working with another team leader for more than a week, but this is her first day to have the team to herself.

You check with her several times during the morning to see how things are going. She speaks shyly without making eye contact and says that "everything is okay." At about noon, one of the LVN/LPNs comes to you and says that the new nurse has not delegated tasks appropriately and is trying to do too much of the work herself. In addition, some of the other members of the team find her unsmiling behavior and lack of eye contact unsettling.

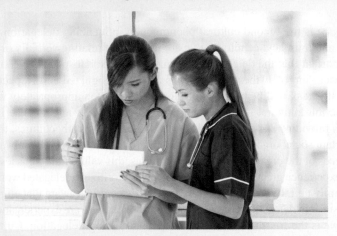

ASSIGNMENT:

Do you feel that you made an appropriate assignment? Because things do not seem to be going well, what should you do now? In a small group, develop a plan of action with the following goals: (a) ensure that patient care is accomplished safely, (b) build self-esteem in the recently hired nurse, and (c) be a cultural bridge to staff.

Integrating Leadership Roles and Management Functions in Delegation

The right to delegate and the ability to provide formal rewards for successful completion of delegated tasks reflect the legitimate authority inherent in the management role. Delegation provides a means of increasing unit productivity. It is also a managerial tool for promoting subordinate accomplishment and enrichment.

Delegation, however, is not easy. It requires high-level management skills because effective delegation involves selecting the right person for the right reason and at the right time and assessing the qualifications, availability, and experience of individuals being delegated to. Novice managers often make delegation errors such as delegating too late, not delegating enough, delegating to the wrong person or for the wrong reason, and failing to provide appropriate supervision and guidance of delegated tasks.

Delegation also requires highly developed leadership skills such as sensitivity to subordinates' capabilities and needs, the ability to communicate clearly and directly, the willingness to support and encourage subordinates in carrying out delegated tasks, and the vision to see how delegation might result in increased personal growth for subordinates as well as increased unit productivity.

With the increased use of NAP in patient care, the need for nurses to have highly developed delegation skills has never been greater. The outcomes associated with the increased use of NAP are not yet known. An increasing number of studies suggest a direct link between decreased RN staffing and declines in patient outcomes, including an increased incidence of patient falls, nosocomial infections, physical restraint use, and medication errors (Huston, 2023).

The challenge continues to be using NAP only to provide personal care needs or nursing tasks that do not require the skill and judgment of the RN. With increasing patient loads and the current nursing shortage, many health care organizations and the RNs who work within them are tempted to allow NAP to perform tasks that should be limited to professional nursing practice. Nurses must remember, however, that the responsibility for assuring that patients are protected and that NAP do not exceed their scope of practice ultimately falls to the RN. When NAP are allowed to encroach into professional nursing care, patients are placed at risk (Huston, 2023).

It is critical that RNs never lose sight of their ultimate responsibility for ensuring that patients receive appropriate, high-quality care. Only RNs have the formal authority to practice nursing, and activities that rely on the nursing process or require specialized skill, expert knowledge, or professional judgment should never be delegated.

To protect their patients and their professional license, RNs must continue to seek current information regarding national efforts to standardize the scope of practice for NAP and professional guidelines regarding what can be safely delegated to the NAP. Using delegation skills appropriately will help to reduce the personal liability associated with supervising and delegating to NAP. It will also ensure that clients' needs are met, and their safety is not jeopardized.

Key Concepts

- Professional nursing organizations and regulatory bodies are actively engaged in clarifying the scope of practice for unlicensed workers and delegation parameters for RNs.
- Delegation is not an option for the manager—it is a necessity.
- Delegation should be used for assigning routine tasks and tasks for which the manager does not have time. It is also appropriate as a tool for problem solving, changes in the manager's own job emphasis, and building capability in subordinates.
- In delegation, managers must clearly communicate what they want to be done, including the purpose for doing so. Limitations or qualifications that have been imposed should be delineated. Although the manager should specify the end product desired, it is important that the subordinate has an appropriate degree of autonomy in deciding how the work is to be accomplished.
- Managers must delegate the authority and the responsibility necessary to complete the task.
- Most delegation errors could be avoided if the five rights of delegation, identified by the ANA and the NCSBN, were followed.

- RNs who are asked to assume the role of supervisor and delegator need preparation to assume these leadership tasks.
- Assuming the role of delegator and supervisor to the NAP increases the scope of liability for the RN. Although the NAP does bear some personal accountability for their actions, this does not negate accountability for the RN who delegated the task(s).
- The RN always bears the ultimate responsibility for ensuring that the nursing care provided by their team members meets or exceeds minimum safety standards.
- Although the Omnibus Budget Reconciliation Act of 1987 established regulations for the education and certification of "certified nurse's aides" (minimum of 75 hours of theory and practice and successful completion of an examination in both areas), no federal or community standards have been established for training the more broadly defined NAP.
- When subordinates resist delegation, the delegator must ascertain why the delegated task was not accomplished and take appropriate action to remove these restraining forces.
- Transcultural sensitivity in delegation is needed to create a productive multicultural work team.

Additional Learning Exercises and Applications

LEARNING EXERCISE 20.5

Need for Immediate Delegation

You are the charge nurse on the 7:00 AM to 3:00 PM shift in an oncology unit. Immediately after report in the morning, you are overwhelmed by the following information:

- The nursing aide reports that Mrs. Jones has become comatose and is moribund. Although this is not unexpected, her family members are not present, and you know that they would like to be notified immediately.
- There are three patients who need 7:30 AM insulin administration. One of these patients had a 6:00 AM blood sugar of 400.
- Mr. Johnson inadvertently pulled out his central line catheter when he was turning over in bed. His wife just notified the ward clerk by the call-light system and states that she is applying pressure to the site.
- The public toilet is overflowing, and urine and feces are pouring out rapidly.
- Breakfast trays arrived 15 minutes ago, and patients are using their call lights to ask why they do not yet have their breakfast.
- The medical director of the unit has just discovered that one of her patients has not been started on a chemotherapeutic drug that she ordered 3 days ago. She is furious and demands to speak to you immediately.

ASSIGNMENT:

The other registered nurses are all very busy with their patients, but you have the following people to whom you may delegate: yourself, a ward clerk, and an intravenous-certified licensed vocational nurse/licensed practical nurse. Decide who should do what and in what priority. Justify your decision.

LEARNING EXERCISE 20.6

Delegating Discipline

You are the registered nurse (RN) supervisor of the oncology unit. One of your closest friends and colleagues is Paula, the RN supervisor of the medical unit. Frequently, you cover for each other in the event of absence or emergency. Today, Paula stops at your office to let you know that she will be gone for 7 days to attend a management workshop on the East Coast. She asks that you check on the unit during her absence. She also asks that you pay particularly close attention to Mary Jones, an employee on her unit. She states that Mary, who has worked at the hospital for 4 years, has been counseled repeatedly about her unexcused absences from work and has recently received a written reprimand specifying that she will be terminated if there is another unexcused absence. Paula anticipates that Mary may attempt to break the rules during her absence. She asks that you follow through on this disciplinary plan in the event that Mary again takes an unexcused absence. Her instructions to you are to terminate Mary if she fails to show up for work this week for any reason.

When you arrive at work the next day, you find that Mary called in sick 20 minutes after the shift was to begin. The hospital's policy is that employees are to notify the staffing office of illness no less than 2 hours before the beginning of their shift. When you attempt to contact Mary by telephone at home, there is no answer.

Later in the day, you finally reach Mary and ask that she come into your office early the next morning to speak about her inadequate notice of sick time. Mary arrives 45 minutes late the next morning. You are already agitated and angry with her. You inform her that she is to be terminated for any rule broken during Paula's absence and that this action is being taken in accord with the disciplinary contract that had been established earlier.

Mary is furious. She states that you have no right to fire her because you are not her "real boss" and that Paula should face her herself. She goes on to say that "Paula told me that the disciplinary contract was just a way of formalizing that we had talked and that I shouldn't take it too seriously." Mary also says, "Besides, I didn't get sick until I was getting ready for work. The hospital rules state that I have 12 sick days each year." Although you feel certain that Paula was very clear about her position in reviewing the disciplinary contract with Mary, you begin to feel uncomfortable with being placed in the position of having to take such serious corrective action without having been involved in prior disciplinary review sessions. You are, however, also aware that this employee has been breaking rules for some time and that this is just one in a succession of absences. You also know that Paula is counting on you to provide consistency of leadership in her absence.

ASSIGNMENT:

• • • • • • • • •

Discuss how you will handle the situation. Was it appropriate for Paula to delegate this responsibility to you? Is it appropriate for one manager to carry out another manager's disciplinary plan? Does it matter that a written disciplinary contract had already been established?

LEARNING EXERCISE 20.7

How Will You Plan This Busy Morning?

You are a staff nurse who functions as a modular leader on a general medical–surgical unit in a small rural hospital. The group for which you are responsible is assigned to care for patients in Rooms 401 through 409, with a maximum capacity of 13 patients.

In your unit, a modular type of patient care organization is employed, using a combination of licensed and unlicensed staff. Each module consists of one registered nurse (RN), one licensed vocational nurse (LVN)/licensed practical nurse (LPN), and one nursing assistive personnel (NAP). The LVN/LPN is intravenous (IV) certified and can maintain and start IVs but cannot hang piggybacks or give IV push medications. The LVN/LPN may give all other medications except IV medications. The RN gives all IV medications. The NAP, with the assistance of their modular team members, generally bathes and feeds patients and provides other care that does not require a license.

The RN, as modular leader, divides up the workload at the beginning of the shift between the three modular team members. In addition, they act as a teacher and resource person for the other members of the module.

(continues on page 530)

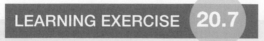

LEARNING EXERCISE **20.7**

How Will You Plan This Busy Morning? (continued)

Today is Wednesday. You have one LVN/LPN and one NAP assigned to work with you—LVN Franklin and NAP Martinez. LVN Franklin is 26 years old and the mother of four preschool children. Her husband is a city bus driver. NAP Martinez is 53 years old and a grandmother with no children living at home. Her husband died 2 years ago. She says that work keeps her "happy." The patient roster this morning is as follows:

Room	Patient	Age	Diagnosis	Condition	Acuity Level
401	Mrs. Jones	33	Mastectomy for breast cancer (CA)	2 days postoperative/fair	II
402	Mrs. Redford	55	Intractable back pain with hypercortisolemia	Good	I
403	Mrs. Worley	76	Abscess following cholesystectomy	2 days postoperative/good	III
404–1	Mrs. Smith	83	Parkinson's, cardiovascular disease, hypertension	Fair	II
404–2	Mrs. Dewey	26	Septicemia post urinary tract infection	Good—home today	I
405–1	Mr. Arthur	71	Metastatic CA	Poor—semi-comatose/ chemotherapy	IV
405–2	Mr. Vines	72	Possible peptic ulcer/ severe anemia	Good—upper gastrointestinal today	II
406–1	Vacant				
406–2	Ms. Brown	83	Abnormal uterine bleeding/dilatation and curettage	To operating room this AM	II
407–1	Mrs. West	41	Myocardial infarction Heparin lock from yesterday/telemetry	Fair	III
408–1	Mr. Niles	21	Open reduction femur (motor vehicle accident)	Fair/3 days postoperative	III
408–2	Mr. Ford	44	Gastrectomy	Fair/1 day postoperative	III
409	Mrs. Land	42	Depression/new onset rectal bleeding/history colon cancer	Fair/colonoscopy today	III

Additional information about patients:

- Mr. Niles is depressed because he believes that his football career is over.
- There have been problems with Mr. Ford's IV and his nasogastric tube. Both will need to be replaced today.
- Mrs. Worley requires frequent changes (every 2 to 3 hours) of the dressings at the laparoscopy site owing to a high volume of serous drainage.
- Mrs. Jones will need instructions regarding her postoperative activities and has begun to talk about her prognosis.

- Mrs. Land began to speak with you yesterday about her husband's recent death.
- The preparation for the colonoscopy will result in Mrs. Land's having frequent toileting needs today.
- Mrs. Smith requires assistance with feeding at mealtime.
- Mr. Arthur is no longer able to turn himself in bed.
- Mr. Vines states that being in the same room with a critically ill patient upsets him, and he has asked to be moved to a new room.

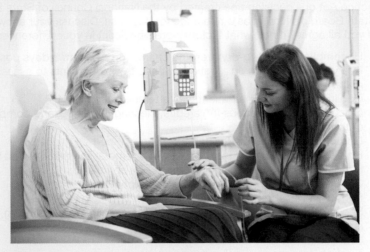

ASSIGNMENT:

How will you make out your assignments this morning? Assign these patients to the LVN/LPN, NAP, and yourself. Be sure to include assessments, procedures, and basic care needs. What will you do if a patient is admitted to your team? Explain the rationale for all your patient assignments. Refer to the sample acuity levels provided to assist in determining patient needs and staffing.

LEARNING EXERCISE 20.8

Evaluating Staffing Safeguards

Interview a middle- or top-level manager of a local health care agency. Determine the staffing mix at their agency. Are there minimum hiring criteria for the nursing assistive personnel (NAP)? Are there written guidelines for determining tasks appropriate for NAP delegation? What educational or training opportunities on delegation are made available to staff who must delegate work assignments on a regular basis?

On the basis of your interview results, write an essay evaluating whether you believe there are adequate safeguards in place at that agency to protect the licensed staff, unlicensed staff, and clients. Would you feel comfortable working in such a facility?

LEARNING EXERCISE 20.9

Deciding Delegation Using the Nurse Practice Act

Which of the following tasks would you be willing to delegate to a nursing assistive personnel or licensed practical nurse/licensed vocational nurse? Use your state's Nurse Practice Act or a decision tree created by the National Council of State Boards of Nursing or a State Board of Nursing as a reference for this case. Discuss your answers in small groups. Did you all agree? If not, what factors were significant in your differences?

1. Uncomplicated wet-to-dry dressing change on a patient 3 days post-hip replacement
2. Every 2 hours checks on a patient with soft wrist restraints to assess circulation, movement, and comfort
3. Cooling measures for a patient with a temperature of 104°F
4. Calculation of intravenous (IV) credits, clearing IV pumps, and completing shift intake/output totals
5. Completing phlebotomy for daily drawing of blood
6. Holding pressure on the insertion site of a femoral line that has just been removed
7. Educating a patient about components of a soft diet
8. Conducting guaiac stool tests for occult blood
9. Performing electrocardiographic testing
10. Feeding a patient with swallowing precautions (high risk of choking post-cardiovascular accident [CVA])
11. Oral suctioning
12. Tracheostomy care
13. Ostomy care

LEARNING EXERCISE 20.10

Reflecting on Negative Delegation Experiences

Write a one-page essay about one of the following situations you have experienced:

- A supervisor asked you to complete a task you believed was beyond your capability.
- A supervisor delegated a task to you but failed to give you adequate authority to carry out the task.
- A supervisor gave such explicit directions on how to complete a delegated task that you felt demoralized.

LEARNING EXERCISE 20.11

Delegating Work in Group Projects

You are a nursing student assigned to work in groups to do a presentation for your leadership/management class. There will be four of you in the work group, and you have been appointed the group leader. The project requires the group to create a 40-minute presentation that examines the controversy around educational entry into practice for nurses. No one in the group has any special expertise about this topic. PowerPoint presentations must be used, handouts must be created, and a written reference list (in American Psychological Association format) must be submitted to your instructor. The presentation counts for 50% of your class grade, so quality of the end product is important. The presentation is due in 4 weeks.

ASSIGNMENT:

Make a list of 10 things you must do to break this task down into smaller parts. Then divide the workload into what you consider to be four equivalent parts. Then develop a timeline for follow-up with group members to make sure all group members are on target to accomplish the delegated tasks.

LEARNING EXERCISE 20.12

When Resistance to Delegation Is Needed

You are a senior nursing student caring for a patient with multiple fractures and a closed head injury in a neurotrauma unit as part of your clinical rotation. You feel challenged in caring for this patient (Mike Schmied) as there is much to learn about the many treatments, medications, and technologies being used as part of his care. As you are in the room providing care to Mr. Schmied, his physician arrives and begins asking you a few questions. You are a little nervous that the staff nurse assigned to care for Mr. Schmied is not present but are pleased that you have been able to answer all the questions she has asked. The physician turns to you as she is leaving the room and issues two orders: one related to the ventilator settings for the patient and one related to his IV fluids. You quickly respond that you are a nursing student and cannot take medical orders, but she simply says, "You are smart, and you heard what I said—just pass it on to the nurse so she can write the order. I'm already late for surgery." With that, she leaves.

ASSIGNMENT:

Decide what you will do next. Is there anything you could have or should have done to minimize the likelihood of the situation occurring? How did differences in power and status affect this delegation?

LEARNING EXERCISE 20.13

Delegating to the Modular Health Care Team

You are a new graduate nurse working on a high-acuity medical unit during the 7:00 AM to 3:30 PM shift. The unit uses modular nursing to provide total patient care to groups of 10 to 12 patients. The staff assigned to work with you on your mini-team today are Ms. Foster, an experienced licensed vocational nurse/licensed practical nurse, and Ms. Grimes, a nursing assistive personnel (NAP) who was called in from the local registry due to short staffing today. Ms. Grimes says she has been an NAP for 2 years and is a first-year student in the local community college nursing program. She has not, however, worked on this unit before and has only worked at the hospital a few times. There is no ward clerk/unit secretary assigned to assist you today. There is one possible admit in the emergency room (rule out pneumonia) who would come to your time, although they said it was likely he would not arrive on the unit until after lunch today. They will call you with report before the transfer is made.

(continues on page 534)

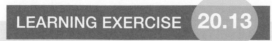

LEARNING EXERCISE **20.13**

Delegating to the Modular Health Care Team (continued)

You are assigned to care for the patients in Rooms 100 to 112. The patients your team will care for include:

- Room 100: vacant (this is the room closest to the nursing station)
- Room 101: Saul Baker, a 73-year-old male, had a cerebrovascular accident 2 days ago. He is conscious but has total left-sided paralysis and is dependent in all activities of daily living. His lungs have become congested today and he was started on intravenous (IV) diuretics (due at 9:00 AM) and IV antibiotics, which are due at 8:00 AM and 12:00 PM. He also receives oxygen (O₂) at 4 L/minute. He needs to be assisted in turning every 2 hours. In addition, his indwelling Foley catheter was accidentally pulled out at change of shift when he was being turned and needs to be replaced. Speech therapy will be in today at 10:00 AM to complete a swallowing study. His home-bound wife has asked to be called about an update in his condition as soon as possible.
- Room 102: Lisa Laffins, a 22-year-old female, was admitted for an exacerbation of her cystic fibrosis. She receives multiple oral medications at 8:00 AM, 10:00 AM, 12:00 PM, and 2:00 PM and IV medications at 8:00 AM and 2:00 PM. Her sputum is thick and has a foul odor, and her breathing continues to be labored. She is highly anxious about this being her fourth hospitalization in 6 months and wants to talk to someone about her prognosis and the new treatment regimes being established. New orders have been written on her chart and are waiting for your review and transcription.
- Room 103: Sam Liggett, a 58-year-old male, was admitted last night to rule out myocardial infarction. His initial cardiac enzymes were negative, but his telemetry is showing frequent ectopy, including premature ventricular contractions. His physician needs to be notified as this is a change in his condition. In addition, his IV site is red and puffy and needs to be restarted. His vital signs are stable.
- Room 104: Ryan Welch, a 25-year-old male, was admitted 2 days ago for complications related to the chemotherapy and radiation he received for his testicular cancer (CA). He is unable to keep food down and is being started today on total parenteral nutrition (TPN) and lipids. He needs to have a second IV started because his TPN and lipids are not compatible with other IV medications he is receiving. He seems depressed and withdrawn and states he was awake almost all last night because of the patient in Room 105. He has asked to be transferred to another room.
- Room 105: Gladys Cooper, a 96-year-old female, was admitted during the night shift for pneumonia from a local convalescent care facility. On admission, she was found to have a stage 4 decubitus on her right hip and two smaller ulcers on her heels. All three wounds require packing and dressing changes today. She is confused and frequently calls out. She also needs to be fed and is a high fall risk. She also needs to be bathed because she was incontinent of stool just before the shift began. She has IV medications due at 9:00 AM, 12:00 PM, and 2:00 PM. Her oral medications are due at 9:00 AM, 10:00 AM, 12:00 PM, and 2:00 PM. She also needs to be assisted to use an incentive spirometry every 4 hours today.
- Room 106: vacant
- Room 107: James Gardner, a 71-year-old male, was admitted for possible bile duct blockage. He is jaundiced, and his stools are clay colored. He is experiencing significant abdominal pain and requested IV pain medication every 2 to 3 hours throughout the night, which brought him only partial relief. He is also complaining of extreme itching, which he says is even worse than the relentless pain. There are no orders for anti-itching medications on his chart. He is scheduled for an endoscopic retrograde cholangiopancreatogram at 8:30 AM this morning and will need to sign his surgical consent and receive his preprocedure medications. He will likely be in the procedure lab from 8:15 AM to 11:15 AM today, and you do not expect his physician to make rounds on the unit until after the procedure.
- Room 108: Patty Baker, a 39-year-old woman, was admitted for severe pelvic inflammatory disease requiring IV antibiotics every 4 hours (8:00 AM and 12:00 PM) and as-needed oral pain medication. She is extremely depressed and has been reaching out to the staff to talk about her fears of never having children, something she has wanted all of her life.

- Room 109: Clarence Verne, an 84-year-old male, was admitted for end-stage metastasis from his lung CA yesterday. He was being cared for at home by his wife but has become too sick for her to care for alone. She has refused hospice care for him and declined to sign a do-not-resuscitate order because she "is not yet ready to let him go." Today, his breathing is extremely labored, and he is confused. He requires intermittent oral suctioning to clear his secretions. He has O_2 at 6 L/minute and is on an IV morphine drip. His physician has shared that he does not believe Mr. Verne will live more than a few more days. Mr. Verne did not void on the night shift, and the nurse on handoff suggests that he likely needs a Foley catheter inserted. There is an order on his chart to insert such a catheter if needed.
- Room 110: Gina Graham, a 55-year-old female, was admitted for intractable back pain 3 days ago. Her traction was removed last night, and she is expected to be discharged at noon today. She will need to have her saline lock removed. She has oral medications ordered for 8:00 AM and 12:00 PM and will need teaching regarding her discharge medications. She also needs to be instructed by physical therapy today about her home activity plan.
- Room 111: vacant
- Room 112: Carol Carson, a 54-year-old female, was admitted 3 days ago for recurrent urinary tract infection and to rule out sepsis. Her white blood cell since admission has been only slightly elevated; however, Ms. Carson continues to complain of burning and frequency, and her urine remains cloudy and positive for blood. The urologist plans to do a cystoscopy at the patient's bedside today about 10:00 AM. He said he will bring his portable scope and all the equipment he will need but will need someone to help him during the actual procedure, something he anticipates will take 20 to 30 minutes. Ms. Carson receives IV antibiotics at 12:00 PM and oral medications at 9:00 AM, 12:00 PM, and 2:00 PM.

Note: All patients require vital signs every 4 hours. Breakfast trays arrive at 8:00 AM, and lunch trays arrive at 12:00 PM. Patients are typically bathed every other day but are offered washcloths to clean up and oral care daily. Staff are expected to take a 30-minute lunch break.

ASSIGNMENT:

Create a plan for your day that includes a time inventory for each member of your mini-team. Determine what tasks you will delegate and to whom you will delegate. Provide a rationale for your choices. As you create your plan, be aware about whether your innate tendency was to overdelegate, underdelegate, or inappropriately delegate. Did you allow time in your plan for the unexpected? Did the fact that Ms. Grimes was a nursing student influence the tasks you delegated to her?

LEARNING EXERCISE 20.14

Delegating at Home

You are a single parent enrolled full time in nursing school. Your children are 16, 13, and 11 years old. It is very difficult to juggle going to school full time, working part time, and raising three children, but you know the payoff in the end will be worth it. As the children have grown older, you have increasingly delegated household chores to them including doing the laundry, mowing the lawn, helping to prepare meals, and cleaning the house. This has worked very well the past few years, although lately, you have returned home to find laundry hampers overflowing, dishes in the sink, and general clutter all around the house. While you understand that the children also have after school activities, homework, and other personal commitments that compete for their time, you are also aware that they are spending more time than ever doing social networking on their computers, talking to their friends on the phone, and isolating themselves in their rooms.

(continues on page 536)

LEARNING EXERCISE 20.14

Delegating at Home (continued)

When you tried to talk to them about the problem several weeks ago, they shrugged their shoulders and said they'd try harder, but there has been no improvement in the situation. Today, when you return home, the situation is worse than ever. You are tempted to set aside the homework you must complete tonight since you simply cannot stand the state the house is in but realize this will not address what is rapidly becoming a significant problem.

ASSIGNMENT:

Decide what you will do. What factors might be contributing to your children's resistance to delegation? Has your delegation been specific enough? Are the desired goals clear? How might you increase oversight of the delegated tasks? Should you create consequences for your children not following through on their delegated tasks? Would doing so increase or decrease their resistance?

REFERENCES

American Nurses Association. (n.d.). *Medication aids, assistants, technicians.* https://www.nursingworld.org/practice-policy/medication-aides–assistants–technicians/

American Nurses Association & National Council of State Boards of Nursing. (n.d.). *Joint statement on delegation.* https://www.ncsbn.org/Delegation_joint_statement_NCSBN-ANA.pdf

Biddle, M. (2021, July 29). *Why some employees resist delegation from their managers.* Phys.org. https://phys.org/news/2021-07-employees-resist.html

California Board of Registered Nursing. (2010). *Unlicensed assistive personnel.* http://www.rn.ca.gov/pdfs/regulations/npr-b-16.pdf

Giger, J. N. (2017). *Transcultural nursing: Assessment and intervention* (7th ed.). Mosby.

Greenwood, B. (2021). *What cannot be delegated to an LPN?* The Nest. http://woman.thenest.com/cannot-delegated-lpn-12251.html

Huston, C. (2023). Unlicensed assistive personnel and the registered nurse (chapter 8). In C. Huston (Ed.), *Professional issues in nursing: Challenges and opportunities* (6th ed., pp. 109–120). Wolters Kluwer.

Kentucky Board of Nursing. (Revised 2018, June). *Decision tree for delegation to unlicensed assistive personnel (UAP).* https://kbn.ky.gov/General/Documents/decision-tree-for-delegation-to-uap.pdf

Lineberry, M., Noland, M., & Wilson, J. F. (2021, April). Intentions of Kentucky school nurses to delegate diabetes-related tasks to unlicensed assistive personnel. *Journal of School Nursing, 37*(2), 99–108. https://doi-org.mantis.csuchico.edu/10.1177/1059840519849098

Meyer-Cuno, D. (2021, November 30). *Life-changing leadership: Delegation.* Forbes. https://www.forbes.com/sites/forbesbooksauthors/2021/11/30/life-changing-leadership-delegation/?sh=1e748de9c6e2

National Association of School Nurses. (2021). *Nursing delegation in the school setting (Position statement adopted June 2019).* Retrieved December 3, 2021, from https://www.nasn.org/advocacy/professional-practice-documents/position-statements/ps-delegation

North Carolina Board of Nursing. (2014, January). *Delegation—Non-nursing functions. Position statement for RN and LPN practice (Revised).* https://www.ncbon.com/vdownloads/position-statements-decision-trees/delegation-non-nursing-functions.pdf

Royal College of Nursing. (2021). *Accountability and delegation in practice.* Retrieved December 3, 2021, from http://rcnhca.org.uk/46-2/accountability-and-delegation/delegation/

Salemme, I. (2021, February 11). *How to delegate tasks with efficiency.* Pipefy. http://www.pipefy.com/best-practices/how-to-delegate-tasks-with-efficiency/

Shasta College. (2021). *Vocational nursing program: General information.* Retrieved December 4, 2021, from https://www.shastacollege.edu/academics/divisions-departments/health-sciences-hsup/health-sciences-programs/vocational-nursing-vn-program/

Thompson, P. (2021, June 3). How to delegate: Tips for delegating tasks at work. *Better Up Blog.* https://www.betterup.com/blog/delegation

21

Conflict, Workplace Violence, and Negotiation

*… Seemingly inconsequential acts of bad behavior can spread through your organization like the flu, taking a financial and emotional toll if left unchecked.—**Christine Pearson***

*… There is an immutable conflict at work in life and in business, a constant battle between peace and chaos. Neither can be mastered, but both can be influenced. How you go about that is the key to success.—**Phil Knight***

*… Workplace violence should not and does not 'come with the territory' of being a nurse.—**Rhonda Collins***

CROSSWALK

This chapter addresses:

- **AACN Essentials Domain 5**: Quality and safety
- **AACN Essentials Domain 6**: Interprofessional partnerships
- **AACN Essentials Domain 7**: Systems-based practice
- **AACN Essentials Domain 9**: Professionalism
- **AACN Essentials Domain 10**: Personal, professional, and leadership development
- **AONL Nurse Executive Competency 1**: Communication and relationship building
- **AONL Nurse Executive Competency 3**: Leadership
- **AONL Nurse Executive Competency 4**: Professionalism
- **AONL Nurse Executive Competency 5**: Business skills
- **ANA Standard of Professional Performance 8**: Advocacy
- **ANA Standard of Professional Performance 9**: Respectful and equitable practice
- **ANA Standard of Professional Performance 10**: Communication
- **ANA Standard of Professional Performance 11**: Collaboration
- **ANA Standard of Professional Performance 12**: Leadership
- **ANA Standard of Professional Performance 18**: Environmental health
- **QSEN Competency**: Teamwork and collaboration
- **QSEN Competency**: Safety

LEARNING OBJECTIVES

The learner will:

- differentiate between qualitative and quantitative conflict and between intrapersonal and interpersonal conflict
- describe the stages of conflict
- seek win–win conflict resolution outcomes whenever possible
- identify the functional and dysfunctional results of various methods of conflict resolution
- select appropriate conflict resolution strategies to solve various conflict situations

- identify the components of effective collaboration
- describe manifestations of workplace violence, incivility, bullying, and mobbing
- identify strategies that might be used to immediately confront and intervene when workplace violence exists
- describe why zero tolerance must be an organizational expectation for workplace violence
- describe strategies that can be used before, during, and after negotiation to increase the likelihood that desired outcomes will be achieved
- identify effective ways to counter commonly used destructive tactics in conflict negotiation
- describe how alternative dispute resolution might be used to resolve conflicts when negotiation has not been successful
- reflect on the challenges as well as rewards in seeking consensus to address group conflict

Introduction

Conflict is generally defined as the internal or external discord that results from differences in ideas, values, or feelings between two or more people. Because work typically involves interpersonal relationships with people having different values, beliefs, backgrounds, and goals, conflict is an expected outcome. Indeed, Cardillo (2021) notes there will always be differing opinions and ways of doing things. Leader-managers must decide which issues they can live with, and which need addressing.

Conflict is also created when there are differences in economic and professional values and when there is competition among professionals. Scarce resources, restructuring, and poorly defined role expectations also are frequent sources of conflict in organizations.

Openly acknowledging that conflict is a naturally occurring and expected phenomenon in organizations reflects a tremendous shift from how sociologists viewed conflict a century ago. The current sociologic view is that organizational conflict should be neither avoided nor encouraged but managed. The leader's role is to create a work environment where conflict may be used as a conduit for growth, innovation, and productivity. When organizational conflict becomes dysfunctional, the manager must recognize it in its early stages and actively intervene so that subordinates' motivation and organizational productivity are not adversely affected.

Leonard (2020) agrees, suggesting that the distinction between constructive and destructive conflict lies in how the conflict is managed to produce positive or negative results. Destructive conflict hinders work performance because people refuse to speak to each other, or they do not have civilized conversations. Thus, it can reduce the morale of an entire department as well as productivity and efficiency. Constructive conflict embraces differing ideas and worldviews, in an effort to move the company toward its goals and mission. Thus, it increases productivity, rather than hampers it (Leonard, 2020).

> Conflict is neither good nor bad, and it can produce growth or destruction, depending on how it is managed.

This chapter presents an overview of growth producing versus dysfunctional conflict in organizations. The history of conflict management, categories of conflict, the conflict process itself, and strategies for successful conflict resolution are discussed. Incivility, workplace violence, bullying, and mobbing are presented as threats to patient and worker safety, and

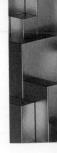

DISPLAY 21.1 **LEADERSHIP ROLES AND MANAGEMENT FUNCTIONS IN CONFLICT RESOLUTION**

Leadership Roles

1. Is self-aware and conscientiously works to resolve intrapersonal conflict
2. Addresses conflict as soon as it is perceived and before it becomes felt or manifest
3. Immediately confronts and intervenes when incivility, bullying, and mobbing occur
4. Seeks a win–win solution to conflict whenever feasible
5. Lessens the perceptual differences that exist between conflicting parties and broadens the parties' understanding about the problems
6. Assists subordinates in identifying alternative conflict resolutions
7. Recognizes and accepts individual differences in team members
8. Uses assertive communication skills to increase persuasiveness and foster open communication
9. Role models honest and collaborative negotiation efforts
10. Encourages consensus building when group support is needed to resolve conflicts

Management Functions

1. Creates a work environment that minimizes the antecedent conditions for conflict
2. Uses appropriately legitimate authority in a competing approach when a quick or unpopular decision needs to be made
3. Facilitates conflict resolution among team members when appropriate
4. Accepts mutual responsibility for reaching predetermined supraordinate goals
5. Establishes a workplace culture that has zero tolerance for incivility, bullying, mobbing, and workplace violence
6. Obtains needed unit resources through effective negotiation strategies
7. Compromises unit needs only when the need is not critical to unit functioning and when higher management gives up something of equal value
8. Is adequately prepared to negotiate for unit resources, including the advance determination of a bottom line and possible trade-offs
9. Addresses the need for closure and follow-up to negotiation
10. Pursues alternative dispute resolution when conflicts cannot be resolved using traditional conflict management strategies

---

strategies for eliminating workplace violence are suggested. This chapter concludes with a discussion of negotiation as a conflict resolution strategy. Leadership roles and management functions necessary for conflict resolution at the unit level are outlined in Display 21.1.

The History of Conflict Management

Early in the 20th century, conflict was considered an indication of poor organizational management, was deemed destructive, and was avoided at all costs. When conflict occurred, it was ignored, denied, or dealt with immediately and harshly. The theorists of this era believed that conflict could be avoided if employees were taught the one right way to do things, and if expressed, employee dissatisfaction was met swiftly with disapproval.

In the mid-20th century, as organizations increasingly recognized that worker satisfaction and feedback were important, conflict was more often accepted passively and perceived as normal and expected. Attention centered on teaching managers how to resolve conflict rather than how to prevent it. Although conflict was still considered primarily dysfunctional, it was believed that conflict and cooperation could happen simultaneously.

The interactionist theorists of the 1970s, however, recognized conflict as a necessity and actively encouraged organizations to promote conflict as a means of producing growth. From

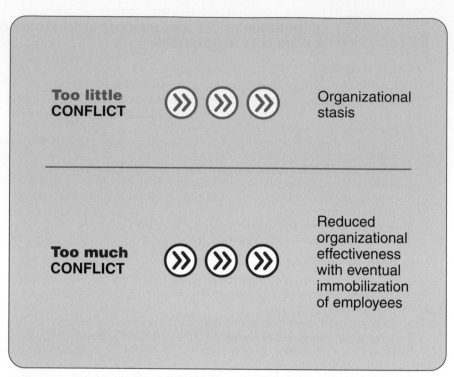

FIGURE 21.1 The relationship between organizational conflict and effectiveness.

this, one can infer that some conflict is desired, although its extent is difficult to know. Perhaps more important than the quantification of conflict is the impact this conflict has on the organization.

> Some level of conflict in an organization appears desirable, although the optimum level for a specific person or unit at a given time is difficult to determine.

Too little conflict results in organizational stasis. Too much conflict reduces the organization's effectiveness and eventually immobilizes its employees (Fig. 21.1). The responsibility for determining and creating an appropriate level of conflict on the individual unit often falls to the leader-manager. Cardillo (2021) notes then that leaders must choose their battles carefully: "If you bring up only the most important issues, you will develop credibility. On the other hand, if you make an issue about everything, you'll be labeled a complainer. Then, when you have a legitimate beef, you likely will be ignored like the fabled boy who cried wolf" (para. 9).

Conflict also has a qualitative nature. A person may be totally overwhelmed in one conflict situation yet can handle several simultaneous conflicts later. The difference is in the quality or significance of that conflict to the person experiencing it. Although *quantitative* and *qualitative* conflicts produce distress at the time they occur, they can lead to growth, energy, and creativity by generating new ideas and solutions. If handled inappropriately, quantitative and qualitative conflicts can lead to demoralization, decreased motivation, and lowered productivity.

Nursing managers can no longer afford to respond to conflict traditionally (i.e., to avoid or suppress it) because this is nonproductive. The ability to understand and deal with conflict appropriately is a critical leadership skill.

LEARNING EXERCISE 21.1

Thinking and Writing about Conflict

Do you generally view conflict positively or negatively?
Does conflict affect you more cognitively, emotionally, or physically?
How was conflict expressed in the home in which you grew up?
Does the way that you handle conflict mirror that of your role models as a child?
Do you believe that you have too much or too little conflict in your life?
Do you feel like you have control over the issues that are now causing conflict in your life?

ASSIGNMENT:

Write a one-page essay, answering one of the questions above.

Intergroup, Intrapersonal, and Interpersonal Conflict

There are three primary categories of conflict: intergroup, intrapersonal, and interpersonal (Fig. 21.2). *Intergroup conflict* occurs between two or more groups of people, departments, and organizations. An example of intergroup conflict might be two political affiliations with widely differing or contradictory beliefs or nurses experiencing intergroup conflict with family and work issues.

Interpersonal conflict happens between two or more people with differing values, goals, and beliefs. *Intrapersonal conflict* occurs within the person. It involves an internal struggle to clarify contradictory values or wants. For managers, intrapersonal conflict may result from the

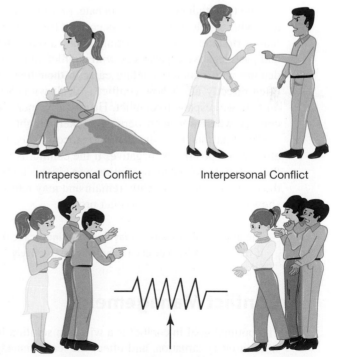

Intrapersonal Conflict   Interpersonal Conflict

FIGURE 21.2 Primary categories of conflict.

Intergroup Conflict

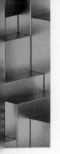

multiple areas of responsibility associated with the management role. Managers' responsibilities to the organization, subordinates, consumers, the profession, and themselves sometimes conflict, and that conflict may be internalized. Being self-aware and conscientiously working to resolve intrapersonal conflict as soon as it is first felt is essential to the leader's physical and mental health.

The Conflict Process

Before managers can or should attempt to intervene in conflict, they must be able to assess its five stages accurately. The first stage in the conflict process, *latent conflict*, implies the existence of antecedent conditions such as short staffing and rapid change. In this stage, conditions are ripe for conflict, although no conflict has actually occurred, and none may ever occur. Much unnecessary conflict could be prevented or reduced if managers examined the organization more closely for antecedent conditions. For example, change and budget cuts almost invariably create conflict. Such events, therefore, should be well thought out so that interventions can be made before the conflicts created by these events escalate.

If conflict progresses, it may develop into the second stage: *perceived conflict*. Perceived or substantive conflict is intellectualized and often involves issues and roles. The person recognizes it logically and impersonally as occurring but does not feel emotionally involved in it. Sometimes, conflict can be resolved at this stage before it is internalized or felt. In an environment characterized by open communication and mutual support, many conflicts can be resolved simply by pointing out that a potential or actual problem exists.

The third stage, *felt conflict*, occurs when the conflict becomes emotionalized. Felt emotions include hostility, fear, mistrust, and anger. This stage is also referred to as *affective conflict*. It is possible to perceive conflict and not feel it (e.g., no emotion is attached to the conflict and the person views it only as a problem to be solved). A person also can feel the conflict but not perceive the problem (e.g., they feel conflict is present but may be unaware of its roots).

In the fourth stage, *manifest conflict*, also called *overt conflict*, action is taken. The action may be to withdraw, compete, debate, or seek conflict resolution. Individuals are uncomfortable with or reluctant to address conflict for many reasons. These include fear of retaliation, fear of ridicule, fear of alienating others, a sense that they do not have the right to speak up, and past negative experiences with conflict situations. Indeed, people often learn patterns of dealing with manifest conflict early in their lives, and family background and experiences often directly affect how conflict is dealt with in adulthood. Gender also may play a role on how we respond to conflict. Historically, men were socialized to respond aggressively to conflict, whereas women were more likely taught to try to avoid conflicts or to pacify them.

The final stage in the conflict process is *conflict aftermath*. There is always conflict aftermath—positive or negative. If the conflict is managed well, people involved in the conflict will believe that their position was given a fair hearing. If the conflict is managed poorly, the conflict issues frequently remain and may return later to cause more conflict. Figure 21.3 shows a schematic of this conflict process.

> The aftermath of conflict may be more significant than the original conflict
> if the conflict has not been handled constructively.

Conflict Management

The optimal goal in conflict is a win–win solution for all involved. This outcome is not possible in every situation, and often, the leader-manager's goal is to manage the conflict in a way that lessens the perceptual differences that exist between the involved parties. A leader

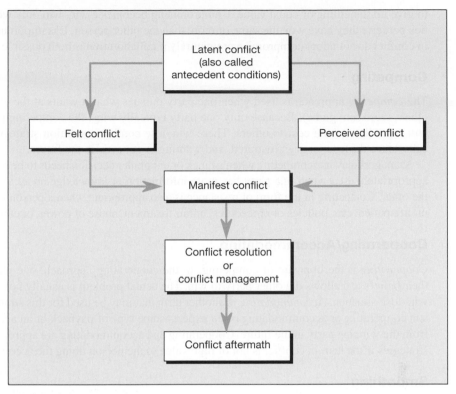

FIGURE 21.3 The conflict process.

recognizes which conflict management or resolution strategy is most appropriate for each situation. Common conflict management strategies are identified in Display 21.2. The choice of the most appropriate strategy depends on many variables, such as the situation itself, the urgency of the decision, the power and status of the players, the importance of the issue, and the maturity of the people involved in the conflict.

> The optimal goal in resolving conflict is creating a win–win solution for all involved.

Compromising

In *compromising*, each party gives up something it wants. Although many see compromise as an optimum conflict resolution strategy, it may result in a lose–lose situation because either or both parties perceive that they have given up more than the other and may therefore feel defeated. For compromising not to result in a lose–lose situation, both parties must be willing

DISPLAY 21.2 COMMON CONFLICT RESOLUTION STRATEGIES

1. Compromising
2. Competing
3. Cooperating/accommodating
4. Smoothing
5. Avoiding
6. Collaborating

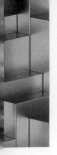

to give up something of equal value. Compromising becomes a win–win only when both parties perceive they have won the same or more than the other person. It is important that parties in conflict do not adopt compromise prematurely if collaboration is both possible and feasible.

Competing

The *competing* approach is used when one party pursues what it wants at the expense of the others (zero sum game). Because only one party typically wins, the competing party seeks to win regardless of the cost to others. These win–lose conflict resolution strategies then typically leave the loser angry, frustrated, and wanting to get even in the future.

Managers may use competing when a quick or unpopular decision needs to be made. It is also appropriately used when one party has more information or knowledge about a situation than the other. Competing in the form of resistance is also appropriate when a person needs to resist unsafe patient care policies or procedures, unfair treatment, abuse of power, or ethical concerns.

Cooperating/Accommodating

Cooperating is the opposite of competing. In the cooperating approach, one party sacrifices their beliefs and allows the other party to win. The actual problem is usually not solved in this win–lose situation. *Accommodating* is another term that may be used for this strategy. The person cooperating or accommodating often expects some type of payback or an accommodation from the winning party in the future. Cooperating and accommodating are appropriate political strategies if the item in conflict is not of high value to the person doing the accommodating.

Smoothing

Smoothing is used to manage a conflict situation. Smoothing occurs when one party in a conflict attempts to pacify the other party or to focus on agreements rather than differences. In doing so, the emotional component of the conflict is minimized. Managers often use smoothing to get someone to accommodate or cooperate with another party. Although it may be appropriate for minor disagreements, smoothing rarely results in resolution of the actual conflict.

Avoiding

In the *avoiding* approach, the parties involved are aware of a conflict but choose not to acknowledge it or attempt to resolve it. Avoidance may be indicated in trivial disagreements, when the cost of dealing with the conflict exceeds the benefits of solving it, when the problem should be solved by people other than you, when one party is more powerful than the other, or when the problem will solve itself. The greatest problem in using avoidance is that the conflict remains, often only to reemerge later in an even more exaggerated fashion.

Collaborating

Collaborating is an assertive and cooperative means of conflict resolution that results in a win–lose solution. In collaboration, all parties set aside their original goals and work together to establish a *supraordinate* or priority common goal. In doing so, all parties accept mutual responsibility for reaching the supraordinate goal.

Although it is very difficult for people truly to set aside original goals, collaboration cannot occur if this does not happen. For example, a married couple experiencing serious conflict over whether to have a baby may first want to identify whether they share the supraordinate goal of keeping the marriage together. A nurse who is unhappy that they did not receive requested days off might meet with their supervisor and jointly establish the supraordinate goal that staffing will be adequate to meet patient safety criteria. If the new goal is truly a jointly set goal, each party will perceive that an important goal has been achieved and that the

LEARNING EXERCISE 21.2

Personal Conflict Solving

It is important for managers to be self-aware regarding how they view and deal with conflict. In your personal life, how do you solve conflict? Is it important for you to win? When was the last time you were able to solve conflict by reaching supraordinate goals with another person? Are you able to see the other person's position in conflict situations? In conflicts with family and friends, are you least likely to compromise values, scarcities, or role expectations?

supraordinate goal is most important. In doing so, the focus remains on problem solving and not on defeating the other party.

Collaboration, however, is rare when there is a wide difference in power between the groups and individuals involved. Many think of collaboration as a form of cooperation, but this is not an accurate definition. In collaboration, problem solving is a joint effort with no superior–subordinate, order-giving–order-taking relationships. True collaboration requires mutual respect; open and honest communication; and equitable, shared decision-making powers.

> Although conflict is a pervasive force in health care organizations, only a small percentage of time is spent in true collaboration.

Collaboration enhances a person's participation in decision making to accomplish mutual goals and therefore is the best method to resolve conflict to achieve long-term benefits. Because it may involve others over whom the manager has no control and because its process is often lengthy, it may not be the best approach for all situations.

LEARNING EXERCISE 21.3

Conflicting Personal, Professional, and Organizational Obligations

You are a registered nurse. You have been working on the oncology unit since your graduation from the state college a year ago. Your supervisor, Mary, has complimented your performance. Lately, she has allowed you to be relief charge nurse on the 3:00 PM to 11:00 PM shift when the regular charge nurse is not there. Occasionally, you have been asked to work on the medical–surgical units when your department has a low census. Although you dislike leaving your own unit, you have cooperated because you felt that you could handle the other clinical assignments and wanted to show your flexibility.

On arriving at work tonight, the nursing office calls and requests that you help out in the busy delivery room. You protest that you do not know anything about obstetrics and that it is impossible for you to take the assignment. Carol, the supervisor from the nursing office, insists that you are the most qualified person; she says to "just go and do the best you can." Your own unit supervisor is not on duty, and the charge nurse says that she does not feel comfortable advising you in this conflict. You feel torn between professional, personal, and organizational obligations.

ASSIGNMENT:

What should you do? Select the most appropriate conflict resolution strategy. Give rationale for your selection and for your rejection of the others. After you have made your choice, read the analysis found in the Appendix.

> **DISPLAY 21.3 COMMON CAUSES OF ORGANIZATIONAL CONFLICT**
>
> - Poor communication
> - Inadequately defined organizational structure
> - Individual behavior (incompatibilities or disagreements based on differences of temperament or attitudes)
> - Unclear expectations
> - Individual or group conflicts of interest
> - Operational or staffing changes
> - Diversity in gender, culture, or age

Managing Unit Conflict

Managing conflict effectively requires an understanding of its origin. Some of the sources of organizational conflict are shown in Display 21.3. Some common causes of unit conflict are unclear expectations, poor communication, lack of clear jurisdiction, incompatibilities or disagreements based on differences of temperament or attitudes, individual or group conflicts of interest, and operational or staffing changes. In addition, not only does diversity in gender, age, and culture influence conflict resolution, it may also create conflict itself. This occurs because of communication difficulties, including language and literacy issues and a growing recognition that some factors are beyond assimilation.

Organizational conflicts can disrupt working relationships, generate a breakdown in trust, and lower productivity. When a team or individuals within a team are in conflict, communication between team members can decline and patient care can suffer as a result. It is imperative, then, that the manager identify the origin of unit conflicts and intervene early to promote cooperative, if not collaborative, conflict resolution.

At times, unit conflict requires that the manager facilitate conflict resolution between others. This does not, however, include the daily disagreements that employees experience at work. Sometimes, however, employees simply cannot or will not resolve these differences and then they can escalate and begin to negatively affect work and other employees. It is at this point that the mediation skills of the leader-managers become critical. The manager may also want to intervene if the relationship with one or both parties is highly significant to them, even if the issue is not.

The following is a list of strategies that a manager may use to facilitate conflict resolution between members in the workplace:

- *Confrontation.* Many times, team members inappropriately expect the manager to solve their interpersonal conflicts. Managers instead can urge subordinates to attempt to handle their own problems by using face-to-face communication to resolve conflicts, as e-mails, answering machine messages, and notes are too impersonal for interpersonal conflicts that can have significant conflict aftermath.
- *Third-party consultation.* Sometimes, managers can be used as a neutral party to help others resolve conflicts constructively. This should be done only if all parties are motivated to solve the problem and if no differences exist in the status or power of the parties involved. If the conflict involves multiple parties and highly charged emotions, the manager may find outside experts helpful for facilitating communication and bringing issues to the forefront.
- *Behavior change.* This is reserved for serious cases of dysfunctional conflict. Educational modes, training development, or sensitivity training can be used to solve conflict by developing self-awareness and behavior change in the involved parties.

- *Responsibility charting.* When ambiguity results from unclear or new roles, it is often necessary to have the parties come together to delineate the function and responsibility of roles. If areas of joint responsibility exist, the manager must clearly define such areas as ultimate responsibility, approval mechanisms, support services, and responsibility for informing. This is a useful technique for elementary jurisdictional conflicts. An example of a potential jurisdictional conflict might arise between the house supervisor and unit manager in staffing or between an in-service educator and unit manager in determining and planning unit educational needs or programs.
- *Structure change.* Sometimes, managers need to intervene in unit conflict by transferring or discharging people. Other structure changes may be moving a department under another manager, adding an ombudsperson, or putting a grievance procedure in place. Often, increasing the boundaries of authority for one member of the conflict will act as an effective structure change to resolve unit conflict. Changing titles and creating policies are also effective techniques.
- *Soothing one party.* This is a temporary solution that should be used in a crisis when there is no time to handle the conflict effectively or when the parties are so enraged that immediate conflict resolution is unlikely. Waiting a few days allows most individuals to deal with their intense feelings and to be more objective about the issues. Regardless of how the parties are soothed, the manager must address the underlying problem later or this technique will become ineffective.

Bullying, Incivility, Mobbing, and Workplace Violence

Definitions

Sometimes, conflict escalates to harmful and even dangerous conduct. The Workplace Bullying Institute (2021, para 2) defines *bullying* as repeated, health-harming mistreatment of one or more employees of an employer: abusive conduct that takes the form of verbal abuse; or behaviors perceived as threatening, intimidating, or humiliating; work sabotage; or in some combination of the above. The American Nurses Association (ANA) defines bullying as "repeated, unwanted, harmful actions intended to humiliate, offend, and cause distress in the recipient" (Colduvell, 2021, para 3). Both definitions imply bullying is abusive conduct that is threatening, humiliating, or intimidating in nature. When it occurs between coworkers, it is known as *horizontal bullying*.

Incivility is another term used to describe mistreatment or discourtesy to another person. It can be overt (physical or verbal) or it can be expressed passive-aggressively through behaviors such as eye-rolling, walking away, and pointing fingers (Ball, 2021).

In addition, interpersonal conflict can be manifested by *mobbing*, when employees "gang up" on an individual. The degree of harm a nurse experiences from bullying or mobbing often depends on the frequency, intensity, and duration of the behavior and/or tactic used. Moreover, what one person considers as a harmful experience, another may not. Therefore, every person's experience with, or perceptions about, violence are unique to that person (Hockley, 2020).

When bullying, incivility, and mobbing occur in the workplace, they are known collectively as *workplace violence*. Hockley (2020) maintains that workplace violence includes physical violence as well as various antisocial behaviors and incidents that lead a person to believe that they have been harmed by the experience. It also includes, but is not limited to, such behaviors as engaging in favoritism, being verbally abusive, sending abusive correspondence, bullying, pranks, and setting workers up for failure. It also includes economic aggression such

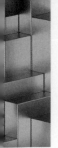

DISPLAY 21.4 MANIFESTATIONS OF WORKPLACE BULLYING

- Backstabbing
- Swearing/yelling/shouting
- Making threats
- Calling names
- Invading personal space
- Threatening gestures
- Constant eye contact
- Withholding information/controlling communication
- Refusing to help
- Finding fault
- Ethnic or racial jokes or slurs
- Sabotage
- Unreasonable workloads/unfair assignments
- Betraying confidence or gossiping
- Humiliation
- Social isolation/exclusion
- Physical harm
- Exclusion and silence
- Eye rolling or other demeaning nonverbal behaviors
- Innuendo
- Cyberbullying

Sources: Hockley, C. (2020). Promoting healthy work environments and civility: Why is this so difficult in nursing? In C. J. Huston (Ed.), *Professional issues in nursing: Challenges and opportunities* (5th ed., pp. 167–181). Wolters Kluwer; Dillon, S. (2021, January 7). *Workplace bullying in nursing: Why it happens and how to confront it.* Bravado Health. https://www.bravadohealth.com/2021/01/07/confronting-nurse-bullying/

as denying workers promotional opportunities. Countless practice settings are hindered by maladaptive social behaviors that victimize nurses and impact patient care (Hockley, 2020). Manifestations of workplace bullying are noted in Display 21.4.

Workplace Violence: Scope of the Problem

Violence against health care workers is a problem worldwide. Indeed, the World Medical Association (WMA, 2020) stated violence against health personnel is "an international emergency that undermines the very foundations of health systems and impacts critically on patient's health." The WMA (2020) also suggests this violence has increased dramatically since the beginning of the COVID-19 pandemic, with health care professionals reporting incidents: threats, insults, and stigmatization from communities and states.

Indeed, a 2021 Workplace Health & Safety survey of registered nurses reports that 44% experienced physical violence at least once during the pandemic from patients, family members, or visitors (Nursing Workplace Violence, 2021). Over two thirds encountered verbal abuse at least once. RNs who provided direct care for patients with COVID-19 experienced more violence than nurses who did not care for these patients. Nurses also faced difficulty reporting these incidents to management (NurseJournal Staff, 2021).

Even before the pandemic, health care workers in the United States had an increased chance of experiencing workplace injury as compared to other professions (Berger & Michelana, 2021). The health care industry leads all other sectors for non-fatal workplace assaults (NurseJournal Staff, 2021; United States Department of Labor [U.S. DOL], n.d.). In fact, workers in health care settings are four times more likely to be assaulted than workers in private industry (Kam, 2021).

Many episodes of violence directed at health care workers come from patients and/or their families. Ladika (2021) notes that aggressive behavior is common in patients experiencing

DISPLAY 21.5 TYPOLOGY OF WORKPLACE VIOLENCE

- Nurse-to-nurse violence (includes nursing students; horizontal violence, lateral violence)
- Patient-to-nurse violence (including visitors)
- Organization-to-nurse violence (vertical downward violence)
- External perpetrators (strangers, criminal intent)
- Third-party violence (other health professionals/family members and significant others as well as other health care workers)
- Impact of mass trauma or natural disasters on nurses (e.g., terrorism, wars, earthquakes, or floods)
- Nurse-to-patient violence
- Personal violence (e.g., intimate partner violence, family violence, interpersonal violence)

Source: Clark, C. M. (2023). Promoting civility and healthy work environments in nursing and health care. In C. J. Huston (Ed.), *Professional issues in nursing: Challenges and opportunities* (6th ed., Chapter 13, pp. 181–197). Wolters Kluwer.

mental health issues or dementia, especially when the need for psychiatric services exceeds the supply. Violent behavior also can be a symptom of head injuries or may occur when people come out of anesthesia. Ladika also notes that family members and loved ones may lash out when they are upset about the lack of appropriate care or because of the pain the patient is suffering.

In addition, patient-to-nurse violence is more likely when patients must stay in the emergency department (ED) for long hours—or even days. Indeed, half of all reported violent incidents in health care settings occur in the ED (Carver & Beard, 2021). Sadly, 40% of ED doctors report having been physically assaulted on the job as do 70% of emergency nurses (Kam, 2021). In addition, although extreme violence may not be tolerated, most ED workers put up with the small acts of abuse, such as verbal assault including curses and threats, and unwelcome sexual advances, on a regular basis.

> Violence and workplace aggression are increasingly being recognized as epidemic in the health care workplace.

Patient-to-nurse violence, however, is not the only type of violence faced by nurses. Nurse-to-nurse violence, nurse-to-patient violence, and third-party violence also occur. Indeed, the types of workplace violence experienced by health care workers are diverse and complex, which only adds to the difficulty in addressing this issue. Nevertheless, it is possible to categorize the types of violence health care workers may experience. These are shown in Display 21.5.

Consequences of Workplace Violence

Unfortunately, cases of workplace violence are likely much higher than reported. Many nurses who experience patient-to-nurse violence do not submit incident reports or have their injuries treated. This does not mean that there are not consequences. Nurses exposed to workplace violence are two to four times more likely to experience posttraumatic stress disorder, anxiety, depression, and burnout than nurses with no exposure (NurseJournal Staff, 2021).

Other medical consequences of workplace violence include an increase in employee health complaints such as neck pain, musculoskeletal complaints, acute pain, fibromyalgia, and cardiovascular symptoms. The emotional/psychological consequences may include increased mental distress, sleep disturbances, fatigue, lack of vigor, depression and anxiety, and adjustment disorders, all of which increase the risk of absenteeism and turnover. It may even lead to increased risk of suicide.

Workplace violence also poses consequences to patient care because the care of an affected nurse often decreases significantly in quality. It is difficult to be patient centered when the

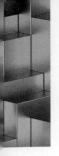

health care worker fears harm from their patients, family members, or colleagues. It is also distracting, which can increase errors. Other damaging consequences include moral distress, burnout, and job dissatisfaction, which can lead to increased turnover.

As a result of these negative worker and patient outcomes, The Joint Commission has called for better protections against workplace violence. It also created "Sentinel Event Alert 59," which addresses violence—physical and verbal—against health care workers to help health care organizations better recognize workplace violence directed toward health care workers and how to better prepare staff to address it, both in real time and afterward (Patient Safety Network, 2021).

Whose Problem Is It?

The responsibility for dealing with workplace violence should initially lie with frontline staff, but the manager must become involved if the conflict is not immediately resolved. In addition, organizations should have a bullying policy in place that clearly describes zero tolerance as the expectation because bullying and incivility impact turnover, productivity, and quality of care. To end abusive behaviors, these policies must be communicated loudly and clearly, and open, respectful communication must be encouraged.

Perhaps most important to ending workplace violence and bullying, however, is that nurses themselves must recognize that verbal abuse, incivility, and bullying are never acceptable behavior. For far too long, the culture in nursing education and clinical has been that bullying is simply part of the job. For example, Dillon (2021) shared the following excerpt from a document given to her daughter on entering nursing school, entitled "Traits of a Successful Nursing Student." The last trait they listed for success was courage: "Some of the situations that nursing students face in clinicals are difficult and challenging. Sometimes verbal abuse occurs as well as patient pain that happens when you are performing a procedure. Nursing students need to find the courage to deal with these situations" (para. 10).

Dillon (2021) notes that although she understands that the school of nursing was trying to prepare students for difficult situations that occur in the profession, she was disheartened to see that they were subliminally planting a seed that implied verbal abuse is normal and to be expected in nursing. "Students who learn early on that abuse is okay have a hard time speaking out against any kind of bullying even that enacted by their peers. The school failed by pointing out a problem without empowering prospective students with solutions" (Dillon, 2021, para. 11).

Kam (2021) agrees, noting that nurses themselves are often conflicted as to what to do when they experience violence at work. They want to help patients and it is easy to excuse the behavior. But workplace violence should not happen, and it should not be allowed to become an expected norm.

> Zero tolerance should be the expectation because bullying and incivility impact turnover, productivity, and quality of care.

Strategies to Address the Problem

Employees need to be given tools that provide information on how to address conflicts and change unacceptable behavior in the workplace. To help address bullying, the ANA has created resources, including a publication, tip cards, fact sheet, and webinars that offer strategies for both individual nurses and organizations to use. The ANA also published a position statement on bullying, incivility, and workplace violence in 2015 that identifies individual and shared roles and responsibilities of RNs and employers to create and sustain a culture of respect, free of incivility, bullying, and workplace violence (ANA, n.d.). Similarly, in 2016, The Joint Commission launched the *Workplace Violence Prevention Resources for Health Care* site.

EXAMINING THE EVIDENCE 21.1

Source: From Esposito, C. L., & Contreras Sollazzo, L. (2021). A time-limited look at whether the New York State Felony D Law or workplace violence programs mitigate violence against nurses in the healthcare setting. *Journal of the New York State Nurses Association, 48*(1), 11–29.

Registered Nurses' and Student Nurses' Perceptions of Workplace Violence Risk

In 2010, the NYS Senate passed legislation strengthening the penalties for individuals who injure or attempt to injure nurses while the nurse is practicing in the line of duty. The Felony D law imposes a penalty for assault on registered nurses (RNs) as a class D felony. This research provided a time-limited look at whether the NYS Felony D law and regulatory anti-workplace violence programs thus far have mitigated the incidence of violence against nurses in the workplace.

In the fall of 2019, the New York State Nurse Association conducted an analysis of the 2019 OSHA logs of five-private-sector hospitals located in Brooklyn, Staten Island, Queens, and the Bronx. The logs revealed a total of 1,508 individuals listed as injured or ill as a result of assault. The total number of reported member cases of workers who had to be away from work as a result of an injury due to an assault was 67 cases, with a collective total of 939 days. Fifteen cases included workers who were away from work for more than 10 days due to a one-injury episode. Among the five facilities, 10% of documented injuries were due to assaults.

Despite more legislative protections and the scope of these illnesses and injuries, only two cases were filed by nurses under the felony assault law. The researchers noted that while advocacy groups say it's time for policymakers and employers to act on this growing but underreported problem, practice is that even with regulatory initiatives, it is more typically perceived as the employer's obligation to ensure a healthy, violence-free work environment.

In addition, ANA's *Code of Ethics for Nurses with Interpretive Statements* states that nurses are required to create an ethical environment and culture of civility and kindness, treating colleagues, coworkers, employees, students, and others with dignity and respect. Nurses must be afforded the same level of respect and dignity as we treat others (ANA, 2015). All RNs and employers in all settings, including practice, academia, and research, must collaborate to create a culture of respect, free of incivility, bullying, and workplace violence (ANA, n.d.).

All health care organizations have a responsibility to establish strategies for preventing workplace violence. In addition, some states are exploring requiring health care organizations to develop more comprehensive workplace violence prevention plans. With the passage of A.B. 30, California became the first state in 2018 to require all acute care hospitals and skilled-nursing facilities to develop and implement such a plan. Other states, such as New York, have enacted stiffer criminal penalties for assaults against health care workers, although evidence suggests the problem continues to be underreported and that the actual filing of criminal complaints is rare (Esposito & Contreras Sollazzo, 2021) (see Examining the Evidence 21.1).

In addition, the federal Occupational Safety and Health Administration (OSHA) has tried to combat violence in emergency rooms by increasing the number of its inspectors dedicated to workplace violence cases and issuing citations when employees are subjected to workplace violence; however, there is no OSHA standard to mitigate workplace violence in health care facilities.

Negotiation

Negotiation in its most creative form is like collaboration and in its most poorly managed form may resemble a competing approach. Negotiation frequently resembles compromise when it

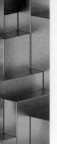

is used as a conflict resolution strategy. During negotiation, each party gives up something, and the emphasis is on accommodating differences between the parties. Few people can meet all of their needs or objectives. Most day-to-day conflict is resolved with negotiation. A nurse who says to another nurse "I'll answer that call light if you'll count narcotics" is practicing the art of negotiation.

Although negotiation implies winning and losing for both parties, there is no rule that each party must lose and win the same amount. Most negotiators want to win more than they lose, but negotiation becomes destructively competitive when the emphasis is on winning at all costs. A major goal of effective negotiation is to make the other party feel satisfied with the outcome. The focus in negotiation should be to create a *win–win* situation.

Many small negotiations take place every day spontaneously and succeed without any advance preparation. However, not all nurses are expert negotiators. If managers wish to succeed in important negotiations for unit resources, they must (a) be adequately prepared, (b) be able to use appropriate negotiation strategies, and (c) apply appropriate closure and follow-up. To become more successful at negotiating, managers need to do several things before, during, and after the negotiation (Display 21.6).

Before the Negotiation

For managers to be successful, they must systematically prepare for the negotiation. As the negotiator, the manager begins by gathering as much information as possible regarding the issue to be negotiated. Because knowledge is power, the more informed the negotiator is, the greater is their bargaining power. Adequate preparation prevents others in the negotiation from catching the negotiator off guard or making them appear uninformed.

In addition, individuals must remember that few negotiations begin at the table. This makes it especially important to know the who, what, when, where, and how of an issue. This is the area where strategies are prepared.

However, another level of preparation is the emotional level, which is the human side of every negotiation and interaction. Remember that the "opponents" you face across the bargaining table are individuals like you. The way the other party perceives you as being fair and open to negotiate often plays a role in the decisions that will be reached in the negotiation.

It is also important for managers to decide where to start in the negotiation. Brodow (2021) notes that successful negotiators are not afraid to ask for what they want. In addition, they should be assertive (not aggressive) because they know that everything is negotiable. He calls this *negotiation consciousness* and suggests that it is what makes the difference between effective negotiators and everybody else.

Because negotiators must be willing to make compromises, they should, however, choose a starting point that is high but not ridiculous. This selected starting point should be at the upper limits of their expectations, realizing that they may need to come down to a more realistic goal. For instance, let us say that you would really like four additional full-time RN positions and a full-time clerical position budgeted for your unit. You know that you could make do with three additional full-time RN positions and a part-time clerical assistant, but you begin by asking for what would be ideal.

It is almost impossible in any type of negotiation to escalate demands; therefore, the negotiator must start at an extreme but reasonable point. It also must be decided beforehand how much can be compromised and what is an acceptable *bottom line* (or the least acceptable resolution). Can the manager accept, at a minimum, one full-time RN position or two or three?

> The very least for which a person will settle is often referred to as the bottom line.

The wise manager also has other options in mind when negotiating for important resources. An alternative option is another set of negotiating preferences that can be used so that managers do not need to use their bottom lines but still meet their overall goal. For instance, you have requested four full-time RN positions and one full-time clerical position. You could get by with three full-time RNs and one part-time clerk. However, you believe strongly that you cannot continue to provide safe patient care unless you are given two RNs and a part-time clerk—your bottom line. However, if the original negotiation is unsuccessful, reopen negotiations by saying that a second option that does not entail increasing the staff would be to float a ward clerk for 4 hours each day, implement a unit-dose system, require housekeeping to pass out linen, and have dietary pass all the patient meal trays. This way, the overall goal of providing more direct patient care by the nursing staff could still be met without adding nursing personnel.

Knowing in advance what you can concede allows you to compromise without feeling that you are giving up and makes it easier for the other party to agree on a workable compromise. Brodow (2021) suggests that "if you depend too much on the positive outcome of a negotiation, you lose your ability to say NO. When you say to yourself, 'I will walk if I can't conclude a deal that is satisfactory,' the other side can tell that you mean business" (para. 10).

If, however, the bottom line is reached, the negotiator should tell the other party that an impasse has been reached and that further negotiation is not possible at this time. Then, the other party should be encouraged to sleep on it and reconsider. The door should always be left open for further negotiation. Another appointment can be made. Both parties should be allowed to save face.

The manager also needs to consider other trade-offs that are possible in these situations. *Trade-offs* are secondary gains, often future oriented, that may be realized as a result of conflict. For example, while attending college, a parent may feel intrapersonal conflict because they are unable to spend as much time as desired with their children. The parent is able to compromise by considering the trade-off: Eventually, everyone's life will be better because of the present sacrifices. The wise manager will consider trading something today for something tomorrow as a means to reach satisfactory negotiations.

The manager also must look for and acknowledge *hidden agendas*—the covert intention of the negotiation. Usually, every negotiation has a covert and an overt agenda. For example, new managers may set up a meeting with their superior with the established agenda of discussing the lack of supplies on the unit. However, the hidden agenda may be that the manager feels insecure and is really seeking performance feedback during the discussion.

Having a hidden agenda is not uncommon and is not wrong by any means. Everyone has them, and it is not necessary or even wise to share these hidden agendas. Managers, however, must be introspective enough to recognize their hidden agendas so that they are not paralyzed if the agenda is discovered and used against them during the negotiation. If the manager's hidden agenda is discovered, they should admit that it is a consideration but not the heart of the negotiation.

For instance, although the hidden agenda for increasing unit staff might be to build the manager's esteem in the eyes of the staff, there may exist a legitimate need for additional staff. If, during the negotiations, the fiscal controller accuses the manager of wanting to increase staff just to gain power, the manager might respond by saying, "It is always important for a successful manager to be able to gain resources for the unit, but the real issue here is an inadequate staff."

> Managers who protest too strongly that they do not have a hidden agenda appear defensive and vulnerable.

During the Negotiation

Because negotiation may be a highly charged experience, the negotiator always wants to appear calm, collected, and self-assured. At least part of this self-assurance comes from having adequately prepared for the negotiation. Part of the preparation should have included learning about the people with whom the manager is negotiating. People come with a variety of personality types, and over the course of their careers, managers will encounter most or all personality types in various negotiations. In addition, the negotiator must remember that concerns about *status* pervade almost every negotiation. Preparation, however, is not enough. In the end, the negotiator must have clarity in their communication, assertiveness, good listening skills, the ability to regroup quickly, and flexibility.

> Negotiation is psychological and verbal. The effective negotiator always appears calm and self-assured.

Brodow (2021) suggests that effective negotiators are like detectives; they ask probing questions and then become quiet. The other negotiator will tell you everything you need to know if you listen. He encourages negotiators to follow the *70/30 Rule*—listen 70% of the time and talk only 30% of the time. In addition, you should encourage the other negotiator to talk by asking lots of *open-ended questions* that cannot be answered with a simple "yes" or "no."

In addition, negotiation requires patience and time. Brodow (2021) notes that being patient in negotiation can be very difficult for Americans. Americans often are in a hurry to complete the negotiation, whereas individuals from Asian, South American, or Middle Eastern cultures will tell you that they look at time differently. They believe that rushing is more likely to cause mistakes and leave money on the table, so whoever can be more flexible about time generally has the advantage (Brodow, 2021).

Strategies commonly used by leaders during negotiation to increase their persuasiveness and foster open communication are shown in Display 21.7.

| DISPLAY 21.7 | STRATEGIES TO INCREASE PERSUASIVENESS AND FOSTER OPEN COMMUNICATION DURING THE NEGOTIATION |

1. Use only factual statements that have been gathered in research.
2. Listen carefully and watch nonverbal communication.
3. Keep an open mind because negotiation always provides the potential for learning. It is important not to prejudge. Instead, a cooperative (not competitive) climate should be established.
4. Try to understand where the other party is coming from. It is probable that one person's perception is different from that of another. The negotiation needs to concentrate on understanding, not just on agreeing.
5. Discuss only the conflict. It is important not to personalize the conflict by discussing the parties involved in the negotiation.
6. Try not to belabor how the conflict occurred or to fix blame for the conflict. Instead, the focus must be on preventing its recurrence.
7. Be honest.
8. Start tough so that concessions are possible. It is much harder to escalate demands in the negotiation than to make concessions.
9. Delay when confronted with something totally unexpected in negotiation. In such cases, the negotiator should respond, "I'm not prepared to discuss this right now" or "I'm sorry, this was not on our agenda; we can set up another appointment to discuss that." If asked a question about something that the negotiator does not know, they should simply say, "I don't have that information at this time."
10. Never tell the other party what you are willing to negotiate totally. You may be giving up too early.
11. Know the bottom line, but try never to use it. If the bottom line is used, the negotiator must be ready to back it up or they will lose all credibility. Negotiations should always result in both sides improving their positions; however, people sometimes have to walk away from the negotiating table if the situation cannot be improved because not every negotiation can result in terms that are agreeable to each party.
12. Take a break if either party becomes angry or tired during the negotiation. Go to the bathroom or make a telephone call. Remember that neither party can effectively negotiate if either is enraged or fatigued.

Destructive Negotiation Tactics

Some negotiators win by using specific intimidating or manipulative tactics. People using these tactics take a competing approach to negotiation rather than a collaborative approach. These tactics might be conscious or unconscious but are used repeatedly because they have been successful for that person. Successful managers do not use these types of tactics, but because others with whom they negotiate may do so, they must be prepared to counter such tactics.

One such tactic is *ridicule*. The goal in using ridicule is to intimidate others involved in the negotiation. If you are negotiating with someone who uses ridicule, maintain a relaxed body posture, steady gaze, and patient smile. Brodow (2021) notes it is very important in negotiation not to take the issues or the other person's behavior personally. All too often, negotiations fail because one or both parties get sidetracked by personal issues unrelated to the negotiation at hand. Successful negotiators focus on solving the problem, which is "How can we conclude an agreement that respects the needs of both parties? Obsessing over the other negotiator's personality, or over issues that are not directly pertinent to making a deal, can sabotage a negotiation. If someone is rude or difficult to deal with, try to understand their behavior and don't take it personally" (Brodow, 2021, para. 16).

Another tactic some people use is *ambiguous* or *inappropriate questioning*. For example, in one negotiating situation, the intensive care unit (ICU) supervisor had requested additional staff to handle open heart surgery patients. During her bargaining, the chief executive officer suddenly said, "I never did understand the heart; can you tell me about the heart?" The supervisor did not fall into this trap and instead replied that the physiology of the heart was irrelevant to the issue. Because people tend to answer an authority figure, it is necessary to be on guard for this type of diversionary tactic.

Flattery is another technique that makes true collaboration in negotiation very difficult. The person who has been flattered may be more reluctant to disagree with the other party in the negotiation, and thus, their attention and focus are diverted. One method that managers can use to discern flattery from other honest attempts to compliment is to be aware of how they feel about the comment. If they feel unduly flattered by a gesture or comment, it is a good indication that they were being flattered. For example, asking for advice or instruction may be a subtle form of flattery, or it may be an honest request. If the request for advice is about an area in which the manager has little expertise, it is undoubtedly flattery. However, exchanging positive opening comments with each other when beginning negotiation is an acceptable and enjoyable practice performed by both parties.

Another destructive technique used in negotiation is *sadness*. Seeing sadness may bring about feelings of empathy and compassion, making it difficult for the negotiator to focus on objective gains. Nurses are also particularly sympathetic to gestures of *helplessness*. Because nursing is a helping profession, the tendency to nurture is high, and managers must be careful not to lose sight of the original intent of the negotiation—securing adequate resources to optimize unit functioning.

Some people win in negotiation simply by rapidly and *aggressively taking over* and controlling the negotiation before other members realize what is happening. If managers believe that this may be happening, they should call a halt to the negotiations before decisions are made. Saying simply, "I need to have time to think this over" is a good method of stopping an aggressive takeover. The manager needs to be aware of destructive negotiation tactics and develop strategies to overcome them because such tactics are antithetical to collaboration.

> Destructive negotiation tactics are never a part of collaborative conflict resolution.

LEARNING EXERCISE 21.4

An Exercise in Negotiation Analysis

You are one of a group of staff nurses who believe that part of your job dissatisfaction results from being assigned different patients every day. Your unit uses a system of total patient care, and the charge nurse makes assignments. Two staff nurses have gone to the charge nurse and requested that each nurse be allowed to pick their own patients based on the previous day's assignment and the ability of the nurse. The charge nurse believes that the staff nurses are being uncooperative because it is the charge nurse's responsibility to see that all the patients get assigned and receive adequate care. Although continuity of care is the goal, many part-time nurses are used on the unit, and not all the nurses are able to care for every type of patient. At the end of the conference, the two nurses are angry, and the charge nurse is irritated. However, the next day, the charge nurse indicates willingness to meet with the staff nurses. The other nurses believe this is a sign that the charge nurse is willing to negotiate a compromise. They plan to get together tonight to plan the strategy for tomorrow's meeting.

ASSIGNMENT:

What are the goals for each party? What could be a possible hidden agenda for each party? What could happen if the conflict escalates? Devise a workable plan that would accomplish the goals of both parties and develop strategies for implementation (see the Appendix for an analysis of these problems).

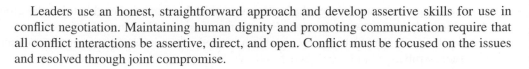

Leaders use an honest, straightforward approach and develop assertive skills for use in conflict negotiation. Maintaining human dignity and promoting communication require that all conflict interactions be assertive, direct, and open. Conflict must be focused on the issues and resolved through joint compromise.

Closure and Follow-Up to Negotiation

Just as it is important to start the formal negotiation with some pleasantries, it is also good to close on a friendly note. Once a compromise has been reached, restate it so that everyone is clear about what has been agreed on. If managers win more in negotiation than they anticipated, they should try to hide their astonishment. At the end of any negotiation, whether it is a short 2-minute conflict negotiation in the hallway with another RN or an hour-long formal salary negotiation, the result should be satisfaction by all parties that each has won something. It is a good idea to follow up formal negotiation in writing by sending a letter or a memo stating what was agreed.

Alternative Dispute Resolution

Many disputes can be solved informally. Occasionally, however, parties cannot reach agreement through negotiation. In these cases, *alternative dispute resolution* (ADR) may be indicated to keep some privacy in the dispute and to avoid expensive litigation. Types of ADR include mediation, fact finding, arbitration, due process hearings, and the use of ombudspersons.

Mediation, which uses a neutral third party, is a confidential, legally nonbinding process designed to help bring the parties together to devise a solution to the conflict. As such, the mediator does not take sides and has no vested interest in the outcome. Instead, the mediator asks questions to clarify the issues at hand (*fact finding*), listens to both parties, meets with parties privately as necessary, and helps to identify solutions both parties can live with.

There are times, however, when mediators are unable to help conflicted parties come to agreement. When this occurs, formal *arbitration* may be used. Unlike mediation, which seeks to help conflicted parties come together to reach a decision themselves, arbitration is a binding conflict resolution process in which the facts of the case are heard by an individual who makes a final decision for the parties in conflict.

Another option for individuals experiencing conflict may be guidance from *ombudspersons*. Ombudspersons generally hold an official title as such within an organization. Their function is to investigate grievances filed by one party against another and to ensure that individuals involved in conflicts understand their rights as well as the process that should be used to report and resolve the conflict.

Seeking Consensus

Consensus means that negotiating parties reach an agreement that all parties can support, even if it does not represent everyone's first priorities. Consensus decision making does not provide complete satisfaction for everyone involved in the negotiation as an initially unanimous decision would, but it does indicate willingness by all parties to accept the agreed-on conditions.

In committees or groups working on shared goals, consensus is often used to resolve conflicts that may occur within the group. To reach consensus often requires the use of an experienced facilitator and having consensus-building skills is a requirement of good leadership.

Building consensus ensures that everyone within the group is heard but that the group will ultimately end up with one agreed-on course of action. Consensual decisions are best used for decisions that relate to a core problem or need a deep level of group support to implement successfully.

Perhaps the greatest challenge in using consensus as a conflict resolution strategy is that like collaboration, it is time consuming. It also requires all of the parties involved in the negotiation to have good communication skills and to be open minded and flexible. It is also important for the leader to recognize when achieving consensus has become unrealistic.

Integrating Leadership Skills and Management Functions in Addressing Conflict, Workplace Violence, and Negotiation

There are many benefits to establishing and maintaining an appropriate amount of conflict in the workplace. The manager who creates a stable work environment that minimizes the antecedent conditions for conflict has more time and energy to focus on meeting organizational and human resource needs. When conflict does occur in the unit, managers must be able to discern constructive from destructive conflict. Conflict that is constructive will result in creativity, innovation, and growth for the unit. When conflict is deemed to be destructive, managers must deal appropriately with that conflict or risk an aftermath that may be even more destructive than the original conflict.

Consistently using conflict resolution strategies with win–lose or lose–lose outcomes will create disharmony within the unit. Leaders who use optimal conflict resolution strategies with a win–win outcome promote increased employee satisfaction and organizational productivity.

Unfortunately, conflict has increasingly erupted in health care settings as workplace violence. Caring for patients and families under significant stress can increase the risk of violence and that certainly appears to be the case with the COVID-19 pandemic. Unfortunately, multiple studies identifying prevalence rates of at least 50% (the percentage is probably much higher due to underreporting by victims) of horizontal bullying and workplace violence exist in nursing. Thus, it is a reasonable assumption that most nurses will experience horizontal bullying, either as the victim, the bully, or a bystander during their career.

Workplace violence cannot be ignored. Nurses must stand up and defend themselves and their coworkers when such behavior occurs. In addition, all nurses must recognize that verbal abuse, incivility, and bullying are never acceptable behavior, and they must be given the tools and training needed to immediately address the problem when it occurs.

Negotiation also requires both management functions and leadership skills. Well-prepared managers know with whom they will be negotiating and prepare their negotiation accordingly. They are prepared with trade-offs, multiple alternatives, and a clear bottom line to ensure that their unit acquires needed resources. Successful negotiation mandates the use of the leadership components of self-confidence and risk taking. If these attributes are not present, the leader-manager has little power in negotiation and thus compromises the unit's ability to secure desired resources. Other attributes that make leaders effective in negotiation are sensitivity to others and the environment and interpersonal communication skills. The leader's use of assertive communication skills, rather than destructive tactics, results in an acceptable level of satisfaction for all parties at the close of the negotiation.

Key Concepts

- Conflict can be defined as the internal discord that results from differences in ideas, values, or feelings of two or more people.
- Because managers have a variety of interpersonal relationships with people with different values, beliefs, backgrounds, and goals, conflict is an expected outcome.
- The most common sources of organizational conflict are communication problems, organizational structure, and individual behavior within the organization.
- Conflict theory has changed dramatically during the last 100 years. Currently, conflict is viewed as neither good nor bad because it can produce growth or be destructive, depending on how it is managed.
- Too little conflict results in organizational stasis, whereas too much conflict reduces the organization's effectiveness and eventually immobilizes its employees.
- Conflict also has a qualitative component, and the impact of a conflict on any individual varies significantly in terms of how it is perceived and handled.
- The three categories of conflict are intrapersonal, interpersonal, and intergroup.
- The first stage in the conflict process is called latent conflict, which implies the existence of antecedent conditions. Latent conflict may proceed to perceived conflict or to felt conflict. Manifest conflict may also ensue. The last stage in the process is conflict aftermath.
- The optimal goal in conflict resolution is creating a win–win solution for everyone involved.
- Common conflict resolution strategies include compromise, competing, accommodating, smoothing, avoiding, and collaboration.
- Bullying is abusive conduct that is threatening, humiliating, or intimidating in nature.

- Incivility is a term used to describe mistreatment or discourtesy to another person. It occurs on a continuum from disruptive behaviors such as eye-rolling and other nonverbal behaviors and sarcastic comments to threatening behaviors, such as intimidation and physical violence.
- In mobbing, employees "gang up" on an individual.
- When bullying, incivility, and mobbing occur in the workplace, it is known as workplace violence.
- Workplace violence impacts the physical, emotional, and socioeconomic health of employees and threatens patient safety.
- All organizations should have bullying policies in place with zero tolerance as the expectation.
- As a negotiator, it is important to win as much as possible, lose as little as possible, and make the other party feel satisfied with the outcome of the negotiation.
- Because knowledge is power, the more informed the negotiator is, the greater is their bargaining power.
- The leader, although able to recognize and counter negotiation tactics, always strives to achieve an honest, collaborative approach to negotiation.
- The manager must know their bottom line but try never to use it.
- Closure and follow-up are important parts of the negotiation process.
- ADR usually involves at least one of the elements of mediation, fact finding, arbitration, and the use of ombudspersons.
- Seeking consensus, a concord of opinion, although time-consuming, is an effective conflict resolution and negotiation strategy.

Additional Learning Exercises and Applications

LEARNING EXERCISE 21.5

Choosing the Most Appropriate Resolution Approach

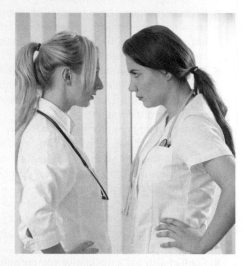

In the following situations, choose the most appropriate conflict resolution strategy (avoiding, smoothing, accommodating, competing, compromising, or collaborating). Support your decision with rationale and explain why other methods of conflict management were not used.

Situation 1

You are a circulating nurse in the operating room. Usually, you are assigned to Room 3 for general surgery, but today, you have been assigned to Room 4, the orthopedic room. You are unfamiliar with the orthopedic doctors' routines and attempt to brush up on them quickly by reading the doctors' preference cards before each case today. So far, you have managed to complete two cases without incident. The next case comes in the room, and you realize that everyone is especially tense; this patient is the wife of a local physician, and the doctors are performing a bone biopsy for possible malignancy. You prepare the biopsy area, and the surgeon, who has a reputation for a quick temper, enters the room. You suddenly realize that you have prepped the area with Betadine, and this surgeon prefers another solution. She sees what you have done and yells, "You are a stupid, stupid nurse."

Situation 2

You are the intensive care unit charge nurse and have just finished an exhausting 8 hours on duty. Working with you today were two nurses who work 12-hour shifts. Each of you were assigned two patients, all with high acuity levels. You are glad that you are going out of town tonight to attend an important seminar because you are certainly tired. You are also pleased that you scheduled yourself an 8-hour shift today and that your replacement is coming through the door. You will just have time to give report and catch your plane.

It is customary for 12-hour nurses to continue with their previous patients and for assignments not to be changed when 8- and 12-hour staff are working together. Therefore, you proceed to give report on your patients to the 8-hour nurse coming on duty. One of your patients is acutely ill with fever of unknown origin and is in the isolation room. It is suspected that he has meningitis. Your other patient is a multiple trauma victim. In the middle of your report, the oncoming nurse says that she has just learned that she is pregnant. She says, "I can't take care of a possible meningitis patient. I'll have to trade with one of the 12-hour nurses." You approach the 12-hour nurses, and they respond angrily, "We took care of all kinds of patients when we were pregnant, and we are not changing patients with just 4 hours left in our shift."

When you repeat this message to the oncoming nurse, she says, "Either they trade or I go home!" Your phone call to the nursing office reveals that because of a flu epidemic, there are absolutely no personnel to call in, and all the other units are already short staffed.

Situation 3

You are the charge nurse on a step-down unit. It is your first day back from a 2-week vacation. The shift begins in 10 minutes, and you sit down to make staffing assignments. The central staffing office has noted that you must float one of your RNs to the oncology unit. When you check the floating roster, you note that Jenny, one of the RNs assigned to work on your unit today, was the last to float (she floated yesterday). That leaves you to choose between Mark and Lisa, your other two RNs. According to the float roster, Mark floated 10 days ago, and Lisa floated last 11 days ago. You tell Lisa that it is her turn to float.

Lisa states that she floated three times in a row while Mark was on vacation for 2 weeks last month. Mark says that vacations should not count and that he should not float because it is not his turn. Lisa says that Jenny should float, as she floated to oncology yesterday and already knows the patients. Jenny says that she agreed to come in and work today (on her day off) to help the unit, and she would not have agreed to do this if she had known that she would have to float. Mark says that it is the last day of a 6-day stretch, and he does not want to float. Jenny says that it is not her turn to float, and she does not want to float willingly.

Situation 4

You are a new nurse working on a busy medical/surgical floor. The mode of patient care delivery used on the unit is team nursing. You have grown increasingly frustrated, however, with a licensed vocational nurse/licensed practical nurse on your team who is unwilling to answer call lights. You have directly observed her both ignore call lights and go out of her way to avoid answering the lights. When you confront her, she always provides an excuse such as she was on her way to do something for another patient or that she did not notice the blinking call light. The result is that you often must run from one end of the hall to the other to answer the call lights because patient safety could be at risk. Your frustration level has risen to the point that you no longer wish to work with this person.

Situation 5

You are a staff nurse on a small telemetry unit. The unit is staffed at a ratio of one nurse for every four patients, and the charge nurse is counted in this staffing because there is a full-time unit secretary and monitor technician to assist at the desk. The charge nurse is responsible for making the daily staffing assignments. Although you recognize that the charge nurse needs to reduce her patient care assignment to have time to perform the charge nurse duties, you have grown increasingly frustrated that she normally assigns herself only one patient, if any, and these patients always have the lowest acuity level on the floor. This has placed a disproportionate burden on the other nurses, who often feel the assignment they are being given may be unsafe. The charge nurse is your immediate supervisor. She has not generally been responsive to concerns expressed by the staff to her about this problem.

Situation 6

You are a junior nursing student who just received the test scores from your pathophysiology exam. You are disappointed because you missed a grade of "A" by two points. In reviewing the test, however, you discovered what you believed to be four questions with either ambiguous or incorrect answers. When you attempted to bring these to the attention of your instructor during the class test review, she told you that she would look at these specific questions for the next test but wasn't willing to change scores at this point. You are both angry and frustrated with your instructor's response.

LEARNING EXERCISE 21.6

Negotiating the Graduation Ceremony

Often, one group is more powerful or has greater status and refuses to relinquish this power position, thus making collaboration impossible. Therefore, negotiating a compromise to a win–win solution, rather than a lose–lose solution, becomes imperative. In the following situation, describe if you could, and how you would, go about negotiating a win–win solution to conflict.

You are a senior member of a traditional on-campus baccalaureate nursing class. Three years ago, your university implemented an online registered nurse (RN)-Bachelor of Science in Nursing (BSN) program. The first students from that program graduated last year, and they held a small, private end-of-program ceremony, separate from the on-campus BSN students.

This year, as a result of ongoing state budget cuts, the school of nursing can no longer subsidize two separate end-of-program ceremonies. This means that the 21 RN-BSN students and the 33 on-campus BSN students must now work together to plan a joint ceremony.

Resistance is high. The two groups of students have spent no time together and do not know each other. The on-campus students have been planning their ceremony since they started the nursing program and have collected additional money each semester to fund a formal dinner and dance reception in the evening and breakfast at one of the nicest hotels in town. Money from the school of nursing would be used to subsidize the cost of a live band and the reception hall. The online students would like to limit the evening reception to cake and punch at the college to reduce the cost because most of them will incur additional travel and lodging costs to attend graduation. However, they would like to have the school of nursing use the funds available to host a "picnic in the park" the following day, to which they can bring their families. Both groups perceive that the other group is trying to control the situation, not being sensitive to needs or wants. Both groups have contacted university officials to complain about the situation, and a number of students are threatening not to attend the ceremony if the two groups must be merged.

You have been appointed as the unofficial spokesperson for the RN-BSN graduates. Joan is the unofficial spokesperson for the on-campus BSN students. You live only 30 miles from campus, so coming to campus to try to resolve the conflict is not a significant hardship.

The faculty member, Alice, who is the liaison for the end-of-program ceremony, has become alarmed at the situation and has contacted both you and Joan. She states that she will cancel the ceremony if the conflict is not resolved. Alice agrees to work with you and Joan to mediate the conflict, but time is of the essence. The semester ends soon, and the on-campus students can get no refund on their reception hall deposit after the end of the current week. Alice wants the conflict resolved in a win–win situation so that no parties leave angry.

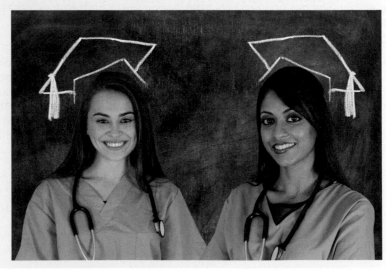

ASSIGNMENT:

Where will you begin? How will you get input from the group that you are representing? Would you plan a face-to-face meeting with Joan to attempt to resolve this conflict? What strategies might you use to help both groups win as much as possible and lose as little as possible? Explain your rationale. Remember, you wish to negotiate a compromise, and although you desire a win–win solution, you are limited in time and may not be able to facilitate a true collaboration. How will you deal with conflicted parties who perceive that they have lost more than they have won? What is your bottom line?

LEARNING EXERCISE 21.7

Behavioral Tactics—Appropriate or Not?

You are a woman who is a unit manager with a master's degree in health administration. You are about to present your proposed budget to the chief executive officer (CEO), who is a man. You have thoroughly researched your budget and have adequate rationale to support your requests for increased funding. Because the CEO is often moody, predicting his response is difficult.

You are also aware that the CEO has some very traditional views about women's role in the workplace, and generally, this does not include a major management role. Because he is fairly paternalistic, he is charmed and flattered when asked to assist "his" nurses with their jobs. Your predecessor, also a woman, was fired because she was perceived as brash, bossy, and disrespectful by the CEO. In fact, the former unit manager was one of a series of nursing managers who had been replaced in the last several years because of these characteristics. From what you have been told, the nursing staff did not share these perceptions.

You sit down and begin to plan your strategy for this meeting. You are aware that you are more likely to have your budgetary needs met if you dress conservatively, beseech the CEO's assistance and support throughout the presentation, and are fairly passive in your approach. In other words, you will be required to assume a traditionally feminine, helpless role. If you appear capable and articulate, you may not achieve your budgetary goals and may not even keep your job. It would probably not be necessary for you to continue to act this way, except in your interactions with the CEO.

ASSIGNMENT:

Are such behavioral tactics appropriate if the outcome is desirable? Are such tactics simply smart negotiation or are they destructively manipulative? What would you do in this situation? Outline your strategy for your budget presentation and present rationale for your choices.

LEARNING EXERCISE 21.8

Your First Budget Presentation

You are the unit manager of the new oncology unit. It is time for your first budget presentation to the administration. You have already presented your budget to the director of nurses, who had a few questions but expressed general agreement. However, it is the policy at Memorial Hospital that the unit manager's budget be presented to the budget committee, consisting of the fiscal manager, the director of nurses, a member of the board of trustees, and the executive director. You know that money is scarce this year because of a new building being constructed, but you really believe that you need the increases you have requested in your budget. Basically, you have asked for the following:

- Replace the 22% aides on your unit with 10% licensed vocational nurses/licensed practical nurses and 12% registered nurses.
- Increase paid educational time by 5% to allow for certification in chemotherapy.
- Provide a new position of clinical nurse specialist in oncology.
- Convert one room into a sitting room and mini-kitchen for patients' families.
- Add shelves and a locked medication box in each room to facilitate primary nursing.
- Provide no new equipment but replace existing equipment that is broken or outdated.

ASSIGNMENT:

Outline your plan. Include your approach what is and what is not negotiable and what arguments you would use. Give a rationale for your plan.

LEARNING EXERCISE 21.9

Handling Staff–Patient Conflict

You are the supervisor of a rehabilitation unit. Two of your youngest female nursing assistants come to your office today to report that a young male patient who is paraplegic has been making lewd sexual comments and gestures when they provide basic care. When you question them about their response to the actions of the patient, they maintain that they normally simply look away and try to ignore him, although they are offended by his actions. They are reluctant to confront the patient directly. Because it is anticipated that this patient may remain on your unit for at least a month, the nursing assistants have asked you to intervene in this conflict by either talking to the patient or by assigning other nurses the responsibility for his care.

ASSIGNMENT:

How will you handle this staff–patient conflict? Is avoidance (assigning different staff to care for the patient) an appropriate conflict resolution strategy in this situation? Will you encourage the nursing assistants to confront the patient directly? What coaching or role playing might you use with them if you choose this approach? Will you confront the patient yourself? What might you say?

LEARNING EXERCISE   21.10

Handling Personal Issues in a Professional Manner

You are a male unit supervisor of a pediatric trauma unit at Children's Hospital. Three years ago, you ended a serious romantic relationship with a nurse named Susan, who was employed at a different hospital in the same city. The breakup was not mutual, and Susan was hurt and angry.

Six months ago, Susan accepted a position as a unit supervisor at Children's Hospital. This has required you and Susan to interact formally at department head meetings and informally regarding staffing and personnel issues on a regular basis. Often, these interactions have been marked by either covert hostility on Susan's part, nonverbal aggression, or sniping comments. When you attempted to confront Susan about her behavior, she stated, "I don't have a problem. You shouldn't flatter yourself."

The situation is becoming increasingly more difficult to "work around," and both staff and fellow unit supervisors have become aware of the ongoing tension. You love your position and do not want to leave Children's Hospital, but it is becoming increasingly apparent that the situation cannot continue as it is.

ASSIGNMENT:

Answer the following questions:
1. How might gender have influenced the latent conditions, perceived or felt conflict, manifest conflict, and conflict aftermath in this situation?
2. What conflict strategies might you use to try to resolve this conflict? Avoidance? Smoothing? Accommodation? Competing? Compromise? Collaboration?
3. Would the use of a mediator be helpful in this situation?

LEARNING EXERCISE   21.11

Choosing the Most Appropriate Resolution Approach

Choose one of the following situations and write a one-page essay, discussing which conflict resolution strategy is most appropriate for this situation. Explain why other conflict resolution strategies were rejected.

Situation 1

You are a registered nurse on a surgical unit. MJ is an orthopedic surgery patient who is 2 days postoperative. Her physician has ordered patient-controlled analgesia (PCA) using morphine as well as as-needed intramuscular (IM) injections of Demerol every 3 to 4 hours. The patient has continued to verbalize a significant amount of pain.

Today, Dr. Jones writes an order for you to give MJ an additional 100 mg Demerol IM now, even though she had 100 mg less than 1 hour ago as well as her PCA. The dose he ordered is contraindicated in your drug handbook. You approach Dr. Jones with your concerns about the safety of such a dose as well as your questioning of the patient's pain level. Dr. Jones interrupts you shortly after you begin and says in a curt, hostile tone, "I am the doctor and I write the medication orders. You are the nurse and your responsibility is to implement my care plan. Give the medication now."

(continues on page 566)

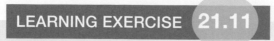

LEARNING EXERCISE 21.11

Choosing the Most Appropriate Resolution Approach (continued)

Situation 2

Today is Wednesday. Julie, a long-time employee on your unit where you are a manager, believes she is entitled to certain privileges regarding scheduling. You have told her to review the policy concerning weekends and days off. Julie believes she deserves every other week-end off, with Friday and Monday off on the weekends she works.

You have been able to meet Julie's request for the last 3 years because other employees preferred working weekends. Your recent employee turnover, however, means that meeting this request is no longer possible. Julie was scheduled to work Monday because of low staffing, but she refused, stating that Monday is her regular day off. You believe you can guarantee each employee 2 days off each week but can't guarantee any specific regular day off. Julie is scheduled to work on Friday.

LEARNING EXERCISE 21.12

When the Conflict Is with a Patient

Sydney Johannson, a 67-year-old man, was admitted to the medical/surgical unit 3 days ago for unresolved nausea, vomiting, and jaundice. A tumor was discovered in his bile duct, and he is scheduled for surgery tomorrow. His probable diagnosis is cancer.

You have been the primary RN caregiver for Mr. Johannson the past 3 days. He is short tempered and verbally abusive to you. He barks orders at you, ridicules almost everything you say, and is never satisfied with the care you give him. You realize that he is sick and frightened, but his behavior is frustrating and obnoxious. You find yourself avoiding going into his room just to avoid his verbal backlash. Today, when you enter his room to adjust his IV and give him his routinely scheduled medications, he makes several derogatory comments about your ethnicity and taunts you about looking like "an overstuffed pillow" and moving "slower than a snail."

ASSIGNMENT:

Decide how you will respond. Is conflict avoidance justified since the patient is sick? Are other conflict resolution strategies more appropriate? Is bullying by a patient any more acceptable than bullying by coworkers? Role play with your peers how you might respond to this patient and what if any limits, you might set in terms of his behavior. How much control do you have over the patient's behavior? What is your bottom line in terms of behavior you will accept from this patient?

REFERENCES

American Nurses Association. (2015). Code of ethics for nurses with interpretive statements.

American Nurses Association. (n.d.). *Violence, incivility, and bullying*. https://www.nursingworld.org/practice-policy/work-environment/violence-incivility-bullying/

Ball, W. S. (2021, October 5). *Civility in nursing and health care*. Nurse Plus. https://nurse.plus/become-a-nurse/civility-in-nursing/

Berger & Michelana. (2021, April 14). *Health care workers more likely to experience workplace injury*. https://www.bergermichelena.com/blog/2021/04/health-care-workers-more-likely-to-experience-workplace-injury/

Brodow, E. (2021, November 12). *Ten tips for negotiating in 2022*. http://www.brodow.com/Articles/NegotiatingTips.html

Cardillo, D. (2021). *Seven strategies for managing conflict*. http://donnacardillo.com/articles/sevenstrategies/

Carver, M., & Beard, H. (2021). Managing violence and aggression in the emergency department. *Emergency Nurse, 29*(6), 32–39. https://doi.org/10.7748/en.2021.e2094

Clark, C. M. (2023). Promoting civility and healthy work environments in nursing and health care. In C. J. Huston (Ed.), *Professional issues in nursing: Challenges and opportunities* (6th ed., Chapter 13, pp. 181–197). Wolters Kluwer.

Colduvell, K. (2021). *Nurse bullying: Stand up and speak out*. Nurse.org. https://nurse.org/articles/how-to-deal-with-nurse-bullying/#:~:text=Bullying%2C%20which%20the%20American%20Nurses%20Association%20%28ANA%29%20defines,reputation%20of%20the%20nursing%20profession%20as%20a%20whole

Dillon, S. (2021, January 7). *Workplace bullying in nursing: Why it happens and how to confront it*. Bravado Health. https://www.bravadohealth.com/2021/01/07/confronting-nurse-bullying/

Hockley, C. (2020). Promoting healthy work environments and civility: Why is this so difficult in nursing? In C. J. Huston (Ed.), *Professional issues in nursing: Challenges and opportunities* (5th ed., pp. 167–181). Wolters Kluwer.

Kam, K. (2021, March 18). *On the front lines: Violence against nurses on the rise. WebMD Health News*. https://www.webmd.com/a-to-z-guides/news/20210318/on-the-front-lines-violence-against-nurses-on-the-rise

Ladika, S. (2021). *Violence against nurses: Casualties of caring*. ManagedcareMag.com. https://www.managed-caremag.com/archives/2018/5/violence-against-nurses-casualties-caring

Leonard, K. (2020, July 8). *Differences between destructive & constructive conflict. Chron*. https://smallbusiness.chron.com/differences-between-destructive-constructive-conflict-1202.html

NurseJournal Staff. (2021, December 21). Nursing workplace violence. *NurseJournal*. https://nursejournal.org/resources/covid-nurse-workplace-violence/#:~:text=A%202021%20research%20study%20published%20in%20Healthcare%20reports,depression%2C%20and%20burnout%20than%20nurses%20with%20no%20exposure

Patient Safety Network. (2021, June 18). *Physical and verbal violence against health care workers*. https://psnet.ahrq.gov/issue/physical-and-verbal-violence-against-health-care-workers

United States Department of Labor. Occupational Safety and Health Administration. (n.d.). *Healthcare*. Retrieved December 19, 2021, from https://www.osha.gov/healthcare

Workplace Bullying Institute. (2021). *What is workplace bullying?* Retrieved December 19, 2021, from https://workplacebullying.org/

World Medical Association. (2020). 73rd World Health Assembly, *Agenda Item 3*: *Covid-19 Pandemic Response*. https://www.wma.net/wp-content/uploads/2020/05/WHA73-WMA-statement-on-Covid-19-pandemic-response-.pdf

22

Collective Bargaining, Unionization, and Employment Laws

… Too few Americans know labor history and how they have benefited from the efforts of unions. We have a 40-hour work week, defined benefits, higher wages, paid vacations and sick leave, largely as the result of union activity in the 20th century.—**Ken Bernstein**

… Organizations with unfair management policies are more likely to become unionized. It is within a manager's power to eliminate some of the needs that staff have for joining unions.—**Carol Huston**

… The labor movement did not diminish the strength of the nation but enlarged it. By raising the living standards of millions, labor miraculously created a market for industry and lifted the whole nation to undreamed of levels of production. Those who attack labor forget these simple truths, but history remembers them.—**Martin Luther King, Jr., speech to AFL-CIO, December 11, 1961**

CROSSWALK

This chapter addresses:

- **AACN Essentials Domain 5:** Quality and safety
- **AACN Essentials Domain 6:** Interprofessional partnerships
- **AACN Essentials Domain 7:** Systems-based practice
- **AACN Essentials Domain 9:** Professionalism
- **AONL Nurse Executive Competency 1:** Communication and relationship building
- **AONL Nurse Executive Competency 2:** A knowledge of the health care environment
- **AONL Nurse Executive Competency 3:** Leadership
- **AONL Nurse Executive Competency 4:** Professionalism
- **AONL Nurse Executive Competency 5:** Business skills
- **ANA Standard of Professional Performance 7:** Ethics
- **ANA Standard of Professional Performance 8:** Advocacy
- **ANA Standard of Professional Performance 9:** Respectful and equitable practice
- **ANA Standard of Professional Performance 10:** Communication
- **ANA Standard of Professional Performance 11:** Collaboration
- **ANA Standard of Professional Performance 12:** Leadership
- **ANA Standard of Professional Performance 15:** Quality of practice
- **ANA Standard of Professional Performance 17:** Resource stewardship
- **ANA Standard of Professional Performance 18:** Environmental health
- **QSEN Competency:** Teamwork and collaboration
- **QSEN Competency:** Quality improvement
- **QSEN Competency:** Safety

LEARNING OBJECTIVES

The learner will:

- identify major legislation that has impacted the ability of nurses to unionize
- identify factors that influence whether nurses join unions
- describe the relationships between national economic prosperity, the existence of nursing shortages and surpluses, and the unionization rates of nurses
- identify the largest unions representing health care employees and nurses in particular
- identify the steps necessary to start a union
- debate philosophically the potential conflicts inherent in having a professional organization also serve as a collective bargaining agent
- reflect on whether going on strike can be viewed as an ethically appropriate action for professional nurses
- explore labor laws regarding overtime and working conditions present in the state in which they live or will seek employment
- explain how equal employment legislation has affected employment and hiring practices
- describe current legislation that seeks to eliminate gender-based differences
- identify how the Civil Rights Act, the Americans with Disabilities Act, and the Age Discrimination and Employment Act have attempted to reduce discrimination in the workplace
- identify strategies for eliminating sexual harassment in the workplace
- identify the purpose of the Occupational Safety and Health Act

Introduction

Collective bargaining, unionization, and employment laws significantly influence the directing phase of the management process. Leader-managers then must understand the interrelationship of unionization and management, the need to adhere to legislation regarding employment practices, and the impact of both on the health care industry.

In addition, leader-managers must be able to see collective bargaining and employment legislation from four perspectives: the organization, the worker, general historical and societal, and personal. Managers who gain this broad perspective will better understand how management and employees can work together cooperatively. Many industrialized countries have adopted an attitude of acceptance and tolerance for the difficulties that may occur in managing under these influences. However, in the United States, some organizations continue to view these forces with at least some resentment and hostility.

The question of whether nurses should participate in collective bargaining has been around since legislation made such organization possible. Advocates on both sides of the issues present earnest, well-reasoned arguments to support their positions. Huston (2020) maintains that the issue at the heart of the debate is whether nursing—long recognized as a caring and altruistic profession—should be a part of collective bargaining efforts to improve working conditions. Yet unions and collective bargaining are very much a part of many nurses' lived experience.

This chapter examines the leadership roles and management functions necessary to create a climate in which organizational goals are not in conflict with unionization and employment legislation. The leadership roles and management functions inherent in dealing with collective bargaining, unionization, and employment laws are shown in Display 22.1.

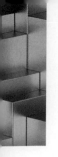

Leadership Roles

1. Is self-aware regarding personal attitudes and values regarding collective bargaining and employment laws
2. Recognizes and accepts reasons why people seek unionization
3. Creates a work environment that is sensitive to employee needs, thereby reducing the need for unionization
4. Maintains an accommodating or cooperative approach when dealing with unions and employment legislation
5. Is a role model for fairness
6. Is nondiscriminatory in all personal and professional actions
7. Examines the work environment periodically to ensure that it is supportive for all members regardless of gender, race, age, disability, or sexual orientation
8. Confronts and addresses immediately sexual harassment in adopting a zero-tolerance approach to the problem
9. Embraces the intent of laws barring discrimination and providing equal opportunity

Management Functions

1. Understands and appropriately implements union contracts
2. Administers personnel policies fairly and consistently
3. Works cooperatively with the personnel department and top-level administration when dealing with union activity
4. Promotes worker identification with management
5. Investigates immediately and fully all complaints regarding violations of the collective bargaining contract and takes appropriate action
6. Creates opportunities for subordinates to have input into organizational decision making to discourage unionization
7. Is alert for discriminatory employment practices in the workplace and intervenes immediately when problems exist
8. Ensures that the unit or department meets state licensing regulations
9. Understands and follows labor and employment laws that relate to the manager's sphere of influence and organization responsibilities
10. Ensures that the work environment is safe
11. Works closely with human resource management to assure the organization follows employment legislation mandates

Unions and Collective Bargaining

Collective bargaining includes activities between organized labor and management regarding employee relations. Such activities include the negotiation of formal labor agreements and day-to-day interactions between unions and management.

A *labor union* (hereafter referred to as a *union*) is an organization of workers, often in a trade or profession, formed to protect their rights and interests and improve their economic status and working conditions through collective bargaining with employers regarding wages, hours, working conditions, and benefits (Huston, 2023). Other terminology associated with unions and collective bargaining is shown in Display 22.2.

Union membership/activity increases during times of high employment and prosperity and decreases during economic recessions and layoffs. It also tends to change in response to work-force excesses and shortages. High demand for nurses is tied directly to a healthy national economy, and historically, this has been correlated with increased union activity. Similarly, when nursing vacancy rates are low, union membership and activity tend to decline.

DISPLAY 22.2 COLLECTIVE BARGAINING TERMINOLOGY

Agency shop—also called an *open shop*. Employees are not required to join the union.

Arbitration—terminal step in the grievance procedure where a third party reviews the grievance, completes fact finding, and reaches a decision. Always indicates the involvement of a third party. Arbitration may be voluntary on the part of management and labor or imposed by the government in a compulsory arbitration.

Collective bargaining—relations between employers, acting through their management representatives, and organized labor.

Conciliation and mediation—synonymous terms that refer to the activity of a third party to help disputants reach an agreement. However, unlike an arbitrator, this person has no final power of decision making.

Fact finding—rarely used in the private sector but used frequently in labor–management disputes that involve government-owned companies. In the private sector, fact finding is usually performed by a board of inquiry.

Free speech—Public Law 101, Section 8, states that "the expressing of any views, argument, or dissemination thereof, whether in written, printed, graphic, or visual form, shall not constitute or be evidence of an unfair labor practice under any provisions of this Act, if such expression contains no threat of reprisal or force or promise of benefit."

Grievance—perception on the part of a union member that management has failed in some way to meet the terms of the labor agreement.

Lockout—closing a place of business by management in the course of a labor dispute for the purpose of forcing employees to accept management terms.

National Labor Relations Board—labor board formed to implement the Wagner Act. Its two major functions are to (a) determine who should be the official bargaining unit when a new unit is formed and who should be in the unit and (b) adjudicate unfair labor charges.

Professionals—professionals have the right to be represented by a union but cannot belong to a union that represents nonprofessionals unless the majority votes for inclusion in the nonprofessional unit.

Strike—concerted withholding of labor supply to bring about economic pressure on employers and cause them to grant employee demands.

Union shop—also called a *closed shop*. All employees are required to join the union and pay dues.

Nurses' perceptions of whether they are valued by their employers have also always had an impact on unionization rates. Nurses join unions when they perceive that management does not listen to them or care about their needs.

> Management that is perceived to be indifferent to the workers' needs provides a fertile ground for union organizers because unions thrive in a climate that perceives the organizational philosophy to be insensitive to the worker.

Historical Perspective of Unionization in America

Unions have been present in America since the 1790s. Skilled craftsmen formed early unions to protect themselves from wage cuts during the highly competitive era of industrialization. For many reasons, however, collective bargaining was slow in coming to the health care industry (Fig. 22.1). Indeed, until labor laws were amended by Executive Order 10988 in 1962, the unionization of health care workers was illegal. This order lifted restrictions preventing public employees from organizing. Therefore, collective bargaining by nurses at city, county, and district hospitals and health care agencies began in the 1960s.

In 1974, Congress amended the *Wagner Act*, extending national labor laws to private, non-profit hospitals; nursing homes; health clinics; health maintenance organizations; and other

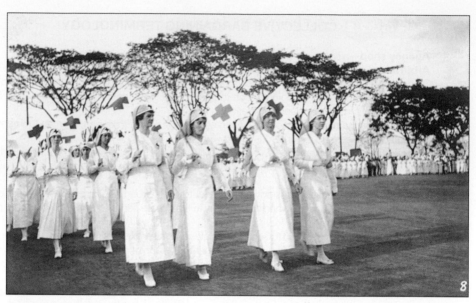

FIGURE 22.1 Historical photo of nurses in uniform marching for a cause. (Used with permission from Shutterstock.com.)

health care institutions. These amendments opened the door to union activity for professions and the public employee sector. Indeed, a review of union membership figures readily shows that, since 1960, most collective bargaining activity in the United States occurred in the public and professional sectors of industry, especially among faculty at institutions of higher education, teachers at primary and secondary levels, and physicians. There have been gradual declines in unionization in the private and blue-collar sectors, however, since membership peaked in the 1950s.

From 1962 through 1989, slow but steady increases occurred in the numbers of nurses represented by collective bargaining agents. In 1989, the National Labor Relations Board (NLRB) ruled that nurses could form their own separate bargaining units, and union activity increased. However, the American Hospital Association immediately sued the American Nurses Association (ANA), and the ruling was halted until 1991 when the Supreme Court upheld the 1989 NLRB decision. Table 22.1 outlines the legislation that led to unionization in health care.

TABLE 22.1 LEGISLATION LEADING TO UNIONIZATION IN HEALTH CARE

Year	Legislation	Effect
1935	National Labor Act/Wagner Act	Gave unions many rights in organizing; resulted in rapid union growth
1947	Taft–Hartley Amendment	Returned some power to management; resulted in a more equal balance of power between unions and management
1962	Kennedy *Executive Order* 10988	Amended the 1935 Wagner Act to allow public employees to join unions
1974	Amendments to Wagner Act	Allowed nonprofit organizations to join unions
1989	National Labor Relations Board ruling	Allowed nurses to form their own separate bargaining units

Effective Labor–Management Relations

Before the 1950s, labor–management relations were turbulent. History books are filled with battles, strikes, mass-picketing scenes, and brutal treatment by management and employees. Over the last three to four decades, however, employers and unions have substantially improved their relationships. Although evidence is growing that contemporary management has come to accept the reality that unions are here to stay, businesses in the United States are still often less comfortable with unions than their counterparts in many other countries. Likewise, unions have come to accept the fact that there are times when organizations are not healthy enough to survive aggressive union demands. The attitudes and philosophies of the leaders in management and the union determine the type of relationship that develops between the two parties in any given organization.

> It is possible to create a climate in which labor and management can work together to accomplish mutual goals.

Faced with the reality of negotiations with a bargaining agent, management has several choices. It may actively oppose the union by using various union-busting techniques, or it may more subtly oppose the union by attempting to discredit it and win employee trust. *Acceptance* also may run along a continuum. Management may accept the union with reluctance and suspicion. Although managers know that the union has legitimate rights, they often believe that they must continually guard against the union encroaching further into traditional management territory.

There is also the type of union acceptance known as *accommodation*. Increasingly common, accommodation is characterized by management's full acceptance of the union, with both the union and the management showing mutual respect. With accommodation, leader-managers create open discussion forums with unions to avoid the problems that occur when communication is poor. Thus, labor and management can establish mutual goals, particularly in the areas of safety, cost reduction, efficiency, elimination of waste, and improved working conditions. Such cooperation represents the most mature and advanced type of labor-management relations.

Unionization in the health care industry will undoubtedly continue. It is important to learn how to deal with this potential constraint to effective management. Managers must learn to work with unions and to develop the art of using unions to assist the organization in building a team effort to meet organizational goals.

Union Representation of Nurses

About 17% of nurses and 12% of other US health care workers are currently covered by a union although the share of hospital workers with union representation declined from above 22% in 1983 to below 15% in 2018, reflecting a decades-long decline in organized labor (Philbrick & Abelson, 2021). This compares to 10.3% of the general population across the United States in 2021 (Bureau of Labor Statistics, 2022). Public sector workers had a union membership rate of 33.9%, more than five times higher than that of private-sector workers (6.1%) (Bureau of Labor Statistics, 2022).

> Nurses are roughly twice as likely to be in a union as are other workers.

Nurses are represented by a multitude of unions. The *California Nurses Association* (CNA)/*National Nurses Organizing Committee* joined with two other nurses' unions (*United American Nurses* [UAN] and the *Massachusetts Nurses Association*) in 2009 to create a new

175,000+ member advocacy association known as *National Nurses United* (NNU, 2010–2021). Although all three unions maintained separate identities, the merger gave these members a greater national voice. NNU is the largest union and professional association of RNs in US history (NNU, 2010–2021).

The *Service Employees International Union* (SEIU) is another large union in the health care industry representing just under 2 million RNs, licensed practical nurses/licensed vocational nurses (LPNs/LVNs), doctors, lab technicians, nursing home workers, and home care workers (Center for Union Facts, 2021a).

In addition, the American Federation of Teachers (AFT) amended their constitution in 1978 to allow the organizing and affiliation of health care workers. The AFT Nurses and Health Professionals division represents more than 200,000 health professionals who practice in a variety of disciplines and settings (AFT, n.d.). The division's membership also includes approximately 15,000 school nurses. The AFT is the second largest nurses' union in the American Federation of Labor–Congress of Industrial Organizations (AFL-CIO) (AFT, n.d.).

Also, in 2013, the National Union of Healthcare Workers, which formed in 2009 when SEIU took control of California local United Healthcare Workers West, affiliated with CNA. Like NNU, this was a strategic alliance and not a merger. Such alliances are becoming increasingly commonplace as unions recognize that increased negotiating power comes with greater membership.

Some of the other unions that represent nurses include the ANA; the National Union of Hospital and Health Care Employees of the Retail, Wholesale, and Department Store Union; the AFL-CIO; the United Steelworkers of America; the American Federation of Government Employees, AFL-CIO; the American Federation of State, County, and Municipal Employees, AFL-CIO; the International Brotherhood of Teamsters; the American Federation of State, County, and Municipal Employees, which operates mostly in the public sector; the "24/7 Frontline Service Alliance"; and the United Automobile Workers.

Union representation also varies by state. The states with the most unions organizing for all industries including health care are Hawaii (22.4%) and New York (22.2%) whereas South Carolina (1.7%) and North Carolina (2.6%) continued to have the lowest (Bureau of Labor Statistics, 2022).

American Nurses Association and Collective Bargaining

One difficult union issue faced by nurse-managers that is not typically encountered in other disciplines stems from the dual role of their professional organization—ANA. ANA exists to advance the nursing profession by fostering high standards of nursing practice; promoting a safe and ethical work environment; bolstering the health and wellness of nurses; and advocating on health care issues that affect nurses and the public (ANA, n.d.). The ANA represents the interests of the nation's 4 million RNs through its constituent member nurses associations, its organizational affiliates, and its subsidiaries.

Yet, the Center for Union Facts (2021b) notes that just under 196,000 RNs belonged to the ANA as of 2018, less than 5% of the RN population. This low membership rate may be occurring in part because the NLRB recognizes the ANA, at most state levels, as a collective bargaining agent. The use of state associations as bargaining agents has been a divisive issue among American nurses. Some nurse-managers believe that they have been disenfranchised by their professional organization because supervisors are not allowed to belong to a union. Other managers recognize the conflicts inherent in attempting to sit on both sides of the bargaining table. For some members of the nursing profession, this issue presents no conflict. Regardless of individual values, however, there does appear to be some conflict in loyalty.

LEARNING EXERCISE 22.1

The Role of the American Nurses Association as a Collective Bargaining Agent

How do you feel about the American Nurses Association's (ANA's) certification as a collective bargaining agent? Do you belong to the state student nurses' association? Why or why not? Do you plan to join your state ANA? What are the primary driving and restraining forces for your decision? Divide into two groups to debate the pros and cons of having the ANA, rather than other unions, represent nurses.

There are no easy solutions to the dilemma created by the dual role held by the ANA. Clarifying issues begins with the manager examining the motivation of nurses to participate in collective bargaining. The manager must at least try to hear and understand the employees' points of view.

Employee Motivation to Join or Reject Unions

Knowing that human behavior is goal oriented, it is important to examine what personal goals union membership fulfills. Nurse-managers often tell each other that health care institutions differ from other types of industrial organizations. This is really a myth because most nurses work in large and impersonal organizations. The nurse frequently feels powerless and vulnerable as an individual alone in a complex institution. It is this vulnerability that often encourages nurses to join unions.

Common Reasons Nurses Join Unions

The reality though is that at least six primary motivations for joining a union exist (Display 22.3). The first is to increase the power of the individual. Wages are typically higher in health care organizations that have been unionized. Indeed, the Bureau of Labor Statistics (2022) notes that among full-time wage and salary workers, nonunion workers had median weekly earnings that were 17% less than workers who were union members ($975 vs. $1,169).

DISPLAY 22.3 UNION MEMBERSHIP: PROS AND CONS

Reasons Nurses Join Unions

1. To increase the power of the individual
2. To increase their input into organizational decision making
3. To eliminate discrimination and favoritism
4. Because of a social need to be accepted
5. Because they are required to do so as part of employment (closed shop)
6. Because they believe it will improve patient outcomes and quality of care

Reasons Nurses Do Not Join Unions

1. A belief that unions promote the welfare state and oppose the American system of free enterprise
2. A need to demonstrate individualism and promote social status
3. A belief that professionals should not unionize
4. An identification with management's viewpoint
5. Fear of employer reprisal
6. The cost of membership dues
7. They are employed in "right-to-work" states that grant workers a choice about whether to belong to a union
8. Fear of lost income associated with a strike or walkout

In addition, employees know that singly, they are much more dispensable. Because a large group of employees is less dispensable, nurses generally increase their bargaining power and reduce their vulnerability by joining a union. This is a particularly strong motivating force for nurses when jobs are scarce, and they feel vulnerable. Indeed, during the massive downsizing and restructuring of the 1990s, collective bargaining priorities shifted from wages and benefits to job security.

This focus shifted again to worker safety when the first US Ebola patient died in Fall 2014 in Dallas. Union leaders argued that hospitals were not providing nurses with adequate training and protective equipment to care for infected patients. The protests succeeded in focusing public awareness on Ebola readiness and safety.

Similarly, unions raised their voices to advocate for worker safety during the COVID-19 pandemic, protesting staffing shortages, inadequate and persistent supplies of protective equipment, limited testing for the virus, and the pressuring of health care workers to work even if they might be sick (Philbrick & Abelson, 2021). In addition, in late 2021, NNU condemned the Centers for Disease Control and Prevention's decision to shorten the recommended isolation period for health care workers who test positive for COVID-19, saying the move could be "dangerous" for both workers and patients (Conley, 2021).

> Although historically, unions focused heavily on wage negotiations, current issues deemed by nurses to be just as or more important are nonmonetary, such as guidelines for staffing, worker safety, float provisions, shared decision making, and scheduling.

When there are nursing shortages, nurses feel less vulnerable, and other reasons to join unions become motivating factors. A second motivator driving nurses toward unionization is the desire to communicate their aims, feelings, complaints, and ideas to others and to have input into organizational decision making.

In addition, because unions emphasize equality and fairness, nurses join them because they need to eliminate discrimination and favoritism. This might be a particularly strong motivator for members of groups that have experienced discrimination, such as women and racial–ethnic minorities. Unions can also help nurses settle grievances more fairly and can provide standard rules for firing, transferring, or laying off nurses that may not exist when employees are hired at will.

Many social factors also act as motivators to nurses regarding union activity. A fourth motivation stems from the social need to be accepted. Sometimes, this social need results from family or peer pressure. Because many working-class families have a long history of strong union ties, children are frequently raised in a cultural milieu that promotes unionization.

A fifth reason why nurses join unions is because the union contract dictates that all nurses belong to the union. This has been a big driving force among blue-collar workers. However, the *closed shop*—or requirement that all employees belong to a union—has never prevailed in the health care industry. Most health care unions have *open shops*, allowing nurses to choose if they want to join the union.

Finally, some nurses join unions because they believe that patient outcomes are better in unionized organizations due to better staffing and supervised management practices, although evidence to support this claim is limited. This is because unions can negotiate for better working conditions, and better working conditions often translate to reduced workloads and mandatory overtime.

Common Reasons Nurses Do Not Join Unions

Just as there are many reasons to join unions, there are also reasons why nurses reject unions (see Display 22.3). Perhaps the strongest reasons are societal and cultural factors. Many people distrust unions because they believe that unions promote the welfare state and undermine the American system of free enterprise. Other reasons for rejecting unions might be a need to demonstrate that nurses can get ahead on their own merits.

Professional employees have also been slow in forming unions for reasons that deal with class and education. They argue that unions were appropriate for the blue-collar worker but not for nurses, the university professor, physician, or engineer. Nurses who reject unions on this basis usually are driven by a need to demonstrate their individualism and social status. Some employees identify with management and thus frequently adopt its viewpoint toward unions. Such nurses, therefore, would reject unions because their values more closely align with management than with workers.

In addition, although employees are protected under the *National Labor Relations Act* (NLRA), many reject unions because of fears of employer reprisal. Nurses who reject unions on this basis could be said to be motivated, most of all, by a need to keep their jobs.

Some employees are reluctant to join unions because of the cost of membership dues. Burger (2021) notes nurses in a collective bargaining unit may pay as much as $90 per month for union representation.

In addition, some employees reject unions simply because they have a right to not belong to a union. The United States is currently composed of 27 "right-to-work" states that grant workers a choice about whether to belong to a union (National Right to Work Legal Defense Foundation, 2022). The right-to-work states as of 2022 are shown in Display 22.4. Prior to June 2018, in the other states and Washington, DC, employees were not required to belong to the union but were required to pay a portion of the union dues that go toward collective bargaining and other nonpolitical union-related activities. These "*fair share*" dues were generally only a small percentage of the union dues.

In June 2018, however, the Supreme Court in *Janus vs. American Federation of State, County, and Municipal Employees* (AFSCME) ruled that nonunion members no longer had to pay their fair share for union representation in collective bargaining negotiations (Rushe, 2018). In a 5-4 decision, the court overturned a previous decision that had protected the right of public sector unions to collect administrative fees from nonmembers, ruling it was inconsistent with the first amendment right to free speech. The case was brought by Mark Janus, a child support specialist at the Illinois Department of Healthcare and Family Services, who was represented by the AFSCME union. Although he was not a union member, 78% of the full union dues were deducted from his paycheck.

The outcome of the Supreme Court decision is that the nonunion public sector workers in more than 20 states who had to pay fair share dues will no longer have to and collective bargaining agents will lose fees from hundreds of thousands of nonmembers as a result. The case will clearly permanently weaken public unions (Rushe, 2018).

Finally, some nurses reject unions out of the fear of lost income associated with a *strike* or *walkout*. Burger (2021) notes that when a union decides to go on strike, many nurses are faced with losing significant wages during the strike as well as their own personal ethical

---

DISPLAY 22.4 RIGHT-TO-WORK STATES IN THE UNITED STATES

Alabama	Iowa	Nevada	Texas
Arizona	Kansas	North Carolina	Utah
Arkansas	Kentucky	North Dakota	Virginia
Florida	Louisiana	Oklahoma	West Virginia
Georgia	Michigan	South Carolina	Wisconsin
Idaho	Mississippi	South Dakota	Wyoming
Indiana	Nebraska	Tennessee	

Source: From National Right to Work Legal Defense Foundation. (2022). *Right to work states*. Retrieved July 11, 2022, from https://www.nrtw.org/right-to-work-states

dilemma of leaving their patients to replacement nurses who are unfamiliar with their patient population. Patient outcomes also decline significantly during a nursing strike and the cost to the organization can be detrimental. Organizations have reported losses of over $46 million to train and replace the nurses for large strikes (Burger, 2021).

Strikes and walkouts are a reality in unions; however, they are closely regulated by law. The NLRA states in part that "employees shall have the right to engage in other concerted activities for the purpose of collective bargaining or other mutual aid or protection." The phrase *other concerted activities* refers to "working to rule," "blue flu" epidemics, work slowdowns, filing a barrage of grievances, participating in informational or recognition picketing, and striking. Unions must, however, give employers and the Federal Mediation and Conciliation Service 10 days' notice of their intent to strike. In doing so, the facility should have a reasonable amount of time to stop admitting patients, transfer existing patients to other facilities, and reduce medical procedures that require nurse-intensive labor. Problems occur when management continues to admit new patients or attempts to maintain normal operations.

It should be noted, however, that nurses do have the option to refuse to participate in strikes or to cross picket lines when strikes occur. They risk derision by their peers in doing so, however, because strikebreakers—commonly known as *scabs*—are viewed as taking the management's side on the issue and may never be fully accepted by their peers after the strike action has ended (Huston, 2020).

The ANA (2015) *Code of Ethics for Nurses with Interpretive Statements* may provide some guidance for nurses weighing their duty to care against the implications of participating in a work stoppage or strike. Provision 2 states, "The nurse's primary commitment is to the patient, whether an individual, family, group, community, or population" (ANA, 2015, p. 5). Interpretive statements under this provision specify that the patient's interests come first, and they address conflicts that may arise when nurses are caring for patients. Provision 5 states, "The nurse owes the same duties to self as to others, including the responsibility to promote health and safety, preserve wholeness of character and integrity, maintain competence, and continue personal and professional growth" (ANA, 2015, p. 21). Thus, if faced with actions that they morally cannot support, nurses have a "right and a duty according to their personal and professional values" to communicate this to the appropriate leaders. Finally, Provision 6 states, "The nurse, through individual and collective effort, establishes, maintains, and improves the ethical environment of the work setting and conditions of employment that are conducive to safe, quality health care" (ANA, 2015, p. 25). Nurses then must consider their own personal and professional values in determining whether striking is ethical.

Averting the Union

Because of the health care industry's movement toward unionization, most nurses will probably be involved with unions in some manner during their careers. Managers who are not employed in a unionized health care organization should anticipate that one or more unions may attempt to organize their nurses.

LEARNING EXERCISE 22.2

Discussing the Pros and Cons of Unions

List the reasons why you would or would not join a union. Share this with others in your group and examine the following questions. Would you feel differently about unions if you were a manager? What influences you the most in your desire to join or reject unions? Have you ever felt discriminated against or powerless in the workplace?

Once managers understand the drives and needs behind joining unions though, they can begin to address those needs and possibly avert some of them. One strategy is to review the current literature and research on nurse satisfaction and dissatisfaction. When managers are aware of the concerns of RNs nationwide, they are better able to assess their own staff's potential for the type of dissatisfaction that can lead to unionization.

LEARNING EXERCISE 22.3

List and Support Your Reasons for or Against Striking

You are a staff nurse in the intensive care unit (ICU) at one of your city's two hospitals. You have worked at this hospital for 5 years and transferred to the ICU 2 years ago. You love nursing but are sometimes frustrated in your job due to a short supply of nurses, excessive overtime demands, and the stress of working with critically ill patients.

The hospital has a closed shop, so union dues are deducted from your pay even though you are not actively involved in the union. The present union contract is up for renegotiation, and the union and management have been unable to agree on numerous issues. When the management made its last offer, the new contract was rejected by the nurses. Now that the old contract has expired, nurses are free to strike if they vote to do so.

You had voted for accepting the management offer; you have two children to support, and it would be devastating to be without work for a long time. Last night, the nurses voted on whether to return to the bargaining table and try to renegotiate with management or to go out on strike. Again, you voted for no strike. You have just heard from your friend that the strike vote won. Now, you must decide if you are going to support your striking colleagues or cross the picket line and return to work tomorrow. Your friends are pressuring you to support their cause. You know that the union will provide some financial compensation during the strike but believe that it will not be adequate to support yourself and your children. You agree with union assertions that the organization has overworked and underpaid you and that it has been generally unresponsive to nursing needs. On the other hand, you believe that your first obligation is to your children.

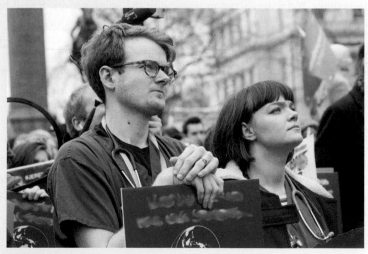

ASSIGNMENT:

List all of the reasons for and against striking. Decide what you will do. Use appropriate rationale from outside readings to support your final decision. Share your thoughts with the class. Take a vote in class to determine how many would strike and how many would cross the picket line.

DISPLAY 22.5 BEFORE THE UNION COMES

1. Know and care about your employees.
2. Establish fair and well-communicated personnel policies.
3. Use an effective upward and downward system of communication.
4. Ensure that all managers are well-trained and effective.
5. Establish a well-developed formal procedure for handling employee grievances.
6. Have a competitive compensation program of wages and benefits.
7. Have an effective performance appraisal system in place.
8. Use a fair and well-communicated system for promotions and transfers.
9. Use organizational actions to indicate that job security is based on job performance, adherence to rules and regulations, and availability of work.
10. Have an administrative policy on unionization.

Clearly, organizations with unfair management policies are more likely to become unionized. Managers can encourage feelings of power by allowing subordinates to have input into decisions that will affect their work. Managers can also listen to ideas, complaints, and feelings and take steps to ensure that favoritism and discrimination are not part of their management style. In addition, the manager can strengthen the drives and needs that make nurses reject unions. By building a team effort, sharing ideas and future plans from upper management with the staff, and encouraging individualism in employees, the manager can facilitate the worker's identification with management.

When nurses begin to show signs of job dissatisfaction and when they feel frustrated, stressed, or powerless, they send a wake-up call to nursing management. Leader-managers must be alert to employment practices that are unfair or insensitive to employee needs and intervene appropriately before such issues lead to unionization. It is critical that they do not ignore issues or try to overwhelm others with power. The rational approach to problem solving must be used. Display 22.5 lists practices the organization may put in place to discourage union activity. If the organization waits until the union arrives, it will be too late to perform these functions.

However, even organizations offering liberal benefit packages and fair management practices may experience union activity if certain social and cultural factors are present. If union activity does occur, managers must be aware of specific employee and management rights so that the NLRA is not violated by managers or employees.

Union-Organizing Strategies

Unions use many strategies to organize health care workers (Display 22.6), including one-on-one and group meetings with union representatives. Other strategies include providing literature about union benefits, writing letters, and otherwise contacting potential union members.

In corporate campaigns, the union often uses public events, political connections, and the local media to bring into question a hospital's quality of care, level of charity work, its tax-exempt status (if nonprofit), and nurse staffing. In addition, unions often file lawsuits against the employer. Labor unions maintain the goal of breaking employer resolve and demonstrate their ability to protect employees by initiating legal action on behalf of employees against targeted employers.

The internet has made information about how to organize a union very accessible to interested workers. E-mail has also proved to be an inexpensive and efficient means of mass communication regarding critical union issues.

DISPLAY 22.6 **SELECT UNION-ORGANIZING STRATEGIES**

1. Meetings (both group and one-on-one)
2. Leaflets and brochures
3. Pressure on the hospital corporation through media and community contacts
4. Political pressure of regional legislators and local lawmakers
5. Corporate campaign strategies
6. Activism of local employees
7. Using lawsuits
8. Bringing pressure from financiers
9. Technology

Steps to Establish a Union

The first step in establishing a union is demonstrating an adequate level of desire for unionization among the employees. The NLRB requires that at least 30% of employees sign an interest card before an election for unionization can be held. Most unions, however, will require between 60% and 70% of the employees to sign interest cards before spending the time and money involved in an organizing campaign. Union representatives have generally been careful to keep a campaign secret until they were ready to file a petition for election. They did this so that they could build momentum without interference from the employer.

After a designated number of cards have been signed, the organization is forced to have an election. At that time, all employees of the same classification, such as RNs, would vote on whether they desire unionization. A choice in every such election is *no representation*, which means that the voters do not want a union. During the election, 50% plus one of the petitioned units must vote for unionization before the union can be recognized. A process like that of certification can also decertify unions. *Decertification* may occur when at least 30% of the eligible employees in the bargaining unit initiate a petition asking to no longer be represented by the union.

It is important to remember that there are differences between organizing in a health care facility and other types of organizations. In general, the solicitation and distribution of union literature is banned entirely in "immediate patient care areas." Middle-level and first-level managers should never, however, independently attempt to deal with union-organizing activity. They should always seek assistance and guidance from upper management and the personnel department.

The entire list of rights for management and labor during the organization and establishment phases of unionization is beyond the scope of this book. Throughout the years, Congress has amended various labor acts and laws so that power is balanced between management and labor. At times, the balance of power has shifted back and forth, but Congress eventually enacts laws that restore the balance. The manager must ensure that the rights of management and employees are protected. The two most sensitive areas of any union contract, once wages have been agreed on, are discipline and the grievance process, which are discussed in Unit VII.

The Manager's Role During Union Organizing

In addition to laws regarding collective bargaining, the manager needs to be aware of one section of the Wagner Act (1935) and the Taft–Hartley Amendment (1947), which deals with unfair labor practices by employers and unions. The original Wagner Act listed and prohibited five unfair labor practices:

1. To interfere with, restrain, or coerce employees in a manner that interfered with their rights as outlined under the act. Examples of these activities are spying on union gatherings, threatening employees with job loss, or threatening to close down a company if the union organizes.

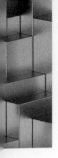

2. To interfere with the formation of any labor organization or to give financial assistance to a labor organization. This provision was included to prohibit "employee representation plans" that were primarily controlled by management.
3. To discriminate regarding hiring, tenure, etc., to discourage union membership
4. To discharge or discriminate against an employee who filed charges or testified before the NLRB
5. To refuse to bargain in good faith

The original Wagner Act gave so much power to the unions that it was necessary in 1947 to pass additional federal legislation to restore a balance of power to labor–management relations. The Taft–Hartley Amendment retained the provisions under the Wagner Act that guaranteed employees the right to collective bargaining. However, the Taft–Hartley Amendment added the provision that employees have the right to refrain from taking part in unions. In addition to that provision, the Taft–Hartley Amendment added and prohibited the following six unfair labor practices of unions:

1. Requiring a self-employed person or an employer to join a union
2. Forcing an employer to cease doing business with another person (This placed a ban on secondary boycotts, which were then prevalent in unions)
3. Forcing an employer to bargain with one union when another union has already been certified as the bargaining agent
4. Forcing the employer to assign certain work to members of one union rather than another
5. Charging excessive or discriminatory initiation fees
6. Causing or attempting to cause an employer to pay for unnecessary services. This prohibited *featherbedding*, a term used to describe union practices that prevented the displacement of workers due to advances in technology

Because the NLRA provides union protections only to employees, a supervisor cannot form or participate in a union. Nurse-managers, as legally defined hospital "supervisors," are spokespersons for the hospital. As such, the NLRB closely monitors what they may say and do. Prohibited managerial activities include threatening employees, interrogating employees, promising employee rewards for cessation of union activity, and spying on employees.

This does not mean that these activities do not occur. For example, in November 2021, the Michigan Nurses Association (MNA) filed an unfair labor practice charge with the National Labor Relations Board (NLRB) against Sparrow Health System. Among the MNA allegations were that hospital executives abandoned the safe staffing concerns process in the caregivers' union contract prior to its expiration; interrogated staff about union activities and attempted to prevent staff from wearing red to show support for their union; and coerced employees' legally protected right to strike including by making bargaining proposals containing a written threat to withdraw proposals on wages, health care, and other economic terms automatically upon notice of a strike (Draugelis & Kelly, 2021). Sparrow denied the allegations.

Similarly, the NLRB issued a formal complaint against Prime Health–East Liverpool City Hospital in December 2021, alleging that the hospital broke federal labor laws in negotiations with the Ohio Nurses Association, the union representing the registered nurses. The NLRB argued that the hospital engaged in bad faith bargaining, refused to provide the union with information about hospital working conditions, unlawfully declared a premature impasse, and implemented unlawful changes to conditions of employment for registered nurses without negotiating with the union (The Review, 2021).

> Employees have a right to participate in union organizing under the NLRA, and managers must not interfere with this right.

There have been some small gains recently, however, in terms of restoring more rights to management. The U.S. Court of Appeals for the District of Columbia Circuit ruled in 2013 that health care organizations do not have to display a list of workers' collective bargaining rights, including the rights of workers to join a union and bargain collectively to improve wages and working conditions. This overturned a ruling scheduled to go into effect in January. The Court said the NLRB violated employers' free speech rights in trying to force them to display the posters or face charges of committing an unfair labor practice.

The Nurse as Supervisor: Eligibility for Protection Under the National Labor Relations Act

The NLRA establishes certain protections for private-sector employees who want to form or join a labor union. These protections do not, however, extend to supervisors. The NLRA defines a supervisor as "any individual having authority, in the interest of the employer, to hire, transfer, suspend, lay off, recall, promote, discharge, assign, reward, or discipline other employees, or responsibly to direct them, or to adjust their grievances, or effectively to recommend such action, if in connection with the foregoing the exercise of such authority is not of a merely routine or clerical nature, but requires the use of independent judgment" (*NLRB Clarifies Definition*, 2022).

However, several 2006 NLRB rulings deemed that *charge nurses* might also be considered supervisors because they are responsible for the coordination and provision of patient care throughout a unit. Even part-time charge nurses were so labeled. The 2006 NLRB decisions—collectively known as the *Kentucky River* cases, after the name of the 2005 Supreme Court decision that sent the issue back to the NLRB—expanded the category of "supervisor" dramatically. The Court found that occasional guidance to other employees was enough to identify someone as a supervisor (*Who Counts as a Supervisor*, 2022):

> The nurses in Kentucky River directed the work of nursing assistants but did not hire, fire, discipline, evaluate, or otherwise play a role in the terms and conditions of the nursing assistants' employment. The NLRB had concluded that these nurses did not exercise sufficient independent judgment to qualify as supervisors, since they simply relied on their "ordinary professional or technical judgment" in directing lower level employees. The Supreme Court, however, categorically rejected the Board's analysis, concluding instead that these nurses clearly met the Act's definition of a supervisory employee because they did "responsibly direct" the work of lower level employees; using independent judgment and exercising their authority in the interest of the employer while doing so. (para. 6)

This finding has been contested legally since that time, and several interpretations have occurred. Reinterpretations by the NLRB are expected in the future.

In addition, the definition of supervisor in nursing came into question with several administrative and court rulings in the early 1990s. These rulings came about because of a case involving four LPNs employed at Heartland Nursing Home in Urbana, Ohio. During late 1988 and early 1989, these LPNs complained to management about what they thought were disparate enforcement of the absentee policy; short staffing; low wages for nurses' aides; an unreasonable switching of prescription business from one pharmacy to another, which increased the nurses' paperwork; and management's failure to communicate with employees (*NLRB v. Health Care & Retirement Corp.*, 1994). Despite assurances from the Vice President for Operations that they would not be harassed for bringing their concerns to headquarters' attention, three of the LPNs were terminated as a result of their actions.

In response to what they perceived to be illegal termination, the LPNs filed for protection under the NLRA. The NLRB ruled that because the LPNs had responsibility to ensure adequate staffing, to make daily work assignments, to monitor the aides' work to ensure proper performance, to counsel and discipline aides, to resolve aides' problems and grievances, to evaluate aides' performances, and to report to management, they should be classified as "supervisors," thereby making them ineligible for protection under the NLRA.

On appeal, the administrative law judge (ALJ) disagreed, concluding that the nurses were not supervisors, and that the nurses' supervisory work did not equate to responsibly directing the aides *in the interest of the employer*, noting that the nurses' focus is on the well-being of the residents rather than on the employer.

In another turnabout, the U.S. Court of Appeals for the Sixth Circuit then reversed the decision of the ALJ, arguing that the NLRB's test for determining the supervisory status of nurses was inconsistent with the statute and that the interest of the patient and the interest of the employer were not mutually exclusive. The court said that, in fact, the interests of the patient are the employer's business and argued that the welfare of the patient was no less the object and concern of the employer than it was of the nurses. The court also argued that the statutory dichotomy the NLRB first created was no more justified in the health care field than it would be in any other business in which supervisory duties are necessary to the production of goods or the provision of services (*NLRB v. Health Care & Retirement Corp.*, 1994).

The court further stated that it was up to Congress to carve out an exception for the health care field, including nurses, should Congress not wish for such nurses to be considered supervisors. The court reminded the NLRB that the courts, and not the board, bear the final responsibility for interpreting the law. After concluding that the board's test was inconsistent with the statute, the court found that the four LPNs involved in this case were indeed supervisors and ineligible for protection under the NLRA (*NLRB v. Health Care & Retirement Corp.*, 1994).

These cases have set precedence and figured in multiple subsequent decisions in both health care and industrial settings, although there have been no further rulings addressing the charge nurse/supervisor status. Hence, the *Kentucky River* ruling is still in effect today, specifying that nurses, on average, with less than 10% to 15% (equal to about one shift per pay period) of their time as charge nurse are considered staff nurses, whereas nurses working more than 15% of their professional time as charge nurses are considered supervisors.

Employment Legislation

Like unionization, the many legal issues involved in recruitment and employment have an impact on the directing function. These potential constraints are present regardless of union presence. The American industrial relations system is regarded as one of the most legalistic in the Western world, and it continues to grow. Few aspects of the employment relationship are free from regulation by either state or federal law. Employment laws discussed here provide a cursory examination of such laws. Many of these regulations relate to specific aspects of personnel management, such as the laws that deal with collective bargaining or the equal employment laws that regulate hiring. Some personnel regulations are discussed in previous chapters, and others are discussed later. The prudent manager will always work closely with human resource management when dealing with employment legislation issues.

Some observers believe that employment and labor–management laws have become so prescriptive that they preclude experimentation and creativity on the part of management. Others believe that, like collective bargaining, the proliferation of employment laws must be viewed from a historical standpoint to understand their need. Regardless of whether one believes such laws and regulations are necessary, they are a fact of each manager's life.

TABLE **22.2 LEGISLATION RELATED TO LABOR LAWS**

Title of Legislation	Regulation
Fair Labor Standards Act (1938); has been amended many times since 1938	Sets minimum wage and maximum hours that can be worked before overtime is paid
Civil Rights Act of 1964 (updated 1977)	Sets equal employment practices Recognizes sexual harassment as a form of sex discrimination
Executive Order 11246 (1965) and Executive Order 11375 (1967)	Sets affirmative action guidelines
Age Discrimination Act (1967) and 1978 amendment	Protects against forced retirement
Rehabilitation Act (1973)	Prohibits discrimination on the basis of disability
Vietnam Veterans Act (1973/1974)	Provides reemployment rights
The Equal Pay Act of 1963	Requires that men and women performing equal work receive equal compensation
California Fair Pay Act (2016)	Companies in California must justify any pay disparities between men and women doing "substantially similar" work. (Prior fair pay legislation only required men and women of the same job title to be paid equally.) Also, legally guaranteed employees the right to ask coworkers about pay without retribution from management

> The feeling that the employer is fair to all will set the stage for the type of team building that is so important in effective management.

Being able to handle management's legal requirements effectively requires a comprehension of labor laws and their interpretation. The leader who embraces the intent of laws barring discrimination and providing equal opportunity becomes a role model for fairness. Labor laws, such as those given in Table 22.2, fall into one of five categories:

1. *Labor standards*. These laws establish minimum standards for working conditions regardless of the presence or absence of a union contract. Included in this set are minimum wage, health and safety, and equal pay laws.
2. *Labor relations*. These laws relate to the rights and duties of unions and employers in their relationship with each other.
3. *Equal employment*. The laws that deal with employment discrimination were introduced in Chapter 15.
4. *Civil and criminal laws*. These are statutory and judicial laws that proscribe certain kinds of conduct and establish penalties.
5. *Other legislation*. Nursing managers have some legal responsibilities that do not generally apply to industrial managers. For instance, licensed personnel are required to have a current, valid license from the state in which they practice. In addition, most states require that employers of nurses report certain types of substance abuse to the state licensing boards. Confidentiality laws also have a significant impact on health care organizations.

Labor Standards

Labor standards are regulations dealing with the conditions of the employee's work, including physical conditions, financial aspects, and the number of hours worked. Regulations may be issued by state and/or federal bodies. When the regulations overlap, the more stringent regulation is likely the one that applies.

> State and federal employment legislation often overlap; as a general rule, the employer must abide by the stricter of the two regulations.

Minimum Wages and Maximum Hours

The overwhelming majority of nonsupervisory employees are covered by the *Fair Labor Standards Act* (FLSA) since the FLSA applies to any business engaged in interstate commerce with yearly sales of $500,000 or more (Sedhom Law Group PLLC, 2021). This law was enacted by Congress in 1938 and established an hourly minimum wage at that time of 25 cents. Since then, the law has been amended numerous times.

It is often said that in addition to putting a "floor under wages," the FLSA also puts a "ceiling over hours." The latter statement, however, is not quite accurate. The FLSA sets a maximum number of hours in any week beyond which a person may be employed only if they are paid an overtime rate. Some states have enacted a law that makes an exception to this weekly rule on overtime. The exception is an 80-hour, 2-week pay period ceiling, after which the employee must receive overtime pay. Overtime pay can be significant, so it is imperative that managers know which standard their organization is using.

Hours worked includes all the time that the employee is required to be on duty. Therefore, mandatory classes, orientation, conferences, etc., must be recorded as duty time and are subject to the overtime rules. The FLSA does not require time clocks but does require that some record be maintained of hours worked.

The FLSA also regulates the minimum amount of overtime pay, which is at least 1.5 times the basic rate. When state and federal laws differ on when overtime pay begins, the stricter rule usually applies. Some union contracts also have stricter overtime pay agreements than the FLSA.

Federal labor laws exempt certain employees from the minimum wage and overtime pay requirements. Executive employees, administrative employees, and professional employees are the three most notable white-collar exemptions. The functions of the position, rather than the title or the fact that employees are paid a monthly wage, differentiate an exempt employee. Certain students, apprentice learners, and other special circumstances also may qualify an employee for an exemption to FLSA regulations. The personnel department in any large organization is particularly helpful to the manager in implementing these labor laws. Managers, however, should have a general understanding of how these laws restrict staffing and scheduling policies.

LEARNING EXERCISE 22.4

Time Clocks

Until the 1950s, most health care organizations did not require that employees use a time clock when arriving at or leaving work for meal breaks. Now, time clocks are the norm for hospitals and some other, but not all, health care organizations.

ASSIGNMENT:

Survey several community hospitals, clinics, student health centers, home health care facilities, and other organizations that employ nurses. How many of them require nurses to use time clocks? How do you feel about professionals being required to use a time clock for meal breaks? Discuss this issue in class and with the nurses you know.

The Equal Pay Act of 1963

The *Equal Pay Act of 1963* requires that men and women performing equal work receive equal compensation. Four equal pay tests exist: *equal skill*, *equal effort*, *equal responsibility*, and *similar working conditions*. This law had a great impact on nursing management when it was enacted. Before 1963, male orderlies were routinely paid a higher wage than female aides performing identical duties. Although this fact seems incredible today, at the time, many managers condoned this widespread practice of blatant wage discrimination. Most health care agencies now call these employees "nursing assistants," whether they are male or female, and all are paid the same wage.

Yet, complaints of pay discrimination based on gender still exist. In 2021, women earned 82 cents for every dollar men made. This 18% difference is the raw gender pay gap. Over the past few decades, this gender pay gap has narrowed, but it's a slow process and at the current rate, the gender pay gap will remain until 2059. Indeed, in 2021, *Equal Pay Day* was March 21; that's how far into 2021 the average American woman had to work (in addition to working all of 2020) to make as much money as the average American man earned in 2020 (Spiggle, 2021).

Some question, however, whether this pay inequity reflects equal work. Some economists have suggested that the more rapid career trajectory and relatively higher pay for male nurses compared with female nurses likely reflects the historical trend that more men are employed full time in their career paths, whereas women tend to have career gaps related to childbearing or childrearing families and often work fewer hours (Huston, 2023). Evidence suggests, however, that the gender pay gap cannot be entirely explained by these differences, even after accounting for non-gender–related worker characteristics.

Spiggle (2021) notes instead, that in the vast majority of jobs, this pay discrepancy probably has multiple explanations, many of which fall into one of two categories described by the Organization for Economic Co-operation and Development (OECD) as "glass ceilings" and "sticky floors." *Glass ceilings* are obstacles that stand in the way of women advancing their careers. An example might include a woman choosing not to apply for a promotion because she knows she needs to work part-time for caregiving responsibilities. In contrast, *sticky floors* are disadvantages women consistently face whether they're just starting their careers or preparing for retirement. For example, a manager may assume women are less competent or qualified in a position and decide to offer a lower salary when making a job offer. The OECD concluded that about 60% of a gender pay gap is the result of a glass ceiling while 40% comes from a sticky floor. Regardless of which category the pay gap explanation falls into, this issue is often subtle and difficult to directly address (Spiggle, 2021).

Wheelwright (2022) notes that Washington, DC pays women the highest median salary and has the smallest wage gap in the nation at 8.1%. The state closest to gender pay parity is Vermont, where woman earn just 10% less than men overall. Wyoming has the largest pay gap, with women earning 34.6% less than men overall (Wheelwright, 2022).

Ethnic pay parity also is lacking. The average income for White Non-Hispanic workers in the United States is $71,125.40 (P.K., 2009–2022). The average for Black earners is $48,761.39 whereas Hispanic or Latino workers average $42,164.96 (P.K., 2009–2022).

Federal legislation known as the *Paycheck Fairness Act* (PFA) was first introduced into Congress in 1997 and has been reintroduced many times since. This bill would require companies to report pay data to the government, give grants for negotiation training, and make class-action lawsuits easier. More and more state legislatures are, however, taking action to strengthen equal pay laws, including California. That state passed the *Fair Pay Act* in 2015 (enacted January 1, 2016), which included some elements of the PFA, such as making it more difficult for employers to justify pay disparities in court (State of California Department of Industrial Relations, 2022).

Equal Employment Opportunity Laws

Under the American free enterprise system, employers have historically been able to hire whomever they desired. Today, a transplanted employer of the 1920s might be shocked to see that racial and ethnic minorities, women, older adults, and people with disabilities have acquired substantial rights in the workplace. The first legislation in employment hiring practices resulted from years of discrimination against underrepresented groups. More recent legislation has been aimed at eliminating discrimination that occurs for other reasons. The *U.S. Equal Employment Opportunity Commission* (USEEOC) website lists the following types of discrimination: age, disability, equal pay/compensation, genetic information, national origin, pregnancy, race/color, religion, retaliation, sex, and sexual harassment (USEEOC, n.d.-a).

> Equal employment opportunities have fostered profound changes in the American workplace. Women, racial and ethnic minorities, and individuals with disabilities have had success in gaining jobs previously denied to them. However, only modest gains in achieving ethnic diversity have occurred in nursing (Huston, 2023).

Although men are a minority in nursing, their minority status appears to have led to advantages rather than discrimination, particularly in hiring and promotion. Indeed, men in nursing often rise more rapidly into management positions and earn more money than their female counterparts (Huston, 2023). Paton (2021) notes that 2021 survey data found that male nurse salaries were on average almost 10% higher than female nurse salaries even when adjusted for factors like hours worked, education, and experience. Male nurses earned an average of $80,000 compared to $72,703 for women, a difference of $7,297 per year (Paton, 2021).

Discrimination involving pregnant employees also interests nurse-managers because nursing is a predominately female profession and because nurses are often exposed to hazardous chemical, radiation, and infectious organisms. The *Pregnancy Discrimination Act*, which amended Title VII of the *Civil Rights Act of 1964*, requires that pregnant employees be treated the same as other employees who are temporarily disabled. Managers should use common sense as well as ethical and humane treatment when dealing with the pregnant employee.

Civil Rights Act of 1964

The *Civil Rights Act of 1964* laid the foundation for equal employment in the United States. The thrust of Title VII of the Civil Rights Act is twofold: It prohibits discrimination based on factors unrelated to job qualifications and it promotes employment based on ability and merit. The areas of discrimination specifically mentioned are race, color, religion, sex, and national origin.

This act was strengthened by President Lyndon Johnson's *Executive Order 11246* in 1965 and *Executive Order 11375* in 1967. These executive orders sought to correct past injustices. Because the government believed that some groups had a long history of being discriminated against, it wanted to build in a mechanism that would assist those groups in "catching up" with the rest of the American workforce. Therefore, it created an affirmative action component. *Affirmative action* plans are not specifically required by law but may be required by court order. In most states, affirmative action plans are voluntary unless government contracts are involved. Some states, such as California, have voted to eliminate affirmative action in the workplace, arguing that it actually resulted in reverse discrimination. Many organizations, however, have voluntarily put an affirmative action plan in place when the plan does not conflict with state regulations.

Affirmative action differs from *equal opportunity*. The United States Equal Employment Opportunity legislation is aimed at preventing discrimination. Affirmative action plans are aimed at actively seeking to fill job vacancies with members from groups who are underrepresented, such as women, ethnic minorities, and individuals with disabilities.

The USEEOC is responsible for enforcing Title VII of the Civil Rights Act, and the investigatory responsibility of the USEEOC is broad. When it finds that a charge of discrimination is justified, the agency attempts to reach an agreement through persuasion and conciliation. When the USEEOC is unable to reach an agreement, it has the power to bring civil action against the employer. When discrimination is found, the courts will order restoration of rightful economic status; this means that the court may order that the employee receives back the pay for up to 2 years. In health care organizations, when discrimination has been found (such as unequal pay for men and women in nursing assistant jobs), financial awards in class action suits have been extraordinarily high. Managers must be alert for any such discriminatory practices. Some states have fair employment legislation that is stricter than the federal act. Again, the stricter regulations always apply.

Age Discrimination and Employment Act

Enacted by Congress in 1967, the purpose of the *Age Discrimination in Employment Act* (ADEA) was to promote the employment of older people based on their ability rather than age. In early 1978, the ADEA was amended to increase the protected age to 70 years. In 1987, Congress voted to remove even this age restriction except in certain job categories.

Although some people are alarmed by the removal of mandatory age retirements, trends continue toward earlier retirement. However, reversal of this trend may have serious consequences for some organizations. It could have a significant impact on organizations that are labor intensive, particularly if those labor-intensive organizations also have demanding physical requirements such as those in nursing.

LEARNING EXERCISE 22.5

Addressing Mary's Failing Health

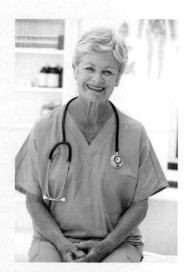

You are the manager of a well-baby newborn nursery. Among your staff is 79-year-old licensed vocational nurse/ licensed practical nurse Mary Jones, who has worked for the hospital for 50 years. No mandatory retirement age exists. This has not been a problem in the past, but Mary's general health is now making this a problem for your unit. Mary has grown physically fragile. Cataracts cloud her vision, and she has hypertension. Last month, she began to prepare a little girl for circumcision because she did not read the armband properly.

Your staff has become increasingly upset over Mary's inability to fulfill her job duties. The physicians, however, support Mary and found the circumcision incident humorous. Last week, you requested that Mary have a physical examination, at hospital expense, to determine her physical ability to continue working.

You were not particularly surprised when she returned with medical approval. Her physician spoke sharply with you. Admitting privately that Mary's health was rapidly failing, the physician told you that working was Mary's only reason for living and left you with these words: "Force Mary to retire and she will die within the year."

ASSIGNMENT:

Using your knowledge of age discrimination, patient safety, employee rights, and management responsibilities, decide on an appropriate course of action for this case. Be creative and think beyond the obvious. Be able to support your decisions.

Sexual Harassment

Although job discrimination related to gender became illegal with the *Civil Rights Act of 1964*, it was not until 1977 that the federal appeals court upheld a claim that a supervisor's verbal and physical advances constituted sexual harassment in the workplace. Since then, sexual harassment has been recognized as a form of sex discrimination that violates Title VII of the *Civil Rights Act*. The recent *#MeToo* and *Time's Up* movements have also emphasized the ubiquity of sexual harassment (Papantoniou, 2021).

The USEEOC (n.d.-b) defines *sexual harassment* as "unwelcome sexual advances, requests for sexual favors, and other verbal or physical conduct of a sexual nature when submission to or rejection of this conduct explicitly or implicitly affects an individual's employment; unreasonably interferes with an individual's work performance; or creates an intimidating, hostile, or offensive work environment" (para. 2).

The USEEOC (n.d.-b) states that sexual harassment can occur in a variety of circumstances including but not limited to the following:

- The victim as well as the harasser may be a woman or a man. The victim does not have to be of the opposite sex.
- The harasser can be the victim's supervisor, an agent of the employer, a supervisor in another area, a coworker, or a nonemployee.
- The victim does not have to be the person harassed but could be anyone affected by the offensive conduct.
- Unlawful sexual harassment may occur without economic injury to or discharge of the victim.
- The harasser's conduct must be unwelcome.

Since the 1977 ruling, allegations of sexual harassment and lawsuits have permeated virtually every type of industry, and the health care system is not immune. Indeed, sexual harassment as well as other types of nonphysical violence are worldwide problems for nurses. Recent studies estimate that 60% of female nurses worldwide report an incident of sexual harassment and a recent systematic review found a pooled prevalence of sexual harassment against female nurses to be 43.2%, which included verbal, nonverbal, psychological, and physical acts (Hope & Munro, 2021).

While a growing body of evidence exists about sexual harassment among female nurses, less is known about the phenomenon among male nurses. Papantoniou (2021) found that 4 in 10 male nurses have experienced sexual harassment at least once in their working lives. The most frequent type of sexual harassment was gender harassment, followed by unwanted sexual attention while only a minority experienced sexual coercion. Young age and limited years of experience were crucial factors that increased the frequency of sexual harassment. The researchers concluded that more channels must be opened for victims to report their experiences, hierarchical organizational structures must be redesigned to foster upward communication, and well-defined policies must be created that encapsulate what sexual harassment is, what the process of reporting is, and that committees are established to assess the complaints of victims and ensure the transparency and confidentiality of the process (see Examining the Evidence 22.1).

In addition, although most discussion about sexual harassment in the health care workplace focuses on employee-to-employee harassment, sexual harassment can also be perpetrated by the patients and families being cared for. Employment laws note that employers must protect their workers from such treatment. Unfortunately, although hospital procedure enables direct care workers to remove themselves from cases where patients are sexually inappropriate, nurses rarely do (Rossheim, 2022). In addition, although sexual harassment

EXAMINING THE EVIDENCE 22.1

Sources: From Papantoniou, P. (2021, August). Are male nurses sexually harassed? A cross-sectional study in the Greek Health System. *BMC Nursing, 20*(1), 1–9. https://doi-org.mantis.csuchico.edu/10.1186/s12912-021-00656-6

Sexual Harassment of Male Nurses

An electronic-based cross-sectional study was conducted using the Sexual Experiences Questionnaire (SEQ) to collect data from 507 male nurses working in Greece's various settings during October and February 2021. Convenience sampling was used due to the sensitive nature of the research topic based on respondents' willingness and availability.

Study results found that 40% of male nurses had experienced sexual harassment at least once in their working lives, and the most common form of sexual harassment faced was gender harassment, followed by unwanted sexual attention. Male doctors and male nurses were the most common perpetrators. Private and younger male nurses with up to 5 years of experience experienced more frequent sexual harassment.

Most cases occurred in the hallway (50%), patient care units (25%) and surgery areas (17%). In most cases, victims ignored the behavior and avoided the harasser (45%), stayed silent (30%), and only 1 in 4 told the harasser to stop. In the cases where victims reported the incident, the organization did not initiate an internal investigation (99%), whereas when it did, the perpetrator was not penalized in all cases.

In addition, multiple regression analyses showed that unwanted sexual attention and sexual coercion were associated with physical and job-related outcomes. Almost 36% of respondents experienced physical problems, while 30% dealt with mental issues due to sexual harassment.

The researchers concluded that sexual harassment has a detrimental impact on nurses' well-being and noted significant concern that the male nurses' failure to report the problem occurred because the nurses perceived accurately that their experiences would not be taken seriously. The researchers suggested that policymakers introduce work ethics and training programs to prevent sexual harassment in clinical settings.

is a difficult issue in any employment setting, many nursing homes have residents who act out inappropriately because of dementia or Alzheimer's disease. Nevertheless, these agencies must take steps to address and minimize the risk of their employees even when it comes from residents.

Recognizing that nurses are uniquely vulnerable to verbal and physical abuse in the workplace, the American Association of Critical-Care Nurses (AACN) released a position statement in 2019 that called for health care facilities to ensure the safety and security of staff, patients, and visitors (Hope & Munro, 2021). Indeed, health care organizations must be alert to sexual harassment and intervene immediately when it is suspected, regardless of the perpetrator. This requires a proactive approach on the part of employers to prevent, detect, and correct instances of harassment. At minimum, organizations must have a plan that outlines temporary steps to deal with such allegations while they are being investigated as well as permanent remedial steps once the investigation has been completed to ensure that the situation does not recur.

Lastly, nurses must take appropriate action when they witness the harassment of others or when they themselves are the targets of such offenses. When one person makes another uncomfortable in the workplace using sexual innuendoes or jokes or invades another's personal space, this behavior should be recognized and confronted as sexual harassment. Unfortunately, underreporting of the problem is common, and nurses often make light of sexually harassing incidents.

LEARNING EXERCISE　22.6

Confronting Sexual Harassment

You are a new female employee at Valley Medical Center's intensive care unit and love your job. Although only 25 years old, you have been a nurse for 4 years, and the last 2 years were spent in a small critical care unit in a rural hospital. You work the 3:00 PM to 11:00 PM shift. Ever since you came to work there, one of the male physicians, Dr. Long, has been especially attentive to you. At first, you were flattered, but more recently, you have become uncomfortable around him. He sometimes touches you and seems to be flirting with you. You have no romantic interest in him and know that he is married. Last night, he asked you to meet him for an after-work drink and you refused. He is a very powerful man in the unit, and you do not want to alienate him, but you are becoming increasingly troubled by his behavior.

Today, you went to your shift charge nurse and explained how you felt. In response, the nurse said, "Oh, he likes to flirt with all the new staff, but he's perfectly harmless." These comments did not make you feel better. At approximately 7:00 PM, Dr. Long came to the unit and cornered you again in a comatose patient's room and asked you out. You said no again, and you are feeling more anxious because of his behavior.

ASSIGNMENT:

Outline an appropriate course of action. What options can you identify? What is your responsibility? What are the driving and restraining forces for action? What support systems for action can you identify? What responsibility does the organization have? Be creative and think beyond the obvious. Be able to support your decisions.

Legislation Affecting Americans with Disabilities

The *Rehabilitation Act of 1973* required all employers with government contracts of more than $25,000 to take affirmative action to recruit, hire, and advance persons with disabilities who are qualified. Similar but less aggressive affirmative action steps were required for other companies doing business with the federal government, with specific requirements depending on the size of the company and the dollar amount of the contract. The Department of Labor was charged with enforcing this act. Although initially, there was very slow progress in getting companies to hire those with disabilities, steady progress has been made.

In 1990, Congress passed the *Americans with Disabilities Act* to eliminate discrimination against Americans with physical or mental disabilities in the workplace and in social life. *Disability* is defined as "any physical or mental impairment that limits any major life activity." This includes people with obvious physical disabilities as well as those with cancer, diabetes, HIV or AIDS, and those recovering from substance use disorders.

Veterans Readjustment Assistance Act

The *Veterans Readjustment Assistance Act* provides employment rights and privileges for veterans for positions that they held before they entered the armed forces. This act was used by some nurses after the Vietnam War and during the nursing surplus after the Persian Gulf War to gain reemployment after military service. There is a lesser need for nurses implementing this act when veterans return from war during a nursing shortage because jobs are readily available.

The Occupational Safety and Health Act

The manager needs to be particularly cognizant of legislation imposed by the Occupational Safety and Health Act (OSHA) and state health licensing boards. The OSHA speaks to the employer's requirements to provide a place of employment that is free from recognized hazards that may cause physical harm. The Department of Labor enforces this act. Because it is impossible for the Department of Labor to physically inspect all facilities, most inspections are brought about by employee complaint or employer request. The act allows fines to be levied if employers continue with unsafe conditions.

Since OSHA's inception, many organizations have vehemently criticized the act and specifically its administration. They have charged that the cost of meeting OSHA standards has excessively burdened American businesses. On the other hand, unions have asserted that the federal government has never staffed or funded OSHA adequately. They have charged that the OSHA has been negligent in setting standards for toxic substances, carcinogens, and other disease-producing agents.

Because the risk of discovery and the fine (if judged guilty) are both low, employers may choose to ignore unsafe working conditions. Nurse-managers are in a unique position to call attention to hazardous conditions in the workplace and should communicate such concerns to a higher authority. Ongoing controversies regarding safety issues include the cost and effectiveness of universal precautions and immunizations against potential bioterrorism. Most states also have occupational and safety regulations. Again, the employer must comply with the more stringent regulations in the case of overlaps.

State Health Facilities Licensing Boards

In addition to health and safety requirements, many state boards have regulations regarding staffing requirements. It is the ultimate responsibility of top-level management to meet the requirements for state licensing. However, all managers are responsible for knowing and meeting the regulations that apply to their unit or department. For example, if the manager of an ICU has a state staffing level that mandates 12 hours of nursing care per patient per day and requires that the ratio of RNs to other staff be 2:1, then the supervisor is obligated to staff at that level or greater. If, during times of short staffing, supervisors are unable to meet this level of staffing, they must communicate this to the upper-level management so that there can be a joint resolution.

The variation in state licensing requirements makes a lengthy discussion of them inappropriate for this book. However, managers must be knowledgeable about state licensing regulations that pertain to their level of supervision.

Integrating Leadership Skills and Management Functions When Working with Collective Bargaining, Unionization, and Employment Laws

Unionization and employment laws will seem less burdensome if managers remember that both primarily protect the rights of patients and employees. If managers perform their jobs well and work for organizations that desire to "do the right thing" by accepting their social responsibility, they need not fear either. If the organization is not unionized, the manager must use the leadership skills of communication, fairness, and shared decision making to ensure that employees do not feel unionization is necessary. The integrated leader-manager is a role model for fairness, knows unit employees well, and sincerely seeks to meet their needs.

When making decisions that deal with unions and employment legislation, the effective leader-manager always seeks to do what is just. In addition, they seek appropriate assistance before finalizing decisions that involve sensitive legal or contractual issues. By using these leadership skills, the manager becomes fairer in personnel management, develops increased self-awareness, and develops an understanding of the average individual's need to seek unionization and of the necessity for employment legislation.

The effective manager maintains the required amount of staffing and ensures a safe working environment. The rights of the organization and the employee are protected as the manager uses personnel policies in a nondiscriminatory and consistent manner. The emphasis is on flexibility and the accommodation of employment legislation and union contracts.

Key Concepts

- The question of whether nurses should participate in collective bargaining has been around since legislation made such organization possible.
- Historically, union activity increases during times of labor shortages and economic upswings.
- Nurses working in unionized organizations appear to have some economic advantage, and their individual vulnerability to arbitrary action on the part of their employer is reduced.
- Union alliances are becoming increasingly commonplace in health care because increased negotiating power comes with greater membership.
- People are motivated to join or reject unions because of their numerous needs and values.
- Although unions historically focused heavily on wage negotiations, current issues that nurses deem just as or more important are nonmonetary, such as guidelines for staffing, float provisions, shared decision making, and scheduling.
- The ANA acts as a professional association for RNs and as a collective bargaining agent. This dual purpose poses a conflict in loyalty for nurses who work in management positions. Even unionized nurses have not been able to agree on the intensity and direction their unions should take, resulting in some state unions breaking off from the ANA.
- In June 2018, the Supreme Court ruled that nonunion members no longer had to pay their "fair share" for union representation in collective bargaining negotiations.
- Under current legislation, nurses with less than 10% to 15% (equal to about one shift per pay period) of their time as charge nurse are considered staff nurses, whereas nurses working more than 15% of their professional time as charge nurses are considered supervisors and, therefore, are ineligible for protection under the NLRA.

- The issues around who can belong to a union, what the definition of "supervisor" is in nursing, and whether strikes and walkouts are ethically justified for nursing professionals add to the complexity of discussion about whether collective bargaining should be a part of professional nursing.
- Although all managers play an important role in establishing and maintaining effective management–labor relationships, the middle-level manager has the greatest influence on preventing unionization in a nonunion organization.
- The relationships health care organizations have developed with their collective bargaining agents vary from direct opposition to collaboration. Creating a climate in which labor and management can work together to accomplish mutual goals is possible.
- Labor relation laws concern the rights and duties of unions and employers in their relationship with each other.
- Labor standards are regulations dealing with the conditions of the employee's work, including physical conditions, financial aspects, and the number of hours worked.
- State and federal employment legislation often overlap; generally, the employer must abide by the stricter of the two regulations.
- Much of the human rights legislation concerning employment practices came about because of documented discrimination in the workplace.
- Sexual harassment and other types of nonphysical violence are worldwide problems for nurses.
- Although some legislation makes the job of managing people more difficult for managers, it has resulted in increased job fairness and more opportunities for women, racial and ethnic minorities, older adults, and individuals with disabilities.

Additional Learning Exercises and Applications

LEARNING EXERCISE 22.7

Writing about Employment Laws

Many employment laws generate emotion. Usually, people feel strongly about at least one of these issues. Select one of the following employment laws and write a 250-word essay on why you support or disapprove of the law. Choose from the *Equal Pay Act of 1963*, equal opportunity laws, affirmative action, sexual harassment, or age discrimination.

LEARNING EXERCISE 22.8

Dilemma Involving an Expired Nursing License

At your long-term care facility, it is a policy that licensed nursing employees have a current, valid nursing license. This is in keeping with the state licensing code. It is always difficult to get people to bring their license in to verify that it is current.

You have just come from a meeting with the director who reminded you that you must not have people performing duties that require a license if the license has expired. You decide to issue a memo stating that you will suspend all employees who have not verified their licenses with you.

Following this, all the licensed vocational nurses/licensed practical nurses (LVNs/LPNs) brought their licenses in for verification. However, one of the LVNs/LPNs has an expired license. When questioned, the nurse admitted that payment for relicensure was not made until after your memo was received. This nurse delayed payment because of a financial crisis. You call the licensing board and learn it will be 2 weeks before the employee will receive the license in the mail or before web verification of the license is possible. Active license status cannot be verified over the telephone.

You consider the following facts. It is illegal to perform duties that require a license without one. The LVN/LPN had prior knowledge of the licensing laws and hospital policy. The LVN/LPN has been a good employee with no record of prior disciplinary action.

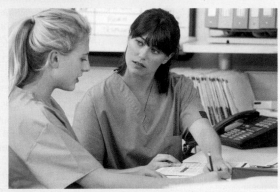

ASSIGNMENT:

Decide what you should do. What alternatives do you have? Provide rationale for your decision.

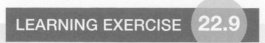

LEARNING EXERCISE 22.9

How Would You Handle This Petition?

Betty Smith, a unit clerk, has come to see you, the nurse-manager of the medical unit, to complain of flagrant discriminatory practices against female employees of University General Hospital. She alleges that women are denied promotional and training opportunities comparable to those made available to men. She shows you a petition with 35 signatures supporting her allegations. Ms. Smith has threatened to forward this petition to the administrator of the hospital, the press, and the Department of Labor unless corrective action is taken at once. Being a woman yourself, you have some sympathy for Ms. Smith's complaint. However, you believe overall that employees at University General are treated fairly, regardless of their gender.

Ms. Smith, a competent employee, has worked on your unit for 4 years. However, she has been creating problems lately. She has been reprimanded for taking too much time for breaks. Personnel evaluations that recommend pay raises and promotions are due next week.

ASSIGNMENT:

How should you handle this problem? Is the personnel evaluation an appropriate time to address the petition? Outline your plan and explain your rationale.

REFERENCES

American Federation of Teachers. (n.d.). *About AFT nurses and health professionals.* https://www.aft.org/healthcare/about

American Nurses Association. (n.d.). *About ANA.* Retrieved July 11, 2022, from https://www.nursingworld.org/ana/about-ana/

American Nurses Association. (2015). *Code of ethics for nurses with interpretive statements.* https://www.nursingworld.org/practice-policy/nursing-excellence/ethics/code-of-ethics-for-nurses/coe-view-only/

Bureau of Labor Statistics. (2022). *Economic news release. Union members summary.* http://www.bls.gov/news.release/union2.nr0.htm

Burger, C. (2021). *Do unions benefit or harm healthcare & nursing industries?* RegisteredNursing.org. https://www.registerednursing.org/articles/do-unions-benefit-harm-healthcare-nursing/

Center for Union Facts. (2021a). *Service employees.* Retrieved July 11, 2022, from https://www.unionfacts.com/union/Service_Employees

Center for Union Facts. (2021b). *American Nurses Association.* Retrieved July 11, 2022, from https://www.unionfacts.com/union/American_Nurses_Association

Conley, J. (2021). *Nurses' union slams CDC guidance shortening isolation period for healthcare workers with Covid-19.* Common Dreams. https://www.commondreams.org/news/2021/12/26/nurses-union-slams-cdc-guidance-shortening-isolation-period-healthcare-workers-covid

Draugelis, J., & Kelly, D. (2021). *Michigan Nurses Association takes legal against Sparrow Hospital, allege federal labor law violations.* WILX. https://www.wilx.com/2021/11/25/michigan-nurses-association-takes-legal-against-sparrow-hospital-allege-federal-labor-law-violations/

Hope, A. A., & Munro, C.L. (2021). Getting to zero sexual harassment in the workplace. *American Journal of Critical Care, 30*(4), 250–252. https://doi-org.mantis.csuchico.edu/10.4037/ajcc2021198

Huston, C. J. (2020). Collective bargaining and the professional nurse. In Huston C. J. (Ed.), *Professional issues in nursing: Challenges and opportunities.* (Chapter 15, 5th ed., pp. 215–229.) Wolters Kluwer.

Huston, C. J. (2023). Diversity in the nursing workforce. In Huston C. J. (Ed.), *Professional issues in nursing: Challenges and opportunities.* (Chapter 9, 6th ed., pp. 121–135.) Wolters Kluwer.

National Labor Relations Board v. Health Care & Retirement Corp., 114 S. Ct. 1778 (1994). http://www.law.cornell.edu/supct/html/92-1964.ZS.html

National Nurses United. (2010–2021). *About National Nurses United.* Retrieved July 11, 2022, from https://www.nationalnursesunited.org/about

National Right to Work Legal Defense Foundation. (2022). *Right to work frequently-asked questions.* http://www.nrtw.org/b/rtw_faq.htm

NLRB clarifies definition of supervisor. (2022). Edited and reviewed by FindLaw Attorney Writers May 05, 2016. Retrieved July 11, 2022, from https://corporate.findlaw.com/litigation-disputes/nlrb-clarifies-definition-of-supervisor.html

Paton, F. (2021). *Nurse salary 2021: How much do registered nurses make?* Nurseslabs. https://nurseslabs.com/nurse-salary/

Philbrick, I. P., & Abelson, R. (2021). Health care unions find a voice in the pandemic. *New York Times.* https://www.nytimes.com/2021/01/28/health/covid-health-workers-unions.html

P.K. (2009–2022). Income by race: Average, top one percent, median, and inequalities. *DQYDJ*. Retrieved July 11, 2022, from https://dqydj.com/income-by-race/

Rossheim, J. (2022). *How nurses can fight sexual harassment*. Monster. https://www.monster.com/career-advice/article/How-Nurses-Can-Fight-Sexual-Harassment

Rushe, D. (2018). Supreme Court strikes blow against unions with 'fair share' ruling. *The Guardian*. https://www.theguardian.com/us-news/2018/jun/27/supreme-court-unions-fair-share-ruling

Sedhom Law Group, PLLC. (2021). *Understanding the Fair Labor Standards Act (FLSA)*. https://www.bespokelaw-firm.com/blog/2021/08/understanding-the-fair-labor-stan-dards-act-flsa/

Spiggle, T. (2021). *The gender pay gap: Why it's still here*. Forbes. https://www.forbes.com/sites/tomspiggle/2021/05/25/the-gender-pay-gap-why-its-still-here/?sh=2f66582d7baf

State of California Department of Industrial Relations. (2022). *California Equal Pay Act*. https://www.dir.ca.gov/dlse/California_Equal_Pay_Act.htm

The Review. (2021). *Federal labor charges issued against East Liverpool City Hospital for violations of union rights*. https://www.reviewonline.com/news/local-news/2021/12/federal-labor-charges-issued-against-east-liverpool-city-hospital-for-violations-of-union-rights/

U.S. Equal Employment Opportunity Commission. (n.d.-a). *Discrimination by type*. Retrieved July 11, 2022, from http://www.eeoc.gov/laws/types/index.cfm

U.S. Equal Employment Opportunity Commission. (n.d.-b). *Facts about sexual harassment*. Retrieved July 11, 2022, from https://www.eeoc.gov/fact-sheet/facts-about-sexual-harassment

Wheelwright, T. (2022). *The gender pay gap across the US in 2022*. Business.org. Retrieved July 11, 2022, from https://www.business.org/hr/benefits/gender-pay-gap/

Who counts as a supervisor under current labor law? (2022). Edited and reviewed by FindLaw Attorney Writers June 07, 2016. Retrieved July 11, 2022, from https://corporate.findlaw.com/litigation-disputes/who-counts-as-a-supervi-sor-under-current-labor-law.html

Roles and Functions in Controlling

23

Quality Control in Creating a Culture of Patient Safety

… Because quality health care is a complex phenomenon, the factors contributing to quality in health care are as varied as the strategies needed to achieve this elusive goal.—Carol Huston

… Too often, the health-care system silences people around a problem.—Dr. Martin Makary

... The proliferation of different and sometimes contradictory hospital report cards is confusing patients. People want reliable information to make informed decisions about their care. Instead, they find a cacophony of contradictory reports and ratings.—Bea Grause, RN, JD, President, Healthcare Association of New York State

CROSSWALK

This chapter addresses:

- **AACN Essentials Domain 2**: Person-centered care
- **AACN Essentials Domain 4**: Scholarship for nursing practice
- **AACN Essentials Domain 5**: Quality and safety
- **AACN Essentials Domain 6**: Interprofessional partnerships
- **AACN Essentials Domain 7**: Systems-based practice
- **AACN Essentials Domain 8**: Information and health care technologies
- **AONL Nurse Executive Competency 1**: Communication and relationship building
- **AONL Nurse Executive Competency 2**: A knowledge of the health care environment
- **AONL Nurse Executive Competency 3**: Leadership
- **AONL Nurse Executive Competency 5**: Business skills
- **ANA Standard of Professional Performance 7**: Ethics
- **ANA Standard of Professional Performance 8**: Advocacy
- **ANA Standard of Professional Performance 10**: Communication
- **ANA Standard of Professional Performance 11**: Collaboration
- **ANA Standard of Professional Performance 12**: Leadership
- **ANA Standard of Professional Performance 13**: Education
- **ANA Standard of Professional Performance 14**: Scholarly inquiry
- **ANA Standard of Professional Performance 15**: Quality of practice
- **ANA Standard of Professional Performance 17**: Resource stewardship
- **ANA Standard of Professional Performance 18**: Environmental health
- **QSEN Competency:** Patient-centered care
- **QSEN Competency:** Teamwork and collaboration
- **QSEN Competency:** Evidence-based practice
- **QSEN Competency:** Quality improvement
- **QSEN Competency:** Safety
- **QSEN Competency:** Informatics

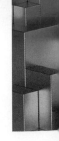

LEARNING OBJECTIVES

The learner will:

- describe the complexity of defining and measuring quality health care
- describe a systematic process (such as FOCUS PDCA) that could be used to initiate a quality improvement process
- determine appropriate criteria or standards for measuring quality
- collect and analyze quality control data to determine whether established standards have been met
- identify appropriate corrective action to be taken when standards have not been met
- differentiate among outcome, structure, and process audits as well as concurrent, retrospective, and prospective audits
- write nursing criteria for process, outcome, and structure audits
- debate the importance of articulating "nursing-sensitive" outcome measures in measuring the quality of health care
- identify the purpose of standardized nursing languages and discuss how creating a common use of terminology/definitions in nursing could improve the quality of patient care
- describe processes used for benchmarking and the identification of best practices
- describe key components of total quality management
- select appropriate quantitative and qualitative tools to measure quality in given situations
- analyze the impact of diagnosis-related groups and the prospective payment system on the quality of care of hospitalized patients
- describe the role of organizations such as The Joint Commission (TJC), the Centers for Medicare & Medicaid Services, the American Nurses Association, the National Committee for Quality Assurance, and the Agency for Healthcare Research and Quality in establishing standards of practice and clinical practice guidelines for health care organizations and health care professionals
- define and provide examples of sentinel events and never events in health care
- describe national efforts such as Health Plan Employer Data and Information Set, ORYX, Core Measures, and the National Database of Nursing Quality Indicators to standardize the collection of quality data and make that data more transparent to providers and consumers
- identify the scope of the problem of medical errors in contemporary health care as well as strategies that have been undertaken to address the problem
- describe characteristics of a "just culture" and discuss why having such a culture is critical to timely and accurate medical error reporting
- identify the four evidence-based standards The Leapfrog Group believes will provide the greatest impact on reducing medical errors
- identify how Lean Six Sigma methodology reduces waste and increases outcome expectations in health care
- analyze (quantitatively and qualitatively) the extent of quality health care gains (if any) that have occurred since the publication of *To Err Is Human*, the first in a series of Quality Chasm reports by the Institute of Medicine
- empower subordinates and followers to participate in *continuous quality improvement* efforts

Introduction

This unit explores controlling as the fifth and final step in the management process. Because the management process—like the nursing process—is cyclic, controlling is not an end in itself; it is implemented throughout all phases of management. During the *controlling* phase of the management process, performance is measured against predetermined standards, and

DISPLAY 23.1 HALLMARKS OF EFFECTIVE QUALITY CONTROL PROGRAMS

1. There must be support from top-level administration.
2. There must be a commitment by the organization in terms of fiscal and human resources.
3. Quality goals reflect search for excellence rather than minimums.
4. Process is ongoing (continuous).

action is taken to correct discrepancies between these standards and actual performance. In health care organizations, the goal of quality control at minimum is to create a culture of patient safety. Optimally, it allows patient health care goals to be met.

Employees who feel that they can influence the quality of outcomes in their work environment experience higher levels of motivation and job satisfaction. Organizations also need some control over productivity, innovation, and quality outcomes. Controlling, then, should not be viewed as a means of determining success or failure, but as a way to learn and grow, both personally and professionally.

Quality control—a specific type of controlling—refers to activities that are used to evaluate, monitor, or regulate services rendered to clients. For any quality control program to be effective, certain components need to be in place (Display 23.1). First, the program needs to be supported by top-level administration; a quality control program cannot merely be an exercise to satisfy various federal and state regulations. In addition, a sincere commitment by the institution, as evidenced by fiscal and human resource support, will be a deciding factor in determining and improving quality of services. Another required component is that developed quality control criteria should be pushed to optimal levels rather than minimally acceptable levels. Finally, the process of quality control must be ongoing; that is, it must reflect a belief that the search for improvement in quality outcomes is continuous and that care can always be improved.

To understand quality control, the manager must become familiar with the process and terminology used in quality measurement and improvement activities. This chapter introduces quality control as a specific and systematic process. Audits are presented as tools for assessing quality. In addition, the historical impact of external forces on the development and implementation of quality control programs in health care organizations is discussed. Key organizations involved in the establishment and monitoring of quality initiatives in the United States are discussed. In addition, quality control strategies, quality measurement tools, benchmarking, and *clinical practice guidelines* (CPGs) are introduced. Finally, strategies for creating a culture of safety are identified, as are the challenges of changing a system that all too often focuses on individual errors rather than on the need to make system-wide changes.

Although controlling is generally defined as a management function, effective quality control requires managers to have skill in both leadership and management. Leadership roles and management functions inherent in quality control are delineated in Display 23.2.

Defining Quality Health Care

Quality measurement and *outcomes accountability* have been buzzwords in health care since the 1980s and continue to be at the forefront of almost every health care agenda today. Indeed, most health care organizations today are striving to become *high-reliability organizations* (HROs). HROs are organizations that perform well (minimal catastrophic error) despite high levels of complexity and the existence of multiple risk factors that encourage error. Achieving this quality designation, however, is both difficult and complex because quality care itself is both difficult to define and even more difficult to achieve.

DISPLAY 23.2 LEADERSHIP ROLES AND MANAGEMENT FUNCTIONS ASSOCIATED WITH QUALITY CONTROL

Leadership Roles

1. Encourages followers to be actively involved in the quality control process
2. Communicates expected standards of care to subordinates clearly
3. Encourages the setting of high standards to maximize quality instead of setting minimum safety standards
4. Embraces and champions quality improvement (QI) as an ongoing process
5. Uses control as a method of determining why goals were not met
6. Is active in communicating quality control findings and their implications to other health professionals and consumers
7. Acts as a role model for followers in accepting responsibility and accountability for nursing actions
8. Uses established professional standards and ethical codes as a guide for practice excellence
9. Distinguishes between clinical standards and resource utilization standards, ensuring that patients receive at least minimally acceptable levels of quality care
10. Supports/actively participates in research efforts to identify and measure nursing-sensitive patient outcomes
11. Creates a work culture that deemphasizes blame for errors and focuses instead on addressing factors that lead to and cause near misses, medical errors, and adverse events
12. Encourages the use of Six Sigma as the benchmark for QI goals
13. Establishes benchmarks that mirror those of best performing organizations and that drive a goal of *continuous quality improvement*
14. Seeks transparency in sharing and translating quality data with consumers

Management Functions

1. Establishes clear-cut, measurable standards of care and determines the most appropriate method for measuring if those standards have been met, in conjunction with other personnel in the organization
2. Selects and uses process, outcome, and structure audits appropriately as quality control tools
3. Collects and accesses appropriate sources of information in data gathering for quality control activities
4. Determines discrepancies between care provided and unit standards and uses *critical event analysis* or *root cause analysis* to determine why standards were not met
5. Uses quality control findings in determining needed areas of staff education or coaching
6. Keeps abreast of current government, accrediting body, and licensing regulations that affect quality control
7. Participates actively in state and national benchmarking and "best practices" initiatives
8. Assesses continually the unit or organizational environment to identify and categorize errors that are occurring and proactively reworks the processes that led to the errors
9. Establishes an environment where research evidence and clinical guidelines based on best practices drive clinical decision making and patient care
10. Is accountable to insurers, patients, providers, and legislative and regulatory bodies for quality outcomes
11. Establishes Lean Six Sigma methodology as a goal for every aspect of QI
12. Complies with external regulatory requirements and data collection related to QI efforts
13. Coordinates efforts to become a high-reliability organization

In 1994, the Institute of Medicine (IOM) defined *health care quality* as the degree to which health services for individuals and populations increase the likelihood of desired health outcomes and are consistent with current professional knowledge (Agency for Healthcare Research and Quality [AHRQ], 2020). Although this classic definition is widely accepted, parts of it merit further examination. The first is the assertion that quality does not exist unless desired health outcomes are attained. Outcomes are only one indicator of quality. Sometimes, patients receive the best possible care with the information available and poor outcomes occur.

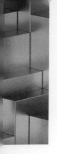

At other times, poor care may still result in good outcomes. Using outcomes alone to measure quality care then is flawed.

> Although outcomes are an important measure of quality care, it is dangerous to use them as the only criteria for quality measurement.

The second implication in the IOM definition is that for care to be considered high quality, it must be consistent with current professional knowledge. Staying current in terms of professional knowledge is difficult for even the most dedicated providers. To complicate the issue even further, how quality of care is defined and measured often differs between providers and patients. Clearly, it is difficult to find a common definition of quality health care that represents the viewpoints of all stakeholders in the health care system.

What is even more difficult, however, is identifying and elucidating the myriad of factors that play a part in determining whether quality health care exists. For example, the IOM further defines quality as having the following properties or domains (AHRQ, 2020):

- **Effectiveness.** Relates to providing care processes and achieving outcomes as supported by scientific evidence.
- **Efficiency.** Relates to maximizing the quality of a comparable unit of health care delivered or unit of health benefit achieved for a given unit of health care resources used.
- **Equity.** Relates to providing health care of equal quality to those who may differ in personal characteristics other than their clinical condition or preferences for care.
- **Patient centeredness.** Relates to meeting patients' needs and preferences and providing education and support.
- **Safety.** Relates to actual or potential bodily harm.
- **Timeliness.** Relates to obtaining needed care while minimizing delays.

Evaluation of this phenomenon then is a complex process.

Quality Control as a Systematic Process

If defining health care quality is problematic, then the measurement of health care quality is even more difficult. To make the process more effective and efficient, the collection of both quantitative and qualitative data is used as well as a specific and systematic process. This process, when viewed simplistically, can be broken down into three basic steps:

1. The criterion or standard is determined.
2. Information is collected to determine if the standard has been met.
3. Educational or corrective action is taken if the criterion has not been met.

The first step, as depicted in Figure 23.1, is the establishment of *control criteria* or *standards*. Measuring performance is impossible if standards have not been clearly established. Not only must standards exist, leader-managers must also see that subordinates know and understand the standards and be aware that their performance will be measured in terms of their ability to meet the established standards.

Many organizations have begun using *benchmarking*—the process of measuring products, practices, and services against best performing organizations—as a tool for identifying desired standards of organizational performance. In doing so, organizations can determine how and why their performance differs from exemplar organizations and use the exemplar organizations as role models for standard development and performance improvement.

> Benchmarking is the process of measuring products, practices, and services against best performing organizations.

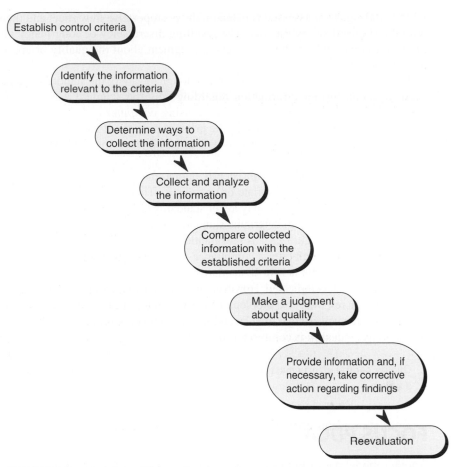

FIGURE 23.1 Steps in auditing quality control.

Many states have initiated a best practices program that invites health care institutions to submit a description of a program or protocol relating to quality improvements (QIs). Experts review the submissions, examine outcomes, and then designate a *best practice*. The difference in performance between top-performing health care organizations and the national average is called the *quality gap*. Although the quality gap is typically small in many industries, it can be significant in health care.

The second step in the quality control process includes identifying information relevant to the criteria. What information is needed to measure the criteria? In the example of postoperative patient care, this information might include the frequency of vital signs, dressing checks, and neurologic or sensory checks. Often, such information is determined by reviewing current research or existing evidence.

The third step is determining ways to collect information. As in all data gathering, the manager must be sure to use all appropriate sources. When assessing quality control of the postoperative patient, the manager could find much of the information in the patient chart. Postoperative flow sheets, the physician orders, and the nursing notes would probably be most helpful. Talking to the patient or family could also yield information.

The fourth step in auditing quality control is collecting and analyzing information. For example, if the standards specify that postoperative vital signs are to be checked every 30 minutes for 2 hours and every hour thereafter for 8 hours, it is necessary to look at how often vital signs were taken during the first 10 hours after surgery. The frequency with which vital signs are assessed is listed on the postoperative flow sheet and then is compared with the standard set by the unit. The resulting discrepancy or congruency gives managers information with which they can make a judgment about the quality or appropriateness of the nursing care.

If vital signs were not taken frequently enough to satisfy the standard, the manager would need to obtain further information regarding why the standard was not met and counsel employees as needed. This is often done using *computer-aided error analysis* (CEA) or through *root cause analysis* (RCA). The primary purpose of RCA is to analyze a problem in terms of what and why it happened as well as taking the steps needed to prevent the problem from recurring.

If organizational goals are consistently unmet, the leader must reexamine those goals and determine if they are inappropriate or unrealistic. There is danger that the leader, who feels pressured to meet these goals, may lower standards to the point where quality is meaningless. This reinforces the need to determine standards first and then evaluate goals accordingly.

The last step in Figure 23.1 is reevaluation. If quality control is measured on 20 postoperative charts and a high rate of compliance with established standards is found, the need for short-term reevaluation is low. If standards are consistently unmet or met only partially, frequent reevaluation is indicated. However, quality control measures need to be ongoing, not put forth simply in response to a problem. Effective leaders ensure that quality control is proactive by pushing standards to maximal levels and by eliminating problems in the early stages before productivity or quality is compromised.

> Quality control efforts must be proactive, not solely as a reaction to a problem.

FOCUS PDCA

Another model put forth to simplify the QI process is *FOCUS PDCA*, which was developed for the health care industry. The meaning of the acronym is detailed in Display 23.3. It's an extension of the classic PDCA methodology, where FOCUS is a set of activities that precedes those used in the PDCA cycle (ISIXSIGMA, 2000–2022). PDCA follows, allowing for a continuous QI cycle to test improvement strategies one by one, in a controlled manner, to measure results and drive further improvements.

DISPLAY 23.3 FOCUS PDCA: A METHOD FOR HEALTH CARE QUALITY IMPROVEMENT

F: Find a process to improve.
O: Organize the effort to work on improvement.
C: Clarify current knowledge of the process.
U: Understand process variation and capability.
S: Select a strategy for continued improvement.

Once the FOCUS process has identified the area for improvement, brought together a team, and found the best possible solution, it's time to implement that solution through PDCA.

P: Plan.
D: Do.
C: Check.[a]
A: Act.

[a]Note that some organizations use the acronym PDSA instead, for plan, do, study, act.

Source: Trindent Consulting. (2022). *Focus PDCA—A lean tool for the healthcare industry.* https://www.trindent.com/focus-pdca-a-lean-tool-for-the-healthcare-industry

The Development of Standards

A *standard* is a level of excellence that serves as a guide for practice. Standards have distinguishing characteristics: They are predetermined, established by an authority, and communicated to and accepted by the people affected by them. Because standards are used as measurement tools, they must be objective, measurable, and achievable. There is no one set of standards. Each organization and profession must set standards and objectives to guide individual practitioners in performing safe and effective care. *Standards of practice* define the scope and dimensions of professional nursing.

The American Nurses Association (ANA) has been instrumental in developing professional standards for almost a century. In 1973, the ANA Congress first established standards for nursing practice, thereby providing a means of determining the quality of nursing that a patient receives, regardless of whether such services are provided by a professional nurse alone or in conjunction with nonprofessional assistants.

> The ANA has played a key role in developing standards for the profession.

Currently, the ANA publishes numerous different standards for nursing practice that reflect different areas of specialty nursing practice. The *Scope and Standards of Practice*—originally published by the ANA in 1991 and revised several times since—provides a foundation for all registered nurses (RNs) in practice. These standards consist of *Standards of Practice* and *Standards of Professional Performance*, as described in this book's preface.

Other developed standards reflect such diverse fields of practice as diabetes nursing, forensic nursing practice, home health nursing practice, gerontologic nursing, correctional nursing, parish nursing, oncology nursing, school nursing, psychiatric–mental health nursing practice, nursing informatics, and public health. All these standards exemplify optimal performance expectations for the nursing profession and have provided a basis for the development of organizational and unit standards nationwide.

Similarly, *organizational standards* outline levels of acceptable practice within the institution. For example, each organization develops a policy and procedures manual that outlines its specific standards. These standards may minimize or maximize in terms of the quality of service expected. Such standards of practice allow the organization to measure unit and individual performance more objectively.

One contemporary effort to establish standards for individual nursing practice has been the development of CPGs. *CPGs* or *standardized clinical guidelines* provide diagnosis-based, step-by-step interventions for providers to follow to promote high-quality care while controlling resource utilization and costs. CPGs, such as those developed by the AHRQ, are developed following an extensive review of the literature and suggest what interventions, in what order, will likely lead to the best possible patient outcomes.

> CPGs reflect evidence-based practice; that is, they should be based on cutting-edge research and best practices.

Not all accepted guidelines, however, are based on evidence. Others are produced by parties with a potential or actual conflict of interest. In addition, some providers avoid CPGs, arguing that they are "cookbook medicine." The reality, however, is that evidence-based CPGs likely serve as the best possible guide in caring for specific patient populations that exists today. This does not mean that providers cannot deviate from evidence-based guidelines; they can and do. However, such deviations should be accompanied by the identification of the unique factors of the individual case that calls for that deviation.

Audits as a Quality Control Tool

Where standards provide the yardstick for measuring quality care, audits are measurement tools. An *audit* is a systematic and official examination of a record, process, structure, environment, or account to evaluate performance. Auditing in health care organizations provides managers with a means of applying the control process to determine the quality of services rendered. Auditing can occur retrospectively, concurrently, or prospectively. *Retrospective audits* are performed after the patient receives the service. *Concurrent audits* are performed while the patient is receiving the service. *Prospective audits* attempt to identify how future performance will be affected by current interventions. The audits most frequently used in quality control include the outcome, process, and structure audits.

Outcome Audit

Outcomes can be defined as the result of care. *Patient-reported outcome measures* (PROMs) attempt to capture whether the services provided actually improved patients' health and sense of well-being (Hostetter & Klein, 2022). Hostetter and Klein (2022) argue that the ultimate measure of health system performance is whether it helps people recover from an acute illness, live well with a chronic condition, and face the end of life with dignity—and people's reports are the only way to gauge success. Thus, PROMs are a critical component of assessing whether clinicians are improving the health of patients.

Outcome audits determine what results, if any, occurred because of specific nursing interventions for patients. These audits assume that the outcome accurately demonstrates the quality of care that was provided. Most experts currently consider outcome measures to be the most valid indicators of quality care, but historical evaluations of hospital care focused on structure and process.

> Outcomes reflect the result of care or how the patient's health status changed as a result of an intervention.

Outcome measurement, however, is not new; Florence Nightingale was advocating the evaluation of patient outcomes when she used mortality and morbidity statistics to publicize the poor quality of care during the Crimean War. In today's era of cost containment, outcome research is needed to determine whether managed care processes, restructuring, and other new clinical practices are producing the desired cost savings without compromising the quality of patient care.

Outcomes are complex, and it is important to recognize that many factors contribute to patient outcomes. There is growing recognition, however, that it is possible to separate the contribution of nursing to the patient's outcome; this recognition of outcomes that are *nursing sensitive* creates accountability for nurses as professionals and is important in developing nursing as a profession. Although outcomes traditionally used to measure quality of hospital care include mortality, morbidity, and length of hospital stay, these outcomes are not highly nursing sensitive. More nursing-sensitive outcome measures for the acute care setting include patient fall rates, nosocomial infection rates, the prevalence of pressure sores, physical restraint use, and patient satisfaction rates.

Process Audit

Process audits measure how nursing care is provided. The audit assumes a connection between the process and the quality of care. For example, a process audit might be used to establish

LEARNING EXERCISE 23.1

Designing an Audit Tool

You are a public health nurse in a small, nonprofit visiting nurse clinic. The nursing director has requested that you chair the newly established quality improvement committee because of your experience with developing audit criteria. Because a review of the patient population indicates that maternal–child visits make up the greatest percentage of home visits, the committee chose to develop a retrospective-process audit tool to monitor the quality of initial postpartum visits. The criteria specified that the clients to be included in the audit had to have been discharged with an infant from a birth center or obstetrical unit following uncomplicated vaginal delivery. The home visit would occur no later than 72 hours after the delivery.

ASSIGNMENT:

Design an audit tool appropriate for this diagnosis that would be convenient to use. Specify percentages of compliance, sources of information, and number of patients to be audited. Limit your process criteria to 20 items. Try solving this yourself before reading the possible solution that appears in the Appendix.

whether fetal heart tones or blood pressures were checked according to an established policy. In a community health agency, a process audit could be used to determine if a parent received instruction about a newborn during the first postpartum visit.

Process audits tend to be task oriented and focus on whether practice standards are being fulfilled. Process standards may be documented in patient care plans, procedure manuals, or nursing protocol statements. Critical pathways and standardized clinical guidelines are examples of efforts to standardize the process of care. They also provide a tool to measure deviations from accepted best practice process standards.

> Process audits are used to measure the process of care or how the care was carried out and assume that a relationship exists between the process used by the nurse and the quality of care provided.

Structure Audit

Structure audits assume that a relationship exists between quality care and appropriate structure. A structure audit includes resource inputs such as the environment in which health care is delivered. It also includes all those elements that exist prior to and separate from the interaction between the patient and the health care worker. For example, staffing ratios, staffing mix, emergency department wait times, and the availability of fire extinguishers in patient care areas are all structural measures of quality of care.

Structural standards, which are often set by licensing and accrediting bodies, ensure a safe and effective environment, but they do not address the actual care provided. An example of a structural audit might include checking to see if patient call lights are in place or if bed rails are raised to reduce the risk of hospitalized patients getting out of bed and falling. It also might examine staffing patterns to ensure that adequate resources are available to meet changing patient needs.

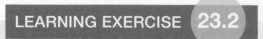

LEARNING EXERCISE 23.2

Identifying Structure, Process, and Outcome Measures

You are a charge nurse on a postsurgical unit. Retrospective survey data reveal that many patients report high levels of postoperative pain in the first 72 hours after surgery. You decide to make a list of possible structure, process, and outcome variables that may be impacting the situation. One of the structure measures you identify is that the narcotic medication carts are located some distance from the patient rooms and that may be contributing to a delay in pain medication administration. One of the process measures you identify is that licensed staff are inconsistent in terms of how soon they make their initial pain assessments on postoperative patients as well as the tools they use to assess pain levels. An outcome measure might be the average wait time from the time a patient requests pain medication until it is administered.

ASSIGNMENT:

Identify at least three additional structure, process, and outcome measures for which you might collect data to resolve this problem. Select at least one of these measures and specifically identify how you would collect the data. Then describe how you would use your findings to increase the likelihood that future practice on the unit will be evidence based.

Standardized Nursing Languages

One means of better identifying nursing-sensitive outcomes has been the development of standardized nursing languages. A *standardized nursing language* provides a consistent terminology for nurses to describe and document their assessments, interventions, and the outcomes of their actions. Sample standardized nursing languages are noted in Display 23.4. Three are discussed in this chapter.

One of the oldest standardized nursing languages is the *Nursing Minimum Data Set* (NMDS). The NMDS—developed by Werley and Lang—represents efforts lasting more than three decades to standardize the collection of nursing data. With the NMDS, a minimum set of items of information with uniform definitions and categories is collected to meet the needs of multiple data users. Thus, it creates a shared language that can be used by nurses in any care delivery setting as well as by other health professionals and researchers. This data then

---

DISPLAY 23.4 SAMPLE STANDARDIZED NURSING LANGUAGES

1. NANDA International (NANDA-I)
2. Nursing Interventions Classification (NIC)
3. Nursing Outcomes Classification (NOC)
4. Clinical Care Classification System (CCC)
5. The Omaha System
6. Perioperative Nursing Data Set (PNDS)
7. International Classification for Nursing Practice (ICNP)
8. Systematized Nomenclature of Medicine-Clinical Terms (SNOMED-CT)
9. Logical Observation Identifiers Names and Codes (LOINC)
10. Nursing Minimum Data Sets (NMDS)
11. Nursing Management Minimum Data Sets (NMMDS)
12. ABC Codes
13. Patient Care Data Set (Retired)

can be used to compare nursing effectiveness, costs, and outcomes across clinical settings and nursing interventions.

Another tool that helps to link nursing interventions and patient outcomes is the *Nursing Interventions Classification* (NIC) developed by the Iowa Interventions Project, College of Nursing, Iowa City, Iowa. The NIC is a research-based classification system that provides a common, standardized language for nurses; it consists of independent and collaborative interventions of nurses in all specialty areas and in all settings. The 565 interventions in NIC (7th ed.) are grouped into 30 classes and 7 domains for ease of use (The University of Iowa College of Nursing, 2022). With diverse classes of care, such as drug management, child bearing, community health promotion, physical comfort promotion, and perfusion management and the domains of interventions, the NIC can be linked with the *North American Nursing Diagnosis Association* taxonomy, the NMDS, and nursing outcomes to improve patient outcomes (The University of Iowa College of Nursing, 2022).

Finally, the International Council of Nurses (ICN) has developed the *International Classification for Nursing Practice* (ICNP), a compositional terminology for nursing practice that is applicable globally. As such, it provides a framework for sharing data about nursing and for comparing nursing practice across settings (ICN, 2022). The ICNP represents the domain of nursing practice as an essential and complementary part of professional health services, necessary for decision making and policy development aimed at improving health status and health care.

Quality Improvement Models

Over the past several decades, the American health care system has moved from a *quality assurance* (QA) model to one focused on QI. The difference between the two concepts is that QA models target currently existing quality; QI models target ongoing and continually improving quality. One model that emphasizes the ongoing nature of QI includes *total quality management* (TQM).

Total Quality Management

TQM, also referred to as *continuous quality improvement*, is a philosophy developed by Edward Deming. TQM assumes that production and service focus on the individual and that quality can always be better. Thus, identifying and doing the right things, the right way, the first time, and problem-prevention planning—not inspection and reactive problem solving—lead to quality outcomes.

> TQM is based on the premise that the individual is the focal element on which production and service depend (i.e., it must be a customer–responsive environment) and that the quest for quality is an ongoing process.

Because TQM is a never-ending process, everything and everyone in the organization are subject to continuous improvement efforts. No matter how good the product or service is, the TQM philosophy says that there is always room for improvement. Customer needs and experiences with the product are constantly evaluated. Workers—not a central QA/QI department—do this data collection, thus providing a feedback loop between administrators, workers, and consumers. Any problems encountered are approached in a preventive or proactive mode so that crisis management becomes unnecessary.

Another critical component of TQM is the empowerment of employees by providing positive feedback and reinforcing attitudes and behaviors that support quality and productivity. Based on the premise that employees have an in-depth understanding of their jobs, believe

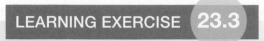

LEARNING EXERCISE 23.3

Deming's 14 Total Quality Management Principles

Think about an organization you have worked in. How many of Deming's 14 principles for total quality management were used in that organization? Do you believe some of the 14 principles are more important than others? Why or why not? Could an organization have a successful quality management program if only some of the principles are used?

they are valued, and feel encouraged to improve product or service quality through risk taking and creativity, TQM trusts the employees to be knowledgeable, accountable, and responsible and provides education and training for employees at all levels. Although the philosophy of TQM emphasizes that quality is more important than profit, the resultant increase in quality of a well-implemented TQM program attracts more customers, resulting in increased profit margins and a financially healthier organization. The 14 quality management principles of TQM as outlined by Deming (1986) are summarized in Display 23.5.

Who Should Be Involved in Quality Control?

Ideally, everyone in the organization should participate in quality control because everyone receives the benefits. Quality control gives employees feedback about their current quality of care and how the care they provide can be improved.

Engagement of frontline staff appears to be especially critical when implementing or sustaining QI efforts such as *Transforming Care at the Bedside* (TCAB)—a national program developed and led by the Robert Wood Johnson Foundation and the Institute for Healthcare Improvement (IHI) from 2003 to 2008 and directed at medical-surgical units (IHI, 2022). TCAB engaged leaders at all levels of the organization, empowered frontline staff to improve care processes, and engaged family members and patients in decision making about their care. Ideas that came out of TCAB were the use of *Rapid Response Teams* to "rescue" patients

---

DISPLAY 23.5 TOTAL QUALITY MANAGEMENT PRINCIPLES

1. Create a constancy of purpose for the improvement of products and service.
2. Adopt a philosophy of continual improvement.
3. Focus on improving processes not on inspection of product.
4. End the practice of awarding business on price alone; instead, minimize total cost by working with a single supplier.
5. Improve constantly every process for planning, production, and service.
6. Institute job training and retraining.
7. Develop the leadership in the organization.
8. Drive out fear by encouraging employees to participate actively in the process.
9. Foster interdepartmental cooperation and break down barriers between departments.
10. Eliminate slogans, exhortations, and targets for the workforce.
11. Focus on quality and not just quantity; eliminate quota systems if they are in place.
12. Promote teamwork rather than individual accomplishments. Eliminate the annual rating or merit system.
13. Educate/train employees to maximize personal development.
14. Charge all employees with carrying out the total quality management package.

Source: Deming, W. E. (1986). *Out of the crisis*. MIT Press.

before a crisis occurred, specific communication models that supported consistent and clear communication among caregivers, liberalized diet plans and meal schedules for patients, and redesigned workspaces that enhanced efficiency and reduced waste (IHI, 2022). The result was an improvement in patient safety indicators.

Many contemporary organizations, however, designate an individual (frequently a nurse) to be their *patient safety officer*. This strategy is risky, as it may create the impression that the responsibility for quality care is not shared. Therefore, although it is impractical to expect full staff involvement throughout the quality control process, as many staff as possible should be involved in determining criteria or standards, reviewing standards, collecting data, or reporting.

Quality control also requires evaluating the performance of all members of the multidisciplinary team. Professionals such as physicians, respiratory therapists, dietitians, and physical therapists contribute to patient outcomes and therefore must be considered in the audit process. Patients should also be actively involved in the determination of an organization's quality of care. It is important to remember, however, that quality care does not always equate with patient satisfaction.

> Patient satisfaction may have little to do with whether a patient's health improved during a hospital stay.

For example, the quality of food, provision of privacy, satisfaction with a roommate, or noisiness of the nursing station may play into a patient's satisfaction with a hospital admission. In addition, patient satisfaction may be adversely affected by long waits for call lights to be answered and for transport to ancillary services such as the radiology department. Even the friendliness of the staff can impact patient satisfaction and perception of quality care. Although these factors are an important component of patient comfort, and therefore quality of care, quality is more encompassing and must always include an examination of whether the patient received the most appropriate treatment from the most appropriate provider in a timely manner.

Quality Measurement as an Organizational Mandate

Organizational accountability for the internal monitoring of quality and patient safety has increased exponentially the last four decades. Most health care organizations today have complete QI programs and are actively working to improve patient outcomes and promote patient safety. Changing government regulations regarding quality control, however, continue to influence QI efforts strongly. Managers must be cognizant of changing government and licensing regulations that affect their unit's quality control and standard setting. This awareness allows the manager to implement proactive rather than reactive quality control.

Although few organizations would debate the significant benefits of well-developed and implemented quality control programs, quality control in health care organizations has evolved primarily from external influences and not as a voluntary monitoring effort. When Medicare and Medicaid (see Chapter 10) were implemented in the mid-1960s, health care organizations had little need to justify costs or prove that the services provided met patients' needs. Reimbursement was based on the costs incurred in providing the service, and no real ceilings were placed on the amount that could be charged for services. Only when the cost of these programs skyrocketed did the government establish regulations requiring organizations to justify the need for services and to monitor the quality of services.

Professional Standards Review Organizations

Professional Standards Review Board legislation (Pub. L. No. 92-603), established in 1972, was among the first of the federal government's efforts to examine cost and quality. *Professional Standards Review Organizations* mandated certification of need for the patient's admission and continued review of care; evaluation of medical care; and analysis of the patient profile, the hospital, and the practitioners.

This new kind of surveillance and the existence of external controls had a huge effect on the industry. Health care organizations began to question basic values and were forced to establish new methods for collecting data, keeping records, providing services, and accounting in general. Because government programs, such as Medicare and Medicaid, represent such a large group of today's patients, organizations that were unwilling or unable to meet these changing needs did not survive financially.

The Prospective Payment System

The advent of *diagnosis-related groups* (DRGs) in the early 1980s added to the ever-increasing need for organizations to monitor cost containment yet guarantee a minimum level of quality (see Chapter 10). As a result of DRGs, hospitals became part of the *prospective payment system* (PPS), whereby providers are paid a fixed amount per patient admission regardless of the actual cost to provide the care. This system has been criticized as promoting abbreviated hospital stays and services leading to a reduced quality of care. Clearly, DRGs have resulted in increased acuity levels of hospitalized patients, a decrease in the length of patient stay, and a perception by some health care providers that patients have been discharged prematurely. All these factors have contributed to health care provider concerns regarding the quality of care they provide.

> Critics of the PPS argue that although DRGs may have helped to contain rising health care costs, the associated rapid declines in length of hospital stay and services provided have likely resulted in declines in quality of care.

The Joint Commission

The Joint Commission (TJC) (formerly known as the *Joint Commission for Accreditation of Healthcare Organizations* [JCAHO])—an independent, not-for-profit organization that accredits more than 22,000 health care organizations and programs in the United States (TJC, 2022d)—has historically had a tremendous impact on planning for quality control in acute

LEARNING EXERCISE 23.4

Quality of Patient Care

How do you define quality of care? Is the quality of your care always what you would like it to be? If not, why not? What factors can you control in terms of providing high-quality care? (Which are internal and which are external?) In your clinical experience, have diagnosis-related groups affected the quality of care provided? If so, how? Do you see differences in the quality of care provided to clients based on their ability to pay for that care or the type of insurance that they have?

care hospitals. TJC was the first to mandate that all hospitals have a QA program in place by 1981. These QA programs were to include a review of the care provided by all clinical departments, disciplines, and practitioners; the coordination and integration of the findings of quality control activities; and the development of specific plans for known or suspected patient problems. Again, in 1982, TJC began to require quarterly evaluations of standards for nursing care as measured against written criteria.

Sentinel Event Reporting

TJC also maintains one of the nation's most comprehensive databases of sentinel events (serious adverse events) by health care professionals and their underlying causes. A *sentinel event* is defined by TJC as a *patient safety event* (an event, incident, or condition that could have resulted or did result in harm to a patient) that results in death, permanent harm, or severe temporary harm (TJC, 2022a). Such events are called "sentinel" because they signal the need for immediate investigation and response. Information from TJC sentinel database is regularly shared with accredited organizations to help them take appropriate steps to prevent medical errors. Sentinel events identified by TJC are shown in Display 23.6.

Another TJC priority is the development of RCA with a plan of correction for the errors that do occur. TJC's (2022a) Sentinel Event Policy provides that organizations that are either voluntarily reporting a sentinel event or responding to TJC's inquiry about a sentinel event submit their related RCA and action plan electronically to TJC whenever such events occur. The sentinel event data are then reviewed, and recommendations are made. TJC defends the confidentiality of the information, if necessary, in court.

Similarly, some organizations use a *failure mode and effects analysis* (FMEA) to examine all possible failures in a design—including sequencing of events, actual and potential risk, points of vulnerability, and areas for improvement (American Society for Quality, 2022). Using FMEA allows organizations to review multiple components and subsystems so that the causes and effects of failures can be identified.

ORYX

In the late 1990s, TJC instituted its *Agenda for Change*—a multiphase, multidimensional set of initiatives directed at modernizing the accreditation process by shifting the focus of accreditation from organizational structure to organizational performance or outcomes. This required the development of clinical indicators to measure the quality of care provided. To further this goal, TJC approved a milestone initiative, known as *ORYX*, in 1997 (TJC, 2022b). This initiative integrated outcomes and other performance measures into the accreditation process with data being publicly reported at a website known as *Quality Check* (https://www.qualitycheck.org/disclaimer/) (TJC, 2022c).

DISPLAY 23.6 SENTINEL EVENTS AS DEFINED BY THE JOINT COMMISSION (2022a)

Sentinel events are patient safety events (not primarily related to the natural course of the patient's illness or underlying condition) that reach a patient and result in any of the following:

- Death
- Permanent harm
- Severe temporary harm (i.e., critical, potentially life-threatening harm lasting for a limited time with no permanent residual but requires transfer to a higher level of care/monitoring for a prolonged period of time, transfer to a higher level of care for a life-threatening condition, or additional major surgery, procedure, or treatment to resolve the condition)

Under ORYX, all organizations accredited by TJC were required to select at least 1 of 60 acceptable performance measurement systems and to begin data collection on specific clinical measures. Organizations could also volunteer for *ORYX Plus*, an effort by TJC to create a national standardized database of 32 performance measures, although this initiative was discontinued in 2009 in favor of core measures reporting. In addition, TJC began collecting data on outcome measures, including the sentinel events overall error rate, the number of reports on possible errors or near misses, hospital readmission rates, and the rate of hospital-acquired infections to better measure quality of care.

Core Measures

TJC also implemented its *Core Measures* program (also called *Hospital Quality Measures*) as part of ORYX in 2002 to better standardize its valid, reliable, and evidence-based data sets. The four areas initially targeted for Core Measures implementation were acute myocardial infarction, pneumonia, heart failure, and the surgical care improvement project. In 2014, performance measurement requirements for accredited general medical-surgical hospitals expanded from four to six core measures. Other core measures have since been added since TJC and CMS periodically redefine the core measures based on the latest evidence and nationwide hospital performance. TJC expects that requirements will continue to increase over time, depending on the national health care environment, emerging national measurement priorities, and hospitals' ever-increasing capability to electronically capture and transmit data.

National Patient Safety Goals

To augment the core measures and promote specific improvements in patient safety, TJC also issues *National Patient Safety Goals* (NPSGs) annually. For example, NPSGs have been created for ambulatory health care, behavioral health care, critical access hospitals, home care, and hospital care. Sample hospital goals for 2022 include using at least two patient identifiers when providing care, treatment, and services; labeling medicines that are not labeled before a procedure; reporting critical results of tests and diagnostic procedures to the right person on a timely basis; and making improvements to ensure that alarms on medical equipment are heard and responded to on time (TJC, 2022e).

Medication Reconciliation

In addition, TJC has recommended the use of a medication reconciliation process to prevent medication errors at patient transition points. *Medication reconciliation* is the process of comparing the medications a patient is taking (or should be taking) with newly ordered medications (TJC, 2022a). This reconciliation is done to avoid medication errors such as omissions, duplications, dosing errors, or drug interactions. It should be done at every transition of care in which new medications are ordered or existing orders are rewritten. The process of medication reconciliation is shown in Display 23.7.

There are numerous studies in the literature that suggest that medication reconciliation can reduce discrepancies in care as well as errors; however, effective implementation in real-world settings is challenging. Most medication reconciliation interventions have focused on attempting to prevent medication errors at hospital admission or discharge, but the most effective and generalizable strategies remain unclear. Medication reconciliation has therefore become an example of a safety intervention that has been effective

---

DISPLAY 23.7 THE FIVE STEPS OF MEDICATION RECONCILIATION

1. Identify medications the patient is currently taking when admitted to the hospital or when seen in an outpatient setting.
2. Identify medication information (e.g., name, dose, route, frequency, purpose).
3. Compare the medication information the patient brought to the care setting with the medications ordered for the patient in the care setting in order to identify and resolve discrepancies.
4. Provide the patient (or family, caregiver, or support person as needed) with written information on the medications the patient should be taking when they are discharged from the hospital or at the end of an outpatient encounter.
5. Explain the importance of managing medication information to the patient when they are discharged from the hospital or at the end of an outpatient encounter.

Source: Paraphrased from The Joint Commission. (2021). *National Patient Safety Goals effective January 2022 for the hospital program*. https://www.jointcommission.org/-/media/tjc/documents/standards/national-patient-safety-goals/2022/npsg_chapter_hap_jan2022.pdf

---

in research settings but has been difficult to implement successfully in general practice (AHRQ, 2019).

Centers for Medicare & Medicaid Services

The *Centers for Medicare & Medicaid Services* (CMS), formerly the Health Care Financing Administration, also plays an active role in setting standards for and measuring quality in health care. With the introduction of the Medicare *Quality Initiatives* in November 2001, a new era of public reporting on quality began. These diverse initiatives encouraged the public reporting of quality measures for nursing homes, home health agencies, hospitals, and kidney dialysis facilities. These data are then made available to consumers on the Medicare website to assist them in making health care choices or decisions.

Medicare also established pay for performance (P4P), also known as *quality-based purchasing*, in the middle of the first decade of the 21st century. Because research conducted in the past decade has suggested little relationship between quality of care provided and the cost of that care, P4P initiatives were created to align payment and quality incentives and to reduce costs through improved quality and efficiency. Multiple P4P programs have been developed and implemented since that time. All provided incentive payments to eligible professionals who satisfactorily reported quality information to Medicare.

Currently, most providers who bill Medicare Part B must participate in one of two tracks in the Quality Payment Program: the *Merit-based Incentive Payment System* (MIPS) or *Alternative Payment Models* (APMs). Providers participating in an APM may be eligible for an incentive payment if they send in data about the care they provide and how the practice used technology. Providers in MIPS receive a negative payment adjustment if the data are not submitted.

Also, as part of the Affordable Care Act (ACA), the CMS has now instituted the *Hospital Value-Based Purchasing* program. In this program, participating hospitals are paid for inpatient acute care services based on the quality of care, not just quantity of the services they provide. Reductions in payment are possible, but it is possible for a hospital to earn back a value-based incentive payment percentage that is less than, equal to, or more than the applicable reduction for that fiscal year (CMS, 2021a). Similarly, the *Readmissions Reduction Program* penalizes hospitals for high readmission rates with lower Medicare reimbursement overall. For purposes of the program, readmission is defined as an admission to a hospital within 30 days of discharge from the same or another hospital.

Hospital Consumer Assessment of Healthcare Providers and Systems Survey

The *Hospital Consumer Assessment of Healthcare Providers and Systems* (HCAHPS) survey is the first national, standardized, publicly reported survey of patients' perspectives of hospital care after discharge. Developed by a partnership between AHRQ and CMS beginning in 2002, the 29 question HCAHPS (pronounced "H-caps") survey instrument measures patients' perceptions of their hospital experience and can be conducted by mail, telephone, mail with telephone follow-up, or active interactive voice recognition (CMS, 2021b).

The HCAHPS survey contains 19 core questions about critical aspects of patients' hospital experiences (communication with nurses and doctors, the responsiveness of hospital staff, the cleanliness and quietness of the hospital environment, communication about medicines, discharge information, overall rating of hospital, and whether they would recommend the hospital). The survey also includes three items to direct patients to relevant questions, five items to adjust for the mix of patients across hospitals, and two items that support congressionally mandated reports. Data collected include how well nurses and doctors communicate with patients, how responsive hospital staff are to patients' needs, how well hospital staff help patients manage pain, how well the staff communicates with patients about medicines, and whether key information is provided at discharge. In addition, the survey addresses the cleanliness and quietness of patients' rooms, the patients' overall rating of the hospital, and whether they would recommend the hospital to family and friends. HCAHPS measures are publicly reported on the CMS *Hospital Compare* website (https://www.hospitalcompare.hhs.gov) for each participating hospital.

Although many hospitals collected information on patient satisfaction for their own internal use, until HCAHPS, there were no common metrics and no national standards for collecting and publicly reporting information about patient experience of care. Since 2008, HCAHPS data have been reported, publicly making valid comparisons possible across hospitals locally, regionally, and nationally, increasing transparency of the quality of hospital care.

Multistate Nursing Home Case Mix and Quality Demonstration

There has also been a major move to develop quality indicators in long-term care settings. One of the most significant efforts has been the *Multistate Nursing Home Case Mix and Quality Demonstration*, funded by the CMS. This demonstration seeks to develop and implement both a case mix classification system to serve as the basis for Medicare and Medicaid payment and a quality-monitoring system to assess the impact of case mix payment on quality and to provide better information to the nursing home survey process.

National Committee for Quality Assurance

Another external force assessing quality control in health care organizations is the *National Committee for Quality Assurance* (NCQA). The NCQA, a private nonprofit organization that accredits managed care organizations, has developed the *Health Plan Employer Data and Information Set* (HEDIS) to compare the quality of care in managed care organizations. HEDIS is used by more than 90% of America's health plans to measure performance on important dimensions of care and service (Office of Disease Prevention and Health Promotion [ODPHP], 2022). For 2021, there were 71 measures across 8 domains of care (ODPHP,

2022; NCQA, 2022). Because so many plans use HEDIS and because the measures are so specifically defined, HEDIS can be used to make comparisons among plans. Future versions are expected to have an even greater number of performance indicators as the growing Medicaid and Medicare segment of the population enrolled in managed care adds more specific performance indicators.

One of the most significant weaknesses of NCQA accreditation, however, is that such accreditation is voluntary. Since 1999, however, Medicare and Medicaid have contracted their managed care plans only with health plans that are accredited by the NCQA. More employers are also adopting this policy with the result that most managed care organizations will need this accreditation in the future to survive fiscally.

National Database of Nursing Quality Indicators

The *National Database of Nursing Quality Indicators* (NDNQI) was founded by the ANA in 2001 to examine the relationships between nursing and patient outcomes by tracking nursing-sensitive quality measures (NDNQI, n.d.-b). Health care organizations participate in the NDNQI program through focused surveys to measure nursing quality, improve nurse satisfaction, strengthen the nursing work environment, assess staffing levels, and improve reimbursement under current P4P policies.

NDNQI is the richest database of nursing performance in the country (NDNQI, n.d.-a). Hospitals can compare performance and job satisfaction levels of individual nursing units to similar units locally, regionally, and nationally, allowing them to develop more effective, finely targeted improvements and also helping them to understand the relationship between the nursing-sensitive quality indicators, staffing data, and RN survey data.

Report Cards

In response to the demand for objective measures of quality, many health plans, health care providers, employer purchasing groups, consumer information organizations, and state governments have begun to formulate health care quality report cards. Most states have laws requiring providers to report some type of data. AHRQ has also been exploring the development of a report card for the nation's health care delivery system.

However, many current report cards do not contain information about the quality of care rendered by specific clinics, group practices, or physicians in a health plan's network. In addition, some critics of health care report cards point out that health plans may receive conflicting ratings on different report cards. This is a result of using different performance measures and how each report card chooses to pool and evaluate individual factors. In addition, report cards may not be readily accessible or may be difficult for the average consumer to understand.

Recent research by Li et al. (2021) suggest that because of the difficulties patients have in knowing how to access and interpret health care quality report cards, many are now using internet reviews to inform their choice of provider (see Examining the Evidence 23.1). The concern here is that these internet reviews primarily reflect subjective patient experiences and not the objective outcome data, more likely to be found on report cards. Li et al. (2021) concluded that it is important to find ways to provide consumers with information that incorporates the advantages of both online ratings and report cards. For policy makers, it is urgent to improve report card systems by making them easier to access and interpret, by working to increase media coverage of report card information, and perhaps by adding attribute measures that patients care about.

EXAMINING THE EVIDENCE 23.1

Source: From Li, X., Chou, S.-Y., Deily, M. E., & Qian, M. (2021). Comparing the impact of online ratings and report cards on patient choice of cardiac surgeon: Large observational study. *Journal of Medical Internet Research, 23*(10), 1–10. https://doi-org.mantis.csuchico.edu/10.2196/28098

Do Online Ratings and Report Cards Influence Patients' Choice of Surgeon?

Patients are increasingly aware that quality information about physicians is available both online and through public report cards. The online reviews are typically written by patients to reflect their subjective experience, and report cards are based on more objective health outcomes.

The aim of this study was to examine the impact of online ratings on patient choice of cardiac surgeon compared to that of report cards. Ratings were obtained from a leading physician review platform, Vitals, which was launched in 2008; and report card scores were obtained from Pennsylvania Cardiac Surgery Reports. The study population was patients who had undergone coronary artery bypass graft (CABG) surgeries in Pennsylvania from 2008 to 2017. Inclusion criteria included surgeons who had received at least one set of report card scores during the study time frame and a sample of 37,354 CABG surgeries performed by 184 surgeons. A total of 1096 reviews for 132 out of 184 surgeons (71.7%) were obtained.

Researchers found that a high online rating had positive and significant effects on patient utility, with limited variation in preferences across individuals, while the impact of a high report card score on patient choice was trivial and insignificant. About 70.13% of patients considered no information on Vitals better than a low rating; the corresponding figure was 26.66% for report card scores. The results also showed that the interaction effect of rating information and a time trend was positive and significant for online ratings, but small and insignificant for report cards.

Researchers offered two possible reasons for the increasing influence of online ratings. First, online ratings are easier to use. If a patient searches for a surgeon, most of the returned links were to physician review websites. In contrast, to access report card scores, patients had to know the scores existed, go to the correct website of the state agency, download the report, understand the meaning of the scores, and read through the report to find the physician they were interested in. Second, online ratings can provide information on things like communication skills, friendliness of the staff, or ease of making an appointment, attributes that patients care about, but which are not available from report cards.

The researchers concluded that a patient's choice of surgeon is affected by both types of rating information; however, over the past decade, online ratings have become more influential, while the effect of report cards has remained trivial. The researchers called for information provision strategies that incorporate the advantages of both online ratings and report cards.

Medical Errors: An Ongoing Threat to Quality of Care

In reviewing the literature on medical errors, medication errors, and adverse events in health care, it is helpful to first define common terms. *Medical errors* are defined by the Encyclopedia of Surgery (2022) as adverse events that could be prevented given the current state of medical knowledge. In addition, the Quality Interagency Coordination Task Force suggests that medical errors are "the failure of a planned action to be completed as intended or the use of a wrong plan to achieve an aim. Errors can include problems in practice, products, procedures, and systems" (Encyclopedia of Surgery, 2022, para. 3).

Medication errors are the most common type of medical error and are a significant cause of preventable adverse events. *Medication errors* are defined by the National Coordinating Council for Medication Error Reporting and Prevention (NCC MERP, 2022) as:

Any preventable event that may cause or lead to inappropriate medication use or patient harm while the medication is in the control of the health care professional, patient, or consumer. Such events may be related to professional practice, health care products, procedures, and systems, including prescribing; order communication; product labeling, packaging, and nomenclature; compounding; dispensing; distribution; administration; education; monitoring; and use. (para. 1)

Finally, *adverse events* are defined as adverse changes in health that occur because of treatment. When medications are involved, these are known as *adverse drug events* (ADEs).

Many studies over the past two decades suggest that medical errors are rampant in the health care system. The most well-known of these studies is likely the 1999 IOM report called *To Err Is Human* (Kohn et al., 2000). This report found that between 44,000 and 98,000 Americans die each year because of medical errors, making medical errors the eighth leading cause of death in this country, even when the lower estimate was used. The IOM study also looked at the type of errors that were occurring. Medication errors stood out as a particularly high risk because these errors can lead to patient injuries, often called ADEs.

Perhaps the most significant contribution of the IOM report, however, was the conclusion that most of these errors did not occur from individual recklessness. Instead, they occurred because of basic flaws in the way that the health delivery system is organized and delivered. The current focus in medical error research is on fixing these flaws and creating and/or fostering environments that minimize the likelihood of errors occurring.

Reporting and Analyzing Errors in a Just Culture

One critical strategy for addressing errors in the health care system is to increase both the mandatory and voluntary reporting of medical errors. At the unit level, organizational cultures must be created that remove blame from the individual and, instead, focus on how the organization itself can be modified to reduce the likelihood of such errors occurring in the future. Only then will health care workers feel they can report the errors and near misses they see occurring every day in their clinical practice.

This does not, however, remove individual practitioner responsibility and accountability to do everything they can to provide safe and competent care. This need to find a middle ground between a blame-free culture, which attributes all errors to system failure and says no individual is held accountable, and an overly punitive culture, where individuals are blamed for all mistakes, has been labeled a *just culture*.

> Ignoring the problem of medical errors, denying their existence, or blaming the individuals involved in the processes does nothing to eliminate the underlying problems.

Legislation is also occurring at the national level to promote both the mandatory and voluntary reporting of medical errors. For example, the *Patient Safety and Quality Improvement Act* was signed into law in 2005. This bill protects medical error information voluntarily submitted to private organizations (*patient safety organizations*) from being subpoenaed or used in legal discovery and generally requires that the information is treated as confidential.

Federal legislation has also been proposed to protect the voluntary reporting of ordinary injuries and "*near misses*"—errors that did not cause harm this time but easily could the next time. This would be like what is done in aviation, in which near misses are confidentially reported and can be analyzed by anyone.

Health care organizations also need to do a better job of identifying what errors are occurring, categorizing those errors, and examining and reworking the processes that led to the errors. It is the leader-manager who bears the responsibility for proactively creating a work environment that minimizes these risks.

The Leapfrog Group

In addition, to help minimize risks to patients, the standards and expectations of oversight groups, insurers, and professional groups have been raised. One such effort is *The Leapfrog Group*, a growing conglomeration of non–health care Fortune 500 company leaders who are committed to modernizing the current health care system. Based on current research, The Leapfrog Group (Leapfrog Hospital Survey, 2020a, 2020b, 2020c, 2020d) has identified four evidence-based standards that they believe will provide the greatest impact on reducing medical errors: *computerized physician–provider order entry* (CPOE), *evidence-based hospital referral*, *intensive care unit physician staffing* (IPS), and the use of *National Quality Forum–endorsed Safe Practices*. These strategies and the evidence supporting their use are described more fully in Table 23.1.

Scientific evidence suggests that The Leapfrog Group initiatives will reduce preventable medical errors. Their implementation is already underway or feasible in the short term; consumers can appreciate their value; and health plans, purchasers, or consumers can easily ascertain their presence or absence in selecting health care providers.

The Leapfrog Group has also endorsed the use of *bar coding* to reduce point-of-care medication errors. As set forth by the U.S. Food and Drug Administration (FDA), all prescription and over-the-counter medications used in hospitals must contain a *national drug code* number, which indicates its dosage forms and strength. The FDA suggests that a bar code system coupled with a CPOE system would greatly enhance the ability of all health care workers to follow the "five rights" of medication administration—that the *right* person receives the *right* drug in the *right* dose via the *right* route at the *right* administration time.

Six Sigma Approach and Lean Manufacturing

Another approach that has been taken to create a culture of patient safety at the institutional level has been the implementation of a *Six Sigma approach*. *Sigma* is a statistical measurement that reflects how well a product or process is performing. Higher sigma values indicate better performance.

Historically, the health care industry has been comfortable striving for three sigma processes (all data points fall within three standard deviations) in terms of health care quality, instead of six (Huston, 2023). This is one reason why health care has more errors than the banking or airline industries, where Six Sigma is the expectation. Organizations should aim for this target by carefully applying the Six Sigma methodology to every aspect of QI. In doing so, patient satisfaction can be increased, and errors can be reduced by process improvement strategies.

> The safety record in health care is a far cry from the enviable record of the similarly complex aviation industry.

In addition, many organizations have adopted principles of *Lean Manufacturing*, a process improvement strategy based on the highly acclaimed Toyota Production System. The focus in Lean Manufacturing is the removal of waste, so that it is possible to produce the right material, in the right amount, at the right time.

Lean Six Sigma results when the Six Sigma approach and Lean Manufacturing are combined. Using a five-step approach to process improvement (Define-Measure-Analyze-Improve-Control [DMAIC]), Lean Six Sigma can improve both the patient experience as well as promote the achievement of desired outcomes (Six Sigma Global Institute, 2019).

TABLE 23.1 **EVIDENCE-BASED LEAPFROG INITIATIVES**

Initiative	Description	Evidence
Computerized physician–provider order entry (CPOE)	CPOE requires primary care providers to enter orders into a computer instead of handwriting them. Because approximately 90% of medication errors occur during manual ordering and transcribing (handwriting and interpreting the prescription), the use of CPOE (electronic prescribing) systems can help eliminate these types of errors. In addition, CPOE integrates medication orders with patient information, such as allergies, laboratory results, and other prescription data. The order is then automatically checked for potential errors or problems such as drug and allergy interactions or drug-to-drug interactions. It also gives providers vital clinical decision support via access to information tools that support a health care provider in decisions related to diagnosis, therapy, and care planning of individual patients.	Research suggests CPOE significantly reduces serious prescribing errors in hospitals by more than 50%. A study at Boston's Brigham and Women's Hospital, demonstrated that CPOE reduced error rates by 55%. Rates of serious medication errors fell by 88% in a subsequent study by the same group. Another study conducted at LDS Hospital in Salt Lake City demonstrated a 70% reduction in antibiotic-related adverse drug events after implementation of decision support for these drugs. In addition, a study at Wishard Memorial Hospital in Indianapolis showed that length of stay fell by 0.9 days, and hospital charges decreased by 13% after implementation of CPOE. A study at Ohio State University also identified substantial reductions in pharmacy, radiology, and laboratory turnaround times, and a reduction in length of stay in one of the two hospitals studied.
Evidence-based hospital referral	Outcomes of high-risk surgeries can vary greatly based on the hospital's skill at performing the procedure. This initiative suggests that patients with high-risk conditions should be treated at hospitals with characteristics shown to be associated with better outcomes. Consumers and health care purchasers should choose hospitals with the best track records. By referring patients needing certain complex medical procedures to hospitals offering the best survival odds based on scientifically valid criteria—such as the number of times a hospital performs a procedure each year or other process or outcomes data—a patient's risk of dying could be significantly reduced. Healthgrades (2021) agrees, noting that the quality of the hospital in which care is received, is a significant predictor of morbidity, mortality, and the achievement of desired patient outcomes.	Leapfrog Hospital Survey (2020c) has identified eleven high-risk procedures for which there is a strong volume–outcome relationship. The procedures are: • Bariatric surgery for weight loss • Esophageal resection for cancer • Lung resection for cancer • Pancreatic resection for cancer • Rectal cancer surgery • Carotid endarterectomy • Open aortic procedures • Mitral valve repair and replacement • Norwood procedure • Total knee replacement • Total hip replacement In addition, a study of cancer surgeries by the California Health Care Foundation found an association between low hospital surgery volume and higher mortality and complication rates for the following cancers: bladder, brain, breast, colon, esophagus, liver, lung, pancreas, prostate, rectum, and stomach.

continues on page 624

TABLE 23.1 (CONTINUED)

Initiative	Description	Evidence
Intensive care unit (ICU) physician staffing (IPS)	Mortality rates in patients admitted to the ICU average 10–20% in most hospitals. Given the high stakes involved, the quality of care delivered in ICUs is particularly important. Unfortunately, evidence suggests that quality varies widely across hospitals. This initiative examines the level of training of ICU medical personnel and suggests that quality of care in hospital ICUs is strongly influenced by (a) whether *intensivists* (doctors with special training in critical care medicine) are providing care and (b) the staff organization in the ICU.	Mortality rates are significantly lower in hospitals with closed ICUs managed exclusively by board-certified intensivists. A systematic review of the existing literature regarding ICU physician staffing and quality found that high-intensity staffing (ICUs where intensivists manage or comanage all patients) versus low-intensity staffing (where intensivists manage or comanage some or none of the patients) is associated with a 30% reduction in hospital mortality and a 40% reduction in ICU mortality. Evidence suggests that more than 54,855 deaths that occur in the ICUs could be avoided if The Leapfrog Group's IPS Safety Standard were implemented in all urban hospitals with ICUs across the United States. Studies have also demonstrated a reduced hospital and ICU length of stay with high-intensity versus low-intensity staffing.
National Quality Forum (NQF)-endorsed Safe Practices	*The NQF-endorsed safe practices cover a range of practices that, if utilized, would reduce the risk of harm in certain processes, systems, or environments of care. Included in the 34 practices are the three initiatives above.* *On the 2018 Leapfrog Hospital Survey, hospitals were asked to report on the following five Safe Practices:* *1. Safe Practice 1: Culture of Safety Leadership Structures and Systems* *2. Safe Practice 2: Culture Measurement, Feedback, and Intervention* *3. Safe Practice 4: Risks and Hazards* *4. Safe Practice 9: Nursing Workforce* *5. Safe Practice 19: Hand Hygiene*	*For the 2018 Leapfrog Hospital Survey, The Leapfrog Group scored hospitals' progress on the five NQF Safe Practices listed here. Each practice area was assigned an individual weight, with the relative weights for each individual safe practice developed by a group of internationally recognized patient safety leaders. Hospitals' overall scores were assigned to performance categories which are publicly reported on The Leapfrog Group website at http://leapfroggroup.org/compare*

Sources: Data from Healthgrades. (2021). *Healthgrades 2021 report to the nation.* https://www.healthgrades.com/quality/healthgrades-2021-report-to-the-nation; Leapfrog Hospital Survey. (2020a, April 1). *Factsheet: ICU physician staffing.* https://www.leapfroggroup.org/sites/default/files/Files/2020%20IPS%20Fact%20Sheet.pdf; Leapfrog Hospital Survey. (2020b, April 1). *Factsheet: NQF safe practices.* https://www.leapfroggroup.org/sites/default/files/Files/2020%20NQF%20Safe%20Practices%20Factsheet.pdf; Leapfrog Hospital Survey. (2020c). *Factsheet: Computerized physician order entry.* https://www.leapfroggroup.org/sites/default/files/Files/2020%20CPOE%20Fact%20Sheet.pdf; Leapfrog Hospital Survey. (2020d). *Factsheet: Inpatient surgery.* https://ratings.leapfroggroup.org/sites/default/files/inline-files/2020%20Surgical%20Volume-Appropriateness%20Fact%20Sheet.pdf; Leapfrog Hospital Survey. (2021, March 19). *Factsheet. Never events.* https://ratings.leapfroggroup.org/sites/default/files/inline-files/2021%20Never%20Events%20Fact%20Sheet.pdf

Reforming the Medical Liability System

Finally, if quality health care is to be achieved, the medical liability system and our litigious society must be recognized as potential barriers to systematic efforts to uncover and learn from mistakes that are made in health care. Organizational cultures need to change for employees and patients to be comfortable in reporting hazards that can affect patient safety without fear of personal risk. Many experts have argued that the culture in health care organizations must shift from one of blame to one in which errors are identified and responded to in a timely manner.

Are We Making Progress?

Quality health care has emerged as a critically important yet underachieved goal in the United States. Among the most significant threats to achieving quality health care are the scope and prevalence of medical errors. Indeed, preventable medical errors are reported to be the third highest cause of death in the United States, following heart disease and cancer, claiming the lives of 250,000 Americans every year. In addition, every year, roughly 12 million Americans are misdiagnosed, a little more than 4,000 surgical errors occur, and an estimated 7,000 to 9,000 patients die from medication errors (Medical Error Statistics, 2020).

In addition, The National Quality Forum (NQF) has issued a list of 29 events that they termed *never events*—serious, preventable medical errors that should never happen (see Display 23.8). Although rare, they happen far more often than most people realize. For example, Leapfrog Hospital Survey (2021) notes that Minnesota has had a mandatory reporting program for never events in place since 2005 and has averaged roughly 100 to 150 reported never events per year.

DISPLAY 23.8 NATIONAL QUALITY FORUM'S 29 SERIOUS REPORTABLE EVENTS/aka NEVER EVENTS

1. Surgery or other invasive procedure performed on the wrong site
2. Surgery or other invasive procedure performed on the wrong patient
3. Wrong surgical or other invasive procedure performed on a patient
4. Unintended retention of a foreign object in a patient after surgery or other invasive procedure
5. Intraoperative or immediately postoperative/postprocedure death in an ASA Class 1 patient
6. Patient death or serious injury associated with the use of contaminated drugs, devices, or biologics provided by the health care setting
7. Patient death or serious injury associated with the use or function of a device in patient care, in which the device is used or functions other than as intended
8. Patient death or serious injury associated with intravascular air embolism that occurs while being cared for in a health care setting
9. Discharge or release of a patient/resident of any age, who is unable to make decisions, to other than an authorized person
10. Patient death or serious injury associated with patient elopement (disappearance)
11. Patient suicide, attempted suicide, or self-harm that results in serious injury, while being cared for in a health care setting
12. Patient death or serious injury associated with a medication error (e.g., errors involving the wrong drug, wrong dose, wrong patient, wrong time, wrong rate, wrong preparation, or wrong route of administration)
13. Patient death or serious injury associated with unsafe administration of blood products
14. Maternal death or serious injury associated with labor or delivery in a low-risk pregnancy while being cared for in a health care setting
15. Death or serious injury of a neonate associated with labor or delivery in a low-risk pregnancy

continues on page 626

DISPLAY 23.8 (CONTINUED)

16. Patient death or serious injury associated with a fall while being cared for in a health care setting
17. Any Stage 3, Stage 4, and unstageable pressure ulcers acquired after admission/presentation to a health care setting
18. Artificial insemination with the wrong donor sperm or wrong egg
19. Patient death or serious injury resulting from the irretrievable loss of an irreplaceable biological specimen
20. Patient death or serious injury resulting from failure to follow up or communicate laboratory, pathology, or radiology test results
21. Patient or staff death or serious injury associated with an electric shock in the course of a patient care process in a health care setting
22. Any incident in which systems designated for oxygen or other gas to be delivered to a patient contains no gas, the wrong gas, or are contaminated by toxic substances
23. Patient or staff death or serious injury associated with a burn incurred from any source in the course of a patient care process in a health care setting
24. Patient death or serious injury associated with the use of physical restraints or bedrails while being cared for in a health care setting
25. Death or serious injury of a patient or staff associated with the introduction of a metallic object into the MRI area
26. Any instance of care ordered by or provided by someone impersonating a physician, nurse, pharmacist, or other licensed health care provider
27. Abduction of a patient/resident of any age
28. Sexual abuse/assault on a patient or staff member within or on the grounds of a health care setting
29. Death or serious injury of a patient or staff member resulting from a physical assault (i.e., battery) that occurs within or on the grounds of a health care setting

Sources: Leapfrog Hospital Survey. (2021). *Factsheet: Never events*. https://ratings.leapfroggroup.org/sites/default/files/inline-files/2021%20Never%20Events%20Fact%20Sheet.pdf; National Quality Forum. (2022). *List of SREs*. https://www.qualityforum.org/Topics/SREs/List_of_SREs.aspx

Clearly, gaps continue to exist between the care that patients should receive and the care they receive. This has been borne out in numerous studies including the follow-up 2001 IOM study *Crossing the Quality Chasm: A New Health System for the 21st Century*. In addition, the IOM released another major study, *Improving Diagnosis in Health Care*, in 2015. This report found that most Americans will experience a misdiagnosis in our lifetimes, sometimes with devastating consequences (IOM, 2015). In fact, 5% of US adults who seek outpatient care each year experience a diagnostic error. Postmortem examination research spanning decades has shown that diagnostic errors contribute to approximately 10% of patient deaths, and medical record reviews suggest that they account for 6% to 17% of adverse events in hospitals (IOM, 2015). Furthermore, diagnostic errors are the leading type of paid medical malpractice claims and are almost twice as likely to have resulted in the patient's death compared with other claims.

The report (IOM, 2015) also suggested that interprofessional–patient communication needs to be improved and that information technology needs to be better integrated into workflow and have better usability. In addition, the report suggested that these diagnostic errors are frequently the result of failings in the health system rather than provider negligence, and its authors criticized the legal system for its punitive structure. They argued that instead, state and federal action is urgently needed to address the medical liability system. The report concluded that without a dedicated focus on improving diagnosis, diagnostic errors will likely worsen as the delivery of health care and the diagnostic process continues to increase in complexity.

Huston (2023) explains that unfortunately, efforts to reduce medical errors over the last three decades have not achieved desired outcomes. Instead, there is a plethora of current research that suggests the health care system continues to be riddled with errors and that patient and worker safety is compromised. Yet, movement toward the IOM goals is occurring, and it is likely that there has never been another time when the public, providers, and government have worked together so closely to achieve a shared health care goal. It is clear then that despite all the interventions that have come out from the IOM studies and the multitude of organizations dedicated to QI in health care, progress in addressing the problem of medical errors is limited, and changes have been incremental at best.

Integrating Leadership Roles and Management Functions with Quality Control

Quality control provides managers with the opportunity to evaluate organizational performance from a systematic, scientific, and objective viewpoint. To do so, managers must determine what standards will be used to measure quality care in their units and then develop and implement quality control programs that measure results against those standards. All managers are responsible for monitoring the quality of the product that their units produce; in health care organizations, that product is patient care. Managers, too, must assess and promote patient satisfaction whenever possible.

The manager, however, cannot operate in a vacuum in determining what quality is and how it should be measured. This determination should come from research-based evidence. Demands for hard data on quality have increased as regulatory bodies, patients, payers, and health care managers have required justification for services provided. Managers must be cognizant of rapidly changing quality control regulations and proactively adjust unit standards to meet these changing needs. Until less than three decades ago, limited attention was given to quality measurement in health care. As we entered the 21st century, however, there was an ever-increasing focus on the quality of care and the standardization of quality data collection and an increased accountability for outcomes from the system level to the individual provider.

Inspiring subordinates to establish and achieve high standards of care is a leadership skill. Leaders are role models for high standards in their own nursing care and encourage subordinates to seek maximum rather than minimum standards. One way that this can be accomplished is by involving subordinates in the quality control process. By studying direct cause–effect relationships, subordinates learn to modify individual and group performance to improve the quality of care provided.

Vision is another leadership skill inherent in quality control. The visionary leader looks at what is and determines what should be. This future focus allows leaders to shape organizational goals proactively and improve the quality of care. Moreover, the integrated leader-manager in quality control must be willing to be a risk taker and to be accountable. In an era of limited resources and cost containment, there is great pressure to sacrifice quality to contain costs. The self-aware leader-manager recognizes this risk and seeks to achieve a balance between quality and cost containment that does not violate professional obligations to patients and subordinates.

Leader-managers are also challenged to address the pervasive problem of medical errors in the health care system. Huston (2023) suggests medical errors are one of the greatest threats to quality health care that exists today but notes that nurses are uniquely positioned to identify, interrupt, and correct medical errors and to minimize preventable adverse outcomes. Only recently, however, have their error recovery strategies been described. Much remains to be done.

Unfortunately, many people believe patient safety is mainly the responsibility of health care providers, hospital leaders, and administrators. These patients must be empowered to be active participants in assuring the care they receive is both safe and appropriate to meet their health care goals.

Sustained public interest will be needed to create the momentum necessary to systematically change the health care system in a way that reduces patients' vulnerability to errors and poor-quality care. In addition, although there has been a great deal of talk about using a systems approach to address the problem of errors, there has been inadequate discussion regarding exactly how this integration is to be accomplished. The bottom line is that significant and continuous reform of the health care system will be needed before the problem shows any resolution (Huston, 2023).

Increasing consumer knowledge and participation in health care will be imperative in this effort. In addition, change agents must be able to successfully address the disconnect that still exists between consumers' perceptions of the quality of their own care and the actual quality provided. This dialogue has only just begun.

Key Concepts

- Controlling is implemented throughout all phases of management.
- Quality control refers to activities that are used to evaluate, monitor, or regulate services rendered to consumers.
- A standard is a predetermined baseline condition or level of excellence that constitutes a model to be followed and practiced.
- Because there is no one set of standards, each organization and profession must set standards and objectives to guide individual practitioners in performing safe and effective care.
- CPGs provide diagnosis-based, step-by-step interventions for nurses to follow in an effort to promote evidence-based, high-quality care and yet control resource utilization and costs.
- Benchmarking is the process of measuring products, practices, and services against those of best performing organizations.
- The difference in performance between top-performing health care organizations and the national average is called the quality gap. Although the quality gap is typically small in industries such as manufacturing, aviation, and banking, wide variation is more common in health care.
- CEA and RCA help to identify not only what and how an event happened but also why it happened, with the end goal being to ensure that a preventable negative outcome does not recur.
- Outcome audits determine what results, if any, followed from specific nursing interventions for patients.
- Process audits are used to measure the process of care or how the care was carried out.
- Structure audits monitor the structure or setting in which patient care occurs (such as the finances, nursing service structure, medical records, and environmental structure).
- There is growing recognition that it is possible to separate the contribution of nursing to the patient's outcome; this recognition of outcomes that are nursing sensitive creates accountability

- for nurses as professionals and is important in developing nursing as a profession.
- Standardized nursing languages provide a consistent terminology for nurses to describe and document their assessments, interventions, and the outcomes of their actions.
- QA models seek to ensure that quality currently exists, whereas QI models assume that the process is ongoing, and that quality can always be improved.
- Quality control in health care organizations has evolved primarily from external forces and not as a voluntary effort to monitor the quality of services provided.
- Critics of the PPS argue that although DRGs may have helped to contain rising health care costs, the associated rapid declines in length of hospital stay and services provided have resulted in declines in quality of care.
- The Joint Commission (TJC) is the major accrediting body for health care organizations and programs in the United States. It also administers the ORYX initiative and collects data on core measures to better standardize data collection across acute care hospitals.
- CMS plays an active role in setting standards for and measuring quality in health care including P4P.
- HCAHPS survey is the first national, standardized, publicly reported survey of patients' perspectives of hospital care. It measures recently discharged patients' perceptions of their hospital experience.
- NCQA, a private nonprofit organization that accredits managed care organizations, also developed the HEDIS to compare quality of care in managed care organizations.
- Ideally, everyone in an organization should participate in quality control activities.
- In response to the demand for objective measures of quality, many health plans, health care providers, employer-purchasing groups, consumer information organizations, and state governments have begun to formulate health care quality report cards.

- A plethora of studies across the past two decades suggests that medical errors continue to be rampant in the health care system.
- A "just culture" deemphasizes blame for errors and focuses instead on addressing factors that lead to and cause near misses, medical errors, and adverse events.
- The Leapfrog Group identified four evidence-based standards that they believe will provide the greatest impact on reducing medical errors: CPOE, evidence-based hospital referral, IPS, and the use of The Leapfrog Group Safe Practices scores.
- The FDA has suggested that a drug bar code system coupled with a computerized order entry system would greatly decrease the risk of medication errors.
- Historically, the health care industry has been comfortable with striving for three sigma processes (all data points fall within three standard deviations) in measuring health care quality; Six Sigma is typically adopted by the highest performing organizations for quality.
- As direct caregivers, staff nurses are in an excellent position to monitor nursing practice by identifying problems and implementing corrective actions that have the greatest impact on patient care.

Additional Learning Exercises and Applications

LEARNING EXERCISE 23.5

Identifying Nursing-Sensitive Outcome Criteria

Some patients get better despite nursing care, not because of it. However, the quality of nursing care can affect patient outcomes tremendously. Do you believe that quality nursing care makes a difference in patients' lives? Identify five criteria that you would use to define *quality nursing care*. These criteria should reflect what you believe nurses do (nursing sensitive) that makes the difference in patient outcomes. Are the criteria you listed measurable?

LEARNING EXERCISE 23.6

Working Short Staffed—Again

You are a staff nurse at Mercy Hospital. The hospital's patient census and acuity have been very high for the last 6 months. Many of the nursing staff have resigned; a coordinated recruitment effort to refill these positions has been largely unsuccessful. The nursing staff is demoralized, and staff frequently call in sick or fail to show up for work. Today, you arrive at work and find that you are again being asked to work shorthanded. You will be the only registered nurse on a unit with 30 patients. Although you have two licensed practical nurses/licensed vocational nurses and two certified nursing assistants assigned to work with you, you are concerned that patient safety could be compromised. A check with the central nursing office confirms that no additional help can be obtained.

You feel that you have reached the end of your rope. The administration at Mercy Hospital has been receptive to

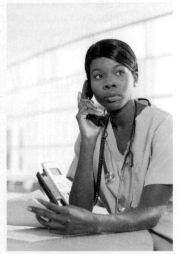

(continues on page 630)

LEARNING EXERCISE 23.6

Working Short Staffed—Again (continued)

employee feedback about the acute staffing shortage, and you believe that they have made some efforts to try to alleviate the problem. You also believe, however, that the efforts have not been at the level they should have been, and that the hospital will continue to expect nurses to work shorthanded until some major force changes things. Although you have thought about quitting, you really enjoy the work that you do and feel morally obligated to your coworkers, the patients, and even your superiors. Today, it occurs to you that you could anonymously phone the state licensing bureau and turn in Mercy Hospital for consistent understaffing of nursing personnel, leading to unsafe patient care. You believe that this could be the impetus needed to improve the quality of care. You are also aware of the action's political risks.

ASSIGNMENT:

Discuss whether you would take this action. What is your responsibility to the organization, to yourself, and to patients? How do you make decisions such as this one, which have conflicting moral obligations?

LEARNING EXERCISE 23.7

Examining Mortality Rates

You have been the nursing coordinator of cardiac services at a medium-sized urban hospital for the last 6 months. Among the hospital's cardiac services are open-heart surgery, invasive and noninvasive diagnostic testing, and a comprehensive rehabilitation program. The open-heart surgery program was implemented a little over a year ago. During the last 3 months, you have begun to feel uneasy about the mortality rate of postoperative cardiac patients at your facility. An audit of medical records shows a unit mortality rate that is approximately 30% above national norms. You approach the unit medical director with your findings. He becomes defensive and states that there have been a few freakish situations to skew the results but that the open-heart program is one of the best in the state. When you question him about examining the statistics further, he becomes very angry and turns to leave the room. At the door, he stops and says, "Remember that these patients are leaving the operating room alive. They're dying on your unit. If you stir up trouble, you are going to be sorry."

ASSIGNMENT:

Outline your plan. Identify areas in your data gathering that may have been misleading or that may have skewed your findings. If you believe action is still warranted, what are the personal and professional risks involved? How well developed is your power base to undertake these risks? To whom do you have the greatest responsibility? What strategies might you employ to bring attention to the problem while reducing your personal risk as a whistleblower?

LEARNING EXERCISE 23.8

Weighing Conflicting Obligations

You are the unit supervisor of a medical-surgical unit. Shauna, a registered nurse on your unit, who graduated 3 years ago from nursing school, has made several small errors in the past few months, all of which she has voluntarily reported. These errors included things like missing medications, giving medications late, and on one occasion, giving medications to the wrong patient. No apparent harm has occurred to her patients as a result of these errors, and on each occasion, Shauna has responded to your coaching efforts with an assertion that she will be more attentive and careful in the future.

Today, however, Shauna came to your office to admit that she flushed a patient's intravenous line with 10,000 units of heparin rather than with the 100 units that was ordered. The vials looked similar, and she failed to notice the dosing on the label. Shauna also failed to have someone co-check her dose before giving it, as required. Shauna reported the error to the patient's physician and filled out the Adverse Incident report form required by the hospital on all medication errors. At this point, the patient is demonstrating no ill effects from the overdosing but will need to be monitored closely for the next 24 hours.

You recognize that Shauna's pattern of repetitive medication errors is placing patients at risk. You have some reservations, however, about dealing with Shauna in a punitive way because she openly reports the errors she makes and because none of her errors until today had really jeopardized patient safety. You are also aware, however, that you have an obligation to make sure that the staff caring for your patients are competent and that patients are protected from harm. You are also attempting to establish a unit culture that encourages open reporting, not "shame and blame," so you are aware that your staff are watching closely how you will respond to yet another error on Shauna's part.

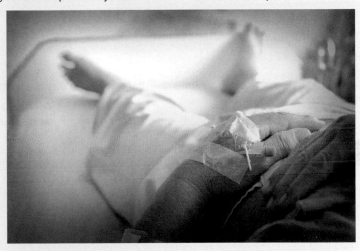

ASSIGNMENT:

What will you do to address this error as well as the errors Shauna has made in the past few months? What options are available to you? What obligations do you have to Shauna, to the organization, and to the patients on your unit? How will you create a culture that encourages the open reporting of errors and yet protects patients from potentially unsafe practitioners?

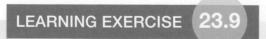

LEARNING EXERCISE 23.9

Avoiding Adverse Events and Medication Errors

Interview the patient safety officer or the manager of the risk management department at your local hospital. Use the following questions as a guide to begin the interview. Present a report to your peers regarding your findings.

1. What are the most common causes of medication errors in this facility?
2. Which medications are more commonly involved in medication errors? What factors has this agency identified that cause these errors to occur?
3. What are the most common adverse events affecting patients? What precipitating factors have been identified as increasing the possibility of these adverse events?
4. What new technologies have been adopted to increase patient safety? Examples might be intravenous smart pumps, bar coding of medications, and computerized physician–provider order entry.
5. How are medication errors or adverse events reported? What safeguards have been built in to encourage voluntary reporting of errors? Do disincentives exist that would discourage someone from reporting such an error?
6. Are staff included in the quality control process? If so, how?
7. For which of The Joint Commission core measures are data being collected? What is the process for this data collection?

LEARNING EXERCISE 23.10

Quality Topics for Group Discussion

ASSIGNMENT:

Select one of the topics below for small- or large-group debate. Generate as many perspectives as possible.

- Support or oppose the proposition that quality in health care should be quantitatively measurable.
- Support or oppose the proposition that public and private sector initiatives during the past three to four decades have been successful in lowering health care costs while maintaining quality.
- Support or oppose the proposition that traditional natural science study designs, such as the experimental method, are the most appropriate models for testing hypotheses about quality and health care delivery.
- Support or oppose the proposition that quality in health care should be measured more by client satisfaction than by traditional outcome measures.
- Support or oppose the proposition that increased use of unlicensed assistive personnel is affecting the quality of patient care negatively.

LEARNING EXERCISE 23.11

Tracking Down an Infection Through Root Cause Analysis

You work in a small, long-term care facility and are often the only registered nurse working on the unit. Many of your patients have indwelling Foley catheters. Recently, several patients have developed bladder infections, after having a unit nosocomial urinary tract infection (UTI) rate of less than 1% for the past year. In fact, the facility has always prided itself on carefully following established evidence-based policies and procedures, both in catheter insertion and in routine catheter care. When you talk to the chief nursing officer about the problem, she asks you to investigate the problem and report back to her. You decide to sit down and make a list of the structure and process indicators you could examine to find the cause of the problem.

ASSIGNMENT:

Identify at least eight process and structure variables you could use to determine the cause(s) of the spike in nosocomially acquired UTIs in the facility. Then develop a quality evaluation plan for one of these variables. What data will you collect? What steps will you implement to carry out this quality audit?

LEARNING EXERCISE 23.12

Is There an Obligation to Report?

You are a new graduate nurse working in an acute care hospital. You are very conscientious about your care but have just discovered you made a mistake today. About 30 minutes ago, you went into Room 1308 to give Lasix to Ms. Sanderson in bed A and Coumadin to Ms. Jarvik in bed B. Just as you handed the Lasix to Ms. Sanderson, the code alarm sounded for one of your patients down the hall. You set down the med pass tray on her overbed table and told her you would be back just as soon as possible. You then responded to the code, which ended successfully several minutes ago. When you return to the room to finish passing your medications, you find Ms. Jarvik's pill cup empty. Ms. Sanderson is confused and does not remember if she took the pill or what she did with it. Ms. Jarvik is also confused and is unaware that she did not receive her intended medication.

When you report to the charge nurse what occurred, she lowers her voice and tells you to "just forget about it. It was one low-dose Coumadin pill and likely wouldn't have any impact on Ms. Sanderson anyway." She goes on to say that if you fill out an Adverse Incident form, that she will have to notify Ms. Sanderson's short-tempered physician as well as the nursing office. The hospital was recently cited for several small infractions by The Joint Commission (TJC) and tensions are running high about all types of medical errors. In addition, she says that a copy of the Adverse Incident form will be placed in your personnel file, which could have ramifications for you in terms of your 3-month performance appraisal as a new nurse. She also says that neither of the patients would ever know that an error occurred.

Finally, she shares that the culture at the hospital around medical errors is "blame and shame," not "report and learn," and asks you to think twice before pursuing the matter. She says that because of the recent TJC sanctions, the hospital is adopting a zero-tolerance approach to preventable errors and your job might even be at stake.

(continues on page 634)

LEARNING EXERCISE 23.12

Is There an Obligation to Report? (continued)

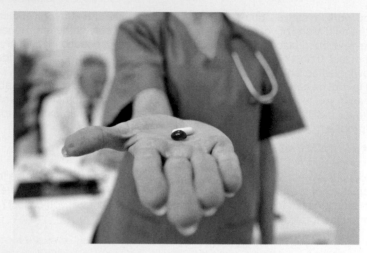

ASSIGNMENT:

What will you do? What alternatives could you consider and what are the driving and restraining forces for each possible choice? What are the relative risks to both patients and the possible costs to you? What is your professional obligation in terms of reporting? Create a cost–benefit table to help you make your choice for action in this situation.

LEARNING EXERCISE 23.13

Using Report Cards to Compare Health Care Institutions

Go to the Healthgrades website (http://www.healthgrades.com/) which has health care report cards for physicians, hospitals, and nursing homes. Review the star ratings for the three hospitals closest to where you live in terms of cardiac, orthopedic, maternity, pulmonary, and transplant care. Then review their patient safety ratings compared to other hospitals in the area as well as to national averages. Did this review influence where you would and would not want to be treated for a specific health care problem? Do most patients access and use the information that is available to them through report cards such as the ones offered by Healthgrades? If not, why not, and what could nurses do to educate the public about the availability of health care report cards?

REFERENCES

Agency for Healthcare Research and Quality. (2019). *Medication reconciliation.* https://psnet.ahrq.gov/primers/primer/1/medication-reconciliation

Agency for Healthcare Research and Quality. (2020). *Understanding quality measurement.* https://www.ahrq.gov/professionals/quality-patient-safety/quality-resources/tools/chtoolbx/understand/index.html

American Society for Quality. (2022). *Failure mode and effects analysis (FMEA).* http://asq.org/learn-about-quality/process-analysis-tools/overview/fmea.html

Centers for Medicare & Medicaid Services. (2021a). *The Hospital Value-Based Purchasing (VBP) program.* https://www.cms.gov/Medicare/Quality-Initiatives-Patient-Assessment-Instruments/Value-Based-Programs/HVBP/Hospital-Value-Based-Purchasing.html

Centers for Medicare & Medicaid Services. (2021b). *HCAHPS: Patients' perspectives of care survey.* https://www.cms.gov/Medicare/Quality-Initiatives-Patient-Assessment-Instruments/HospitalQualityInits/HospitalHCAHPS

Deming, W. E. (1986). *Out of the crisis.* MIT Press.

Encyclopedia of Surgery. (2022). Medical errors. In *Encyclopedia of surgery.* Retrieved July 11, 2022, from http://www.surgeryencyclopedia.com/La-Pa/Medical-Errors.html

Healthgrades. (2021). *Healthgrades 2021 Report to the Nation.* https://www.healthgrades.com/quality/healthgrades-2021-report-to-the-nation

Hostetter, M., & Klein, S. (2022). *Using patient-reported outcomes to improve health care quality.* The Commonwealth Fund. https://www.commonwealthfund.org/publications/newsletter-article/using-patient-reported-outcomes-improve-health-care-quality

Huston, C. J. (2023). Medical errors: An ongoing threat to quality health care. In C. J. Huston (Ed.), *Professional issues in nursing: Challenges and opportunities.* (Chapter 15, 6th ed., pp. 212–228.) Wolters Kluwer.

Institute for Healthcare Improvement. (2022). *Transforming care at the bedside.* http://www.ihi.org/Engage/Initiatives/Completed/TCAB/Pages/default.aspx

Institute of Medicine. (2015). *Improving diagnosis in health care.* Retrieved July 11, 0222, from http://www.nationalacademies.org/hmd/Reports/2015/Improving-Diagnosis-in-Healthcare

International Council of Nurses. (2022). *About ICNP.* Retrieved December 28, 2021, from https://www.icn.ch/what-we-do/projects/ehealth-icnptm/about-icnp

ISIXSIGMA. (2000–2022). *Find, organize, clarify, understand, select (FOCUS–PDCA).* https://www.isixsigma.com/dictionary/find-organize-clarify-understand-select-focus-pdca/

The Joint Commission. (2021). *National Patient Safety Goals® effective January 2022 for the hospital.* https://www.jointcommission.org/-/media/tjc/documents/standards/national-patient-safety-goals/2022/npsg_chapter_hap_jan2022.pdf

The Joint Commission. (2022a). *Sentinel event.* https://www.jointcommission.org/resources/patient-safety-topics/sentinel-event/

The Joint Commission. (2022b). *Reporting.* https://www.jointcommission.org/facts_about_oryx_performance_measurement_systems/

The Joint Commission. (2022c). *Quality check.* https://www.qualitycheck.org/

The Joint Commission. (2022d). *Facts about The Joint Commission.* http://www.jointcommission.org/about_us/fact_sheets.aspx

The Joint Commission. (2022e). *Hospital: 2022 National Patient Safety Goals.* 2022, from https://www.jointcommission.org/standards/national-patient-safety-goals/hospital-national-patient-safety-goals/

Kohn, L. T., Corrigan, J. M., & Donaldson, M. S. (2000). *Executive summary.* In L. T. Kohn, J. M. Corrigan, & M. S. Donaldson (Eds.), *To err is human: Building a safer health system* (pp. 1–6). http://www.nap.edu/openbook.php?record_id=9728&page=R1

Leapfrog Hospital Survey. (2020a). *Factsheet: ICU physician staffing.* https://www.leapfroggroup.org/sites/default/files/Files/2020%20IPS%20Fact%20Sheet.pdf

Leapfrog Hospital Survey. (2020b). *Factsheet: NQF safe practices.* https://www.leapfroggroup.org/sites/default/files/Files/2020%20NQF%20Safe%20Practices%20Factsheet.pdf

Leapfrog Hospital Survey. (2020c). *Factsheet: Computerized physician order entry.* https://www.leapfroggroup.org/sites/default/files/Files/2020%20CPOE%20Fact%20Sheet.pdf

Leapfrog Hospital Survey. (2020d). *Factsheet: Inpatient surgery.* https://ratings.leapfroggroup.org/sites/default/files/inline-files/2020%20Surgical%20Volume-Appropriateness%20Fact%20Sheet.pdf

Leapfrog Hospital Survey. (2021). *Factsheet: Never events.* https://ratings.leapfroggroup.org/sites/default/files/inline-files/2021%20Never%20Events%20Fact%20Sheet.pdf

Medical Error Statistics. (2020). My Medical Score. https://mymedicalscore.com/medical-error-statistics/

National Committee for Quality Assurance. (2022). *HEDIS measures and technical resources.* https://www.ncqa.org/hedis/measures/

National Coordinating Council for Medication Error Reporting and Prevention. (2022). *About medication errors.* http://www.nccmerp.org/about-medication-errors

National Database of Nursing Quality Indicators. (n.d.-a). *How is NDNQI used?* https://nursingandndnqi.weebly.com/how-is-ndnqi-used.html

National Database of Nusring Quality Indicators. (n.d.-b). *NDNQI nursing-sensitive indicators.* https://nursingandndnqi.weebly.com/ndnqi-indicators.html

Office of Disease Prevention and Health Promotion. (2022). *Healthcare effectiveness data and information set.* https://www.healthypeople.gov/2020/data-source/healthcare-effectiveness-data-and-information-set#:~:text=The%20Healthcare%20Effectiveness%20Data%20and%20Information%20Set%20%28HEDIS%29,of%2071%20measures%20across%208%20domains%20of%20care

Six Sigma Global Institute. (2019). *What is DMAIC?* https://www.6sigmacertificationonline.com/what-is-dmaic/?gclid=EAIaIQobChMIxITSx67x-AIVRBB9Ch3s-dAT3EAAYAiAAEgLoPPD_BwE

The University of Iowa College of Nursing. (2022). *CNC. NIC overview.* https://nursing.uiowa.edu/cncce/nursing-interventions-classification-overview

Performance Appraisal

*… it is a paradoxical but profoundly true and important principle of life that the most likely way to reach a goal is to be aiming not at that goal itself but at some more ambitious goal beyond it.—**Arnold Toynbee***

*… performance stands out like a ton of diamonds. Non-performance can always be explained away.—**Harold S. Geneen***

*… Nothing raises hackles as fiercely as a change in performance feedback methods, especially when they may affect compensation decisions.—**Susan Heathfield***

CROSSWALK

This chapter addresses:

- **AACN Essentials Domain 1:** Knowledge for nursing practice
- **AACN Essentials Domain 5:** Quality and safety
- **AACN Essentials Domain 6:** Interprofessional partnerships
- **AACN Essentials Domain 7:** Systems-based practice
- **AACN Essentials Domain 10:** Personal, professional, and leadership development
- **AONL Nurse Executive Competency 1:** Communication and relationship building
- **AONL Nurse Executive Competency 2:** A knowledge of the health care environment
- **AONL Nurse Executive Competency 3:** Leadership
- **AONL Nurse Executive Competency 5:** Business skills
- **ANA Standard of Professional Performance 10:** Communication
- **ANA Standard of Professional Performance 11:** Collaboration
- **ANA Standard of Professional Performance 12:** Leadership
- **ANA Standard of Professional Performance 13:** Education
- **ANA Standard of Professional Performance 15:** Quality of practice
- **ANA Standard of Professional Performance 17:** Resource stewardship
- **QSEN Competency:** Teamwork and collaboration
- **QSEN Competency:** Safety

LEARNING OBJECTIVES

The learner will:

- identify and use appropriate performance appraisal tools for measuring professional nursing performance
- identify factors that increase the likelihood that a performance appraisal will develop and motivate staff
- avoid the halo effect, horns effect, Matthew effect, and central tendency errors in conducting performance appraisals
- recognize subjectivity as an ever-present limitation of the performance appraisal process
- gather data for performance appraisals in a systematic manner that is fair and objective

- develop an awareness of biases that influence a person's ability to complete a fair and objective performance appraisal
- differentiate between performance appraisal tools such as rating scales, checklists, essays, self-appraisal, management by objectives, and 360-degree reviews
- identify strategies to help employees complete objective, accurate, and growth-producing self-appraisals as part of the performance appraisal process
- provide feedback regarding peer performance in a constructive and assertive manner
- describe the challenges inherent in implementing peer review for performance appraisal
- differentiate between advocacy in peer review and providing constructive feedback to promote employee growth
- identify strategies that can be used before, during, and after the performance appraisal to increase the likelihood of a positive outcome
- describe coaching techniques that promote ongoing employee growth in work performance
- encourage employee involvement in the performance appraisals of their managers whenever possible

Introduction

One critical part of the controlling function of performance management is determining how well employees carry out the duties of their assigned jobs. This is typically done through *performance appraisals*. Performance appraisals let employees know the level of their job performance as well as any expectations that the organization may have of them. Performance appraisals also generate information for salary adjustments, promotions, transfers, disciplinary actions, and terminations.

> In performance appraisals, actual performance, not intent, is evaluated.

Performance appraisal, however, is not easy. None of the manager's actions is as personal as appraising the work performance of others. Indeed, Kerr (2022) notes that next to disciplining an employee, performance evaluation is likely the most dreaded task a manager faces. Because work is an important part of one's identity, people are very sensitive to opinions about how they perform. "According to Gregorio Billikopf, an adviser with the University of California, Davis, when a supervisor becomes an 'expert' on a worker's performance, employees will often become resistant or even defensive. However, creating a positive environment, involving the employee in the process, and discussing performance goals can help mitigate some of the challenges of performance evaluations" (Kerr, 2022, para. 1).

Sherman and Cohn (2021) agree, arguing that constructive feedback is a gift, since professional colleagues rarely offer the kind of feedback needed to develop, although it often is not perceived that way, at least initially. Soliciting and learning from feedback is not easy, but it is necessary. The goal should be the development of a growth mindset, whereby an individual recognizes feedback as the opportunity to improve skill sets and achieve new learning. Indeed, when used correctly, performance appraisal can be one of the greatest tools an organization has to develop and motivate staff. It can also encourage staff and increase retention and productivity; however, in the hands of an inept or inexperienced manager, the appraisal process may significantly discourage and demotivate workers.

In addition, because a manager's opinions and judgments are used for far-reaching decisions regarding the employee's work life, they must be determined in an objective, systematic, and formalized manner as possible. Using a formal system of performance review reduces,

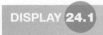

DISPLAY 24.1   LEADERSHIP ROLES AND MANAGEMENT FUNCTIONS ASSOCIATED WITH PERFORMANCE APPRAISAL

Leadership Roles

1. Uses the performance appraisal process to motivate employees and promote growth
2. Uses appropriate techniques to reduce the anxiety inherent in the performance appraisal process
3. Involves employees in all aspects of performance appraisal
4. Is aware of own biases and prejudices in the performance appraisal process
5. Develops employee trust by being honest and fair when evaluating performance
6. Encourages peer review among professional staff
7. Uses performance appraisal interviews to facilitate two-way communication
8. Provides ongoing support to employees who are attempting to correct performance deficiencies
9. Uses coaching techniques that promote employee growth in work performance
10. Individualizes performance goals and the appraisal interview as needed to meet the unique needs of a culturally diverse staff
11. Role models risk taking in seeking feedback from subordinates and colleagues regarding own work performance to promote self-growth

Management Functions

1. Uses a formalized system of performance appraisal
2. Gathers fair and objective data throughout the evaluation period to use in employee's performance appraisals
3. Uses the appraisal process to determine staff education and training needs
4. Bases performance appraisal on documented standards
5. Is as objective as possible in performance appraisal
6. Includes suggestions for growth in performance appraisals as well as recognitions of employee accomplishments
7. Maintains appropriate documentation of the appraisal process
8. Follows up on identified performance deficiencies
9. Conducts the appraisal interview in a manner that promotes a positive outcome
10. Provides frequent informal feedback and coaching on work performance throughout the evaluation cycle to promote employee success

but does not eliminate, the appraisal's subjectivity. In addition, the more professional a group of employees is, the more complex and sensitive the evaluation process becomes. The skilled leader-manager who uses a formalized system for the appraisal is better able to build a team approach to patient care.

This chapter focuses on the relationship between performance appraisal and motivation and discusses how performance appraisals can be used to determine the developmental needs of the staff. Emphasis is placed on appropriate data gathering and the types of performance appraisal tools available. The performance appraisal interview is explored, and strategies are presented for reducing appraiser bias and increasing the likelihood that the appraisal itself will be growth producing. Finally, performance management is introduced as an alternative to the traditional annual performance appraisal. The leadership roles and management functions inherent in successful performance appraisal are shown in Display 24.1.

Using the Performance Appraisal to Motivate Employees

Although systematic employee appraisals have been used in management since the 1920s, using the appraisal as a tool to promote employee growth did not begin until the 1950s.

This evolution of performance appraisals is reflected in its changing terminology. At one time, the appraisal was called a *merit rating* and was tied closely to salary increases. More recently, it was termed *performance evaluation*, but because the term *evaluation* implies that personal values are being placed on the performance review, that term is used infrequently. Some organizations continue to use both terms or others, such as *competency assessment*, *effectiveness report*, and *service rating*. Most health care organizations, however, use the term *performance appraisal* because this term implies an appraisal of how well employees perform the duties of their job as delineated by the job description or some other prespecified criteria.

The desired time frame for performance appraisals has also changed over time. Some organizations still conduct an annual review, but it is increasingly being replaced, or at least supplemented, by *pulse surveys* (short questions asked frequently and tracked over time) and other types of reviews throughout the year. Qualtrics (2022) suggests this has occurred because traditional annual and formal performance reviews tended to become overblown, with too much information in them to be manageable, or to be a fair evaluation of an employee's efforts.

Another important point to consider, if the appraisal is to have a positive outcome, is how the employee views the appraisal. Indeed, many employees and even some managers view the appraisal process with mistrust, perceiving either that it can be unfair or meaningless.

Management research, however, has shown that various factors influence whether the appraisal ultimately results in increased motivation and productivity. Some of these factors (Display 24.2) include the following:

- The employee must believe that the appraisal is based on a standard to which other employees in the same classification are held accountable. This standard must be communicated clearly to employees at the time they are hired and may be a job description or an individual goal set by staff for the purpose of performance appraisal.
- The employee must believe that the appraisal tool adequately and accurately assesses performance criteria directly related to their job.
- The employee should have some input into developing the standards or goals on which their performance is judged. This is imperative for the professional employee.
- The employee must know in advance what happens if the expected performance standards are not met.
- The employee needs to know how information will be obtained to determine performance. The appraisal tends to be more accurate if various sources and types of information are solicited. Sources could include peers, coworkers, nursing care plans, patients, and personal observation. Employees should be told which sources will be used and how such information will be weighted.

DISPLAY 24.2 FACTORS INFLUENCING EFFECTIVE PERFORMANCE APPRAISAL

Appraisal should be based on a standard.
The appraisal tool must adequately and accurately assess job performance.
Employee should have input into development of the standard.
Employee must know the standard in advance.
Employee must know the sources of data gathered for the appraisal.
Appraiser should be someone who has observed the employee's work.
Appraiser should be someone who the employee trusts and respects.
Employer support and clarity of expectations are critical to the employee perceiving the appraisal as fair.

- The appraiser should be one of the employee's direct supervisors. For example, the charge nurse who works directly with the staff nurse should be involved in the appraisal process and interview. It is appropriate and advisable in most instances for the unit supervisor also to be involved. However, employees must believe that the person doing the major portion of the review has directly observed their work.
- The performance appraisal is more likely to have a positive outcome if the appraiser is viewed with trust and professional respect. This increases the chance that the employee will view the appraisal as a fair and accurate assessment of their work performance.
- Employees' perception of fairness in the performance appraisal may be contingent on how well they feel they were supported by their supervisors as well as the transparency that existed between the employee and the manager in terms of expectations.

> If employees believe that the appraisal is based on their job description rather than on whether the manager approves of them personally, they are more likely to view the appraisal as relevant.

The importance of all these factors was clear in research completed by Bindels et al. (2021) of a performance appraisal protocol that used a multisource feedback tool and a peer coaching approach to discuss performance appraisal data with physicians. The research found that professional development could be supported when the appraisal process involved three characteristics: the appraisal process was appreciative and explored developmental opportunities; coaches were trustworthy and skilled; and the physician had control over the disclosure of the appraisal output (see Examining the Evidence 24.1).

EXAMINING THE EVIDENCE 24.1

Source: From Bindels, E., Boerebach, B., Scheepers, R., Nooteboom, A., Scherpbier, A., Heeneman, S., & Lombarts, K. (2021, August 12). Designing a system for performance appraisal: Balancing physicians' accountability and professional development. *BMC Health Services Research, 21*(1), 1–12. https://doi-org.mantis.csuchico.edu/10.1186/s12913-021-06818-1

Solution-Focused Coaching to Improve Physician Performance

Using a design-based research approach, a Dutch hospital-based research group drafted and implemented a performance appraisal protocol for physicians (n = 17), selecting a multisource feedback tool, codeveloping and piloting a coaching approach, implementing a planning tool, recruiting peer coaches, and facilitating their training and peer group debriefings. The protocol included a 2-hour peer-to-peer or professional coach conversation based on the principles of appreciative inquiry and solution-focused coaching.

For most participants, the review/coaching session did not reveal new insights about their performance. Rather, it confirmed existing ideas, or was instrumental in rendering, accepting, or internalizing the feedback received. The session did, however, deepen their insights in their developmental opportunities and improvement goals. For all participants, at least one improvement goal was formulated.

Characteristics that appeared crucial and non-negotiable for the facilitation of professional development were an appreciative and development-oriented performance appraisal process, the trustworthiness and skills of the peer coaches, and a nondisclosed appraisal output. Both expertise and confidentiality of the peer coach were considered of special importance because of the potential sensitivity of the topics that were discussed during the coaching session.

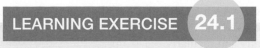

LEARNING EXERCISE 24.1

Writing about Performance Appraisals

During your lifetime, you probably have had many performance appraisals. These may have been evaluations of your clinical performance during nursing school or as a paid employee. Reflect on these appraisals. How many of them encompassed the eight recommendations listed in Display 24.2? How did the inclusion or exclusion of these recommendations influence your acceptance of the results?

ASSIGNMENT:

Select one of the eight recommendations about which you feel strongly. Write a three-paragraph essay about your personal experience as it relates to these recommendations.

Strategies to Ensure Accuracy and Fairness in the Performance Appraisal

If the goal of the performance appraisal is to satisfy the requirements of the organization, then the performance appraisal is largely a waste of time. The performance appraisal does provide an opportunity to document specific criteria for salary increases, promotions, or disciplinary actions, but it should also involve ongoing communication, setting achievable goals with clear expectations, and having a plan of action for the next period.

> A performance appraisal wastes time if it is merely an excuse to satisfy regulations and the goal is not employee growth.

Indeed, if the employee views the appraisal as valuable, valid, and growth producing, it can have many positive effects. Information obtained during the performance appraisal can be used to develop the employee's potential, to assist the employee in overcoming difficulties that they have in fulfilling the job's role, to point out strengths of which the employee may not be aware, and to aid the employee in setting goals. However, because inaccurate and unfair appraisals are negative and can demotivate, it is critical that the manager use strategies that increase the likelihood of a fair and accurate appraisal.

Although some subjectivity is inescapable, the following strategies will assist the manager in arriving at a fairer and more accurate assessment:

1. *The appraiser should develop an awareness of their own biases and prejudices.* This helps to guard against subjective attitudes and values influencing the appraisal. The appraiser must always recognize, though, that all employee reviews involve some subjectivity.
2. *Consultation should be sought frequently.* Another manager should be consulted when a question about personal bias exists and in many other situations. For example, it is very important that new managers solicit assistance and consultation when they complete their first performance appraisals. Even experienced managers may need to consult with others when an employee is having great difficulty fulfilling the duties of the job. Consultation must also be used when employees work several shifts so that information can be obtained from all shift supervisors.
3. *Data should be gathered appropriately.* Many different sources should be consulted about employee performance, and the data gathered needs to reflect the entire time period of the appraisal. Frequently, managers gather data and observe an employee just

before completing the appraisal, which gives an inaccurate picture of performance. Because all employees have periods when they are less productive and motivated, data should be gathered systematically and regularly.

4. *Accurate record keeping is another critical part of ensuring accuracy and fairness in the performance appraisal.* Information about subordinate performance (both positive and negative) should be recorded and not trusted to memory. The recording of both positive and negative performance behavior throughout the performance period is also known as *critical incident* recording. The manager should make a habit of keeping notes about observations, others' comments, and their periodic review of charts and nursing care plans. Taking regular notes on employee performance is a way to avoid the *recency effect*, which favors appraisal of recent performance over less recent performance during the evaluation period.

> When ongoing anecdotal notes are not maintained throughout the evaluation period, the appraiser is more apt to experience the recency effect, where recent issues are weighed more heavily than past performance.

5. *Collected assessments should contain positive examples of growth and achievement and areas where development is needed.* Nothing delights employees more than discovering that their immediate supervisor is aware of their growth and accomplishments and can cite specific instances in which good clinical judgment was used. Too frequently, collected data concentrate on negative aspects of performance.

6. *Some effort must be made to include the employee's own appraisal of their work.* Self-appraisal may be performed in several appropriate ways. Employees can be instructed to come to the appraisal interview with some informal thoughts about their performance, or they can work with their managers in completing a joint assessment.

7. The appraiser needs to guard against three common pitfalls of assessment: the *halo effect*, the *horns effect*, and *central tendency*. The halo effect occurs when the appraiser lets one or two positive aspects of the assessment or behavior of the employee unduly influence all other aspects of the employee's performance. The horns effect occurs when the appraiser allows some negative aspects of the employee's performance to influence the assessment to such an extent that other levels of job performance are not accurately recorded.

   The manager who falls into the central tendency trap is hesitant to risk true assessment and therefore rates all employees as average. These appraiser behaviors lead employees to discount the entire assessment of their work. Transtutors (2007–2022) suggests that to minimize the occurrence of central tendency error, a manager can temporally separate the performance dimensions; increase the number of scale points; use items that appear desirable on their face but differ in terms of their relevance to the job; and rate employees from "top to bottom."

8. *Reviewers need to guard against a bias known as the Matthew effect.* The *Matthew effect* is said to occur when employees receive the same appraisal results, year after year. Those who performed well early in their employment are likely to do well. Those who struggled will continue to struggle. In other words, no matter how hard an employee works to improve, their past appraisals prejudice any chance for future improvement (Kerr, 2022).

   Often, the Matthew effect is compared with the adage "the rich get richer and the poor get poorer." Thus, past appraisals prejudice an employee's future attempts to improve. Kerr (2022) notes that supervisors can overcome this bias if they are aware of it and are willing to adjust their performance evaluations accordingly.

9. Performance appraisals should always include asking the employee how the organization or the manager can make work easier to achieve better quality, greater volume, and improved outcomes.

Display 24.3 provides a summary of management strategies for successful performance appraisals.

DISPLAY **24.3** **MANAGEMENT STRATEGIES FOR SUCCESSFUL PERFORMANCE APPRAISALS**

Develop self-awareness regarding own biases and prejudices.
Use appropriate consultation.
Gather data adequately over time.
Keep accurate anecdotal records for the length of the appraisal period.
Collect positive data and identify areas where improvement is needed.
Include employee's own appraisal of their performance.
Guard against the halo effect, horns effect, central tendency trap, and Matthew effect.
Ask the employee how the organization or the manager can help the employee be successful.

LEARNING EXERCISE 24.2

Planning an Employee's First Performance Appraisal

Mrs. Jones is a new licensed vocational nurse (LVN)/licensed practical nurse (LPN) and has been working the 3:00 PM to 11:00 PM shift on the long-term care unit where you are the evening charge nurse. It is time for her 3-month performance appraisal. In your facility, each employee's job description is used as the standard of measure for performance appraisal. Essentially, you believe that Mrs. Jones is performing her job well, but you are somewhat concerned because she still relies on the registered nurses even for minor patient care decisions. Although you are glad that she does not act completely on her own, you would like to see her become more independent. The patients have commented favorably to you on Mrs. Jones's compassion and on her follow-through on all their requests and needs.

Mrs. Jones gets along well with the other LVNs/LPNs, and you sometimes believe that they take advantage of her hardworking and pleasant nature. On a few occasions, you believe that they inappropriately delegated some of their work to her. When preparing for Mrs. Jones's upcoming evaluation, what can you do to make the appraisal as objective as possible? You want Mrs. Jones's first evaluation to be growth producing.

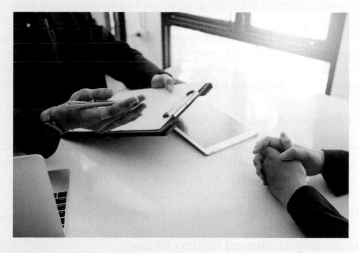

ASSIGNMENT:

Plan how you will proceed. What positive forces are already present in this scenario? What negative forces will you have to overcome? Support your plan with readings from references at the end of this chapter.

Performance Appraisal Tools

Since the 1920s, many appraisal tools have been developed, all of which have been popular at different times. Since the early 1990s, The Joint Commission (TJC) has been advocating the use of an employee's job description as the standard for performance appraisal. It is important, however, to make sure the job description is current and truly reflects the work the employee is assigned to do. TJC also suggests that employers must be able to demonstrate that employees know how to plan, implement, and evaluate care specific to the ages of the patients they care for. This continual refinement of critical *competencies* for professional nursing practice has a tremendous impact on the tools used in the appraisal process.

It is important to remember, however, that competence assessments are not the same as performance evaluations. A *competence assessment* examines one's knowledge or ability to complete a specific task or skill; a *performance evaluation* evaluates execution of a task or tasks.

> A competence assessment evaluates whether an individual has the knowledge, education, skills, or experience to perform the task, whereas a performance evaluation examines how well that individual actually completes that task.

The effectiveness of a performance appraisal system is only as good as the tools used to create those assessments. An effective competence assessment tool should allow the manager to focus on the priority measures of performance. The following is an overview of some of the appraisal tools commonly used in health care organizations.

Trait Rating Scales

A *trait rating scale* is a method of rating a person against a set standard, which may be the job description, desired behaviors, or personal traits. The trait rating scale has been one of the most widely used of the many available appraisal methods. Rating personal traits and behaviors is the oldest type of rating scale. Many experts argue, however, that the quality or quantity of the work performed is a more accurate performance appraisal method than the employee's personal traits and that trait evaluation invites subjectivity. Rating scales are also subject to central tendency and halo- and horns-effect errors and thus are not used as often today as they were in the past. Instead, many organizations use two other rating methods, namely, the job dimension scale and the *behaviorally anchored rating scale* (BARS). Table 24.1 shows a portion of a trait rating scale with examples of traits that might be expected in an employee.

Job Dimension Scales

Job dimension scales require that a rating scale be constructed for each job classification. The rating factors are taken from the context of the written job description. Although job dimension scales share some of the same weaknesses as trait scales, they do focus on job requirements rather than on ambiguous terms such as "quantity of work." Table 24.2 shows an example of a job dimension scale for an industrial nurse.

Behaviorally Anchored Rating Scales

BARS, sometimes called *behavioral expectation scales*, overcome some of the weaknesses inherent in other rating systems. As in the job dimension method, the BARS technique requires that a separate rating form be developed for each job classification. Then, as in the job dimension rating scales, employees in specific positions work with management to delineate key areas of responsibility. However, in BARS, many specific examples are defined for each area

TABLE **SAMPLE TRAIT RATING SCALE**

Job Knowledge

Significant gaps in essential knowledge needed to perform job/high level of supervision is required	Knowledge to perform job is often limited or inadequate/ requires supervision	Knowledge is generally adequate to meet job expectations but needs ongoing coaching/support	Knowledge base is well developed/ performs job expectations with minimal coaching and support	Job knowledge is extensive/works independently with minimal supervision
1	2	3	4	5

Judgment

Decision making is poor/unsafe	Decision making is variable and at times, flawed	Decision making is generally sound	Quality of decision making is good Demonstrates risk taking appropriately	Decision making is complex, timely, and of high quality Demonstrates risk taking and innovation
1	2	3	4	5

Attitude

Resents suggestions, no enthusiasm, new ideas accepted reluctantly	Disengaged but cooperative and accepting	Generally cooperative and accepting of new ideas	Cooperative and open to new ideas Demonstrates team building skills	Cooperative and open to new ideas Demonstrates leadership in team building
1	2	3	4	5

of responsibility; these examples are given various degrees of importance by ranking them from 1 to 9. If the highest ranked example of a job dimension is being met, it is less important that a lower ranked example is not.

Appraisal tools firmly grounded in desired behaviors can be used to improve performance and keep employees focused on the vision and mission of the organization. However, because separate BARS are needed for each job, the greatest disadvantage in using this tool with large numbers of employees is the time and expense. In addition, BARS are primarily applicable to physically observable skills rather than to conceptual skills. Yet, this is an effective tool because it focuses on specific behaviors, allows employees to know exactly what is expected of them, and reduces rating errors.

TABLE **SAMPLE JOB DIMENSION RATING SCALE FOR AN INDUSTRIAL NURSE**

Job Dimension	Rating Scale				
Renders first aid and treats job-related injuries and illnesses	5	4	3	2	1
Holds fitness classes for workers	5	4	3	2	1
Teaches health and nutrition classes	5	4	3	2	1
Performs yearly physicals on workers	5	4	3	2	1
Keeps equipment in good working order and maintains inventory	5	4	3	2	1
Keeps appropriate records	5	4	3	2	1
Dispenses medication as needed	5	4	3	2	1

Rating scale interpretation: 5 = excellent; 4 = good; 3 = satisfactory; 2 = fair; 1 = poor.

Although all rating scales are prone to weaknesses and interpersonal bias, they do have some advantages. Many may be purchased, and although they must be individualized to the organization, there is little need for expensive worker hours to develop them. Rating scales also force the rater to look at more than one dimension of work performance, which eliminates some bias.

Checklists

There are several types of *checklist* appraisal tools. The *weighted scale*, the most frequently used checklist, is composed of many behavioral statements that represent desirable job behaviors. Each of these behavior statements has a weighted score attached to it. Employees receive an overall performance appraisal score based on behaviors or attributes. Often, merit raises are tied to the total point score (i.e., the employee needs to reach a certain score to receive an increase in pay).

Another type of checklist, the *forced checklist*, requires the supervisor to select an undesirable and a desirable behavior for each employee. Both desirable and undesirable behaviors have quantitative values, and the employee again ends up with a total score on which certain employment decisions are made.

Another type of checklist is the *simple checklist*. The simple checklist comprises numerous words or phrases describing various employee behaviors or traits. These descriptors are often clustered to represent different aspects of one dimension of behavior, such as assertiveness or interpersonal skills. The rater is asked to check all those that describe the employee on each checklist. A major weakness of all checklists is that there are no set performance standards. In addition, specific components of behavior are not addressed. Checklists do, however, focus on a variety of job-related behaviors and avoid some of the bias inherent in the trait rating scales.

Essays

The *essay appraisal method* is often referred to as the *free-form review*. The appraiser describes in narrative form an employee's strengths and areas where improvement or growth is needed. Although this method can be unstructured, it usually calls for certain items to be addressed. This technique does appropriately force the appraiser to focus on positive aspects of the employee's performance. However, a greater opportunity for personal bias undoubtedly exists. In addition, it is time-consuming, and some appraisers simply write better than others.

Many organizations combine various types of appraisals to improve the quality of their review processes. Because the essay method does not require exhaustive development, it can quickly be adapted as an adjunct to any type of structured format. This gives the organization the ability to decrease bias and focus on employee strengths.

Self-Appraisals

Employees are increasingly being asked to submit written summaries of their work-related accomplishments and productivity as part of the *self-appraisal* process. Self-appraisal is not easy, however, for many employees because they confuse arrogance with confidence and mitigate what they have accomplished (Bortz, 2022). Other employees try to gloss over their weaknesses—but managers are looking for honest and open self-reflection (Bortz, 2022). The key then is for employees to view self-appraisal as an opportunity to honestly showcase their accomplishments as well as identify areas of potential growth.

Self-assessment is also an important part of *reflective practice*. Reflective practice is defined by Patel and Metersky (2022) as a cognitive skill that demands a conscious effort

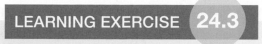

LEARNING EXERCISE 24.3

The Challenges of Self-Appraisal

What is your comfort with self-appraisal as a method of performance review? When you use self-appraisal, are your self-perceptions like those of the individual completing your review? If not, why not? Have you ever intentionally deflated your self-appraisal scores to avoid disappointment with the evaluation outcome? Have you ever artificially inflated your scores in a hope to positively sway the appraiser to give you higher marks? If so, was either of these strategies successful?

ASSIGNMENT:

Write a one- to two-page essay responding to these questions.

to look at a situation with an awareness of one's own beliefs, values, and practice enabling that person to learn from experience and incorporate that learning in improving patient care outcomes.

Clearly, there are advantages and disadvantages to using self-appraisal as a method of performance review. Although introspection and self-appraisal result in growth when the person is self-aware, even mature people require external feedback and performance validation. Some employees look forward to their annual performance review in anticipation of positive feedback. Asking these employees to perform their own performance appraisal would probably be viewed negatively rather than positively.

> Some employees look on their annual performance review as an opportunity
> to receive positive feedback from their supervisor, especially if the employee
> receives infrequent praise on a day–to–day basis.

In addition, managers may wish to complete the performance appraisal tool before reading the employee's self-analysis, or they should view the self-appraisal as only one data source that should be collected when evaluating worker performance. When self-appraisal is not congruent with other data available, the manager may wish to pursue the reasons for this discrepancy during the appraisal conference. Such an exchange may provide valuable insight regarding the worker's self-awareness and ability to view themselves objectively.

Employees may also be asked to submit portfolios as part of the self-appraisal process. These portfolios often contain examples of continuing education, professional certifications, awards, and recognitions the manager may not be fully aware of. The portfolio also generally includes the employee's goals and an action plan for accomplishing these goals.

Management by Objectives

Management by objectives (MBO) is an excellent tool for determining an individual employee's progress because it incorporates both the employee's assessments and the goals of the organization. The focus in this chapter, however, is on how these concepts are used as an effective performance appraisal method rather than on their use as a planning technique.

Although infrequently used in health care, MBO is an excellent method to appraise the performance of the employee in a manner that promotes individual growth and excellence by focusing on performance outcomes.

The following steps delineate how MBO can be used effectively in performance appraisal:

1. The employee and supervisor meet and agree on the principal duties and responsibilities of the employee's job. This is done as soon as possible after beginning employment.
2. The employee sets short-term goals and target dates in cooperation with the supervisor or manager, and the manager guides the process so that it relates to the position's duties.
3. It is important that the subordinate's goals do not conflict with the goals of the organization. In setting these goals, the manager must remember that one's values and beliefs simply reflect a single set of options among many. This is especially true in working with a multicultural staff. Professional expectations and values can vary greatly among cultures, and the manager must be careful to resist judgmental reactions and allow for cultural differences in goal setting.
4. Both parties agree on the criteria that will be used for measuring and evaluating the accomplishment of goals. In addition, a time frame is set for completing the objectives, which depends on the nature of the work being planned. Common time frames used in health care organizations vary from 1 month to 1 year.
5. Regularly, but more than once a year, the employee and supervisor meet to discuss progress. If the employee meets or exceeds the set objectives, then they have demonstrated an acceptable level of job performance.
6. Some modifications can be made to the original goals if both parties agree. Major obstacles that block completion of objectives within the stipulated time frame are identified. In addition, the resources and support needed from others are identified.
7. The manager's role is supportive, assisting the employee to reach goals by coaching and counseling.
8. During the appraisal process, the manager determines whether the employee has met the goals.
9. The entire process focuses on outcomes and results and not on personal traits.

One of the many advantages of MBO is that the method creates a vested interest in the employee to accomplish goals because employees can set their own goals. In addition, defensive feelings are minimized, and a spirit of teamwork prevails.

MBO as a performance appraisal method, however, also has its disadvantages. Highly directive and authoritarian managers find it difficult to lead employees in this manner. Also, the marginal employee may attempt to set easily attainable goals. In addition, set objectives may hinder innovation, and the process, when done well, takes time. TalentLyft (2022) suggests another disadvantage that MBO emphasizes the setting of goals to attain objectives, rather than working on a systematic plan to do so.

LEARNING EXERCISE   24.4

Using Management by Objectives as a Part of Performance Appraisal

It is time for Nancy Irwin's annual performance appraisal. She is a registered nurse on a postsurgical unit, dealing with complex trauma patients requiring high-level nursing intensity. You are the evening charge nurse and have worked with Ms. Irwin for 2 years since she graduated from nursing school. Last year, in addition to the regular 1 to 5 rating scale for job expectations, all of the charge nurses added a management by objectives (MBO) component to the performance appraisal form. In collaboration with their charge nurse, each employee developed five goals that were supposed to have been carried out over a 1-year period.

In reviewing Ms. Irwin's performance, you use several sources, including your written notes and her charting, and your conclusion is that with her strengths and weaknesses, overall, she is a better-than-average nurse. However, you believe that she has not grown much as an employee over the past 6 months. This observation is confirmed by a review of the following:

Objective	Result
1. Conduct a mini in-service or patient-care conference twice monthly for 12 months	Met goal for the first 2 months. In the last 10 months, she conducted only six conferences
2. Attend five educational classes related to work; at least one of these will be given by an outside agency	Attended one surgical nursing wound conference in the city and one in-house conference on total parenteral nutrition
3. Become an active member of a nursing committee at the hospital	Became an active member of the Policies and Procedures Committee and regularly attends meetings
4. Reduce the number of late arrivals at work by 50% (from 24 per year to 12)	First 3 months: not late; second 3 months: three late arrivals; third 3 months: six late arrivals; last 3 months: six late arrivals
5. Ensure that all patients discharged have discharge instructions documented in their charts	Anecdotal notes show that Ms. Irwin still frequently forgets to document these nursing actions

ASSIGNMENT:

As Ms. Irwin's charge nurse, what can you do to ensure that the current appraisal results in greater growth for her? What went wrong with last year's MBO plan? Devise a plan for the performance appraisal. Try solving this yourself before reading the possible solution that appears in the Appendix.

Peer Review

When peers rather than supervisors carry out monitoring and assessing work performance, it is referred to as *peer review*. Most likely, the manager's review of the employee is not complete unless some type of peer review data is gathered. Peer review provides feedback that can promote growth. It can also provide learning opportunities for the peer reviewers.

> The concept of collegial evaluation of nursing practice is closely related to maintaining professional standards.

Although the prevailing practice in most organizations is to have managers evaluate employee performance, there is much to be said for collegial review. Peer review is widely used in medicine and academe; however, health care organizations have been slow to adopt peer review for the following five reasons:

1. Staff are often poorly oriented to the peer review method and many first-level managers, including team leaders, have had little training on how to conduct a growth-producing performance appraisal.
2. Peer review is viewed as very threatening when inadequate time is spent orienting employees to the process and when necessary support is not provided throughout the process.
3. Peers often feel uncomfortable sharing feedback with people with whom they work closely. To avoid potential conflict, they omit needed suggestions for improving the employee's performance. Thus, the review becomes more advocacy than evaluation.
4. Peer review is viewed by many as more time-consuming than traditional superior–subordinate performance appraisals.

5. Because much socialization takes place in the workplace, friendships often result in inflated evaluations, or interpersonal conflict may result in unfair appraisals.
6. Because peer review shifts the authority away from management, the insecure manager may feel threatened.

Peer review has its shortcomings, as evidenced by some university teachers receiving unjustified tenure or the failure of physicians to maintain adequate quality control among some individuals in their profession. In addition, peer review involves much risk taking, is time consuming, and requires a great deal of energy. However, nursing as a profession should be responsible for setting the standards and then monitoring its own performance. Because performance appraisal may be viewed as a type of quality control, it seems reasonable to expect that nurses should have some input into the performance evaluation process of their profession's members.

Peer review can be carried out in several ways. The process may require the reviewers to share the results only with the person being reviewed, or the results may be shared with the employee's supervisor and the employee. The review would never be shared only with the employee's supervisor. The results may or may not be used for personnel decisions. The number of observations, number of reviewers, qualification and classification of the peer reviewer, and procedure need to be developed for each organization. If peer review is to succeed, the organization must overcome its inherent difficulties by doing the following before implementing a peer review program:

- Peer review appraisal tools must reflect standards to be measured, such as the job description.
- Staff must receive a thorough orientation to the process before its implementation. The role of the manager should be clearly defined.
- Ongoing support, resources, and information must be made available to the staff during the process.
- Data for peer review need to be obtained from predetermined sources, such as observations, charts, and patient care plans.
- A decision must be made about whether anonymous feedback will be allowed. This is controversial and needs to be addressed in the procedure.
- Decisions must be reached on whether the peer review will affect personnel decisions and, if so, in what manner.

Peer review has the potential to increase the accuracy of performance appraisal. It can also provide many opportunities for increased professionalism and learning. The use of peer review in nursing should continue to expand as nursing increases its autonomy and professional status. Display 24.4 provides a summary of types of performance appraisal tools.

DISPLAY 24.4 SUMMARY OF PERFORMANCE APPRAISAL TOOLS

Trait rating scales: rates an individual against some standard
Job dimension scales: rates the performance on job requirements
Behaviorally anchored rating scales: rates desired job expectations on a scale of importance to the position
Checklists: rates the performance against a set list of desirable job behaviors
Essays: a narrative appraisal of job performance
Self-appraisals: an appraisal of performance by the employee
Management by objectives: employee and management agree on goals of performance to be reached
Peer review: assessment of work performance carried out by peers
360-degree evaluation: Assessment by all individuals within the sphere of influence of the individual being appraised.

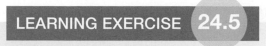

LEARNING EXERCISE 24.5

Addressing Megan's Change in Behavior

Even in organizations that have no formal peer review process, professionals must take some responsibility for colleagues' work performance, even if informally. The following scenario illustrates the need for peer involvement.

You have worked at Memorial Hospital since your graduation from nursing school. Your school roommate, Megan, has also worked at Memorial since her graduation. For the first year, you and Megan were assigned to different units, but you were both transferred to the oncology unit 6 months ago. You and Megan work the 3 PM to 11 PM shift, and it is the policy for the charge nurse duties to alternate among three RNs assigned to the unit on a full-time basis. Both of you are among the nurses assigned to rotate to the charge position. You have noticed lately that when Megan is in charge, her personality seems to change; she barks orders and seems tense and anxious.

Megan is an excellent clinical nurse, and many of the staff seek her out in consultation about patient care problems. You have, however, heard several of the staff grumbling about Megan's behavior when she is in charge. As Megan's good friend, you do not want to hurt her feelings, but as her colleague, you feel a need to be honest and open with her.

ASSIGNMENT:

A very difficult situation occurs when personal and working relationships are combined. Describe what, if anything, you would do.

The 360-Degree Evaluation

An adaptation of peer review, and a newer addition to performance appraisal tools, the *360-degree evaluation*, includes an assessment by all individuals within the sphere of influence of the individual being appraised. For example, a 360-degree evaluation of a ward clerk or unit secretary might include feedback from the nursing staff, from patients, and from staff from other departments who interact with that individual on a regular basis. In addition, most 360-degree feedback tools include a self-assessment.

Getting feedback from multiple individuals provides a broader, more accurate perspective of the employee's work performance. This divergent thinking suggests that involving additional individuals in the appraisal process provides unique and valuable perspectives that might otherwise not be considered. "When done properly, 360-degree evaluation is highly effective as a development tool. The feedback process gives people an opportunity to provide anonymous feedback to a coworker that they might otherwise be uncomfortable giving. Feedback recipients gain insight into how others perceive them and have an opportunity to adjust behaviors and develop skills that will enable them to excel at their jobs" (Custom Insight, 2022, para. 6). When done haphazardly or because everyone else is doing it, 360-degree feedback could create a disaster requiring months and possibly years to recover (Heathfield, 2021). For example, in poorly planned and executed 360-degree evaluations, employees could be deluged with nonconstructive feedback, anonymity of responses could be lost, and a spirit of team cohesion could be destroyed.

In most 360-degree evaluations, somewhere between 8 and 12 people fill out an anonymous online feedback form that asks questions covering a broad range of workplace competencies (Custom Insight, 2022). The feedback forms include questions that are measured on a rating scale and ask raters to provide written comments.

When implementing this type of evaluation, it's best to assure other employees that what they share will remain strictly confidential. Likewise, the evaluator should explain to each employee that their performance will be evaluated by many people, including those who know their work best.

LEARNING EXERCISE **24.6**

The 360-Degree Evaluation

Think of a role you have held which was important to you and which you worked hard at to be successful. This could be a personal role such as being a parent, romantic partner, or a specific job you have held in the past or at present. Identify at least six individuals you would have chosen to complete a 360-degree evaluation of you in that role. Why did you select these individuals? Might their perceptions have been in conflict? Would these individuals have been likely to give you honest appraisal feedback? If so, how might their feedback have altered how you approached the role or the goals you were trying to achieve?

Strategies for Planning and Executing a Successful Performance Appraisal Interview

The most accurate and thorough appraisal will fail to produce growth in employees if the information gathered is not used appropriately. Many appraisal interviews have negative outcomes because the manager views them as a time to instruct employees only on what they are doing wrong rather than looking at strengths as well.

Managers often dislike the appraisal interview more than the actual data gathering. One of the reasons managers dislike the appraisal interview is because of their own negative experiences when they have been judged unfairly or criticized personally. Indeed, some managers are so uncomfortable with conducting performance appraisals that they find reasons not to do them at all.

Clearly, both parties in the appraisal process tend to be anxious before the interview; thus, the appraisal interview remains an emotionally charged event. For many employees, past appraisals have been traumatizing. Although little can be done to eliminate the often-negative emotions created by past experiences, the leader-manager can manage the interview in such a manner that people will not be traumatized further.

Feedback, perhaps the greatest tool a manager has for changing behavior, must be given in an appropriate manner. There is a greater chance that the performance appraisal will have a positive outcome if certain conditions are present before, during, and after the interview.

Before the Interview

- Make sure that the conditions mentioned previously have been met (e.g., the employee knows the standard by which their work will be evaluated), and they have a copy of the appraisal form.
- Select an appropriate time for the appraisal conference. Do not choose a time when the employee has just had a traumatic personal event or is too busy at work to take the time needed for a meaningful conference.
- Give the employee 2 to 3 days of advance notice of the scheduled appraisal conference so that they can prepare mentally and emotionally for the interview.
- Be prepared mentally and emotionally for the conference yourself. If something should happen to interfere with your readiness for the interview, it should be canceled and rescheduled.
- Schedule uninterrupted appraisal time. Hold the appraisal in a private, quiet, and comfortable place. Forward your telephone calls to another line and ask another manager to answer any pages that you may have during the performance appraisal.

- Plan a seating arrangement that reflects collegiality rather than power. Having the person seated across a large desk from the appraiser denotes a power–status position; placing the chairs side by side denotes collegiality.

During the Interview

- Greet the employee warmly, showing that the manager and the organization have a sincere interest in their growth.
- Begin the conference on a pleasant, informal note.
- Conduct the conference in a nondirective and participatory manner. Input from the employee should be solicited throughout the interview; however, the manager must recognize that employees from some cultures may be hesitant to provide this type of input. In this situation, the manager must continually reassure the employee that such input is not only acceptable but also desired.
- Ask the employee to comment on their progress since the last performance appraisal.
- Although it's important to be as positive as possible, it's also essential to be honest (Team MyHub, 2021). If an employee is not performing well in an aspect of their job, you must tell them so; however, be constructive and identify specific ways that they can turn things around. Seek a balance of positives and negatives whenever possible.
- Avoid surprises in the appraisal conference. The effective leader coaches and communicates informally with staff on a continual basis, so there should be little new information at an appraisal conference.
- When dealing with an employee who has several problems—either new or long-standing—do not overwhelm them at the conference with excessive criticism. If there are too many problems to be addressed, select the major ones.
- Use positive encouragement and affirmation as much as possible during the appraisal interview because they are crucial to improving worker performance. "Billikopf calls these 'good-will deposits,' and says without them, 'withdrawals cannot be made'" (Kerr, 2022).
- Listen carefully to what the employee has to say and give them your full attention.
- Focus on the employee's performance and not on their personal characteristics.
- Avoid vague generalities, either positive or negative, such as "your skills need a little work" or "your performance is fine." Be prepared with explicit performance examples. Be liberal in the positive examples of employee performance; use examples of poor performance sparingly. Use several examples only if the employee has difficulty with self-awareness and requests specific instances of a problem area.
- When delivering performance feedback, be straightforward and state concerns directly so as not to retard communication or cloud the message.
- Never threaten, intimidate, or use status in any manner. Differences in power and status interfere with the ability of professionals to form meaningful and constructive relationships. This is not to say that managers should not maintain an appropriate authority–power gap with their employees; it simply suggests that power and status issues should be minimized as much as possible so that the performance appraisal can appropriately focus on the subordinate's performance and needs.
- Let the employee know that the organization and the manager are aware of their uniqueness, special interests, and valuable contributions to the unit. Remember that all employees make some special contribution to the workplace.
- Make every effort to ensure that there are no interruptions during the conference. It is important employees feel as though they are being listened to and their views matter (Team MyHub, 2021).

- Use terms and language that are clearly understood and carry the same meaning for both parties. Avoid words that have a negative connotation. Do not talk down to employees or use language that is inappropriate for their level of education.
- Mutually set realistic and achievable goals for further growth or improvement in the employee's performance. Vague or unachievable goals are counterproductive (Team MyHub, 2021). Decide how goals will be accomplished and evaluated and what support is needed. Make sure it is clear how you as the manager and the organization can support the employee to achieve their personal development and career goals (Team MyHub, 2021).
- Use coaching techniques throughout the conference.
- Plan on being available for employees to return retrospectively to discuss the appraisal review further. There is frequently a need for the employee to return for elaboration if the conference did not go well or if the employee was given unexpected new information. This is especially true for the new employee.

> Indirectness and ambiguity are more likely to inhibit communication than enhance it, leaving the employee unsure about the significance of the message.

After the Interview

- Both the manager and the employee need to sign the appraisal form to document that the conference was held and that the employee received the appraisal information. This does not mean that the employee is agreeing to the information in the appraisal; it merely means that the employee has read the appraisal. An example of such a form is shown in Figure 24.1. There should be a place for comments by both the manager and the employee.
- End the interview on a pleasant note.
- Document the goals for further development that have been agreed on by both parties. The documentation should include target dates for accomplishment, support needed, and when goals are to be reviewed. This documentation is often part of the appraisal form.
- If the interview reveals specific long-term coaching needs, the manager should develop a method of follow-up to ensure that such coaching takes place.

Performance Management

Some experts in human resource management have suggested that annual performance appraisals should be replaced by ongoing *performance management*. In performance management, appraisals are eliminated, and the manager places their efforts into ongoing coaching, mutual goal setting, and the leadership training of subordinates. This focus requires the manager to spend more regularly scheduled face-to-face time with subordinates.

In contrast to the annual performance review, which is often linked to an employee's hire date, the performance management calendar is generally linked to the organization's business calendar. This way, performance planning is coordinated throughout the entire organization, as strategic goals for the year can be identified and subordinates' roles to achieve those goals can be openly discussed and planned. Some organizations, however, view performance management as a continuous cycle. Regardless, all performance-managed organizations identify role-based competency expectations for every employee, regardless of job description. Then, employees can determine how these qualities translate into performance in specific jobs.

Performance appraisal form

Name: _____

Unit: _____

Prepared by: _____

Reason (merit, terminal, end of probation, general reviews): _____

Date of appraisal conference: _____

Comments by employee:

Employee's signature: _____

(Signature of employee denotes that the appraisal has been read. It does not signify acceptance or agreement. Space is provided for any comments the employee wishes to make.) Comments by appraiser.

(These comments are to be written at the time of the appraisal conference and in the presence of the employee.)

Employee's signature (Date)

Evaluator's signature (Date)

FIGURE 24.1 Performance appraisal documentation form.

Coaching: A Mechanism for Informal Performance Appraisal

Coaching is described as a transfer of skills and knowledge from one person to another to achieve agreed on outcomes. In other words, *coaching* conveys the spirit of leaders' and managers' roles in informal day-to-day performance appraisals, which promote improved work performance and team building. Coaching can guide others into increased competence, commitment, and confidence as well as help them to anticipate options for making vital connections between present and future plans.

> Day-to-day feedback regarding performance is one of the best methods for
> improving work performance and building a team approach.

Coaching does not, however, replace the need for self-motivation on the part of the employee. Instead, leader-managers meet with employees regularly to discuss aspects of their performance. Both individuals determine the agenda with the goal of an environment of learning that can span the personal and professional aspects of the employee's experience. Employees can discuss challenges they are encountering and get new ideas and information about how to deal with situations from someone who often has experienced the same problems and issues. This shared connection between the manager and the employee makes the employee feel validated and part of a larger team. When coaching is combined with informal performance appraisal, the outcome is usually a positive modification of behavior. For this to occur, however, the leader must establish a climate in which there is a free exchange of ideas.

Becoming an Effective Coach

The following tactics will assist managers in becoming more effective coaches:

- Be specific, not general, in describing behavior that needs improvement.
- Be descriptive, not evaluative, when describing what was wrong with the work performance.
- Be certain that the feedback is not self-serving but meets the needs of the employee.
- Direct the feedback toward behavior that can be changed.
- Use sensitivity in timing the feedback.
- Make sure that the employee has clearly understood the feedback and that the employee's communication has also been clearly heard.

When employees believe that their manager is interested in their performance and personal growth, they will have less fear of the work performance appraisal. When that anxiety is reduced, the formal performance interview process can be used to set mutual performance goals.

LEARNING EXERCISE 24.7

The New Nurse as Coach

You have just completed your 6-month probation as a new nurse, and while you are beginning to feel comfortable in this new role, you feel there is still much you need to learn. You also know that your self-confidence is not yet what you want it to be.

A new nursing assistive personnel began working on your unit about 3 weeks ago. She has asked the charge nurse to be assigned to your team whenever possible. She is a hard worker and a quick learner, and you enjoy having her on your team.

Today, she comes to you and shares that her goal is to be a registered nurse (RN) and that she is currently taking her prenursing courses at the local university and hopes to apply to the nursing program next year. She asks if you would be willing to "take her under your wing" and teach her more about what being a professional RN is all about. You are flattered that she thinks of you as a role model but are not sure that you have either the time or the skill level yet to be an effective coach for her.

ASSIGNMENT:

How will you respond to her request? What factors will you consider in making your decision? What are the potential driving and restraining forces for both accepting and denying her request? How much knowledge and experience are needed to be an effective coach?

When Employees Appraise Their Manager's Performance (Upward Appraisals)

Upward appraisals occur when employees review their supervisors. These meetings allow managers to improve communication and relationships with their teams and contribute to a collaborative, equal work environment (Buckley, 2021). Indeed, establishing a feedback culture begins with the leader modeling behavior that values input and minimizes defensive responses (Sherman and Cohn, 2021). Often, upward appraisals occur through a 360-degree evaluation process.

In addition, organizations may conduct focus group discussions about management effectiveness (Mayhew, 2022). When focus groups are used, an experience-qualified employee relations specialist facilitates the discussion so that it does not dissolve into a gripe session. Instead, employees are encouraged to speak with respectful candor about how well they believe managers are performing (Mayhew, 2022). In addition, employers may use employee opinion surveys to determine the overall level of job satisfaction in the workplace.

Leader-managers should view the trend for upward appraisals positively because employee feedback provides the same opportunities for growth in leadership or management positions that subordinates have with traditional performance appraisals. In addition, this process may provide the supervisor with feedback from employees who might not otherwise be able to do so. It does, however, require that the leader-manager trust their subordinates and believe their feedback is meant to be constructive.

> "The best nurse leaders are learners. They take the information they receive and use it to improve" (Sherman & Cohn, 2021, p. 16).

Integrating Leadership Roles and Management Functions in Conducting Performance Appraisals

Performance appraisal is a major responsibility in the controlling function of management. The ability to conduct meaningful, effective performance appraisals requires an investment of time, effort, and practice on the part of the manager. Although performance appraisal is never easy, if used appropriately, it produces growth in the employee and increases productivity in the organization.

To increase the likelihood of successful performance appraisal, managers should use a formalized system of appraisal and gather data about employee performance in a systematic manner, using many sources. The manager should also attempt to be as objective as possible, using established standards for the appraisal. The result of the appraisal process should provide the manager with information for meeting training and educational needs of employees. By following up conscientiously on identified performance deficiencies, employees' work problems can be corrected before they become habits.

Integrating leadership into this part of the controlling phase of the management process provides an opportunity for sharing, communicating, and growing. The integrated leader-manager is self-aware regarding their biases and prejudices. This self-awareness leads to fairness and honesty in evaluating performance. This, in turn, increases trust in the manager and promotes a team spirit among employees.

The leader also uses day-to-day coaching techniques to improve work performance and reduce the anxiety of performance appraisal. When anxiety is reduced during the appraisal interview, the leader-manager can establish a relationship of mutual goal setting, which has a greater potential to result in increased motivation and corrected deficiencies. The result of the integration of leadership and management is a performance appraisal that facilitates employee growth and increases organizational productivity.

Key Concepts

- The employee performance appraisal is a sensitive and important part of the management process, requiring much skill.
- Because of past experiences, performance appraisal interviews are highly charged, emotional events for most employees and even managers.
- When accurate and appropriate appraisal assessments are performed, outcomes can be positive and employee growth can result.
- Performance appraisals are used to determine how well employees are performing their job. Therefore, appraisals measure actual behavior and not intent.
- Job descriptions often produce objective criteria for use in the performance appraisal.
- There are many different types of appraisal tools and methods, and the most appropriate one to use varies with the type of appraisal to be done and the criteria to be measured.
- The employee must be involved in the appraisal process and view the appraisal as accurate and fair to result in employee growth.
- Peer review as a performance appraisal tool has great potential for developing professional accountability but is often difficult to implement because it requires risk taking to avoid becoming simply an exercise of advocacy.
- Self-appraisal is not easy for many employees because they often undervalue their own accomplishments or feel uncomfortable giving themselves high marks in many areas.

- MBO has been shown to increase productivity and commitment in employees.
- Unless the appraisal interview is carried out in an appropriate and effective manner, the appraisal data will be useless.
- Showing a genuine interest in the employee's growth and seeking their input at the interview will increase the likelihood of a positive outcome from the appraisal process.
- Performance appraisals should be signed to show that feedback was given to the employee.
- Informal work performance appraisals are an important management function.
- In performance management, appraisals are eliminated. Instead, the manager places their efforts into ongoing coaching, mutual goal setting, and the leadership training of subordinates.
- Leaders should routinely use day-to-day coaching to empower subordinates and improve work performance.
- Workplaces are increasingly encouraging employees to provide feedback regarding the quality of their supervision. An upward appraisal occurs when employees review their supervisors.
- Leader-managers must invest time and resources to develop a feedback-based culture, communicate the true purpose of performance reviews, and build trust in the process.

Additional Learning Exercises and Applications

LEARNING EXERCISE 24.8

Requesting Feedback from Employees

You are the director of a home health agency. You have just returned from a management course and have been inspired by the idea of requesting input from your subordinates about your performance as a manager. You realize that there are some risks involved but believe that the potential benefits from the feedback outweigh the risks. However, you want to provide some structure for the evaluation, so you spend some time designing your appraisal tool and developing your plan.

ASSIGNMENT:

What type of tool will you use? What is your overall goal? Will you share the results of the appraisal with anyone else? How will you use the information obtained? Would you have the appraisal forms signed or have them be anonymous? Who would you include in the group that is evaluating you? Be able to support your ideas with appropriate rationale.

LEARNING EXERCISE 24.9

Making Appraisal Interviews Less Traumatic

You are the new night-shift charge nurse in a large intensive care unit composed of an all-RN staff. When you were appointed to the position, your supervisor told you that there had been some complaints regarding how the previous charge nurse handled evaluation sessions. Not wanting to repeat the mistakes, you draw up a list of things that you could do to make the evaluation interviews less traumatic. Because the evaluation tool appears adequate, you believe that the problems must lie with the performance appraisal interview itself. At the top of your list, you write that you will make sure each employee has advance notice of the evaluation.

ASSIGNMENT:

How much advance notice should you give? What additional criteria would you add to the list to help eliminate much of the trauma that frequently accompanies performance appraisal (even when the appraisal is very good)? Add six to nine items to the list. Explain why you think that each of these would assist in alleviating some of the anxiety associated with performance appraisals. Do not just repeat the guidelines listed in this chapter. You may make the guidelines more specific or use references for assistance in developing your own list.

LEARNING EXERCISE 24.10

Helping a Seasoned Employee Grow

Patty Brown is a licensed vocational nurse/licensed practical nurse who has been employed in your skilled nursing facility for 10 years. She is an older woman and is very sensitive to criticism. Her work is generally of high quality, but in reviewing her past performance appraisals, you notice that during the last 10 years, at least seven times, she has been rated unsatisfactory for not being on duty promptly and eight times for not attending mandatory staff development programs. Because you are Patty's supervisor, you would like to help her grow in these two areas. You have given Patty a copy of the evaluation tool and her job description and have scheduled her appraisal conference for a time when the unit will be quiet. You can conduct the appraisal in the conference room.

ASSIGNMENT:

How would you conduct this performance appraisal? Outline your plan. Include how you would begin. What innovative or creative way would you attempt to provide direction or improvement in the areas mentioned? How would you terminate the session? Be able to give rationale for your decisions.

LEARNING EXERCISE 24.11

Could This Conflict Have Been Prevented?

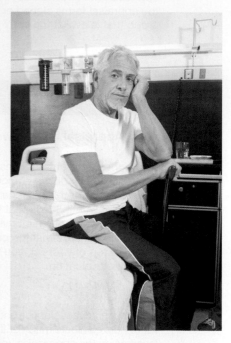

Mr. Reilly, a 60-year-old automobile salesman, was admitted with severe back pain. As his primary care nurse, you have established a rapport with Mr. Reilly. He has a type A personality and has been very critical of much of his hospitalization. He was also very upset by the level and duration of his pain following his laminectomy. You agreed to ambulate him on your shift three times (at 4:00 PM, 7:00 PM, and 10:30 PM) so that he would need to be ambulated only once during the day shift. He does not care for many of the day staff and feels that you help to ambulate him better than anyone else. You noted the ambulating routine on his nursing orders.

Yesterday, Joan Martin, a day nurse, believed that his bowel sounds were somewhat diminished. She urged him to ambulate more on the day shift, but he refused to do so. (The doctor had ordered ambulation q.i.d.) When Mr. Reilly's physician visited, Nurse Martin told him that Mr. Reilly ambulated only once on the shift. She did not elaborate further to the doctor. The physician proceeded to talk very sternly with Mr. Reilly, telling him to get out of bed three times today. Nurse Martin did not mention this incident to you in the report.

By the time you arrived on duty and received the handoff report, Mr. Reilly was very angry. He threatened to sign himself out against medical advice. You talked with his doctor, got the order changed, and finally managed to calm Mr. Reilly down. You then wrote a nursing order that read, "Nurse Martin is not to be assigned to Mr. Reilly again." When Joan Martin came on duty this morning, the night shift pointed out your notation. She was very angry and went to see the head nurse.

ASSIGNMENT:

Should you have done anything differently? If so, what? Could the evaluation of clinical performance by you and Nurse Martin have been done in a manner that would not have resulted in conflict? If you were Nurse Martin, what could you have done to prevent the conflict? Be able to discuss this case in relation to professional trust, peer review, and assertive communication.

LEARNING EXERCISE 24.12

Addressing Casey's Errors in Judgment

You are a senior baccalaureate nursing student. This is your sixth week of a medical-surgical advanced practicum. Your instructor assigns two students to work together in caring for four to six patients. The students alternate fulfilling leader and follower roles and providing total patient care. This is the second full day that you have worked as a team with Casey.

Last week, when you were assigned with Casey, she was the leader and made numerous errors in judgment. She got a patient up who was on strict bed rest. She made a medication error by giving a medication to the wrong patient. She gave a pain medication too soon because she forgot to record the time in the medication record, and she frequently did not seem to know what was wrong with her patients.

Today, you have been the leader and have observed her contaminate a dressing and forget to check armbands twice when she was giving medications. When you asked her about checking the placement of the nasogastric tube, she did not know how to perform this skill. You have heard some of the other students complain about Casey.

ASSIGNMENT:

What is your obligation to Casey, to your patients, your fellow students, the clinical agency, and your instructor? Outline what you would do. Provide the rationale for your decisions.

LEARNING EXERCISE 24.13

Fighting Central Tendency Error

You are a nursing student who is completing your maternal/child clinical practicum. Your final clinical evaluation is scheduled for tomorrow. You are an excellent student and you worked very hard during this clinical rotation. You were shocked during your midterm evaluation to see that the instructor gave you mostly "averages" on the evaluation form with a few "above averages." You had scored yourself with all "above averages" and several "outstandings."

When your instructor noted the discrepancies, she simply said, "There's always room for improvement, and besides, it's only the middle of the rotation." She seemed a bit perturbed when she saw the "outstandings" you had given yourself, suggesting that you might be a bit too self-confident about your skills. She suggested you "try to be more self-aware."

You have since learned that almost all the students in the clinical practicum earned average marks on their midterm evaluations even though there clearly was a broad continuum in terms of the level at which different students met the course objectives. You are also aware that written comments are required on the behalf of the instructor for any marks of "outstanding" or "objective not met" and you wonder if this is influencing her reluctance to grant high marks to students.

ASSIGNMENT:

You need to prepare your self-evaluation for tomorrow's final clinical evaluation. You truly believe that you met almost all of the course objectives at the "outstanding" level with a few "above averages." You do not, however, want to experience another evaluation where your marks are significantly higher than your instructors or to be subjected to the consternation of your instructor for another "inflated self-evaluation." Decide what you will do. If your marks are significantly different than your instructor's at the final conference, what, if anything will you do?

REFERENCES

Bortz, D. (2022). How to complete a self-evaluation for a performance review. *Monster.* https://www.monster.com/career-advice/article/performance-assessment-self-evaluation

Buckley, D. (2021, October 5). *How to conduct employee performance appraisals (with types).* Indeed. https://www.indeed.com/career-advice/career-development/employee-performance-appraisals#:~:text=An%20upward%20appraisal%20occurs%20when%20employees%20review%20their,can%20contribute%20to%20a%20collaborative%2C%20equal%20work%20environment

Custom Insight. (2022). *What is 360 degree feedback?* https://www.custominsight.com/360-degree-feedback/what-is-360-degree-feedback.asp

Heathfield, S. M. (2021). *360 degree feedback: See the good, the bad and the ugly.* The Balance. https://www.thebalancecareers.com/360-degree-feedback-information-1917537

Kerr, M. (2022). *Challenges of employee performance evaluations.* Hearst. https://smallbusiness.chron.com/challenges-employee-performance-evaluations-1867.html

Mayhew, R. (2022). *An employee evaluation of a manager.* Hearst. https://smallbusiness.chron.com/employee-evaluation-manager-1927.html

Patel, K. M., & Metersky, M. (2022, July). Reflective practice in nursing: A concept analysis. *International Journal of Nursing Knowledge, 33(3),* 180–187. doi: 10.1111/2047-3095.12350

https://pubmed.ncbi.nlm.nih.gov/34626459/#:~:text=Conclusions%3A%20Reflective%20practice%20is%20a%20cognitive%20skill%20that,It%20also%20leads%20to%20knowledge%20development%20in%20nursing

Qualtrics. (2022). *Your ultimate guide to employee performance reviews.* https://www.qualtrics.com/experience-management/employee/performance-appraisal/

Sherman, R. O., & Cohn, T. M. (2021, May). Benefits of feedback for nurse leaders. *American Nurse Journal, 16(5),* 14–16.

TalentLyft. (2022). *What is management by objective (MBO)?* https://www.talentlyft.com/en/resources/what-is-management-by-objective-mbo

Team MyHub. (2021, August 11). *100 useful performance review example phrases.* https://www.myhubintranet.com/performance-review-example-phrases/

Transtutors. (2007–2022). *To minimize the occurrence of central tendency error you may: temporally separate the performance . . . Questions and answers.* https://www.transtutors.com/questions/to-minimize-the-occurrence-of-central-tendency-error-you-may-temporally-separate-the-8010686.htm#:~:text=To%20minimize%20the%20occurrence%20of%20central%20tendency%20error,bottom%22%20Dec%2030%202021%208%3A14%20AM%20Expert%27s%20Answer

25

Problem Employees: Rule Breakers, Marginal Employees, and Those with Substance Use Disorder

*… as patient advocates, nurse leaders must help ensure fitness for duty.—**Richard Hader***

*… difficult employees can make you question why you became a manager in the first place.—**Mark Pipkin***

*… A person who has been punished is not less inclined to behave in a given way; at best, he learns how to avoid punishment.—**B.F. Skinner***

CROSSWALK

This chapter addresses:

- **AACN Essentials Domain 5:** Quality and safety
- **AACN Essentials Domain 7:** Systems-based practice
- **AACN Essentials Domain 9:** Professionalism
- **AACN Essentials Domain 10:** Personal, professional, and leadership development
- **AONL Nurse Executive Competency 1:** Communication and relationship building
- **AONL Nurse Executive Competency 2:** A knowledge of the health care environment
- **AONL Nurse Executive Competency 3:** Leadership
- **AONL Nurse Executive Competency 4:** Professionalism
- **AONL Nurse Executive Competency 5:** Business skills
- **ANA Standard of Professional Performance 7:** Ethics
- **ANA Standard of Professional Performance 8:** Advocacy
- **ANA Standard of Professional Performance 10:** Communication
- **ANA Standard of Professional Performance 11:** Collaboration
- **ANA Standard of Professional Performance 12:** Leadership
- **ANA Standard of Professional Performance 13:** Education
- **ANA Standard of Professional Performance 15:** Quality of practice
- **ANA Standard of Professional Performance 16:** Professional practice evaluation
- **ANA Standard of Professional Performance 18:** Environmental health
- **QSEN Competency:** Teamwork and collaboration
- **QSEN Competency:** Safety

LEARNING OBJECTIVES

The learner will:

- differentiate between constructive and destructive discipline
- identify factors that must be present to foster a climate of self-discipline in employees
- identify the "hot stove" rules described by McGregor to make discipline as fair and growth producing as possible

- describe the steps typically followed in progressive discipline
- seek to eliminate rules that are outdated or no longer appropriate in the environments in which they function
- compare how the disciplinary process may vary between unionized and nonunionized organizations
- analyze situations in which discipline is required and identify appropriate strategies for constructively modifying behavior
- determine appropriate levels of discipline for rule breaking in specific situations
- develop strategies that assist marginal employees to be contributing members of the workforce
- describe the risk factors that result in an increased risk of substance use disorder (SUD) in the nursing profession
- identify common methods of drug diversion used by nurses in the care of patients
- identify behaviors and actions that may signify SUD in an employee or colleague
- recognize the reporting of SUD suspicions as both a moral and professional obligation
- analyze how personal feelings, values, and biases regarding SUD may alter one's ability to confront and/or help the impaired employee
- recognize the importance of the manager not assuming the role of counselor or treatment provider for employees with SUD

Introduction

Employees' perceptions vary as to what they owe the organization and what they owe themselves. At times, organizational and individual needs, wants, and responsibilities are in conflict. The coordination and cooperation needed to meet organizational goals require leader-managers to control individual subordinates' urges that are counterproductive to these goals. Subordinates do this by self-control. Managers do this by enforcing established rules, policies, and procedures. Leaders do this by creating a supportive and motivating climate and by coaching.

Despite the best efforts of all parties, however, problem employees are everywhere, and every organization has them. At best, they limit productivity; at worst, they can be a threat to the stability of the work environment. Hills (2021) agrees with this, noting that problem employees can take a significant toll on you, the rest of your staff, your patients, and your bottom line. In addition, even if numbers are small, problem employees can consume significant managerial time, attention, and energy.

Problem behavior can assume many forms, including blatant insubordination such as an employee refusing to perform a task, chronic attendance issues, or showing disrespect to coworkers or others. Highly problematic behavior is often subtler but equally serious. This includes behavior such as undermining fellow team members and creating an unwelcome or hostile workplace.

When employees are unsuccessful in meeting organizational goals, managers must attempt to identify the reasons for this failure and counsel employees accordingly. Underachieving employees may require reengagement or efforts to create a more motivating environment (see Chapter 18). If employees fail, however, because they are unwilling to follow rules or established policies and procedures, or they are unable to perform their duties adequately despite assistance and encouragement, the manager has an obligation to take disciplinary action.

Progressive discipline is inappropriate, however, for employees who are impaired due to disease or degree of ability. These employees have special needs that require active coaching, support, and, often, professional counseling to maintain productivity. For employees to be managed most appropriately, managers must be able to distinguish between employees in need of discipline and those who are impaired.

Regardless of the cause, however, supervisors should promptly address inappropriate conduct and poor work performance. Delay only exacerbates such situations. The disenchantment of a single employee can spread, affecting otherwise satisfied and highly valued employees. When someone is not performing well, everyone knows it. And when management refuses to act, employees may perceive that their leaders lack the resolve necessary to make the organization successful.

> Not disciplining an employee who should be disciplined jeopardizes an organization's morale.

This chapter focuses on discipline, coaching, and referral as tools in addressing problem employees, promoting subordinates' growth, and meeting organizational goals. The normal progression of steps taken in disciplinary action and strategies for administering discipline fairly and effectively are delineated. Formal and informal grievances are discussed.

This chapter also focuses on two types of employees with special needs: the marginal employee and the employee with substance use disorder (SUD). *Marginal employees* are those employees who disrupt unit functioning because the quantity or quality of their work consistently meets only minimal standards at best. Employees with *SUD* use nicotine, alcohol, or other illicit substances to an excess that leads to social, academic, and occupational impairment (Jahan & Burgess, 2022). Traditional discipline is not effective in addressing either of these types of employees.

This chapter identifies the challenges inherent in working with marginal employees and those with SUD and presents managerial strategies to address the problem. In addition, the chapter profiles diversion practices and identifying behaviors common to nurses with SUD. Steps in the recovery process and the reentry of the nurse with SUD into the workforce are also discussed. Leadership roles and management functions appropriate for use with problem employees are shown in Display 25.1.

DISPLAY 25.1 LEADERSHIP ROLES AND MANAGEMENT FUNCTIONS IN DEALING WITH PROBLEM EMPLOYEES

Leadership Roles

1. Recognizes and reinforces the intrinsic self-worth of each employee and the role of successful work performance in maintaining a positive self-image
2. Encourages employees to be self-disciplined in conforming to established rules and regulations
3. Understands group norms and works within those norms to mold group behavior
4. Assists employees to identify with organizational goals, thus increasing the likelihood that the standards of conduct deemed acceptable by the organization will be accepted by its employees
5. Is self-aware regarding the power and responsibility inherent in having formal authority to set rules and discipline employees
6. Serves in the role of coach in performance deficiency coaching or problem-centered coaching
7. Assures that the rights and the responsibilities of both the manager and the employee are considered in addressing worker grievances
8. Is self-aware regarding values, biases, and beliefs about SUD
9. Uses active listening as a support tool in working with impaired subordinates but recognizes own limitations in counseling and refers impaired employees to outside experts for appropriate counseling
10. Examines the work environment for stressors that contribute to SUD and eliminates those stressors whenever possible
11. Keeps patient safety first and foremost when considering how best to intervene with problem employees
12. Recognizes that all employees have intrinsic worth and assists them in reaching their maximal potential

continues on page 666

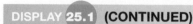

DISPLAY 25.1 **(CONTINUED)**

Management Functions

1. Clearly discusses all written rules and policies with subordinates, explains the rationale for the existence of the rules and policies, and encourages questions
2. Clearly identifies the performance expectations for all employees and confronts employees when those expectations are not met
3. Uses formal authority as judiciously as possible so that subordinates can invoke self-discipline
4. Uses formal authority to administer discipline using a progressive model when employees continue to fail to meet expected standards of achievement
5. Investigates thoroughly the situation before employee discipline is administered
6. Consults with either a supervisor or the Human Resources department before dismissing an employee
7. Maintains clear, objective, and comprehensive written records regarding the problem employee's behavior and attempts to counsel
8. Uses organizational transfers appropriately
9. Seeks out and completes extensive education about SUD in the work setting; provides these same opportunities to staff
10. Acts as a resource to impaired employees regarding professional services or agencies that provide counseling and support services
11. Collects and records adequate objective data when suspicious of employee SUD
12. Focuses employee confrontations on performance deficits and not on the cause of the underlying problem or addiction
13. Works with the rule breaker, marginal employee, or employee with SUD to develop a remedial plan for action; ensures that the employee understands the performance expectations of the organization and the consequences of not meeting these expectations

Constructive Versus Destructive Discipline

Discipline involves training or molding the mind or character to bring about desired behaviors. Discipline is often considered a form of punishment but is not quite the same thing as punishment. *Punishment* is an undesirable event that follows unacceptable behavior.

Punishment, however, has long been a part of standard employment disciplinary strategies. Scientific management theory viewed discipline as a necessary means for controlling an unmotivated and self-centered workforce. Because of this traditional philosophy, managers primarily used threats and fear to control behavior. This "big stick" approach to management focused on eliminating all behaviors that could be considered to conflict with organizational goals. Although this approach may succeed on a short-term basis, it is usually demotivating and reduces long-term productivity because people will achieve goals only up to the level that they believe is necessary to avoid punishment. This approach is also destructive because discipline is often arbitrarily administered and is unfair either in the application of rules or in the resulting punishment.

In contrast, discipline can also be a powerful motivator for behavior change because it has an educational component as well as a corrective one. *Positive* or *constructive discipline* seeks to explain to the employee what positive actions the employer is looking for, opting to focus on the wanted behaviors and outcomes instead of the problems. The idea is to provide motivation for employees to improve.

When discipline is *constructive*, it can assist employee growth. In fact, the word *discipline* comes from the Latin term *disciplina*, which means teaching, learning, and growing. In constructive discipline, punishment may be applied for improper behavior, but it is carried out in a supportive and corrective manner. Employees are reassured that the punishment given is because of their actions and not because of who they are. This can have the effect of improving employee morale, even in the face of needing to improve performance.

LEARNING EXERCISE 25.1

Thinking about Growth-Producing Versus Destructive Discipline

Think back to when someone in authority such as a parent, teacher, or boss set limits or enforced rules in such a way that you became a better child, student, or employee. What made this disciplinary action growth producing instead of destructive? What was the most destructive disciplinary action that you ever experienced? Did it modify your behavior in any way?

> Constructive discipline uses discipline as a means of helping the employee grow, not as a punitive measure.

Self-Discipline and Group Norms

Organizations need people who are self-disciplined for excellence, not punished into compliance. Indeed, the highest level and most effective form of discipline is *self-discipline*. When employees feel secure, validated, and affirmed in their essential worth, identity, and integrity, self-discipline is forthcoming.

Ideally, all employees have adequate self-control and are self-directed in their pursuit of organizational goals. However, this is not always the case. Instead, *group norms* (group-established standards of expected behavior that are enforced by social pressure) often influence individual behavior and make self-discipline difficult. The leader, who understands group norms, can work within those norms to mold group behavior. This modification of group norms, in turn, affects individual behavior and thus self-discipline.

Although self-discipline is internalized, the leader plays an active role in developing an environment that promotes self-discipline in employees. It is impossible for employees to have self-control if they do not understand the acceptable boundaries for their behavior, nor can they be self-directed if they do not understand what is expected of them. Therefore, managers must clearly discuss all written rules and policies with subordinates, explain the rationale for the existence of the rules and policies, and encourage questions.

> Self-discipline is possible only if subordinates know the rules and accept them as valid.

Self-discipline also requires an atmosphere of mutual trust. Managers must believe that employees are capable of and actively seek self-discipline. Likewise, employees must respect their managers and perceive them as honest and trustworthy. Employees lack the security to have self-discipline if they do not trust their managers' motives. Finally, for self-discipline to develop, formal authority must be used judiciously. If formal discipline is quickly and widely used, subordinates do not have the opportunity to invoke self-discipline.

Fair and Effective Rules

Several guidelines must be followed if discipline is to be perceived by subordinates as growth producing. This does not imply that subordinates enjoy being disciplined or that discipline should be a regular means of promoting employee growth. However, discipline, if implemented correctly, should not permanently alienate or demoralize subordinates. McGregor (1967) developed

DISPLAY 25.2	MCGREGOR'S HOT STOVE RULES FOR FAIR AND EFFECTIVE DISCIPLINE

Four elements must be present to make discipline as fair and growth producing as possible:
1. Forewarning
2. Immediate consequences
3. Consistency
4. Impartiality

four rules to make discipline as fair and growth producing as possible (Display 25.2). These rules are called "hot stove" rules because they can be applied to someone touching a hot stove.

1. All employees must be *forewarned* that if they touch the hot stove (break a rule), they will be burned (punished or disciplined). They must know the rule beforehand and be aware of the punishment.
2. If the person touches the stove (breaks a rule), there will be *immediate consequences* (getting burned). All discipline should be administered immediately after rules are broken.
3. If the person touches the stove again, they will again be burned. Therefore, there is *consistency*; each time the rule is broken, there are immediate and consistent consequences.
4. If any other person touches the hot stove, they also will get burned. Discipline must be *impartial*, and everyone must be treated in the same manner when the rule is broken.

Most rule breaking is not enforced using McGregor's rules. For example, many people exceed the speed limit when driving. In general, people are aware of speed limit regulations, and signs are posted along the roadway as reminders of the rules; thus, there is *forewarning*. There is no, however, *immediacy*, *consistency*, or *impartiality*. Many people exceed the speed limit for long periods before they are stopped and disciplined, or they may never be disciplined at all. Likewise, a person may be stopped and disciplined one day and not the next even though the same rule is broken. Finally, the punishment is inconsistent because some people are punished for their rule breaking, but others are not. Even the penalty varies among people.

Imagine what would happen if automobiles were developed that alarmed every time a driver exceeded the speed limit and then transmitted this rule violation to local law enforcement so that a speeding ticket could be issued. The incidence of speeding would decrease dramatically. In addition, drivers would likely accept greater accountability for the speeding tickets they received because they would have been forewarned of the consequences of breaking the speed limit rule, and they would know that this rule would be enforced consistently and impartially for all drivers.

If a rule or regulation is worth having, it should be enforced. When rule breaking is allowed to go unpunished, other people tend to replicate the behavior of the rule breaker. Likewise, the average worker's natural inclination to obey rules can be dissipated by lax or inept enforcement policies because employees develop contempt for managers who allow rules to be disregarded. The enforcement of rules using McGregor's hot stove method keeps morale from breaking down and allows structure within the organization.

An organization should, however, have as few rules and regulations as possible. A leadership role involves regularly reviewing all rules, regulations, and policies to see if they should be discarded or modified in some way. If managers find themselves spending much of their time enforcing one rule, it would be wise to reexamine the rule and consider whether there is something wrong with the rule or how it is communicated.

Rule Breakers and Outdated Rules

Part 1: Think back to "rule breakers" you have known. Were they a majority or minority in the group? How great was their impact on group behavior? What characteristics did they have in common? Did the group modify the rule breaker's behavior, or did the rule breaker modify group behavior?

Part 2: Rules quickly become outdated and need to be deleted or changed in some way. Think of a policy or rule that needs to be updated. Why is the rule no longer appropriate? What could you do to update this rule? Does the rule need to be replaced with a new one?

Discipline as a Progressive Process

Managers have the formal authority and responsibility to take progressively stronger forms of discipline when employees fail to meet expected standards of achievement. However, inappropriate discipline (too much or too little) can undermine the morale of the whole team. Determining appropriate disciplinary action, then, is often difficult, and many factors must be considered.

Discipline is generally administered using a progressive model. Except in limited circumstances, employees should be given the opportunity to correct problems. This is especially true in unionized organizations. However, even in nonunionized organizations, managers should have a disciplinary procedure that is written and well-communicated.

> Action must be taken when employees continue undesirable conduct, either by breaking rules or by not performing their job duties adequately.

In general, the first step of the progressive disciplinary process is an *informal reprimand* or *verbal admonishment*. This reprimand includes an informal meeting between the employee and the manager to discuss the broken rule or performance deficiency. The manager suggests ways in which the employee's behavior might be altered to keep the rule from being broken again. Often, an informal reprimand is all that is needed for behavior modification.

The second step is a *formal reprimand* or *written admonishment*. If rule breaking recurs after verbal admonishment, the manager again meets with the employee and issues a written warning about the behaviors that must be corrected. This written warning is very specific about what rules or policies have been violated, the potential consequences if behavior is not altered to meet organizational expectations, and the plan of action that the employee is expected to take to achieve expected change.

Both the employee and the manager should sign the warning to signify that the problem or incident was discussed. The employee's signature does not imply that the employee agrees with everything on the report, only that it has been discussed. The employee must be allowed to respond in writing to the reprimand, either on the form or by attaching comments to the disciplinary report; this allows the employee to air any differences in perception between the manager and the employee. One copy of the written admonishment is then given to the employee, and another copy is retained in the employee's personnel file. Figure 25.1 presents a sample written reprimand form.

The third step in progressive discipline is usually a *suspension from work*, either with or without pay. If the employee continues the undesired behavior despite verbal and written warnings, the manager should remove the employee from their job for a brief time, generally a few days to several weeks. Such a suspension gives the employee the opportunity to reflect on the behavior and to plan how they might modify the behavior in the future.

The last step in progressive discipline is *involuntary termination* or *dismissal*. Many people terminate their employment voluntarily before reaching this step, but the manager cannot

Name of employee _____

Position _____

Date of hire _____

Person completing report _____

Position _____

Date report completed _____

Date of incident(s) _____

Time _____

Description of incident(s):

Prior attempts to counsel employee regarding this behavior (cite date and results of disciplinary conferences):

Disciplinary contract (plan for correction) and time lines:

Consequences of future repetition:

Employee comments (additional documentation or rebuttal may be attached):

Date/Signature of individual making the report

Date/Signature of employee

Date and time of follow-up appointment to review contract:

FIGURE 25.1 Sample written reprimand form.

count on this happening. Termination should always be the last resort when dealing with poor performance. However, if the manager has given repeated warnings and rule breaking or policy violations continue, then the employee should be dismissed. Although this is difficult and traumatic for the employee, the manager, and the unit, the cost in terms of managerial and employee time and unit morale of keeping such an employee is enormous.

When using progressive discipline, the steps are followed only for repeated infractions of the same. At the end of a predesignated period, the slate is wiped clean. For example, although an employee may have previously received a formal reprimand for unexcused absences, discipline for a first-time offense of tardiness should begin at the first step of the process. Also, remember that although discipline is generally administered progressively, some rule breaking is so

TABLE 25.1 GUIDE TO PROGRESSIVE DISCIPLINE

Offense	First Infraction	Second Infraction	Third Infraction	Fourth Infraction
Gross mistreatment of a patient	Dismissal			
Discourtesy to a patient	Verbal admonishment	Written admonishment	Suspension	Dismissal
Insubordination	Written admonishment	Suspension	Dismissal	
Use of intoxicants while on duty	Dismissal			
Neglect of duty	Verbal admonishment	Written admonishment	Suspension	Dismissal
Theft or willful damage of property	Written admonishment	Dismissal		
Falsehood	Verbal admonishment	Written admonishment	Dismissal	
Unauthorized absence	Verbal admonishment	Written admonishment	Dismissal	
Abuse of leave	Verbal admonishment	Written admonishment	Suspension	Dismissal
Violation of safety rules	Written admonishment	Suspension	Dismissal	
Inability to maintain work standards	Written admonishment	Suspension	Dismissal	
Excessive unexcused tardiness[a]	Verbal admonishment	Written admonishment	Suspension	

[a]The first, second, and third infractions do not mean the first, second, and third time an employee is late but the first, second, and third time that unexcused tardiness becomes excessive as determined by the manager.

serious that the employee may be suspended or dismissed with the first infraction. Table 25.1 presents a progressive discipline guide for managers.

> When using progressive discipline in all but the most serious infractions, the slate should be wiped clean at the end of a predesignated period.

LEARNING EXERCISE 25.3

Deciding on Disciplinary Action

You are a supervisor in a neurologic care unit. One morning, you receive a report from the night-shift registered nurses, Nurse Caldwell and Nurse Jones. Neither of the nurses reports anything out of the ordinary, except that a young patient with head injury has been particularly belligerent and offensive in his language. This young man was especially frustrating because he appeared rational and then would suddenly become abusive. His language was particularly vulgar. You recognize that this is fairly normal behavior in a patient with a head injury, but yesterday morning, his behavior was so offensive to his neurosurgeons that one of them threatened to wash his mouth out with soap.

(continues on page 672)

LEARNING EXERCISE 25.3

Deciding on Disciplinary Action (continued)

After both night nurses leave the unit, you receive a phone call from the house night supervisor who relates the following information: When the supervisor made the usual rounds to the neuro unit, Nurse Caldwell was on a coffee break and Nurse Jones was in the unit with two licensed vocational nurses/licensed practical nurses. Nurse Jones reported that Nurse Caldwell became very upset with the patient with head injury because of his abusive and vulgar language and had taped his mouth shut with a 4-in piece of adhesive tape. Nurse Jones had observed the behavior and had gone to the patient's bedside and removed the piece of tape and suggested that Nurse Caldwell go get a cup of coffee.

The supervisor observed the unit several times following this, and nothing else appeared to be remiss. Stating that no harm had come to the patient, Nurse Jones was reluctant to report the incident but believed that perhaps one of the supervisors should counsel Nurse Caldwell. You thank the night supervisor and consider the following facts in this case:

- Nurse Caldwell has been an excellent nurse but is occasionally judgmental.
- Nurse Caldwell is a very religious young woman and has led a rather sheltered life.
- Taping a patient's mouth with a 4-in piece of adhesive tape is very dangerous, especially for someone with questionable chest and abdominal injuries and neurologic injuries.
- Nurse Caldwell has never been reprimanded before.

You call the physician and explain what happened. The physician believes that no harm was done and notes that it is up to you to determine if and how to discipline the employee. He does, however, express significant concern about her judgment to safely care for patients.

You phone the nurse and arrange for a conference with her. She tearfully admits what she did. She states that she lost control. She asks you not to fire her, although she agrees this is a dischargeable offense. You consult with the administration, and everyone agrees that you should be the one to decide the disciplinary action in this case.

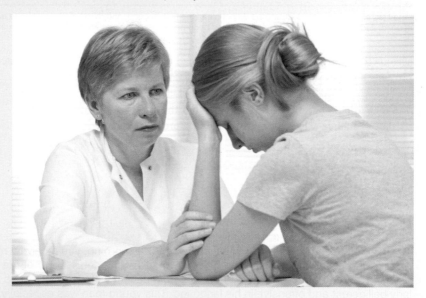

ASSIGNMENT:

Decide what you would do. You have a duty to your patients, the hospital, and your staff. List at least four possible courses of action. Select from among these choices and justify your decision.

Disciplinary Strategies for the Manager

It is vital that managers recognize their power in evaluating and correcting employees' behavior. Because a person's job is very important to them—often as a part of self-esteem and as a means of livelihood—disciplining or taking away a person's job is a very serious action and should not be undertaken lightly. The manager can implement several strategies to increase the likelihood that discipline will be fair and produce growth.

Mayhew (2022) recommends that in preparing to discipline employees, the manager's first step should be to obtain the employee's personnel file materials and review the file documents for a better understanding of past performance and workplace behavior. Determine whether the employee has demonstrated similar behavior in the past, who addressed the previous issues, and how they were resolved. Also be alert for any personal bias you or others may have that is influencing the determination of whether discipline is needed. Hills (2021) concurs, noting if accusers are biased against an employee, a chain of attitudes and actions can be set into motion that unintentionally cause the poor job performance you want to avoid.

Then the manager must thoroughly investigate the situation that has prompted the employee discipline. A supervisor must investigate all allegations of misconduct even if the misconduct is anonymously reported or initially appears to have no basis. The manager might ask the following questions: Was the rule clear? Did this employee know that they were breaking a rule? Is culture a factor in this rule breaking? Has this employee been involved in a situation like this before? Were they disciplined for this behavior? What was their response to the corrective action? How serious or potentially serious is the current problem or infraction? Who else was involved in the situation? Does this employee have a history of other types of disciplinary problems? What is the quality of this employee's performance in the work setting? Have other employees in the organization also experienced the problem? How were they disciplined? Could there be a problem with the rule or policy? Were there any special circumstances that could have contributed to the problem in this situation? What disciplinary action is suggested by organization policies for this type of offense? Has precedent been established? Will this type of disciplinary action keep the infraction from recurring? The wise manager will ask all these questions so that a fair decision can be reached regarding an appropriate course of action.

Another strategy that the manager should use is to always consult with either a supervisor or the Human Resources department before dismissing an employee. Most organizations have very clear policies about which actions constitute grounds for dismissal and how that dismissal should be handled.

> Disciplinary problems, if unrecognized or ignored, generally do not go away; they only get worse.

To protect themselves from charges of willful or discriminatory termination, managers should carefully document the behavior that occurred and any attempts to counsel the employee. The accuracy of your documentation can mean the difference between time in the courtroom and a good, clean break from a poor employee. Managers also must be careful not to discuss with one employee the reasons for discharging another employee or to make negative comments about past employees, which may discourage other employees or reduce their trust in the manager.

Performance Deficiency Coaching

Performance deficiency coaching is another strategy that the manager can use to create a disciplined work environment. This type of coaching may be ongoing or problem centered.

DISPLAY **25.3** PERFORMANCE DEFICIENCY COACHING SCENARIO

Coach: I am concerned that you have been regularly coming into report late. This interrupts the other employees who are trying to hear report and creates overtime because the night shift must stay and repeat report on the patients you missed. It also makes it difficult for your modular team members to prioritize their plan of care for the day if the entire team is not present and ready to begin at 7:00 AM. Why is this problem occurring?

Employee: I've been having problems lately with an unreliable babysitter and my car not starting. It seems like it's always one thing or another, and I'm upset about not getting to work on time, too. I hate starting my day off behind the eight ball.

Coach: This hospital has a long-standing policy on attendance, and it is one of the criteria used to judge work performance on your performance appraisal.

Employee: Yes, I know. I'm just not sure what I can do about it right now.

Coach: What approaches have you tried in solving these problems?

Employee: Well, I'm buying a new car, so that should take care of my transportation problems. I'm not sure about my babysitter, though. She's young and not very responsible, so she'll call me at the last minute and tell me she's not coming. I keep her, though, because she's willing to work the flexible hours and days that this job requires, and she doesn't charge as much as a formal daycare center would.

Coach: Do you have family in the area or close friends you can count on to help with childcare on short notice?

Employee: Yes, my mother lives a few blocks away and is always glad to help, but I couldn't count on her on a regular basis.

Coach: There are employment registry lists at the local college for students interested in providing childcare. Have you thought about trying this option? Often, students can work flexible hours and charge less than formal daycare centers.

Employee: That's a good idea. In fact, I just heard about a childcare referral service that also could give me a few ideas. I'll stop there after work. I realize that my behavior has affected unit functioning, and I promise to try to work this out as soon as possible.

Coach: I'm sure these problems can be corrected. Let's have a follow-up visit in 2 weeks to see how things are going.

Problem-centered coaching is less spontaneous and requires more managerial planning than *ongoing coaching*. In performance deficiency coaching, the manager actively brings areas of unacceptable behavior or performance to the attention of the employee and works with them to establish a plan to correct deficiencies. Because the role of a coach is less threatening than that of an enforcer, the manager becomes a supporter and a helper. Performance deficiency coaching helps employees, over time, to improve their performance to the highest level of which they are capable. As such, the development, use, and mastery of performance deficiency coaching should result in improved performance for all. The scenario depicted in Display 25.3 is an example of performance deficiency coaching.

LEARNING EXERCISE **25.4**

Writing a Performance Deficiency Coaching Plan

You are the professional staff coordinator of a small, outpatient urgent care clinic. Historically, the clinic is busiest on weekend evenings. Many also come to the clinic on weekends to take care of nonemergency medical needs that were not addressed during regular physician office hours. Jane has been a registered nurse at the clinic since it opened 2 years ago. She is well liked by all the employees and provides a sense of humor and lightheartedness in what is usually a highly stressful environment.

Jane, however, has a reputation for being a "party animal." She is known to begin party-ing after work on Friday night and close down the bars Saturday morning. During the last 3 months, Jane has called in sick five of the seven Saturday evenings that she was scheduled to work. The other employees have worked understaffed on what is generally the busiest night of the week, and they are becoming angry. They have asked you to talk to Jane or to staff an additional employee on those Saturday evenings that Jane is assigned to work.

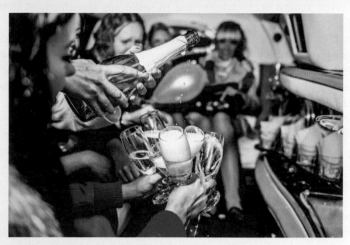

ASSIGNMENT:

You have decided to begin performance deficiency coaching with Jane. Write a possible coaching scenario that includes the following:

- The problem stated in behavioral terms
- An explanation to the employee of how the problem is related to organizational functioning
- A clear statement of the possible consequences of the unwanted behavior
- A request for input from the employee
- Employee participation in the problem solving
- A plan for follow-up on the problem

Disciplining the Unionized Employee

It is essential that all managers be fair and consistent in disciplining employees regardless of whether a union is present. The presence of a union does, however, usually entail more pro-cedural, legalistic safeguards in administering discipline and a well-defined grievance process for employees who believe that they have been disciplined unfairly. If the employee is cov-ered by a collective bargaining agreement, managers should refer to the applicable collective negotiations agreement to ascertain the requirements for notification of the union (Rutgers University Human Resources, 2022). For example, the employee may request that a steward be present if they are being questioned and have a reasonable belief that the answer to such questions will result in discipline (Rutgers University Human Resources, 2022). In addition, usually, the manager of nonunionized employees has greater latitude in selecting which disci-plinary measure is appropriate for a specific infraction. Although this gives the manager more flexibility, discipline among employees may be inconsistent.

On the other hand, unionized employees generally must be disciplined according to spe-cific, preestablished steps and penalties within an established time frame. For example, the union contract may be very clear that excessive unexcused absences from work must be disci-plined first by a written reprimand, then a 3-day work suspension, and then termination. This type of discipline structure is generally fairer to the employee but allows the manager less flexibility in evaluating each case's extenuating circumstances.

Another aspect of discipline that may differ between unionized and nonunionized employees is following *due process* in disciplining union employees. Due process means that management must provide union employees with a written statement outlining disciplinary charges, the resulting penalty, and the reasons for the penalty. Employees then have the right to defend themselves against such charges and to settle any disagreement through formal grievance hearings.

Another difference between unionized and nonunionized employee discipline lies in the *burden of proof*, which typically is the responsibility of the employee without union membership but is the responsibility of the manager of the employee who belongs to a union. This means that managers who discipline union employees must keep detailed records regarding misconduct and counseling attempts.

> In disciplinary situations with nonunionized employees, the burden of proof typically falls on the employee. With union employees, the burden of proof for the wrongdoing and need for subsequent discipline generally falls on management.

Another common difference between unionized and nonunionized employees is that most nonunion employees are classified as *at-will*, meaning that they are subject to dismissal "at the will" of the employer. The at-will doctrine, which is applicable in many states, permits an employer to terminate employment for any or no reason and at the discretion of the supervisor. In states that do not subscribe to the employment-at-will doctrine or in organizations that have union representation for employees, employers must have good and legal cause to dismiss an employee.

It must be noted, however, that even when the employment-at-will doctrine is applicable, there are numerous exceptions, and an employer must be knowledgeable of each exception. Such exceptions where at-will dismissal would not apply might include when employment is being terminated based on membership in a protected legal group such as race, sex, pregnancy, national origin, religion, disability, age, or military status.

The contract language used by unions regarding discipline may be quite specific or quite general. Most contracts recognize the right of management to discipline, suspend, or dismiss employees for just cause. *Just cause* can be defined as having appropriate rationale for the actions taken. For just cause to exist, the manager must be able to prove that the employee violated established rules, that corrective action or penalty was warranted, and that the penalty was appropriate for the offense. These contracts also generally recognize the right of the employee to submit grievances when they believe that these actions have been taken unfairly or are discriminatory in some way.

Managers are responsible for knowing all union contract provisions that affect how discipline is administered on their units. Managers also should work closely with others employed in human resources or personnel positions in the organization. These professionals generally prove to be invaluable resources in dealings with union employees.

The Disciplinary Conference

When coaching is unsuccessful in modifying problem behavior, the manager must take more aggressive steps and use more formal measures, such as a *disciplinary conference*. After thoroughly investigating an employee's offenses, managers must confront the employee with their findings. This occurs in the form of a disciplinary conference. The following steps are generally part of the disciplinary conference.

Reason for Disciplinary Action

Begin by clearly specifying why the employee is being disciplined. Do not bring hearsay or judgments into the conversation or you can find yourself squabbling over details, no matter how big or small (Hills, 2021). Point to data and quantify when you can.

In addition, the manager must not be hesitant or apologetic about the need for discipline because the role of the manager includes both the authority and the responsibility for evaluating employee performance and suggesting appropriate action for improved or acceptable performance. Despite this, novice managers, however, often feel uncomfortable with the disciplinary process and may provide unclear or mixed messages to the employee regarding the nature or seriousness of a disciplinary problem.

> In the disciplinary conference, managers must assume the authority given to them by their role.

Employee's Response to Disciplinary Action

Give the employee the opportunity to explain why the rule was not followed. Allowing employees feedback in the disciplinary process ensures them recognition as human beings. It also reassures them that the ultimate goal is to be fair and promote their growth. Ask the employee whether they believe the performance problem or behavioral issue is resolvable and whether they have suggestions for improvement (Mayhew, 2022).

Rationale for Disciplinary Action

Explain the disciplinary action that you are going to take and why you are going to take it. Although the manager must keep an open mind to new information that may be gathered in the second step, preliminary assessments regarding the appropriate disciplinary action should already have been made. This discipline should be communicated to the employee. The employee who has been counseled at previous disciplinary conferences should not be surprised at the punishment, as the consequences of continued undesired behavior should have been discussed at the last conference.

Clarification of Expectations for Change

Present a *performance improvement plan* to be sure employee expectations for remediation are clear. This plan should include the expected behavioral change as well as the steps needed to achieve this change. Be clear whether the employee and the supervisor share responsibility for improving the employee's work performance (Mayhew, 2022). For example, if the employee's poor performance is based on not having proper training or skills, share what resources will be provided to help the employee improve.

Also explain the consequences of failure to change. Again, do not be apologetic or hesitant; otherwise, the employee will be confused about the seriousness of the issue. Because they may lack self-control, employees who have repeatedly broken rules need firm direction. It must be very clear to the employee that timely follow-up will occur. Finally, it is important to make sure you've been understood. Have the employee repeat back to you what you've said, what needs to change, why, by when, and what will happen if the poor performance or the specific behavior continues (Hills, 2021).

Agreement and Acceptance of Action Plan

Get agreement and acceptance of the plan. Give support and let the employee know that you are interested in them as a person. Remember, too, that the leader-manager administers discipline to promote employee growth rather than to impose punishment. Although the expected standards must be very clear, leaders impart a sense of genuine concern for and desire to help the employee grow. This approach helps the employee to recognize that the discipline is directed at the offensive behavior and not at the individual. The leader-manager must be cautious, however, not to relinquish the management role in an effort to nurture and counsel. The leadership role is to provide a supportive environment and structure so that the employee can make the necessary changes.

The Environment for Discipline

Besides understanding what should be covered in the disciplinary conference, the leader-manager must be sensitive to the environment in which discipline is given. Although the employee must receive feedback about their rule breaking or inappropriate behavior as soon as possible after it has occurred, the manager should implement discipline privately, never in front of patients or peers. If more than an informal admonishment is required, the manager should inform the employee of the unacceptable action and then schedule a formal disciplinary conference later.

> All discipline, even informal admonishments, should be conducted in private.

Timing and Conference Length

All formal disciplinary conferences should be scheduled in advance at a time agreeable to both the employee and the manager. Both will want time to reflect on the situation that has occurred. Allowing time for reflection should reduce the situation's emotionalism and promote employee self-discipline because employees often identify their own plan for keeping the behavior from recurring.

In addition to privacy and advance scheduling, the length of the disciplinary conference is important. It should not be so long that it degenerates into a debate nor so short that both the employee and the manager cannot provide input. If the employee seems overly emotional or if great discrepancies exist between the manager and the employee's perceptions, an additional conference can be scheduled. Employees often need time to absorb what they have been told and to develop a plan that is not defensive. In addition, conducting disciplinary conferences can be as stressful for the manager as it is for the employee, especially when the unit manager is relatively new or inexperienced in this role.

Closure

On ending the disciplinary conference, provide the employee with a copy of the disciplinary action and place a copy of the documentation in the personnel file. Inform the employee about company policy concerning disciplinary action and the length of time disciplinary action forms remain in an employee's file before they can be removed (Mayhew, 2022).

The Termination Conference

When it is apparent that a progressive disciplinary approach has failed and that the necessary change in behavior has not been achieved, managers often need to terminate the employee. At this point, the disciplinary conference becomes a termination conference. Although many of the principles are the same, the termination conference differs from a disciplinary conference in that planning for future improvement is eliminated. The following steps should be followed in the termination conference:

1. *Calmly state the reasons for dismissal.* The manager must not appear angry or defensive. Although managers may express regret that the outcome is termination of employment,

they must not dwell on this or give the employee reason to think that the decision is not final. The manager should be prepared to give examples of the behavior in question.

2. *Explain the employment termination process.* State the date on which employment is terminated as well as the employee's and organization's role in the process.

3. *Ask for employee input.* Termination conferences are always tense; raw, spontaneous, emotional reactions are common. Listen to the employee but do not allow yourself to be drawn emotionally into their anger or sorrow. Always stay focused on the facts of the case and attempt to respond without reacting.

4. *Identify any follow-up that will occur.* The manager should inform the employee what, if any, references will be supplied to prospective employers. Finally, it is usually best to allow the employee who has been dismissed to leave the organization immediately. If the employee continues to work on the unit after dismissal has been discussed, it can be demoralizing for all the employees who work on that unit.

Grievance Procedures

Growth can only occur when employees perceive that feedback and discipline are fair and just. When employees and managers perceive "fair" and "just" differently, the discrepancy can usually be resolved by a more formal means called a *grievance procedure*. The grievance procedure is essentially a statement of wrongdoing or a procedure to follow when one believes that a wrong has been committed. This procedure is not limited to resolving discipline discrepancies; employees can use it any time they believe that they have not been treated fairly by management. This chapter, however, focuses specifically on grievances that result from the disciplinary process. Most grievances or conflicts between employees and management can be resolved informally through communication, negotiation, compromise, and collaboration. In general, even informal resolution has well-defined steps that should be followed.

Formal Process

If the employee and management cannot resolve their differences informally, a formal grievance process begins. The steps of the formal grievance process are generally outlined in all union contracts or administrative policy and procedure manuals. In general, these steps include the progressive lodging of formal complaints up the chain of command. If resolution does not occur at any of these levels, a formal hearing is usually held. A group of people is impaneled—much in the same way as a jury to decide what should be done. Such groups are often at risk for favoring the individual employee over the all-powerful institution. This tendency reinforces the need for the manager to have clear, objective, and comprehensive written records regarding the problem employee's behavior and attempts to counsel.

Arbitration

If the differences cannot be settled through a formal grievance process, the matter may finally be resolved in a process known as arbitration. In *arbitration*, both sides agree on the selection of a *professional mediator* who will review the grievance, complete fact finding, and interview witnesses before coming to a decision.

Although grievance procedures extract a great deal of time and energy from both employees and managers, they serve several valuable purposes. Grievance procedures can settle some problems before they escalate into even larger ones. The procedures are also a source of data to focus attention on ambiguous contract language for labor–management negotiation later.

> Perhaps the most important outcome of a grievance is the legitimate opportunity that it provides for employees to resolve conflicts with their superiors.

Employees who are not given an outlet for resolving work conflicts become demoralized, angry, and dissatisfied. These emotions affect unit functioning and productivity. Even if the outcome is not in the favor of the person filing the grievance, the employee will know that the opportunity was given to present the case to an objective third party, and the chances of constructive conflict resolution are greatly increased. In addition, managers tend to be fairer and more consistent when they know that employees have a method of redress for arbitrary managerial action.

Rights and Responsibilities in Grievance Resolution

Employees and managers have some separate and distinct rights and responsibilities in grievance resolution, but many rights and responsibilities overlap. Although it is easy to be drawn into the emotionalism of a grievance that focuses on one's perceived rights, the manager and employee must remember that they both have rights and that these rights have concomitant responsibilities. For example, although both parties have the right to be heard, both parties are equally responsible to listen without interrupting. The employee has the right to a positive work environment but has the responsibility to communicate needs and discontent to the manager. The manager has the right to expect a certain level of productivity from the employee but has the responsibility to provide a work environment that makes this possible. The manager has the right to expect employees to follow rules but has the responsibility to see that these rules are clearly communicated and fairly enforced.

Both the manager and the employee must show goodwill in resolving grievances. This means that both parties must be open to discussing, negotiating, and compromising and must attempt to resolve grievances as soon as possible. The most significant goal of the grievance resolution should not be to win but to seek a resolution that satisfies both the person and the organization.

In many cases, the manager can eliminate or reduce their risk of being involved in a grievance by fostering a work environment that emphasizes clear communication and fair, constructive discipline. Employees can also eliminate or reduce their risk of being involved in a grievance by being well informed about the labor contract, policies and procedures, and organizational rules. If both the employee and the employer recognize their rights and responsibilities, the incidence of grievances in the workplace should decrease. When mutual problem solving, negotiation, and compromise are ineffective at resolving conflicts, the grievance process can provide a positive and growth-producing resolution to disciplinary conflict.

Transferring Employees

A *transfer* may be defined as a reassignment to another job within the organization. In a strict business sense, a transfer usually implies similar pay, status, and responsibility. Because of the variety of positions available for nurses in any health care organization, coupled with the lack of sufficient higher-level positions available, two additional terms have come into use: lateral transfer and downward transfer.

A *lateral transfer* describes one staff person moving to another unit, to a position with a similar scope of responsibilities, within the same organization. A *downward transfer* occurs when someone takes a position within the organization that is below their previous level. It may be in a nurse's interest to consider a downward transfer because it can increase the chances of long-term career success.

Downward transfers also should be considered when nurses are experiencing periods of stress or role overload. Self-aware nurses often request such transfers. In some circumstances, the manager may need to intervene and use a downward transfer to alleviate temporarily a nurse's overwhelming stress. Another type of downward transfer may accommodate employees in the later stages of their career. In many cases, valued employees who wish to reduce their career roles may be accommodated by a manager's assistance with locating a suitable position for their talent and stature in the profession.

> Managers often assist employees who desire a reduced or different role in their careers to locate a position that will use their talents and still allow them a degree of status.

These *accommodating transfers* generally allow someone to receive a similar salary but with a reduction in energy expenditure. For example, a long-time employee might be given a position as ombudsperson to use their expertise and knowledge of the organization and at the same time assume a status position that is less physically demanding.

Finally, there is the *inappropriate transfer*. Some managers solve unit personnel problems by transferring problem employees to another unsuspecting department. Such transfers are harmful in many ways. They contribute to decreased productivity, are demotivating for all employees, and are especially destructive for the employee who is transferred.

This is not to say that employees who do not "fit" in one department will not do well in a different environment. Before such transfers, however, both the manager and the employee must speak candidly regarding the employee's capabilities and the manager's expectations. All types of transfers should be individually evaluated for appropriateness.

> It is not uncommon for an employee to struggle in one department yet improve their performance in a new department or unit.

The Marginal Employee

Marginal employees are another type of problem employee; however, traditional discipline is generally not constructive in modifying their behavior. This is because marginal employees often make tremendous efforts to meet competencies yet usually manage to meet only minimal standards at best. All organizations have at least a few such employees. Managing these employees then is often a frustrating and tiring task.

> Marginal employees usually do not warrant dismissal, but they contribute very little to overall organizational efficiency.

Managers typically try multiple strategies to deal with marginal employees. One common strategy is simply to transfer the employee to another department, section, or unit. Although some marginal employees may be more successful on one unit than another, more commonly, the problem is simply transferred from one unit to another, and the marginal employee experiences yet another failure.

Other managers choose to dismiss marginal employees or attempt to talk them into early retirement or resignation. Again, this does little to help the marginal employee succeed. Other managers simply choose to ignore the problem and attempt to "work around" the employee. This is not always possible, however, and the result is frequently resentment from coworkers who must carry the burden of finishing work the marginal employee was unable to accomplish.

The most time-intensive option in dealing with marginal employees is *coaching*. With this strategy, the manager attempts to improve the marginal employee's performance through active coaching and counseling. Although this strategy holds the greatest promise for personal growth in the marginal employee, there is no guarantee that the employee's performance will improve or that the end results will justify the time and energy costs to the manager. The strategy chosen for dealing with the marginal employee often varies with the level of the manager. Ignoring the problem is a passive response and is more frequently used by low-level managers. High-level managers tend to employ the more active measures of coaching, transferring, and dismissal.

The nature of the organization also plays a role in determining what strategy is used to deal with the marginal employee. Government-controlled organizations are more likely to use passive measures, whereas managers in nongovernmental organizations are more likely to use active measures. The size of the organization also influences how managers deal with the marginally productive employee. In larger organizations, the trend has been toward passive managerial coping strategies with marginal employees.

It is important for the manager to remember that each person and situation is different and that the most appropriate strategy depends on many variables. Looking at past performance will help determine if the employee is tired, needs educational or training opportunities, is unmotivated, or just has very little energy and only marginal skills for the job. If the latter is true, then the employee may never become more than a marginal employee, no matter what management functions and leadership skills are brought into play.

Learning Exercise 25.5, which has been solved for the reader (see Appendix), depicts alternatives that managers may consider in dealing with the marginal employee.

LEARNING EXERCISE 25.5

The Marginal Employee

You are the supervisor of a long-term acute care hospital. There are 35 beds on your unit that are usually full. It is an extremely busy unit, and your nursing staff needs high-level assessment and communication skills for providing patient care. Because the nursing care needs on this floor are unique and because you use primary nursing, it has been very difficult in the past to find outside staffing when additional staffing is required. Although you have been able to keep the unit adequately staffed on a day-to-day basis, there are two open positions for registered nurses (RNs) on your unit that have been unfilled for almost 3 months.

Historically, your staff members have been excellent employees. They enjoy their work and are highly productive. Unit morale has been exceptionally good. However, in the last 3 months, the staff has begun complaining about Judy, a full-time employee who has been with the unit for about 4 months. Judy has been an RN for approximately 15 years. References from former employers identified Judy's work as competent, although little other information was given. At Judy's 6-week and 3-month performance appraisals, you coached her regarding her barely adequate work habits, assessment and communication skills, and decision making. Judy responded that she would attempt to work on improving her performance in these areas because working with this unit was one of her highest career goals.

Although Judy has been receptive to your coaching and has verbalized to you her efforts to improve her performance, there has been little observable difference in her behavior. You have slowly concluded that Judy is probably currently working at the highest level of her capability and that she is a marginal employee at best. The other nurses believe that Judy is not carrying her share of the workload and have asked that you remove her from the unit.

ASSIGNMENT:

Use the traditional problem-solving process to help you resolve this issue. Compare your solution to the one in Appendix.

The Impaired Employee/Substance Use Disorder

In this chapter, impairment in nursing refers to the nurse being unable to perform their professional responsibilities and duties consistent with expected nursing standards. This chapter focuses on nurses who are impaired due to SUD.

> Nursing administrators may face no management problem more costly or emotionally draining than that of nurses whose practice is impaired by substance use disorder.

Prevalence of SUD in Nursing

Modlin and Montes (1964) first documented SUD in the health professions in studies in the late 1940s, although public recognition of the problem did not really begin until the early 1980s. Despite this relatively recent examination of the problem of substance use in nursing, there is little doubt that SUD has been around as long as alcohol and drugs have been.

Huston and Lillibridge (2023) note, however, that efforts to quantify the prevalence of SUD in nursing are fraught with problems including the stigma, shame, and denial commonly associated with substance use. Estimates often suggest the prevalence of SUD in nursing mirrors or slightly exceeds statistics from the general population. The National Council of State Boards of Nursing agrees, but notes that increased access to controlled substances may contribute to higher incidences of drug dependence (Nyhus, 2021).

How many nurses struggle with SUD? The Recovery Village (2022) estimates that approximately 10% to 15% of nurses are impaired by or recovering from SUD, including alcohol addiction, a figure commonly found in the literature. Similarly, Taylor (2020) notes that SUD is the principal cause of professional impairment for certified registered nurse anesthetists (CRNAs), with one of every 10 experiencing addiction to drugs or alcohol. Some researchers, however, suggest the numbers are higher.

> Given current estimates of impaired nursing practice, it is likely that at least 1 out of every 10 nurses you work with will struggle with a substance use problem.

Nurses turn to drugs or alcohol for many reasons. Co-occurring disorders, such as depression and posttraumatic stress disorder, and genetics contribute to substance use as do fatigue and stress (Gonzales, 2020). Some nurses are subject to workplace bullying and verbal abuse, contributing to stress and feelings of powerlessness. All these issues place nurses at greater risk.

In addition, some nurses believe they are invulnerable; that as caregivers, they can safely self-diagnose and self-medicate. Compounding the problem is that health care providers have relatively easy access to controlled substances and other drugs of abuse.

One common difference, however, between health professionals with SUD and other people with addictions is that health professionals often obtain their drugs of choice through channels such as legitimate prescriptions that were written for them or diversionary measures on the job rather than purchasing them illegally on the street. This is because health professionals have greater access to undiverted medications themselves.

Drug Diversion

Drug *diversion* occurs when medication is redirected from its intended destination for personal use, sale, or distribution to others. Thus, it includes drug theft and use of tampering (adulteration or substitution). The risk of diversion to patients is unrelieved pain, inadequate care from impaired health care workers, and risk of infections such as hepatitis C from contaminated syringes (Nyhus, 2021).

COMMON METHODS OF DRUG DIVERSION

- Administration of only partial doses for patients
- Removal of PRN medications designated for patients or pulling duplicate doses
- Removal of medications designated for a discharged patient
- Removal of fentanyl patches
- Removal of medication without an order
- Creating false verbal orders
- Removal under a colleague's sign-on
- Substitution of a noncontrolled substance (like saline) for a controlled substance
- Theft of patient medications brought from home
- Failure to waste when indicated or falsely noting the wasting of entire doses
- Stealing from sharps containers

Morris (2020) suggests there are many ways in which drugs can be diverted by health care providers, including removing medications of discharged patients; taking medications from pumps, drips, or discarded vials in sharps containers; removing larger doses of medication when a smaller dose is available; not documenting administration or waste of medications; utilizing unnecessary overrides to obtain medications; or stealing medications for personal use from a lockbox or cabinet, never intending to administer them to patients. The methods continue with theft of home medications, removal under a colleague's sign-in, diluting a dose with water or saline, removal of duplicate doses, and substitution of a dose with other medication, water, or saline (Morris, 2020). Display 25.4 lists some of the common methods of drug diversion.

Strategies to address the problem of drug diversion include strict adherence to best practices regarding the observed wasting of controlled substances and using controlled substances in doses that minimize the need to waste at all. In addition, providers should avoid wide range orders for controlled substances that can promote waste and be alert for recurrent documentation that suggests a provider is wasting large amounts of narcotics.

Nyhus (2021) suggests that drug diversion in health care is a serious matter; however, convincing nurses of this is challenging because the problem is substantially underestimated, undetected, and underreported. It is a felony, however, that can result in criminal prosecution and loss of licensure. Indeed, Nyhus (2021) notes that the outcomes of drug diversion are commonly damaged careers, civil and criminal penalties, infectious disease outbreaks, severe patient harm, and death. In addition, health care organizations bear the burden of fines for failed safeguards, loss of eligibility for Medicare reimbursement, and compromised public trust.

Commonly Misused or Abused Drugs

Although alcohol is the most frequently misused substance, *opioid pain relievers*, such as Vicodin or OxyContin; *stimulants* for treating attention deficit hyperactivity disorder, such as Adderall, Concerta, or Ritalin; and *central nervous system depressants* for relieving anxiety, such as Valium or Xanax, are the three classes of prescription drugs mostly commonly misused (National Institute on Drug Abuse, 2020). Barbiturates may also replace alcohol in the workplace so that the employee may feel a similar effect without having alcohol detectable on their breath. Indeed, nearly 7% of nurses use prescription drugs for nonmedical purposes, a rate higher than the national average (Gonzales, 2020).

It is the overuse of opioids, however, that has become a leading cause of injury and death due to drug overdose in the United States. The National Institute on Drug Abuse (2021) notes that in 2019, nearly 50,000 people in the United States died from opioid-involved overdoses. In addition, roughly 21% to 29% of patients prescribed opioids for chronic pain misuse them and between 8% and 12% develop an opioid use disorder (National Institute on Drug Abuse, 2021).

In addition, over the past few years, the opioid death toll has been exacerbated by other synthetic opioids, most notably illicit fentanyl and heroin. About 80% of people who use heroin first misused prescription opioids (National Institute on Drug Abuse, 2021). Clearly, the misuse of and addiction to opioids—including prescription pain relievers, heroin, and synthetic opioids such as fentanyl—is a serious national crisis that affects public health as well as social and economic welfare (National Institute on Drug Abuse, 2021).

Recognizing the Employee with Substance Use Disorder

Although most nurses have finely tuned assessment skills for identifying patient problems, they may be less sensitive to behaviors and actions that may signify SUD in their coworkers. In addition, it may be difficult to find a balance between vigilance and being overly suspicious. An isolated incident may not indicate SUD directly, but the occurrence of several incidents should be documented.

Sensitivity to others and to the environment is a leadership skill. The profile of the nurse with SUD may vary greatly, although several behavior patterns and changes are noted frequently. These behavior changes can be grouped into three primary areas: personality/behavior changes, job performance changes, and time and attendance changes. Display 25.5 shows characteristics of these categories.

As the employee progresses further into drug and alcohol dependency, managers can more easily recognize these behaviors. Typically, in the earliest stages, the employee uses the

---

DISPLAY 25.5 CHARACTERISTIC CHANGES IN EMPLOYEES WITH SUD

Changes in Personality or Behaviors
- Increased irritability with patients and colleagues, often followed by extreme calm
- Social isolation; eats alone, avoids unit social functions
- Extreme and rapid mood swings
- Euphoric recall of events or elaborate excuses for behaviors
- Unusually strong interest in narcotics or the narcotic cabinet
- Sudden dramatic change in personal grooming or any other area
- Forgetfulness ranging from simple short-term memory loss to blackouts
- Change in physical appearance, which may include weight loss, flushed face, red or bleary eyes, unsteady gait, slurred speech, tremors, restlessness, diaphoresis, bruises and cigarette burns, jaundice, and ascites
- Extreme defensiveness regarding medication errors

Changes in Job Performance
- Difficulty meeting schedules and deadlines
- Illogical or sloppy charting
- High frequency of medication errors or errors in judgment affecting patient care
- Frequently volunteers to be medication nurse
- Has a high number of assigned patients who complain that their pain medication is ineffective in relieving their pain
- Consistently meeting work performance requirements at minimal levels or doing the minimum amount of work necessary
- Judgment errors
- Sleeping or dozing on duty
- Complaints from other staff members about the quality and quantity of the employee's work
- Disappears from the work area for long periods of time or may spend long periods of time in the bathroom or around the medication cart

continues on page 686

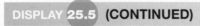

DISPLAY 25.5 (CONTINUED)

Changes in Attendance and Use of Time

- Increasingly absent from work without adequate explanation or notification; most frequent absence on a Monday or Friday
- Long lunch hours
- Excessive use of sick leave or requests for sick leave after days off
- Frequent calling in to request compensatory time
- Arriving at work early or staying late for no apparent reason
- Consistent lateness
- Frequent disappearances from the unit without explanation

addictive substance primarily for pleasure, and although the alcohol or drug use is excessive, it is primarily recreational and social. Thus, substance use usually does not occur during work hours, although some secondary effects of its use may be apparent.

As addiction deepens, the employee develops tolerance to the substance and must use greater quantities more frequently to achieve the same effect. At this point, the person has made a conscious lifestyle decision to use drugs or alcohol. There is a high use of defense mechanisms, such as justifying, denying, and bargaining about that choice. Often, the employee in this stage begins to use the substance both at and away from work. Work performance generally declines in the areas of attendance, judgment, quality, and interpersonal relationships. An appreciable decline in unit morale, resulting from an unreliable and unproductive worker, becomes apparent.

In the final stages of SUD, the employee must continually use the substance, even though they no longer gain pleasure or gratification. Physically and psychologically addicted, the employee generally harbors a total disregard for self and others. Because the need for the substance is so great, the employee's personal and professional lives focus on the need for drugs or alcohol, and the employee becomes unpredictable and undependable in the work area. Assignments are incomplete or not done at all, charting may be sloppy or illegible, and frequent judgment errors occur. Because the employee in this stage must use the substance frequently, signs of drug use during work hours may be seen. Narcotic vials are missing. The employee may be absent from the unit for brief periods with no plausible excuse. Mood swings are excessive, and the employee often looks physically ill.

The bottom line is that employees with SUD should be removed from the work setting long before they reach this stage. The reality, however, is that the identification of SUD is often very difficult. Nursing school courses generally focus on the physiologic effects of alcohol and other drugs, dealing little with the psychological process of addiction and even less with SUD in nurses. Because of this limited knowledge, many nurses feel ill prepared to deal with SUD and choose to ignore it or hope it will go away. Indeed, research by Trinkoff et al. (2021) found that despite being able to accurately identify signs and symptoms of SUD, only 50% of nurses expressed confidence in their ability to identify colleagues with potential SUD and only 44% said they would report a nurse with a SUD to the state board (see Examining the Evidence 25.1). This compromises patient safety and violates professional behavior expectations.

Indeed, if a Board of Nursing finds that an employee's impairment was well known to other licensees and no report was made, the Board may move to also investigate the compliance to the Nurse Practice Act of all those who knew but did not come forward to protect the public. In addition, the American Nurses Association (2015) Code of Ethics (Code 3.6) suggests that the nurse must be vigilant in protecting the public and intervening when a colleague's practice appears to be impaired.

Trinkoff et al. (2021) note that education is needed to stress the benefits of recognition and assistance for nurses with SUDs, as opposed to an incorrect belief that letting SUDs go unaddressed is preferable for the affected nurse. Creating a culture of safety and accountability could help nurses feel more comfortable reporting signs of SUDs among their coworkers.

EXAMINING THE EVIDENCE 25.1

Source: From Trinkoff, A. M., Yoon, J. M., Selby, V. L., Storr, C. L., Edwin, H. S., & Baek, H. (2021, October). Registered nurses' awareness of workplace signs, actions, and interventions for nurses with substance use disorder. *Journal of Nursing Regulation, 12*(3), 20–29. https://www.sciencedirect.com/science/article/abs/pii/S2155825621001137

Recognizing and Reporting SUD in Nursing Colleagues

A mixed modes survey (online, mailed) was conducted between November 2020 and February 2021, with randomly selected RNs in nine states being contacted up to six times. Of the 1,215 surveys returned (31% response rate), 1,170 were included in the analyses. Measures of potential workplace signs of SUD (seven items), actions one would take (seven items), and attitudes toward RN SUD interventions (ten items) were assessed, and prevalence of these items was described.

Most RNs (82%) correctly selected frequent medication errors, medication wasting, and frequent absences/breaks as potential signs of substance use problems, yet only half felt confident in their ability to identify a colleague with SUD. Although the majority (93%) would tell a supervisor, higher proportions of younger (aged <45 years) and Asian nurses reported feeling unsure of what to do and were more afraid to get involved with nurse substance use problems than older nurses and nurses of other races/ethnicities. One of the concerns expressed by most nurses (58.5%) was their worry that a colleague with a SUD could be fired or punished.

Overall, 44% said they would report a nurse with a SUD to the state board, with adult primary care (65%), administration (62%), and multi-specialty (57%) having the highest proportion of those agreeing they would report to the board. The lowest proportion of those agreeing they would report to the board were the specialties of psychiatry (33%), case management (33%), and palliative care and oncology (33%).

Variation in recognition and actions were also found for workplace factors. Charge nurses were more likely to think that nurses with a potential SUD should have their license revoked than those in the reference group (educators/researchers). Yet, most nurses reported favorable opinions of a nurse's ability to succeed in treatment and to re-enter practice, and they preferred supportive over punitive descriptions of impaired nurses.

The researchers concluded that education is needed to stress the benefits of recognition and assistance for nurses with SUD, as opposed to an incorrect belief that letting SUD go unaddressed is preferable for the affected nurse. Creating a culture of safety and accountability could help nurses feel more comfortable reporting signs of SUD among their coworkers.

> Nurses have both a legal and moral imperative to report suspected SUD in a colleague to protect patient safety.

Confronting the Employee with Substance Use Disorder

Unlike most alcoholics or intravenous narcotic users, health care professionals do not achieve tacit peer acceptance of their addictive behavior. Thus, physicians and nurses are much less likely to admit, even to colleagues, that they are using—much less that they are addicted to—a controlled substance. Frequently, they deny their impairment even to themselves.

This self-denial is perpetuated because nurses and managers traditionally have been slow to recognize and reluctant to help these colleagues. Huston and Lillibridge (2023) agree, noting that it is a difficult and often traumatic experience for a nurse to report an impaired peer. The important considerations are that patients are not harmed, the nurse is helped, and the provider is protected.

The first step in dealing with the impaired employee actually occurs before the confrontation process. In the data- or evidence-gathering phase, the manager collects as much hard evidence as possible to document suspicions of SUD in the employee. All behavior, work performance, and time and attendance changes presented in the displays in this chapter should be noted objectively and recorded in writing. If possible, a second person should be asked to validate the manager's observations. In suspected drug addiction, the manager also may examine unit narcotic records for inconsistencies and check to see that the amount of narcotic the nurse signed out for each patient is the same as the amount ordered for that patient.

Griffith et al. (2021) suggest that when a suspicion is reported, the leader-manager may also choose to follow up with coworkers and obtain separate witness statements from those who interacted with the nurse during the alleged impairment. Additional details may be given regarding the nurse's physical appearance or behaviors indicative of SUD. These witnesses should submit their own statements, either handwritten or by e-mail, describing their observations as close to the event as possible. If handwritten, the witness statement should be legible, dated, and signed with their name printed on the document. In addition, patients may be interviewed regarding their pain management and potential receipt of medications, and this information should be compared to the documentation in the medical record. In addition, the leader-manager may want to inspect surrounding areas, such as bathrooms and wastebaskets, where the nurse was at the time and document any abnormal findings.

Because few nurses drink alcohol while on duty, managers must observe for more subtle clues, such as the smell of alcohol on the employee's breath. If the organization's policy allows for it, the manager may wish to require an employee suspected of SUD to undergo immediate drug or alcohol testing. If the employee refuses to cooperate, the organization's policy for documenting and reporting this incident should be followed.

> Proving alcohol impairment is often more difficult than detecting drug impairment, as an employee may be able to hide alcoholism more easily than drug addiction.

If at any time the manager suspects that an employee is impaired and thus presents a potential hazard to patient safety, the employee must be immediately removed from the work environment. The manager should decisively and unemotionally tell the employee that they will not be allowed to return to the work area because of the manager's perception that the employee is impaired. The manager should arrange for the employee to be taken home so that they do not drive while impaired. A formal meeting to discuss this incident should be scheduled within the next 24 hours.

This type of direct confrontation between the manager and the employee is the second phase in dealing with the employee suspected of SUD. Although some employees admit their problem when directly confronted, most use defense mechanisms (including denial) because they may not have admitted the problem to themselves. Indeed, individuals with a history of substance use have often become quite good at deception regarding their drug use.

Denial and anger should be expected in the confrontation. If the employee denies having a problem, documented evidence demonstrating a decline in work performance should be shared. The manager must be careful to keep the confrontation focused on the employee's performance deficits and not allow the discussion to be directed to the cause of the underlying problem or addiction. These are issues and concerns that the manager is unable to address. The manager also must be careful not to preach, moralize, scold, or blame.

Confrontation always should occur before the problem escalates too far. However, in some situations, the manager may have only limited direct evidence but still may believe that the employee should be confronted because of rapidly declining employee performance or unit morale. There is, however, a greater risk that confrontation at this point may be unsuccessful in terms of helping the employee. If direct confrontation is unsuccessful, it may have been too early; the employee may not have been desperate enough or may still be in denial. In these situations, job performance will probably continue to be marginal or unsatisfactory, and progressive discipline may be necessary. If the employee continues to deny SUD and work performance continues to be unsatisfactory despite repeated constructive confrontation, dismissal may be necessary.

The last phase of the confrontation process is outlining the organization's plan or expectations for the employee in overcoming SUD. This plan is like the disciplinary contract in that it is usually written down and clearly outlines the rehabilitative measures that should be undertaken by the employee and consequences if remedial action is not sought. Although the employee is generally referred informally by the manager to outside sources to help deal with the impairment, the employee is responsible for correcting their work deficiencies. Timelines are included in the plan, and the manager and employee must agree on and sign a copy of the contract.

The Manager's Role in Assisting the Employee with SUD

Clearly, the incidence of SUD in health professionals is substantial. On a personal level, a person suffers from an illness that may go undetected and untreated for many years. On a professional level, the employee with SUD affects the entire health care system. Nurses with impaired skills and judgment jeopardize patient care. The impaired nurse also compromises teamwork and continuity as colleagues attempt to pick up the slack for their impaired team member. The personal and professional cost of SUD demands that nursing leaders and managers recognize these employees as early as possible and intervene.

Because of the general nature of nursing, many managers find themselves wanting to nurture the impaired employee, much as they would any other person who is sick. However, this nurturing can quickly become enabling. The employee who already has a greatly diminished sense of self-esteem and a perceived loss of self-control may ask the manager to participate actively in their recovery. This is one of the most difficult aspects of working with the impaired employee. Others who have greater expertise and objectivity should assume this role.

> The manager must be very careful not to assume the role of counselor or treatment provider for the impaired nurse.

LEARNING EXERCISE 25.6

Personal Reflection on SUD

Write a two-page essay that speaks to the following: Has your personal or professional life been affected by a person with SUD? In what ways have you been affected? Has it colored the way that you view SUD and impairment? Do you believe that you can separate your personal feelings about SUD from the actions that you must take as a manager in working with impaired employees? Have you ever suspected a work colleague of SUD? What, if anything, did you do about it? If you did suspect a colleague, would you approach them with your suspicions before talking to the unit manager? Describe the risks involved in this situation.

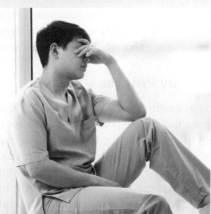

LEARNING EXERCISE 25.7

Working Under the Influence

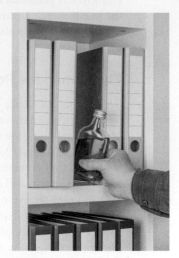

There have been rumors for some time that Mr. Clark, one of the night nurses on the unit you supervise, has been coming to work under the influence of alcohol. Fellow staff have reported the odor of alcohol on his breath, and one staff member stated that his speech is often slurred. The night supervisor states that she believes, "This is not my problem," and your night charge nurse has never been on duty when Mr. Clark has shown this behavior. This morning, one of the patients whispered to you that he thought Mr. Clark had been drinking when he came to work last night. When you question the patient further, he states, "Mr. Clark seemed to perform his nursing duties okay, but he made me nervous." You have decided that you must talk with Mr. Clark. You call him at his home and ask him to come to your office at 3:00 PM.

ASSIGNMENT:

Determine how you are going to approach Mr. Clark. Outline your plan and provide rationale for your choices. What flexibility have you built into your plan? How much of your documentation will be shared with Mr. Clark?

The manager also must be careful not to feel the need to diagnose the cause of the SUD or to justify its existence. Protecting patients must be the top priority, taking precedence over any tendency to protect or excuse subordinates. The manager's role is to clearly identify performance expectations for the employee and to confront the employee when those expectations are not met. This is not to say that the manager should not be humanistic in recognizing the problem as a disease and not a disciplinary problem or that they should be unwilling to refer the employee for needed help. Although the manager may suggest appropriate help or refer the impaired employee to someone, a manager's primary responsibility is to protect patients and then to see that the employee becomes functional again and can meet organizational expectations before returning to work.

The manager can play a vital role in creating an environment that decreases the chances of SUD in the work setting. This may be done by controlling or reducing work-related stressors whenever possible and by providing mechanisms for employee stress management. The manager also should control drug accessibility by implementing, enforcing, and monitoring policies and procedures related to medication distribution. Finally, the manager should provide opportunities for the staff to learn about substance abuse, its detection, and available resources to help those who are impaired.

The Recovery Process

Although most authorities suggest different names or numbers of steps in the recovery process, they do agree that certain phases or progressive observable behaviors suggest that the person is recovering from SUD. In the first phase, the impaired employee continues to deny the significance or severity of the SUD but does reduce or suspend substance use to appease family, peers, or managers. These employees hope to reestablish their substance use in the future.

In the second phase, as denial subsides, the impaired employee begins to see that the addiction is having a negative impact on their life and begins to want to change. Frequently, people in this phase are buoyed with hope and commitment but lack maturity about the struggles they will face. This phase generally lasts for about 3 months.

During the third phase, the person examines their values and coping skills and works to develop more effective coping skills. Frequently, this is done by aligning themselves with support groups that reinforce a substance-free lifestyle. In this stage, the person realizes how sick they were in the active stage of the disease and is often fraught with feelings of humiliation and shame.

In the last phase, people gain self-awareness regarding why they developed SUD, and they develop coping skills that will help them deal more effectively with stressors. As a result of this, self-awareness, self-esteem, and self-respect increase. When this happens, the person can decide consciously whether they wish to or should return to the workplace.

State Board of Nursing Treatment Programs

Although SUD can impair nurses' physical, psychological, social, and professional functioning, the problem was largely ignored until the late 1970s and early 1980s. Since that time, assistance occurs primarily in the form of *diversion programs* (also called *intervention or peer assistance* programs). A diversion program is generally a voluntary, confidential program for nurses whose practice may be impaired due to SUD.

The goal of a diversion program is to protect the public by early identification of impaired nurses and by providing these nurses access to appropriate intervention programs and treatment services. Public safety is protected by immediate suspension of practice, when needed, and by ongoing careful monitoring of the nurse.

Several factors have led state boards to adopt diversion programs. First, a punitive system creates barriers to reporting and keeps impaired nurses from getting help. Nurse colleagues or practitioners who suspect a nurse is impaired may well hesitate to report something that could cost a nurse their job and license. In addition, from an employer's standpoint, the fear of litigation often makes it easier to dismiss a nurse without charges of misconduct. But this practice leaves the nurse, who is at risk for self-harm and for harming patients, free to seek work elsewhere. A board investigation can take months to 2 years, during which time the nurse in question may be able to continue working without restraint. Moving to another state will not, however, allow the nurse to avoid disciplinary action, and states typically consider this in granting license reciprocity.

Diversion programs are voluntary and confidential. Besides helping the nurse with recovery, the programs aid the employers and staff in coping with employee substance use. Impaired nurses who refuse participation in diversion programs are subject to disciplinary review by their State Board of Nursing and possible license revocation. Nurse leader-managers should advocate for those who are impaired so that they receive appropriate assistance, treatment, and access to fair institutional and legal processes.

LEARNING EXERCISE 25.8

Researching Your State Board of Nursing's Recovery Program

Determine if your State Board of Nursing offers some type of recovery program for nurses with SUD. You may either call the board or use the internet. Research the following questions:

- Is the program voluntary and confidential?
- What is the rate of recidivism?
- What types of monitoring mechanisms are in place?
- What is the duration of the program?
- Are nurses allowed to continue practicing while completing the treatment program?
- Are there practice restrictions?

   ASSIGNMENT:

   Write a one-page report of your findings.

The fear of being ostracized by their colleagues has kept many nurses from seeking help even though they knew they were addicted to drugs. Indeed, negative and stigmatizing attitudes continue to surround most individuals experiencing drug and alcohol dependency, and this is accentuated for the nursing professional, who is often held to an even higher standard of behavior. Huston and Lillibridge (2023) suggest that while nursing is a profession known for its caring nature toward others, we often fail to care for ourselves. Huston and Lillibridge (2023) go on to say that employers must create positive work environments, know their employees so that confrontation can occur early, increase awareness about substance abuse so that nurses are not afraid to ask for help, ensure that an *Impaired Practice Policy* is in place, and provide a process that facilitates reentry into practice following recovery.

The Impaired Employee's Reentry to the Workplace

Because nurses with SUD recover at varying rates, predicting how long this process will take is difficult. Many experts believe that impaired employees must devote at least 1 year to their recovery without the stresses of drug availability, overtime, and shift rotation. Success in reentering the workforce depends on factors such as the extent of the recovery process and individual circumstances.

> Although managers must show a genuine personal interest in their employee's rehabilitation, their primary role is to be sure that the employee understands the organization's right to insist on unimpaired performance in the workplace.

For the employee, return to work usually entails a comprehensive return-to-work agreement or contract with the organization. These *last chance agreements* (LCAs) outline the terms and conditions under which the nurse can return to work. Bettinardi-Angres (2020, p. 8) notes that these "LCAs are gifts to recovering nurses from employers and/or state because it prevents their termination and avoids disciplinary action against their licenses if they adhere to the terms. Most state [boards] will honor the LCA and allow the nurse to continue to practice if there is compliance with all recommendations."

In addition, though standardized guidelines do not exist for reentry guidelines, there are some general guidelines that should be considered by all employers when a recovered nurse returns to work (Display 25.6). Mandatory drug testing, however, does invoke questions about privacy rights and generally should not be implemented without advice from human resources personnel or legal counsel.

Humanistic leaders recognize the intrinsic self-worth of each individual employee and strive to understand the unique needs these workers have. If the leader genuinely cares about

---

DISPLAY 25.6 COMMONLY ACCEPTED REENTRY GUIDELINES FOR THE RECOVERING NURSE

- No psychoactive drug use will be tolerated.
- The employee should be assigned to day shift for the first year.
- The employee should be paired with a successfully recovered nurse whenever possible.
- The employee should be willing to consent to random urine screening with toxicology or alcohol screens.
- The employee must give evidence of continuing involvement with support groups such as Alcoholics Anonymous and Narcotics Anonymous. Employees should be encouraged to attend meetings several times each week.
- The employee should be encouraged to participate in a structured aftercare program.
- The employee should be encouraged to seek individual counseling or therapy as needed.

DISPLAY 25.7	ISSUES TO CONSIDER WHEN THE RECOVERED NURSE RETURNS TO WORK

- Should the nurse returning to work following rehabilitation have their practice limited or restricted in some way, such as no exposure to the drug of choice or no access to controlled substances for a period of time?
- How long does the board of nursing have a right to invade the privacy of a recovered nurse?
- Where does the organizational responsibility end?
- Who bears the cost if the recovered nurse is not able to return to work at full capacity?
- Can confidentiality be maintained?
- Should the nurse be allowed to work in stressful practice areas?
- Should the nurse initially be allowed to work fulltime?

and shows interest in each employee, employees learn to trust, and the helping relationship has a chance to begin.

In addition, there are important questions that must be asked or things that must be considered before return to work (Display 25.7). These issues include whether the nurse's practice is limited or restricted in some way, how long the nursing board has a right to invade the nurse's privacy to ensure that recovery is ongoing, where organizational responsibility ends, and who bears the cost if the recovered nurse is not able to return to work at full capacity.

Managers have the responsibility to be proactive in identifying and confronting employees with SUD. Prompt and appropriate intervention by managers is essential for positive outcomes. Organizations have an ethical responsibility to actively assist these employees to return as productive members of the workforce.

Integrating Leadership Roles and Management Functions When Dealing with Problem Employees

The leader recognizes that all employees have intrinsic worth and assists them in reaching their maximal potential. Because individual abilities, achievement drives, and situations vary, the leader recognizes each employee as an individual with unique needs and intervenes according to those specific needs. In some situations, such as frequent rule breaking, discipline may be the most effective tool for ensuring that employees succeed.

In the case of the employee with SUD, there is a need to balance the concern for patient safety with concern for the health of the employee (Huston & Lillibridge, 2023). Assisting the employee to get the treatment needed is a primary leadership responsibility. Effective management, however, demands that organizations take an active role in ensuring patient safety by immediately removing employees with SUD from the work setting. Yet, leader-managers also have a responsibility to help these employees deal with their disease so that they can return to the workforce in the future as productive employees.

Constructive discipline then requires leadership and management skills. In administering discipline, the leader actively shapes group norms and promotes self-discipline. The leader also is a supporter, motivator, enabler, and coach. The humanistic attributes of the leadership role make employees want to follow the rules of the leader and thus the organization. In dealing with the marginal employee, the leader serves more as a coach and resource person than as a counselor, disciplinarian, or authority figure.

The manager, however, must enforce established rules, policies, and procedures, and although good managerial practice greatly reduces the need for discipline, some employees still need external direction and discipline to accomplish organizational goals. Discipline allows employees to clearly understand the expectations of the organization and the penalty for failing to meet those expectations. The manager's primary obligation is to see that patient safety is assured and that productivity is adequate to meet unit goals. The manager uses the authority inherent in their position to provide positive and negative sanctions for employee behavior to meet these goals.

The effective leader-manager blends these unit productivity needs and human resource needs; however, selecting and implementing appropriate strategies to meet both goals is difficult. The leader-manager believes that each employee has the potential to be a successful and valuable member of the unit and intervenes accordingly to meet each employee's special needs.

Key Concepts

- It is essential that managers can distinguish between employees who need progressive discipline and those who have SUD or who are marginal employees so that the employee can be managed in the most appropriate manner.
- Discipline is a necessary and positive tool in promoting subordinate growth.
- The optimal goal in constructive discipline is assisting employees to behave in a manner that allows them to be self-directed in meeting organizational goals.
- To ensure fairness, rules should include McGregor's "hot stove" components of forewarning, immediate application, consistency, and impartiality.
- If a rule or regulation is worth having, it should be enforced. When rule breaking is allowed to go unpunished, groups generally adjust to and replicate the low-level performance of the rule breaker.
- As few rules and regulations as possible should exist in the organization; all rules, regulations, and policies should be regularly reviewed to see if they should be deleted or modified in some way.
- Except for the most serious infractions, discipline should be administered in progressive steps, which include verbal admonishment, written admonishment, suspension, and dismissal.
- In performance deficiency coaching, the manager actively brings areas of unacceptable behavior or performance to the attention of the employee and works with them to establish a short-term plan to correct deficiencies.
- The grievance procedure is essentially a statement of wrongdoing or a procedure to follow when one believes that a wrong has been committed. All employees should have the right to file grievances about disciplinary action that they believe has been arbitrary or unfair in some way.
- The presence of a union generally entails more procedural, legalistic safeguards for administering discipline and a well-defined grievance process for employees who believe that they have been disciplined unfairly.
- Because SUD is a disease, traditional progressive discipline is inappropriate because it cannot result in employee growth.
- The profile of the impaired nurse may vary greatly, although typically, behavior changes are seen in three areas: personality/behavior changes, job performance changes, and time and attendance changes.
- Nurses and managers traditionally have been slow to recognize and respond to colleagues impaired by SUD.
- Confronting an employee who is suspected of SUD should always occur before the problem escalates and before patient safety is jeopardized.
- The manager should not assume the role of counselor or treatment provider or feel the need to diagnose the cause of the employee with SUD. The manager's role is to clearly identify performance expectations for the employee and to confront the employee when those expectations are not met.
- The goal of a diversion program is to protect the public by early identification of impaired nurses and by providing these nurses access to appropriate intervention programs and treatment services.
- Strategies for dealing with marginal employees vary with management level, the nature of the health care organization, and the current prevailing attitude toward passive or active intervention.

Additional Learning Exercises and Applications

LEARNING EXERCISE 25.9

Determining an Appropriate Action When Proof Is Unavailable

You are the supervisor of a pediatric acute care unit. One of your patients, Joey, is a 5-year-old boy who sustained 30% third-degree burns, which have been grafted and are now healing. He has been a patient in the unit for approximately 2 months. His mother stays with him nearly all the waking hours and generally is supportive of both him and the staff.

In the last few weeks, Joey has begun expressing increasing frustration with basic nursing tasks, has frequently been uncooperative, and, in your staff's opinion, has become very manipulative. His mother is frustrated with Joey's behavior but believes that it is understandable given the trauma he has experienced. She has begun working with the staff on a mutually acceptable behavior modification program.

Although you have attempted to assign the same nurses to care for Joey as often as possible, it is not possible today. This lack of continuity is especially frustrating because the night shift has reported frequent tantrums and uncooperative behavior. The nurse whom you have assigned to Joey is Monica. She is a good nurse but has lacked patience in the past with uncooperative patients. During the morning, you are aware that Joey is continuing to act out. Although Monica begins to look more and more harried, she states that she is handling the situation appropriately.

When you return from lunch, Joey's mother is waiting at your office. She furiously reports that Joey told her that Monica hit him and told him he was "a very bad boy" after his mother had gone to lunch. His mother believes that physical punishment was totally inappropriate, and she wants this nurse to be fired. She also states that she has contacted Joey's physician and that he is on his way over.

You call Monica to your office where she emphatically denies all the allegations. Monica states that during the lunch hour, Joey refused to allow her to check his dressings and that she followed the behavior modification plan and discontinued his television privileges. She believes that his accusations further reflect his manipulative behavior. You then approach Joey, who tearfully and emphatically repeats the story that he told to his mother. He is consistent about the details and swears to his mother that he is telling the truth. None of your staff was within hearing range of Joey's room at the time of the alleged incident. When Joey's doctor arrives, he demands that action be taken.

ASSIGNMENT:

Determine your action. You do not have proof to substantiate either Monica's or Joey's story. You believe that Monica is capable of the charges but are reluctant to implement any type of discipline without proof. What factors contribute the most to your decision?

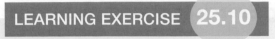

LEARNING EXERCISE 25.10

What Type of Discipline Is Appropriate?

Susie has been a registered nurse on your medical-surgical unit for 18 months. During that time, she has been competent in terms of her assessment and organizational skills and her skills mastery. Her work habits, however, need improvement. She frequently arrives 5 to 10 minutes late for work and disrupts report when she arrives. She also frequently extends her lunch break 10 minutes beyond the allotted 30 minutes. Her absence rate is twice that of most of your other employees. You have informally counseled Susie about her work habits on numerous past occasions. Last month, you issued a written reprimand about these work deficiencies and placed it in Susie's personnel file. Susie acknowledged at that time that she needed to work on these areas but that her responsibilities as a single parent were overwhelming at times and that she felt demotivated at work. Every day this week, Susie has arrived 15 minutes late. The staff are complaining about Susie's poor attitude and have asked that you take action.

You contemplate what additional action you might take. The next step in progressive discipline would be a suspension without pay. You believe that this action could be supported given the previous attempts to counsel the employee without improvement. You also realize that many of your staff are closely watching your actions to see how you will handle this situation. You also recognize that suspending Susie would leave her with no other means of financial support and that this penalty is somewhat uncommon for the offenses described. In addition, you are unsure if this penalty will make any difference in modifying Susie's behavior.

ASSIGNMENT:

Decide what type of discipline, if any, is appropriate for Susie. Support your decision with appropriate rationale. Discuss your actions in terms of the effects on you, Susie, and the department.

LEARNING EXERCISE 25.11

Discipline and Insubordination

You are the coordinator of a small, specialized respiratory rehabilitation unit. Two other nurses work with you. Because all the staff are professionals, you have used a very democratic approach to management and leadership. This approach has worked well, and productivity has always been high. The nurses work out schedules so that there are always two nurses on duty during the week, and they take turns covering the weekends, at which time there is only one registered nurse (RN) on duty. With this arrangement, it is possible for three nurses to be on duty 1 day during the week, if there is no holiday or other time off scheduled by either of the other two RNs.

Several months ago, you told the other RNs that the state licensing board was arriving on Wednesday, October 16, to review the unit. It would, therefore, be necessary for both to be on duty because you would be staying with the inspectors all day. You have reminded them several times since that time and checked the schedule just 4 days ago to make sure everything was covered.

Today is Tuesday, October 15, and you are staying late preparing files for the impending inspection. Suddenly, you notice that one of your staff has changed the schedule in the last day or two and that only one of the RNs is scheduled to work on Wednesday. Alarmed, you phone Mike, the RN who is scheduled to be off. You remind him about the inspection and state that it will be necessary for him to come to work. He says that he is sorry that he forgot about the inspection but that he has scheduled a 3-day cruise and has paid a large, nonrefundable deposit. After a long talk, it becomes obvious to you that Mike is unwilling to change his plans. You say to him, "Mike, I feel this borders on insubordination. I really need you on the 16th, and I am requesting that you come in. If you do not come to work, I will need to take appropriate action." Mike replies, "I'm sorry to let you down. Do what you have to do. I need to take this trip, and I will not cancel my plans."

ASSIGNMENT:

What action could you take? What action should you take? Outline some alternatives. Assume that it is not possible to float in additional staff because of the specialty expertise required to work in this department. Decide what you should do. Give rationale for your decision. Did ego play a part in your decision?

LEARNING EXERCISE 25.12

SUD and the Student Nurse

You are a senior student in a nursing program. You are aware that there are several students in your class who smoke marijuana on an almost daily basis. All of them passed their mandatory drug test on entering the nursing program either by using extensive cleansing methods to obscure the test findings or by temporarily stopping their use of the drug. Once the drug tests cleared, they immediately resumed their drug use.

While these students do not use drugs while they are in clinical, you know that some have used marijuana less than 8 hours before their clinical day began. You worry that this drug use could result in some residual impairment of judgment and potentially place patients at risk of harm, although you have not personally witnessed this occurring.

You consider reporting these students to your instructor, knowing that doing so would likely result in them being re-tested for drugs without any advance warning. A positive drug test could mean removal from the nursing program. You also consider directly confronting your peers to express your concern about their drug use and the resultant potential harm to patients but know that they will likely see you as a troublemaker and resent your interference in their lives. You also know, that should you decide to report their behavior to your instructor after this confrontation, that it may be obvious that it was you who turned them in. Finally, you are considering sending an anonymous letter to your instructor with the drug-using students' names, suggesting that their drug tests be repeated.

ASSIGNMENT:

Determine what you will do. What would be the pros and the cons of all three alternatives you are currently considering? Should other alternatives be considered? What is your primary objective in this case? Does your chosen solution achieve your primary objective?

R E F E R E N C E S

American Nurses Association. (2015). *Code of ethics for nurses with interpretive statements.*

Bettinardi-Angres, K. (2020). Nurses with substance abuse disorder: Promoting successful treatment and reentry, 10 years later. *Journal of Nursing Regulation, 11*(1), 5–11. https://www.journalofnursingregulation.com/article/S2155-8256(20)30054-5/fulltext

Gonzales, M. (2020, February 26). *Nurses and addiction.* DrugRehab.com. https://www.drugrehab.com/addiction/nurses/

Griffith, S. A., Parris, M. K., Griswold, B., Go, R. A., Matthes, A., & VanHouten, M. (2021, October). Investigating a nurse with suspected substance use disorder: Guidance for nurse leaders and hospital administration. *Journal of Nursing Regulation, 12*(3), 61–67. https://doi-org.mantis.csuchico.edu/10.1016/S2155-8256(21)00117-4

Hills, L. (2021, June/July). How to manage problem employees. *Podiatry Management, 40*(5), 103–112.

Huston, C., & Lillibridge, J. (2023). Substance use disorder in nursing practice. In C. J. Huston (Ed.), *Professional issues in nursing: Challenges and opportunities* (6th ed., Chapter 18, pp. 262–273). Wolters Kluwer.

Jahan, A. R., & Burgess, D. M. (2022, May 5). *Substance use disorder. StatPearls (Internet).* National Library of Medicine. https://www.ncbi.nlm.nih.gov/books/NBK570642/

Mayhew, R. (2022). *How to conduct an effective disciplinary interview.* Chron. http://smallbusiness.chron.com/conduct-effective-disciplinary-interview-10327.html

McGregor, D. (Ed.). (1967). *The professional manager.* McGraw-Hill.

Modlin, H. C., & Montes, A. (1964). Narcotics addiction in physicians. *American Journal of Psychiatry, 121*, 358–365.

Morris, L. (2020). A real situation: Drug diversion in nursing. *AAACN Viewpoint, 42*(1), 8–9.

National Institute on Drug Abuse. (2020, June). *Misuse of prescription drugs research report.* https://www.drugabuse.gov/publications/research-reports/misuse-prescription-drugs/summary

National Institute on Drug Abuse. (2021, March 11). *Opioid overdose crisis.* https://www.drugabuse.gov/drugs-abuse/opioids/opioid-overdose-crisis

Nyhus, J. (2021, May). Drug diversion in healthcare: Prevention and detection for nurses. *American Nurse Journal, 16*(5), 23–27.

Recovery Village. (2022, April 22). *When nurses abuse drugs: A look at the issues.* https://www.therecoveryvillage.com/drug-addiction/related-topics/nurses/

Rutgers University Human Resources. (2022). *Employee discipline—information for supervisors.* http://uhr.rutgers.edu/uhr-units-offices/office-labor-relations/employee-discipline-information-supervisors/staff-employee

Taylor, L. (2020, June). Substance abuse and misuse identification and prevention: An evidence-based protocol for CRNAs in the workplace. *AANA Journal, 88*(3), 213–221. https://www.aana.com/docs/default-source/aana-journal-web-documents-1/substance-abuse-and-misuse-identification-and-prevention-an-evidence-based-protocol-for-crnas-in-the-workplace-aana-journal-june-2020.pdf?sfvrsn=76d8a5a1_6

Trinkoff, A. M., Yoon, J. M., Selby, V. L., Storr, C. L., Edwin, H. S., & Baek, H. (2021, October). Registered nurses' awareness of workplace signs, actions, and interventions for nurses with substance use disorder. *Journal of Nursing Regulation, 12*(3), 20–29. https://doi-org.mantis.csuchico.edu/10.1016/S2155-8256(21)00113-7

Solutions to Selected Learning Exercises

The following are possible solutions for challenging situations presented in various Learning Exercises throughout the book.

LEARNING EXERCISE 9.6

A Busy Day at the Public Health Agency

Here is how one nurse handled interruptions and still had time for lunch.

Time	Task	Rationale
8:00 AM	Assign lunch breaks: 11:30–12:30—receptionist 12:30–1:30—clerical worker 12:00–1:00—you	Because you have a lunch engagement at noon, make sure other employees know when their lunch times must be.
	Finish reports	Because reports are due tonight, this would be the immediate task to accomplish. Plan to finish these by 9:00 AM.
8:30 AM	Supervisor's request	Ask her when she needs the information. Tell her that an estimate using primary diagnoses is now available, but that an accurate figure including secondary diagnoses will not be available until you have time to go through your 150 family case files, which will be next week.
9:00 AM	Client with pregnant daughter	The pregnancy takes priority over the chest clinic drop-ins. Ask the receptionist to start the paperwork on drop-ins while you spend 30 minutes with the mother.
9:30 AM	Public health physician's phone call	Delegate this to the receptionist.
9:30 AM	Dental clinic referral	Delegate this duty to the clerical worker.
10:00 AM	Client call	Because this person is confused and you do not have available information, ask him to come at 10:00 AM tomorrow with his bills.
10:45 AM	Families with food vouchers	Ask receptionist to finish paperwork and interviews on the families. Then quickly review information and sign vouchers. These families should not have had such a long wait. Make a note to find out what happened and later counsel office staff about the delay.
11:45 AM	Drug call	Talk with the client. Make a referral to a local drug clinic and make an appointment with a part-time psychiatrist at the clinic. Do not get too involved on the phone with the client because it is better to make the appropriate referrals.

LEARNING EXERCISE 12.3

Cultures and Hierarchies

Below is an analysis of how one might approach a problem involving a nonnursing department but affecting the nurses' work and the nursing staff.

Analysis: Data Assessment

1. A copy of the organizational chart was given to you when you were hired. The formal structure is a line-and-staff organization. The housekeeping department head is below the nursing director and the nursing section supervisor but at the same level as the immediate clinic supervisor. The housekeeping department head reports directly to the maintenance and engineering department head.
2. The county administrator has stated that she has an open-door policy. You do not know if this means that bypassing department heads is acceptable or merely that the administrator is interested in the employees. An important reason for not skipping intermediate supervisors when communicating is that they must know what is going on in their departments. A manager's position, value, and status are strengthened if they serve as a vital and essential link in the vertical chain of command.
3. You have twice attempted to talk with your immediate supervisor; however, it is unclear from the information given whether you followed up regarding your supervisor's action on the complaint.
4. You are a new employee and therefore probably do not know how the formal or informal structure works. This newness might render the complaints less credible.
5. Possible risks include creating trouble for the housekeeping staff or their immediate supervisor, being labeled a troublemaker by others in the organization, and alienating your immediate supervisor.
6. Before proceeding, you need to assess your own values and determine what is motivating you to pursue this issue.

Alternatives for Action

There are many choices available to you.

1. You can do nothing. This is often a wise choice and should always be an alternative for any problem solving. Some problems solve themselves if left alone. Sometimes, the time is not right to solve the problem.
2. You can talk with the county health administrator. Although this involves some risk, it is possible that the administrator will take action. At the very least, you will have unburdened your problem on someone.
3. You can talk directly with the individual housekeepers by using "I" messages, such as, "I get angry when the housekeeping staff take naps, and the bathrooms are dirty." Perhaps, if feelings and frustrations were shared, you would learn more about the problem. Maybe there is a reason for their behavior; maybe they only socialize during their breaks. This alternative involves some risk: The housekeepers might look on you as a troublemaker.
4. Have all the evening staff sign a petition and give it to the immediate supervisor. Forming a coalition often produces results. However, the supervisor could view this action as overreacting or meddlesome and might feel threatened.
5. Go to the housekeeping staff's department head and report them. In this way, you are saving some time and going right to the person who is in charge. However, this might be unfair to the housekeepers and certainly will create some enemies for you.
6. Follow up with the immediate supervisor. You could request permission to take action yourself and ask how best to proceed. This would involve your immediate supervisor and keep her informed. However, it also shows that you are willing to take risks and devote some personal time and energy to solve the problem.

Selecting an Alternative

This problem has no right answer. Under certain conditions, various solutions could be used. Under most circumstances, it is fairer to others and more efficient for you to select the third alternative listed. However, because you are new and have little knowledge of the formal and informal organizational structure, your wisest choice would be Alternative 6. New employees need to seek guidance from their immediate supervisors.

For this follow-up session with the supervisor to be successful, you need to do the following:

1. Talk with the supervisor during a quiet time.
2. Admit to personally "owning" the problem without involving colleagues.
3. Acknowledge that legitimate reasons for the housekeepers' actions may exist.
4. Request permission to talk directly with the housekeepers. Role-play an appropriate approach with the supervisor.

You must accept the consequences of your actions. However, your attempt to correct the problem may motivate your supervisor to pursue the problem directly with the housekeeping staff's supervisor. If this is the action your supervisor takes, you should ask to speak with the housekeeping staff directly first. If, after talking with the housekeeping staff, you decide a problem still exists and you elect to address that problem, then you should return to your immediate supervisor before proceeding.

Analysis of the Problem Solving

Would you have solved this problem differently? What are some other alternatives that could have been generated? Have you ever gone outside the chain of command and had a positive experience as a result?

LEARNING EXERCISE 13.6

A Shifting of Power

This is the strategy that Sally Jones used to solve the conflict between her and Bob Black. In analyzing this case, one must forego feelings of resentment regarding Bob's obvious play for control and power. In truth, what real danger does his "empire building" pose for the director of nursing? Is Sally just ridding herself and her staff of clerical duties and interruptions?

A certain amount of power is inherent in the ability to hire. Employees develop a loyalty to the person who hires them. Because Sally Jones or her designee will still actually make the final selection, Bob's proposal should result in little loss of loyalty or power.

Let us look at what the real Sally Jones did to solve this conflict. When she was able to see that Bob was not stripping her of any power, Sally could use some very proactive strategies. Here was a chance for her to appear compromising, thereby increasing her esteem in the chief executive officer's (CEO's) eyes and gaining political clout in the organization.

When she met with Jane Smith and Bob, Sally began by complimenting Bob on his ideas. Then she suggested that because nurses were in the habit of coming to the nursing department to apply for positions and because human resources offices were rather cold and formal places, stationing the new personnel clerk in the nursing office would be more convenient and inviting. Sally knew that the human resources department lacked adequate space and that the nursing office had some extra room. She went on to say that because some of her unit clerks were very knowledgeable about the hospital organization, Bob might want to interview several of them for the new position. Although an experienced unit clerk would be difficult to replace, Sally said she was willing to make this sacrifice for the new plan to succeed.

(continues on page 702)

LEARNING EXERCISE 13.6

A Shifting of Power (continued)

The CEO, very impressed with Sally's generous offer, turned to Bob and said, "I think Sally has an excellent idea. Why don't you hire one of her clerks and station them in the nursing office?" Jane then said to Sally, "Now, do we understand that the clerk will be Bob's employee and will work under him?"

Sally agreed with this because she felt she had just pulled off a great power play. Let us examine what Sally won in this political maneuver.

1. She gained by not competing with Bob, therefore not making him her enemy.
2. She gained by impressing the CEO with her flexibility and initiative.
3. She gained a new employee.

Although the new employee would be working for Bob with the salary charged to his cost center, the clerk would be Sally's former employee. Because the clerk would be working in the nursing office, she would have some allegiance to Sally. In addition, the clerk would be doing all the work that Sally and her assistants had been doing and at no cost to the nursing department.

When Sally first received Bob's memo, she was angry; her initial reaction was to talk to the CEO privately and complain about Bob. Fortunately, she did not do this. It is nearly always a political mistake for one manager to talk about another behind their back and without their knowledge. This generally reflects unfavorably on the employee, with a loss of respect from the supervisor.

Another option Sally had was to compete with Bob and be uncooperative. Although this might have delayed centralizing the personnel department, in the end, Bob undoubtedly would have accomplished his goal and Sally would not have been able to reap such a great political victory.

The later effects of this political maneuver were even more rewarding. The personnel clerk remained loyal to Sally. Bob became less adversarial and more cooperative with Sally on other issues. The CEO gave her a sly grin later in the week and said, "Great move with Bob Black." This case might be concluded by saying that this is an example of someone being given a lemon and then making lemonade.

LEARNING EXERCISE 21.3

Conflicting Personal, Professional, and Organizational Obligations

The following are some conflict resolution strategies you could have used when the nursing office supervisor (Carol), who considers you to be competent and responsible, asked you to help cover the workload in the delivery room. Although this supervisor believes you can do the job, you think that you do not know enough about labor and delivery nursing to be effective.

Analysis

You need to examine your goal, the supervisor's goal, and a goal on which you can both agree. Your goal might be protection of your license and doing nothing that would bring harm to a patient. Carol's goal might be to provide assistance to an understaffed unit. A possible supraordinate goal would be for neither you nor Carol to do anything that would bring risk or harm to the organization.

The following conflict resolution strategies were among your choices:

Accommodating. Accommodating is the most obvious wrong choice. If you really believe you are unqualified to work in the delivery room, this strategy could be harmful to patients and your career. Such a decision would not meet with your goal or the supraordinate goal.

Smoothing or avoiding. Because you have little power and no one is available to intervene on your behalf, you are unable to choose either of these solutions. The problem cannot be avoided nor will you be able to smooth the conflict away.

Compromising. You might be able to negotiate a compromise. For instance, you might say, "I cannot go to the delivery room, but I will float to another medical-surgical area if there is someone on another medical-surgical unit who has OB experience." Alternatively, you could compromise by stating, "I feel comfortable working postpartum and will work in that area if you have a qualified nurse from postpartum that can be sent to the delivery room." It is possible that either solution could end the conflict, depending on the availability of other personnel and how comfortable you would feel in the postpartum area. Often, someone attempting to solve problems, such as the supervisor in this case, becomes so overburdened and stressed that other alternatives are not apparent to them.

Collaborating. If time allows and the other party is willing to adopt a common goal, this is the preferred method of dealing with conflict. However, the power holder must view the other as having something important to contribute if this method of conflict management is to be successful. Perhaps you could convince Carol that the hospital and she could be at risk if an unqualified registered nurse (RN) was assigned to an area requiring special skills. Once the supraordinate goal is adopted, you and Carol would be able to find alternative solutions to the problem. There are always many more ways to solve a problem than any one person can generate.

Competing. Normally, competing is not an attractive alternative for resolving conflicts, but sometimes, it is the only recourse. Before using competition as a method to manage this conflict, you need to examine your motives. Are you truly unqualified for work in the delivery room, or are you using your lack of experience as an excuse not to float to an unfamiliar area that would cause you anxiety? If you are truly convinced that you are unqualified, then you possess information that the supervisor does not have (a criterion necessary for the use of competing as a method of conflict resolution). Therefore, if other methods for solving the conflict are not effective, you must use competition to solve the conflict. You must win at the expense of the supervisor's losing. You risk much when using this type of resolution. The supervisor might fire you for insubordination or, at best, she may view you as uncooperative. The most appropriate method for using competition in this situation is an assertive approach. An example would be repeating firmly but nonaggressively, "I cannot go to the delivery room to work because I would be putting patients at risk. I am unqualified to work in that area." This approach is usually effective. You must not work in an area where patient safety would be at risk. It would be morally, ethically, and legally wrong for you to do so. (Note: The legal implications of this case are discussed in Chapter 5.)

LEARNING EXERCISE 21.4

An Exercise in Negotiation Analysis

Analysis

A charge nurse's goal is to be sure that all patients receive safe and adequate care. However, some hidden agendas may exist. One might be that the charge nurse does not want to relinquish any authority or does not want to devote energy to the change that has been proposed. The staff nurses have goals of job satisfaction and providing more continuity of care; however, their hidden agenda is probably the need for more autonomy and control of the work setting.

If the conflict is allowed to escalate, the staff nurses could begin to disrupt the unit because of their dissatisfaction, and the charge nurse could transfer some of the "ringleaders" or punish them in some other way. The charge nurse is wise in reconsidering these nurses' request. By demonstrating a willingness to talk and negotiate the conflict, the staff will view the charge nurse as cooperative and interested in their job satisfaction.

The staff nurses must realize that they are not going to obtain everything they want in this conflict resolution, nor should they expect that result. To demonstrate their interest, they should develop some sort of workable policy and procedure for patient care assignments, recognizing that the charge nurse will want to modify their procedure. Once the plan is developed, the nurses need to plan their strategy for the coming meeting. The following may be their outline:

1. Select as a spokesperson a member of the group who has the best assertive skills but whose approach is not abrasive or aggressive. This keeps the group from appearing overpowering to the charge nurse. The other group members will be at the meeting lending their support but will speak only when called on by the group leader. Preferably, the spokesperson should be someone whom the charge nurse knows well and whose opinion is respected.
2. The designated leader of the group should begin by thanking the charge nurse for agreeing to the meeting. In this way, the group acknowledges the authority of the charge nurse.
3. There should be a sincere effort by the group to listen to the charge nurse and to follow modifications to their plan. They must be willing to give up something as well, perhaps some modification in the staffing pattern.
4. As the meeting progresses, the leader of the group should continue to express the goal of the group—to provide greater continuity of patient care—rather than focus on how unhappy the group is with the present system.
5. At some point, the nurses should show their willingness to compromise and offer to evaluate the new plan periodically.

Ideally, the outcome of the meeting would be some sort of negotiated compromise in patient care assignment, which would result in more autonomy and job satisfaction for the nurses, enough authority for the charge nurse to satisfy ongoing responsibilities, and increased continuity of patient care assignment.

LEARNING EXERCISE   23.1

Designing an Audit Tool

When writing audit criteria, first define the patient population as clearly as possible so that information can be retrieved quickly. In this case, eliminate patients who had complicated births, births of newborns with illnesses or disabilities, cesarean births, and home births as these patients will need more assessment and teaching. The performance expectations should be set at 100% compliance with an allowance made for reasonable exceptions. One hundred percent is recommended because if any of these criteria are not recorded in the patient's record, remedial actions should be taken.

Select the patient's record as the most objective source of information. It should be assumed that if criteria were not charted, they were not met. Audit 30 charts to give the agency enough data to make some assumptions but not too many as to make it economically burdensome to review records. An audit form that could be developed follows:

Nursing Audit Form for Visiting Nurses

Nursing diagnosis: Initial home visit within 72 hours after uncomplicated vaginal delivery, with healthy newborn, occurring in a birth center or obstetrical facility
Source of information: Patient's record
Expected compliance: 100%, unless specific exceptions are noted
Number of records to be audited: 30

After the audit committee reviews the records, a summary should be made of the findings. A summary could look like this:

Summary of Audit Findings

Nursing diagnosis: Initial home visit, within 72 hours after uncomplicated delivery with healthy newborn occurring in a birth center or obstetrical facility
Number of records audited: 30
Date of audit: 7/6/2023
Summary of findings: 100% compliance in all areas except recording of mother's temperature (50% compliance) and of newborn's temperature (70% compliance)
Suggestions for improving compliance: Remind nurses to record temperature of mother and infant in record, even if normal. Time might be a factor in initial home visit because temperatures for both were generally recorded on subsequent visits. Committee agrees that temperatures on mother and baby should be taken during first home visit and suggests an in-service and staff meeting regarding this area of noncompliance.
Signed, Chair of the Committee _____

The summaries should be forwarded to the individual responsible for quality improvement, in this case the director of the agency. At no time should individual public health nurses be identified as not having met the criteria. Quality improvement must always be separated from performance appraisal.

LEARNING EXERCISE 24.4

Using Management by Objectives as a Part of Performance Appraisal

Analysis

This case could have several different approaches, depending on whether motivation or change theory or another rationale was being implemented to support the decisions. A manager may employ several different theories to increase productivity. However, this case will be solved by using only performance appraisal techniques to demonstrate that they can also serve as an effective method to control productivity.

There are several aspects that seem to stand out in the information presented in this case. First, it appears that Ms. Irwin is a person who needs to be reminded. She functions well in Objective 3 because she received monthly reminders of the meetings, and because she worked with a group of people, she was able to make a real contribution to this committee. The similarities among the other four objectives are that (a) they all required Ms. Irwin to work alone to accomplish them and (b) there were no built-in reminders.

Rather than viewing this performance appraisal critically, the charge nurse should expend her energy in developing a plan to help Ms. Irwin succeed in the coming months. Nothing is as depressing or demotivating to an employee as failure. The following plan concentrates only on the management by objective (MBO) portion of Ms. Irwin's performance appraisal and does not center on the rating scale of job performance.

Prior to the Interview

1. Ask Ms. Irwin to review her objectives from last year and to come prepared to discuss them.
2. Set a convenient time for you and Ms. Irwin and allow adequate time and privacy.

Rationale

1. Gives the employee opportunity for individual problem solving and personal introspection
2. Demonstrates respect for the employee's time and need for privacy

At the Interview

1. Begin by complimenting Ms. Irwin on meeting Objective 3. Ask her about her work on the committee, what procedures she is working on, and so forth.
2. Review each of the other four objectives and ask for Ms. Irwin's input. Withhold any evidence or criticism at this point.
3. Ask Ms. Irwin if she sees a pattern.

4. Tell Ms. Irwin that MBO often works better if objectives are reviewed on a timelier basis and ask how she feels about this.

5. Suggest that she keeps her unmet four objectives and add one new one.

6. Work with Ms. Irwin in developing a reminder or check point system that will assist her in meeting her objectives.

7. Do not sympathize or excuse her for not meeting objectives.
8. End on a note of encouragement and support: "I know that you are capable of meeting these objectives."

Rationale

1. Shows interest in and support of the employee

2. Allows the employee to make her own judgments about her performance

3. Guides the employee into problem solving on her own
4. This is an offer to assist the employee in achieving improved performance and is not a punitive measure. It allows the employee to have input.
5. Employees should be encouraged to meet objectives unless they were stated poorly or were unrealistic.
6. Again, this helps the employee to succeed. Do not simply tell employees that they should do better; help them to identify how to do better.
7. The focus should remain on growth and not on the status quo.
8. Employees often live up to their manager's expectations of them, and if those expectations are for growth, then the chances are greater that it will occur.

LEARNING EXERCISE 25.5

The Marginal Employee

As the nursing supervisor of a 35-bed unit in a 400-bed hospital, this is how you may solve the problems posed by a marginal employee (Judy) on your staff.

1. *Identify the problem*. The marginal performance of one employee is affecting unit morale.
2. *Gather data to analyze the causes and consequences of the problem*. The following information should be gathered and considered:

   - Judy has been a registered nurse (RN) for 15 years and probably has always been a marginal employee.
   - Judy states she is highly motivated to work with this unit.
   - Judy has been coached on several occasions regarding how she might improve her performance, and no improvement is evident.
   - It is difficult to recruit and retain staff nurses for this unit.
   - The unit is already short of two full-time RN positions.
   - Judy's performance is not unsatisfactory, it is only marginal.
   - The other nurses on the floor considered Judy's performance to be disruptive enough to ask you to remove her from the floor.

3. *Identify alternative solutions.*

   Alternative 1—Terminate Judy's employment.
   Alternative 2—Transfer Judy to another floor.
   Alternative 3—Continue coaching Judy and help her identify specific and realistic goals about her performance.
   Alternative 4—Do nothing and hope the problem resolves itself.
   Alternative 5—Work with the other staff nurses to create a work environment that will make Judy want to be transferred from the unit.

4. *Evaluate the alternatives.*

   Alternative 1—Although this would provide a rapid solution to the problem, there are many negative aspects to this alternative. Judy, although performing at a marginal level, has not done anything that warrants discipline or termination. Although some staff members have requested her removal from the unit, this action could be viewed as arbitrary and grossly unfair by a silent minority. Thus, employees' sense of security and unit morale could decrease even more. In addition, it would be difficult to fill Judy's position.
   Alternative 2—This alternative would immediately remove the problem from the supervisor and would probably please the staff. This alternative merely transfers the problem to a different unit, which is counterproductive to organizational goals. This might be an appropriate alternative if the supervisor could show that Judy could be expected to perform at a higher level on another unit. It is difficult to predict how Judy would feel about this alternative. Judy is probably aware of the other staff's frustration with her, and a transfer would provide at least temporary shelter from her colleagues' hostility. In addition, although Judy would be pleased that she was not dismissed, she would appropriately view the transfer as her failure. This recognition is demoralizing, and the opportunity for her to fulfill a long-term career goal would be denied.
   Alternative 3—This alternative requires a long-term and time-consuming commitment on the part of the manager. There is inadequate information in the case to determine whether the supervisor can make this type of commitment. In addition, there is no guarantee that setting short-term, specific, and realistic goals will improve Judy's work performance. It should, however, increase Judy's self-esteem and reinforce her supervisor's interest in her as a person. It also retains an RN who is difficult to replace. This alternative does not address the staff's dissatisfaction.

(continues on page 708)

LEARNING EXERCISE 25.5

The Marginal Employee (continued)

> Alternative 4—There are few positive aspects to this alternative other than that the supervisor would not have to expend energy at this point. The problem, however, will probably snowball, and unit morale will get worse.
>
> Alternative 5—Although most would agree that this alternative is morally corrupt, there are some advantages. Judy would voluntarily leave the unit, and the supervisor and staff would not have to deal with the problem. The disadvantages are similar to those cited in Alternative 1.

5. *Select the appropriate solution.* As in most decisions with an ethical component, there is no one right answer, and all the alternatives have desirable facets. Alternative 3 probably presents the least number of undesirable attributes. The cost to the supervisor is in time and effort. There is little to lose in attempting this plan to increase employee productivity because there are no replacements to fill the position anyway. Losing Judy by dismissal or transfer merely increases the workload on the other employees due to short staffing. It also cannot help the employee.

6. *Implement the solution.* In implementing Alternative 3, the supervisor should be very clear with Judy about her motives. She also must be sure that the goals they set are specific and realistic. Although the staff may continue to verbalize their unhappiness with Judy's performance, the supervisor should be careful not to discuss confidential information about Judy's coaching plan with them. The manager should, however, reassure the staff that she is aware of their concerns and that she will follow the situation closely.

7. *Evaluate the results.* The supervisor elected to review Judy's problem solving 6 months after the plan was implemented. She found that although Judy was satisfied with her performance and appreciative of her supervisor's efforts, her performance had not improved appreciably. Judy continued to be a marginal employee but was meeting minimal competency levels. The supervisor did find, however, that the staff seemed more accepting of Judy's level of ability and rarely verbalized their dissatisfaction with her anymore. In general, unit morale increased again.

Note: Page numbers followed by *d* indicate displays, those followed by *f* indicate figures, and those followed by *t* indicate tables.